Massachusetts General Hospital Psychiatry Update and Board Preparation

Notice

Massachusetts General Hospital Psychiatry Update and Board Preparation

Second Edition

Editors

Theodore A. Stern, M.D.
Chief, The Avery D. Weisman, M.D., Psychiatry Consultation Service
Massachusetts General Hospital
Professor of Psychiatry, Harvard Medical School
Boston, Massachusetts

John B. Herman, M.D.
Director of Clinical Services
Director of Post-Graduate Education, Department of Psychiatry
Massachusetts General Hospital
Medical Director, EAP
Partners HealthCare, Inc.
Assistant Professor of Psychiatry, Harvard Medical School
Boston, Massachusetts

McGraw-Hill
Medical Publishing Division

New York Chicago San Francisco Lisbon London Madrid Mexico City Milan New Delhi San Juan Seoul Singapore Sydney Toronto

The McGraw-Hill Companies

Massachusetts General Hospital Psychiatry Update and Board Preparation, Second Edition

1 2 3 4 5 6 7 8 9 0 CUS/CUS 0 9 8 7 6 5 4 3

ISBN 0-07-141000-7

This book was set in Times Roman by Pine Tree Composition.
The editors were Marc Strauss and Michelle Watt.
The production supervisor was Catherine Saggese.
Project management was provided by Pine Tree Composition.
The index was prepared by Erica Orloff.

This book is printed on acid-free paper.

Library of Congress Cataloging-in-Publication Data

The Massachusetts General Hospital psychiatry update and board preparation / edited by Theodore A. Stern, John B. Herman.—2nd ed.
p. ; cm.
Rev. ed. of: Psychiatry update and board preparation / editors, Theodore A. Stern, John B. Herman. c2000.
Includes bibliographical references and index.
ISBN 0-07-141000-7
1. Psychiatry—Examinations, questions, etc. I. Title: Psychiatry update and board preparation. II. Stern, Theodore A. III. Herman, John B. IV. Massachusetts General Hospital. V. Psychiatry update and board preparation.
[DNLM: 1. Mental Disorders—therapy—Examination Questions. 2. Psychiatry—Examination Questions. WM 18.2 M414 2004]
RC457.P785 2004
616.89'076—dc21

2003051023

Massachusetts General Hospital
Psychiatry
Update and Board Preparation

Notice

Massachusetts General Hospital Psychiatry Update and Board Preparation

Second Edition

Editors

Theodore A. Stern, M.D.

Chief, The Avery D. Weisman, M.D., Psychiatry Consultation Service
Massachusetts General Hospital
Professor of Psychiatry, Harvard Medical School
Boston, Massachusetts

John B. Herman, M.D.

Director of Clinical Services
Director of Post-Graduate Education, Department of Psychiatry
Massachusetts General Hospital
Medical Director, EAP
Partners HealthCare, Inc.
Assistant Professor of Psychiatry, Harvard Medical School
Boston, Massachusetts

McGraw-Hill
Medical Publishing Division

New York Chicago San Francisco Lisbon London Madrid Mexico City
Milan New Delhi San Juan Seoul Singapore Sydney Toronto

The McGraw-Hill Companies

Massachusetts General Hospital Psychiatry Update and Board Preparation, Second Edition

1 2 3 4 5 6 7 8 9 0 CUS/CUS 0 9 8 7 6 5 4 3

ISBN 0-07-141000-7

This book was set in Times Roman by Pine Tree Composition.
The editors were Marc Strauss and Michelle Watt.
The production supervisor was Catherine Saggese.
Project management was provided by Pine Tree Composition.
The index was prepared by Erica Orloff.

This book is printed on acid-free paper.

Library of Congress Cataloging-in-Publication Data

The Massachusetts General Hospital psychiatry update and board preparation / edited by Theodore A. Stern, John B. Herman.—2nd ed.
p. ; cm.
Rev. ed. of: Psychiatry update and board preparation / editors, Theodore A. Stern, John B. Herman. c2000.
Includes bibliographical references and index.
ISBN 0-07-141000-7
1. Psychiatry—Examinations, questions, etc. I. Title: Psychiatry update and board preparation. II. Stern, Theodore A. III. Herman, John B. IV. Massachusetts General Hospital. V. Psychiatry update and board preparation.
[DNLM: 1. Mental Disorders—therapy—Examination Questions. 2. Psychiatry—Examination Questions. WM 18.2 M414 2004]
RC457.P785 2004
616.89'076—dc21

2003051023

To life-long learners everywhere, and especially to those hard-working and hard-learning course participants who, for 25 years, have held us true to the mission: speak straight and teach clearly.

T.A.S.
J.B.H.

. . . and to my son, Tommy, whose ability to learn, and whose sense of humor, has been a joy to behold.

T.A.S.

Contents

Contributors

Robert S. Abernethy III, M.D. [58]
Psychiatrist
Massachusetts General Hospital
Assistant Professor of Psychiatry
Harvard Medical School
Boston, Massachusetts

Annah N. Abrams, M.D. [4, 5]
Clinical Assistant in Psychiatry
Massachusetts General Hospital
Instructor in Psychiatry
Harvard Medical School
Boston, Massachusetts

Hans R. Agrawal, M.D. [82]
4th Year Resident in Psychiatry
Massachusetts General Hospital and McLean Hospital
Clinical Fellow in Psychiatry
Harvard Medical School
Boston, Massachusetts

Schahram Akbarian, Ph.D., M.D. [41, 42]
Assistant Professor of Psychiatry, University of Massachusetts
Medical School/Brudnick Neuropsychiatric Research Institute
Clinical Assistant in Psychiatry
Massachusetts General Hospital
Assistant Professor of Psychiatry
Harvard Medical School
Boston, Massachusetts

Anne W. Alonso, Ph.D. [62]
Psychologist, Department of Psychiatry
Massachusetts General Hospital
Director, Center for Psychoanalytic Studies
and the Center for Group Therapy
Professor of Psychology, Department of Psychiatry
Harvard Medical School
Boston, Massachusetts

Menekse Alpay, M.D. [33, 40]
Clinical Assistant in Psychiatry
Massachusetts General Hospital
Instructor in Psychiatry
Harvard Medical School
Boston, Massachusetts

Jonathan E. Alpert, M.D., Ph.D. [51]
Assistant Psychiatrist and Associate Director
Depression Clinical and Research Program
Massachusetts General Hospital
Assistant Professor of Psychiatry
Harvard Medical School
Boston, Massachusetts

Lee Baer, Ph.D. [64, 67]
Psychologist and Director of Research
Obsessive Compulsive Disorders Clinic
Massachusetts General Hospital
Associate Professor of Psychology
Harvard Medical School
Boston, Massachusetts

Alexa Bagnell, M.D. [1]
Assistant Professor of Psychiatry
Dalhousie University
Halifax, Nova Scotia, Canada

B. J. Beck, M.S.N., M.D. [9, 75, 79, 80]
Clinical Assistant in Psychiatry
Massachusetts General Hospital
Medical Director, Mental Health/Social Services
East Boston Neighborhood Health Center
Clinical Instructor in Psychiatry
Harvard Medical School
Boston, Massachusetts

Anne E. Becker, M.D., Ph.D. [21]
Director, Adult Eating and Weight Disorders Program
Massachusetts General Hospital
Assistant Professor of Psychiatry and Medical Anthropology
Departments of Psychiatry and Social Medicine
Harvard Medical School
Boston, Massachusetts

Eugene V. Beresin, M.D. [2]
Psychiatrist and Director, Child and Adolescent Residency
Training Program in Psychiatry
Massachusetts General Hospital and McLean Hospital
Associate Professor of Psychiatry
Harvard Medical School
Boston, Massachusetts

Mark A. Blais, Psy.D. [31, 32, 59]
Associate Psychologist
Massachusetts General Hospital
Associate Professor of Psychology, Department of Psychiatry
Harvard Medical School
Boston, Massachusetts

Jeff Q. Bostic, M.D., Ed.D. [1]
Clinical Associate in Psychiatry
Massachusetts General Hospital
Assistant Clinical Professor of Psychiatry
Harvard Medical School
Boston, Massachusetts

Rebecca W. Brendel, M.D., J.D. [72, 76]
Chief Resident, Consultation-Liaison Psychiatry
4th Year Resident in Psychiatry
Massachusetts General Hospital and McLean Hospital
Clinical Fellow in Psychiatry
Harvard Medical School
Boston, Massachusetts

Cristina M. Brusco, M.D. [17]
Columbia Presbyterian–Eastside Psychiatric Associates
New York, New York

Ned H. Cassem, M.D., Ph.L., S.J. [40, 52, 70, 72]
Psychiatrist
Department of Psychiatry
Massachusetts General Hospital
Professor of Psychiatry
Harvard Medical School
Boston, Massachusetts

M. Cornelia Cremens, M.D., M.P.H. [65]
Assistant Psychiatrist and Geriatric Psychiatrist
Beacon Hill Senior Health Practice
Massachusetts General Hospital
Instructor in Psychiatry
Harvard Medical School
Boston, Massachusetts

John W. Denninger, M.D., Ph.D. [39]
Chief Resident in Psychopharmacology
4th Year Resident in Psychiatry
Massachusetts General Hospital and McLean Hospital
Clinical Fellow in Psychiatry
Harvard Medical School
Boston, Massachusetts

Benita Dieperink, M.D. [26]
Hennepin Women's Mental Health Program
Hennepin County Medical Center
Clinical Assistant Professor of Psychiatry
University of Minnesota Medical School
Minneapolis, Minnesota

Darin D. Dougherty, M.D. [29]
Assistant Director, Psychiatric Neuroimaging Group
Massachusetts General Hospital
Assistant Professor of Psychiatry
Harvard Medical School
Boston, Massachusetts

William E. Falk, M.D. [7]
Psychiatrist and Codirector
Geriatric Neurobehavioral Clinic
Massachusetts General Hospital
Assistant Professor of Psychiatry
Harvard Medical School
Boston, Massachusetts

Maurizio Fava, M.D. [30, 46]
Psychiatrist and Director
Depression Clinical and Research Program
Massachusetts General Hospital
Professor of Psychiatry
Harvard Medical School
Boston, Massachusetts

Christine Finn, M.D. [68]
Clinical Associate in Psychiatry
Massachusetts General Hospital
Harvard Partners Center for Genetics and Genomics
Clinical Instructor in Psychiatry
Harvard Medical School
Boston, Massachusetts

John K. Findley, M.D. [73]
Clinical Associate in Psychiatry
Massachusetts General Hospital
Clinical Instructor in Psychiatry
Harvard Medical School
Boston, Massachusetts

Anne K. Fishel, Ph.D. [60]
Assistant in Psychology
Massachusetts General Hospital
Assistant Clinical Professor of Psychology
Department of Psychiatry
Harvard Medical School
Boston, Massachusetts

Alice W. Flaherty, M.D. [41, 42]
Director, Fellowship Training in Movement Disorders
Department of Neurology
Massachusetts General Hospital
Consultant, Deparment of Neurology
McLean Hospital
Harvard Medical School
Boston, Massachusetts

Jean A. Frazier, M.D. [5]
Assistant in Psychiatry and Director
Psychotic Disorders Program for Children and Adolescents
Massachusetts General Hospital and McLean Hospital
Assistant Professor of Psychiatry
Harvard Medical School
Boston, Massachusetts

Cristina Galardy, M.D., Ph.D. [57]
4th Year Resident in Psychiatry
Massachusetts General Hospital and McLean Hospital
Clinical Fellow in Psychiatry
Harvard Medical School
Boston, Massachusetts

Anna Georgiopoulos, M.D. [46]
Resident in Child and Adolescent Psychiatry
Massachusetts General Hospital and McLean Hospital
Clinical Fellow in Psychiatry
Harvard Medical School
Boston, Massachusetts

Edith S. Geringer, M.D. [17, 79]
Psychiatrist and Co-Director
Primary Care Psychiatry Unit
Massachusetts General Hospital
Instructor in Psychiatry
Harvard Medical School
Boston, Massachusetts

S. Nassir Ghaemi, M.D. [14, 48]
Director of the Bipolar Research Program
Cambridge Hospital
Assistant Professor of Psychiatry
Harvard Medical School
Cambridge, Massachusetts

Donald C. Goff, M.D. [12, 45, 74]
Psychiatry and Director
Psychotic Disorders Program
Massachusetts General Hospital
Associate Professor of Psychiatry
Harvard Medical School
Boston, Massachusetts

Lee E. Goldstein, M.D., Ph.D. [65]
Clinical Assistant in Psychiatry
Massachusetts General Hospital
Assistant Professor of Psychiatry
Harvard Medical School
Boston, Massachusetts

Gary L. Gottlieb, M.D., M.B.A. [65, 81]
Psychiatrist and Chairman, Partners Psychiatry and Mental Health System
Partners HealthCare System
President, Brigham and Women's Hospital
Professor of Psychiatry
Harvard Medical School
Boston, Massachusetts

Donna B. Greenberg, M.D. [71]
Psychiatrist and Director
Medical Student Education
Department of Psychiatry
Massachusetts General Hospital
Associate Professor of Psychiatry
Harvard Medical School
Boston, Massachusetts

James L. Griffith, M.D. [61]
Director, Residency Training Program
Department of Psychiatry and Behavioral Sciences
George Washington University Medical Center
Washington, D.C.

James E. Groves, M.D. [59]
Psychiatrist
Massachusetts General Hospital
Associate Clinical Professor of Psychiatry
Harvard Medical School
Boston, Massachusetts

Stephan Heckers, M.D. [6, 34, 36, 43]
Assistant Psychiatrist
Assistant Director of Psychiatric Neuroimaging Research
Massachusetts General Hospital
Assistant Professor of Psychiatry
Harvard Medical School
Boston, Massachusetts

David C. Henderson, M.D. [12, 45, 78]
Assistant Psychiatrist
Massachusetts General Hospital
Director, Clozapine Clinic
Freedom Trail Clinic
Assistant Professor of Psychiatry
Harvard Medical School
Boston, Massachusetts

John B. Herman, M.D. [57]
Director of Clinical Services
Director of Post-Graduate Education
Department of Psychiatry
Massachusetts General Hospital
Medical Director, EAP
Partners HealthCare, Inc.
Assistant Professor of Psychiatry
Harvard Medical School
Boston, Massachusetts

Jeff C. Huffman, M.D. [52]
Fellow in Consultation Psychiatry
Graduate Assistant in Psychiatry
Massachusetts General Hospital
Clinical Fellow in Psychiatry
Harvard Medical School
Boston, Massachusetts

Dan V. Iosifescu, M.D. [15, 44]
Assistant in Psychiatry
Massachusetts General Hospital
Instructor in Psychiatry
Harvard Medical School
Boston, Massachusetts

Robert W. Irvin, M.D. [77]
Clinical Assistant in Psychiatry
McLean Hospital
Instructor in Psychiatry
Harvard Medical School
Boston, Massachusetts

Joshua A. Israel, M.D. [46]
Assistant Clinical Professor of Psychiatry
University of California at San Francisco
San Francisco, California

Michael S. Jellinek, M.D. [81]
Psychiatrist and Chief, Child Psychiatry Service
Senior Vice-President for Administration
Massachusetts General Hospital
President, Newton-Wellesley Hospital
Professor of Psychiatry and Pediatrics
Harvard Medical School
Boston, Massachusetts

John N. Julian, M.D. [8]
Clinical Associate in Psychiatry
Massachusetts General Hospital
Clinical Instructor in Psychiatry
Harvard Medical School
Boston, Massachusetts

Ali Kazim, M.D. [76]
Clinical Assistant Professor of Psychiatry
BioMed Psychiatry & Human Behavior
Brown University Medical Center
Providence, Rhode Island

M. Elyce Kearns, M.D., M.P.H. [3]
Assistant Psychiatrist
Massachusetts General Hospital
Instructor in Psychiatry
Harvard Medical School
Boston, Massachusetts

Shahram Khoshbin, M.D. [37, 38]
Neurologist
Brigham and Women's Hospital
Associate Professor of Neurology
Harvard Medical School
Boston, Massachusetts

Helen G. Kim, M.D. [26, 71]
Hennepin Women's Mental Health Program
Hennepin County Medical Center
Clinical Assistant Professor of Psychiatry
University of Minnesota Medical School
Minneapolis, Minnesota

Sara I. Kulleseid, M.D. [64]
Clinical Assistant in Psychiatry
Massachusetts General Hospital
Instructor in Psychiatry
Harvard Medical School
Boston, Massachusetts

Laura Kunkel, M.D. [12, 45]
Clinical and Research Fellow in Psychiatry
Massachusetts General Hospital
Clinical Fellow in Psychiatry
Harvard Medical School
Boston, Massachusetts

Bandy X. Lee, M.D. [82]
Former Resident in Psychiatry
Massachusetts General Hospital
Clinical Fellow in Psychiatry
Harvard Medical School
Boston, Massachusetts

Carl D. Marci, M.D. [81]
Clinical Assistant in Psychiatry
Massachusetts General Hospital
Instructor in Psychiatry
Harvard Medical School
Boston, Massachusetts

John D. Matthews, M.D. [11, 13, 63]
Psychiatrist and Director
Inpatient Psychiatry Service
Massachusetts General Hospital
Assistant Professor of Psychiatry
Harvard Medical School
Boston, Massachusetts

Dominic J. Maxwell, M.D. [57]
Former Resident in Psychiatry
Massachusetts General Hospital
Clinical Fellow in Psychiatry
Harvard Medical School
Boston, Massachusetts

Edward Messner, M.D. [82]
Psychiatrist
Massachusetts General Hospital
Associate Clinical Professor of Psychiatry
Harvard Medical School
Boston, Massachusetts

David Mischoulon, M.D., Ph.D. [30, 53]
Assistant in Psychiatry
Depression Clinical and Research Program
Massachusetts General Hospital
Assistant Professor of Psychiatry
Harvard Medical School
Boston, Massachusetts

Anne E. Moylan, M.D. [11]
Clinical Instructor in Psychiatry
McLean Hospital
Harvard Medical School
Boston, Massachusetts

Dana Diem Nguyen, M.A. [78]
Senior Research Coordinator
Department of Psychiatry
Massachusetts General Hospital
Boston, Massachusetts

Andrew A. Nierenberg, M.D. [53]
Psychiatrist and Associate Director
Depression Clinical and Research Program
Massachusetts General Hospital
Associate Professor of Psychiatry
Harvard Medical School
Boston, Massachusetts

Dennis K. Norman, Ed.D. [32]
Psychologist and Chief of Psychology
Massachusetts General Hospital
Associate Professor of Psychology, Department of Psychiatry
Harvard Medical School
Boston, Massachusetts

Edward R. Norris, M.D. [39, 52]
Staff, Consultation-Liaison Service
Department of Psychiatry and Behavorial Science
Emory University
Atlanta, Georgia

Sheila M. O'Keefe, Ed.D. [31]
Assistant Psychologist
Massachusetts General Hospital
Instructor in Psychology, Department of Psychiatry
Harvard Medical School
Boston, Massachusetts

Rafael D. Ornstein, M.D. [16, 19]
Assistant in Psychiatry
Massachusetts General Hospital
Instructor in Psychiatry
Harvard Medical School
Boston, Massachusetts

Michael W. Otto, Ph.D. [63]
Psychologist and Director, Cognitive-Behavorial Therapy Program
Massachusetts General Hospital
Associate Professor of Psychiatry, Department of Psychiatry
Harvard Medical School
Boston, Massachusetts

George Papakostas, M.D. [13]
Assistant in Psychiatry
Massachusetts General Hospital
Instructor in Psychiatry
Harvard Medical School
Boston, Massachusetts

Lawrence Park, M.D. [33, 47]
Assistant in Psychiatry
Director, Acute Psychiatry Service
Massachusetts General Hospital
Instructor in Psychiatry
Harvard Medical School
Boston, Massachusetts

Roy H. Perlis, M.D. [7, 14, 54]
Assistant in Psychiatry
Massachusetts General Hospital
Instructor in Psychiatry
Harvard Medical School
Boston, Massachusetts

Roger K. Pitman, M.D. [16]
Clinical Associate in Psychiatry
Massachusetts General Hospital
Professor of Psychiatry
Harvard Medical School
Boston, Massachusetts

Mark H. Pollack, M.D. [15, 44]
Psychiatrist and Director
Anxiety Disorders Program
Clinical Psychopharmacology and Behavior Therapy Unit
Massachusetts General Hospital
Associate Professor of Psychiatry
Harvard Medical School
Boston, Massachusetts

Alicia D. Powell, M.D. [24, 74]
Clinical Associate in Psychiatry
Massachusetts General Hospital
Clinical Instructor in Psychiatry
Harvard Medical School
Boston, Massachusetts

Laura M. Prager, M.D. [73]
Psychiatrist
Massachusetts General Hospital
Clinical Instructor in Psychiatry
Harvard Medical School
Boston, Massachusetts

Daniel G. Price, M.D. [48]
Attending Inpatient Psychiatrist
Maine Medical Center
Graduate Assistant in Psychiatry
Massachusetts General Hospital
Boston, Massachusetts

Jefferson B. Prince, M.D. [50]
Assistant in Psychiatry
Massachusetts General Hospital
Director, Child Psychiatry
North Shore Medical Center
Salem, Massachusetts
Instructor in Psychiatry
Harvard Medical School
Boston, Massachusetts

John Querques, M.D. [27, 70]
Clinical Assistant in Psychiatry
Massachusetts General Hospital
Instructor in Psychiatry
Harvard Medical School
Boston, Massachusetts

Paula K. Rauch, M.D. [4]
Psychiatrist and Director
Pediatric Consultation Liaison Service
Massachusetts General Hospital
Assistant Professor of Psychiatry
Harvard Medical School
Boston, Massachusetts

Scott L. Rauch, M.D. [29, 83]
Psychiatrist and Associate Chief of Psychiatry for Neuroscience Research
Massachusetts General Hospital
Associate Professor of Psychiatry
Harvard Medical School
Boston, Massachusetts

Nadine Recker Rayburn, M.D. [63]
Department of Psychology
Massachusetts General Hospital
Boston, Massachusetts

Brad H. Reddick, M.D. [28, 72]
Former Resident in Psychiatry
Massachusetts General Hospital
Clinical Fellow in Psychiatry
Harvard Medical School
Boston, Massachusetts

John A. Renner, Jr., M.D. [10]
Associate Psychiatrist
Massachusetts General Hospital
Chief, Substance Abuse Treatment Program and Associate Chief, Psychiatry Service
Veterans Administration Medical Center
Boston, Massachusetts
Associate Professor of Psychiatry
Boston University School of Medicine
Clinical Instructor in Psychiatry
Harvard Medical School
Boston, Massachusetts

Gary S. Sachs, M.D. [49]
Psychiatrist and Director
Harvard Bipolar Research Program
Massachusetts General Hospital
Assistant Professor of Psychiatry
Harvard Medical School
Boston, Massachusetts

Martin A. Samuels, M.D., F.A.A.N., F.A.C.P. [35, 39, 41, 42]
Chairman, Department of Neurology
Brigham and Women's Hospital
Professor of Neurology
Harvard Medical School
Boston, Massachusetts

Kathy M. Sanders, M.D. [23, 77]
Psychiatrist and Director
Adult Residency Training Program in Psychiatry
Massachusetts General Hospital and McLean Hospital
Assistant Professor of Psychiatry
Harvard Medical School
Boston, Massachusetts

Adam J. Savitz, Ph.D., M.D. [49]
Weill Medical College of Cornell University
White Plains, New York

Steven C. Schlozman, M.D. [19, 58]
Clinical Associate in Psychiatry
Massachusetts General Hospital
Clinical Instructor in Psychiatry
Harvard Medical School
Boston, Massachusetts

Ronald Schouten, M.D., J.D. [55, 56, 69]
Psychiatrist and Director
Law and Psychiatry Service
Massachusetts General Hospital
Associate Professor of Psychiatry
Harvard Medical School
Boston, Massachusetts

Linda C. Shafer, M.D. [20]
Psychiatrist and Director
Human Sexuality/Sexual Dysfunction Program
Massachusetts General Hospital
Instructor in Psychiatry
Harvard Medical School
Boston, Massachusetts

Janet C. Sherman, Ph.D. [32]
Assistant Psychologist and Clinical Director
Psychology Assessment Center
Massachusetts General Hospital
Assistant Professor of Neurology and Psychiatry
Harvard Medical School
Boston, Massachusetts

Lois S. Slovik, M.D. [61]
Psychiatrist
Director, Family Therapy Training
Massachusetts General Hospital
Assistant Clinical Professor of Psychiatry
Harvard Medical School
Boston, Massachusetts

Patrick Smallwood, M.D. [22, 25]
Director, Consultation-Liaison Psychiatry
University of Massachusetts Medical Center
Worchester, Massachusetts

Steven R. Smith, Ph.D. [31]
Psychologist
Massachusetts General Hospital
Clinical Fellow in Psychology
Harvard Medical School
Boston, Massachusetts

Jordan W. Smoller, M.D., M.S. [68]
Assistant in Psychiatry
Massachusetts General Hospital
Assistant Professor of Psychiatry
Harvard Medical School
Boston, Massachusetts

Theodore A. Stern, M.D. [18, 22, 28, 52, 54, 70]
Psychiatrist and Chief
The Avery D. Weisman, M.D., Psychiatry Consultation Service
Massachusetts General Hospital
Professor of Psychiatry
Harvard Medical School
Boston, Massachusetts

Paul Summergrad, M.D. [81]
Psychiatrist and Director
Psychiatry Network
Partners HealthCare System, Inc.
Massachusetts General Hospital
Associate Professor of Psychiatry
Harvard Medical School
Boston, Massachusetts

Owen S. Surman, M.D. [64, 73]
Psychiatrist and Psychiatric Consultant for the Transplant Unit
Massachusetts General Hospital
Associate Professor of Psychiatry
Harvard Medical School
Boston, Massachusetts

Mason S. Turner-Tree, M.D. [49]
Associate Psychiatrist
Chemical Dependency Recovery Program
Kaiser Permanente Medical Center
San Francisco, California

Adele C. Viguera [18, 26]
Assistant in Psychiatry
Associate Director, Perinatal and Reproductive Psychiatry
Clinical Research Program
Massachusetts General Hospital
Assistant Professor of Psychiatry
Harvard Medical School
Boston, Massachusetts

Anthony P. Weiss, M.D. [35, 47]
Graduate Assistant in Psychiatry
Massachusetts General Hospital
Instructor in Psychiatry
Harvard Medical School
Boston, Massachusetts

Charles A. Welch, M.D. [47]
Psychiatrist and Director
Somatic Therapies Consultation Service
Massachusetts General Hospital
Instructor in Psychiatry
Harvard Medical School
Boston, Massachusetts

Jonathan L. Worth, M.D. [27]
Psychiatrist and Director, Robert B. Andrews
(HIV Psychiatry) Unit and Director, Outpatient Psychiatry
Massachusetts General Hospital
Instructor in Psychiatry
Harvard Medical School
Boston, Massachusetts

Albert S. Yeung, Sc.D., M.D. [66]
Assistant in Psychiatry
Staff Member, MGH Depression Clinical and Research Program
Massachusetts General Hospital
Instructor in Psychiatry
Harvard Medical School
Boston, Massachusetts

Preface

In 1976 Tom Hackett, M.D. (Chief of Psychiatry, MGH, 1975–1988) inspired our department to embark upon a mission which then seemed bold if not quixotic: to offer a national audience a two-week, comprehensive review of psychiatry. One hundred thirty-two trusting souls attended that first course, launching what was to become America's most respected, academically based postgraduate educational program in psychiatry.

As we have grown in size and reputation through the years, so, too, has the variety and frequency of our courses. Every year over 2,000 clinicians from across the country and around the world return to Boston to study and learn in the rigorous and engrossing atmosphere of the medical classroom.

Our flagship course, *Psychiatry: A Comprehensive Review and Board Preparation,* has graduated over 10,000 participants in the quarter century since its inauguration and has set the standard for our field. Given each year shortly before the American Board of Psychiatry and Neurology Part I examinations, this course has been continuously refined and refreshed to reflect psychiatry's rapidly evolving knowledge base.

Through the years those who have attended our course have urged us to create a companion text (with board-style sample test questions) as a tool to aid in their studies and to serve as a basic reference source in everyday clinical practice. As the ABPN recertification examination approaches its 2004 launch, such requests have increased.

This book represents our ongoing response to that encouragement. Like the course itself, its creation has been a team effort, inspired of appreciation for course participants, our partners in life-long learning. One hundred and three authors have created 83 chapters and 400 annotated questions.

Thoroughly indexed, it is designed to allow for quick access to specific areas of inquiry while providing a broad, in-depth review of accepted standards in our field.

T.A.S.
J.B.H.

Acknowledgments

Like our courses, the contents of this highly refined resource were mined from the rich ore of a mountain of collaborators, too massive to recognize by name. Through the years, scores of faculty and friends have contributed lectures, curbside consultations, and course ideas in the effort to improve on the previous years' offerings. Course Directors have included Bill Anderson, M.D., Jon Borus, M.D., Ned Cassem, M.D., Gene Beresin, M.D., Rob Abernethy, M.D., Paula Rauch, M.D., and our current Chief of Psychiatry, Jerry Rosenbaum. Course Coordinators Heidi Mann and Gail Dickson have been the engines driving the entire enterprise from its infancy. Without them we would not have prospered. We are grateful to the able hands at Harvard Medical School's Department of Continuing Education, particularly Norm Shostak, Nancy Bennett, Ph.D., and Steve Goldfinger, M.D. Marlisa Clapp, gifted graphic designer, has brought our courses a new clean "look." Jim Groves, M.D., designed the round Bullfinch medallion that has become our department's logo. Erica Orloff, our excellent indexer, dedicated countless hours to our project. At McGraw-Hill we thank Marc Strauss, Michelle Watt, Michael Medina, Susan Noujaim, Catherine Saggese, Peter McCurdy, Marty Wonsiewicz, and Joe Hefta (for his help getting this project off the ground) and allowing us to complete this entire book in less than one year. We are also indebted to Laura L. Stephens of the MGH's Office of General Counsel who ably steered us through legal currents. John Morton, Barbara Burns, and Sara Nadelman contributed mightily with administrative, typing, and organizational support, and Cynthia Soreff Mortlock provided substantive assistance with typing of hundreds of questions and answers. To our colleagues and co-authors, who did yeoman's work at a maniacal pace, we owe special thanks.

SECTION I

Test-Taking Strategies

Chapter 1

Test-Taking Strategies and Combating Test Anxiety

JEFF Q. BOSTIC AND ALEXA BAGNELL

I. Overview

The Board exam is not designed to fail candidates. Instead, it allows candidates to demonstrate that they understand the core terminology and knowledge of psychiatry (Part I) and that they know how to be sensitive to patients as they arrive at a differential diagnosis and to plan safe, reasonable treatment (Part II). Each candidate has had at least four years of training which should prepare one for this task; the Board Examination aims to assure that candidates have the required skills of an appropriate (not perfect), practicing psychiatrist.

II. Part I (The Written Examination)

A. Components of the Exam

The exam is divided into two sessions (or booklets), one in the morning and the second after lunch. The first question booklet covers psychiatry and neurology mixed together and is usually given in the morning session. After lunch, the second question booklet addresses psychiatry. Each question booklet includes approximately 200 questions, and candidates may skip about the test booklets as there are not timed subsections during these two sessions (but candidates cannot return to the morning booklet if they finish the afternoon booklet early). **The examination questions are multiple choice (usually five choices), and the Board has attempted to employ only Type A (five choices), matching, and clinical vignette items, and to *eliminate* the Type E items** (A = 1, 2, and 3 are correct; B = 1 and 3, C = 2 and 4; D = 4 only; E = all are correct).

1. **Psychiatry. Approximately 300 items will address fundamental psychiatry knowledge.**
   a. Development and the life cycle
   b. Neurobiological and psychosocial aspects of psychopathology
   c. Diagnostic procedures
   d. Psychiatric disorders and co-morbid disorders
   e. Pharmacological and non-pharmacological treatments
   f. Special topics in psychiatry (suicide, dangerousness, ethics, mental health delivery systems, history of psychiatry, and community, consultation-liaison, emergency, and forensic psychiatry)
2. **Neurology. Approximately 100 mostly multiple-choice (up to five answer choices) items will address neurology knowledge.**
   a. Basic science aspects of neurological disorders (cellular and molecular neurobiology, neuroanatomy, neuropathology, and neurophysiology)
   b. Incidence/risk of neurological disorders
   c. Diagnostic procedures (history, neurological evaluation, neurochemistry, neuroelectrophysiology, neuroradiology, and neuropsychological testing)
   d. Clinical evaluation and management of neurological disorders

B. Preparation

To become a hurdler, hurdle. To become a test-taker, take tests. Nothing prepares one better to do a task than practice. Taking written tests such as the **PRITE** (Psychiatry Residency in Training Examination) or review tests is helpful, and educational research clarifies that **familiarity with a testing format predicts success better than studying longer or harder.** The more the real test-taking situation can be simulated, the more likely success will occur in the real situation.

1. **Study recent (within the past five years) textbooks and review articles** that best capture the content of the exam.
2. **Study over a longer time (three months) with smaller material** (10 pages). This strategy is more effective and also diminishes test anxiety more than studying intensively during a shorter interval (30 pages per night the last month).
3. **Make study plans** known and even "write contracts" with oneself or others (spouses, colleagues) to increase both study time and scores on multiple-choice examinations.
4. Studying with others improves enjoyment of studying, but does not improve test performance, self-confidence, or test anxiety.
5. **Devise your own multiple-choice questions at varying levels of complexity** to score better on these type of exams. Some questions assess basic facts whereas others require higher levels of synthesis or analysis.
6. **Construct the same types of multiple-choice questions in other subject areas** (e.g., spouse's work, child's academic courses). This reinforces the metacognitive skills associated with test-taking which generalizes across all subjects.
7. **Take two to three practice examinations in the mornings with the same time constraints as the actual examination;** this optimally simulates the real test-taking situation. The first exam should be taken early in the preparation process (months before the exam), and subsequent tests about 3–4 weeks before the actual exam.

C. Test-Taking Skills

1. **Approach the test systematically**

a. **Make the setting predictable.** Familiarity with the test site enhances comfort while taking an exam. To **minimize distractions by others or outside noises,** candidates should select a seat toward the middle of a row and closer to the front of the room.

b. **Scan the entire examination section before beginning;** this improves one's pace and diminishes anxiety.

c. **Pace yourself. People who finish faster do not score higher than people who finish slower, so proceed at your own pace.** Most people actually answer questions more quickly as the test progresses and as the task becomes more familiar; being behind initially warrants little concern. A pace that allows 5–10 minutes at the end for review of difficult questions is optimal.

2. **Focus on key words in both item *stems* (i.e., the question) and in *answers*** to clarify the purpose of each question. Determine what is the *important* information or concept being sought in each question.

a. **Stem options.** Often keywords in the stem provide clues about what is being sought in the answer.

i. Example: Which of the following medications would be the most appropriate monotherapy for a depressed psychotic patient? (a) fluoxetine, (b) nortriptyline, (c) paroxetine, (d) amoxapine, (e) amitriptyline. Careful reading of the stem indicates that only one medication must address depression and psychosis, but also that no specific diagnosis is provided. Thus, the best answer is (d), since this could be a psychotic patient now depressed, as well as a patient with an affective disorder.

b. **Deductive reasoning strategies are based on choosing the *best* answer to each question.** Similar answers may be present, thereby eliminating multiple answers. Board questions have often employed this strategy in having multiple answers pertaining to symptoms of anticholinergic crisis or neuroleptic malignant syndrome.

i. Example: The preceding example illustrates this since choices (a) and (c) are both serotonin reuptake inhibitor antidepressants and choices (b) and (e) are both tricyclics. Only choice (d) is substantially different from the other choices.

ii. Example: Rimfodine is used to treat (a) psychiatric disorders complicated by a thought disorder, (b) psychotic disorders, (c) depression with psychotic features, (d) impaired reality testing, or (e) anxiety disorders. Answers (a)–(d) all indicate treatment of psychosis, making (e) the best answer. (No drug named rimfodine exists.)

c. **Specific determiners, such as "always" or "never," are less likely to be correct than are choices that include words such as "sometimes, often, or rarely."** Still, Board questions may include correct answers with "all" or "never." Similarly, answers with "sometimes," "often," or "may" are more often correct.

d. **Since many issues in psychiatry remain ambiguous, longer answers with more qualifiers are often correct.**

3. **Avoid making mistakes**

a. **Circle correct answers on the test booklet, and fill them in on the answer sheets to enhance rapid review of items;** preferred strategies include stopping at every tenth item to fill in or at least check at every ten items that test book answers correspond to correct answer sheet items.

b. **For items to be revisited if time permits, circle the entire question in the test book** and make a small line to the left of the number on the answer sheet to allow rapid location of these items.

4. **Increase accuracy levels**

a. **Change answers.** Even when instructed not to change answers, college students *scored better when they went back and changed answers.* The more rapidly one completes a test, the more reasonable it is to go back and change an answer. In addition, changing answers benefited medical students on multiple-choice exams when they changed their answers because they recalled new information (oftentimes, subsequent test items aided recall useful for earlier items) or re-read the question more carefully.

b. If extra time remains, **go back and review answers.** When allowed to review answers, approximately 45% of students change answers, more often to right than wrong by a ratio of over 2:1.

5. **Analyze items perceived as difficult**

a. **Consider why this particular item is important enough to be on the exam.**

b. **Return later to difficult items** to allow information from other items to clarify answers and to allow the item to be read afresh.

c. **Since each item counts the same, proceed to simpler items (e.g., matching) rather than spending excessive time trying to reason through one item.**

6. **Guess**

a. There are **no penalties for guessing**; at least a 20% chance of guessing the correct answer is preferable to 0% (not filling in anything).

b. There is **no pattern to use when guessing** (e.g., always choosing "B"); instead, attempt to eliminate wrong choices to increase the probability of choosing a correct answer.

D. Test Anxiety (Part I)

Among medical students, test anxiety was *positively* related to academic success. **On written exams, test anxiety is most impairing for those who also have *negative mood* (dreading the exam and feeling inadequate for months).** As a result, efforts to both improve optimism toward the exam and efforts to decrease test anxiety are necessary. **Test anxiety does not usually intensify throughout exams, but rather diminishes from the halfway point.**

1. **Weeks before the examination**

a. **Engage in relaxation training (deep muscle techniques);** this improves test scores, although it is less effective for reducing "state" anxiety. That is, relaxation techniques are preferred *before* exams rather than during the exam. If one "freezes up" during the exam, a brief (less than one minute) exercise may be helpful.

b. **Performance improves when an examination is perceived as an opportunity for self-growth and demonstration of knowledge.** Examination performance decreases when the examination is perceived as a *threat* to the individual's aptitude or self-esteem. Accordingly, studying information of one's selected profession should be perceived as valuable and time spent that will improve patient care.

2. **The night before the examination**

a. Aerobic exercise diminishes test anxiety; **plan *light* aerobic exercise the night before an exam.**

b. **Studying the night before the examination is not usually helpful; familiarity with the format of the test is preferable.** If studying cannot be avoided, a broad review of the major psychiatric diagnoses and treatments is preferred to reading journal articles or a review of the PRITE examinations.

c. **Soothing music helps reduce anxiety** the night before, but appears less effective than exercise when the actual exam is confronted the next day.

3. **The morning of the examination**

a. **Eat a normal breakfast;** this is preferable to eating nothing or to eating something atypical.

b. **Drink the same amount of caffeine as one normally drinks** (to avoid increased anxiety but also to prevent withdrawal discomfort). No formal research has been conducted on the use of caffeine, alcohol, or nicotine to enhance Board performance. Still, initiating use (or abuse) of a substance is not perceived as beneficial prior to the exam. Similarly, deciding to stop smoking immediately prior to the exam will not diminish anxiety.

c. Study on the morning of the test makes candidates less confident and more anxious; impairments in test-taking performance exceed any benefits from attempted learning.

4. **During the examination**

a. Unlike many standardized tests, the items are *not* arranged in order of difficulty. **Candidates should not become demoralized if the first items appear difficult.**

b. **Focus on the external (task at hand) cues, and selectively ignore internal responses that interfere with task performance.** Negative self-cognitions during an exam do not stimulate the test-taker to "dig deeper," and these attributions are consistently associated with worse performance. Comparing oneself to other examinees during the exam has an even more negative impact on test performance.

c. Positive self-talk (e.g., "You can do it" or "You've always beaten tests") has not been shown to improve performance and may diminish focus on test items.

d. **If anxiety becomes overwhelming, use foods or snacks to put one at ease.** Chewing gum improved test performance for anxious college students.

e. **During breaks, discussion of test items increases anxiety.** Truth does not occur by consensus, and negative effects on confidence outweigh the benefits of any knowledge item clarification.

f. **Eat lunch with friendly, familiar others (who do not discuss test items).** Greasy or fatty foods may cause tiredness and should be avoided. Similarly, sugar snacks or candy bars are preferred in the afternoon session rather than in morning sessions.

III. Part II (The Oral Examination)

Of the candidates who have passed Part I, 88% will ultimately pass Part II.

A. Components of the Exam

There are two components of the oral exam: a videotape interview and a "live" patient interview. The day before your exams you will be informed of your schedule for these two interviews.

1. **Videotape interview. A 30-minute videotape of a patient interview that candidates watch (in a room with usually six to ten other candidates);** after watching the video, each candidate goes into a room to present the case to two or three examiners. The videotapes are excerpts from longer interviews done by non-candidates, and do *not* represent a model for candidates to employ during the live interviews.

a. **Most candidates perform better on the videotape examination,** where the examination focuses on the candidate's ability to organize and present information; **here they can show how they formulate and plan treatment based on available information.**

2. **Patient interview.** A "live" interview where each candidate meets and interviews an adult psychiatric patient (inpatient or outpatient) for 30 minutes, and then presents that case to two or three examiners.

a. **Essential to the patient examination is to balance the differing agendas of the patient, the examiners, and the candidate during the interview.** Throughout the interview, consideration of this balance helps prevent the candidate from under- or overcontrolling the interview and ensures that all parties are treated respectfully.

i. **The candidate's agenda is to take the information the patient provides and to *start* treatment planning,** mindful of establishing a treatment alliance so that the patient and candidate can work together.

ii. **The patient's agenda is to tell his or her story to someone who appears compassionate and helpful.** Most important, one should show respect for the patient's agenda. This allows the candidate to demonstrate the sensitivity that distinguishes them from other medical professionals. **The most conspicuous deficiency observed in candidates who fail the live patient interview is their inability to follow the affective and informational cues of the patient.** So, it is essential not to allow the candidate's agenda (i.e., seeking clinical information to formulate a diagnosis and plan) to dominate the patient's agenda.

iii. **The Board examiner's agenda is to *impartially* ensure that the candidate is sensitive to the patient's plight, so that a treatment alliance can occur, and that the candidate's plan is safe and reasonable.** Their job is to focus on the candidate as a clinician and to avoid being biased by personality factors. The specific Part II grading criteria are summarized in Figure 1-1.

B. Preparation

1. **Plan a format to organize and present information.** Most candidates devise a comfortable but complete list of categories, such as identifying information (**ID**); history of present illness (**HPI**); substance abuse (**SA**); past psychiatric history (**P**); past medical history (**PMHx**); developmental/social history (**D/S**); family history (**FHx**); mental status examination (**MSE**) with appearance, mood, sensorium, intellect, thought (**AMSIT**); formulation (**FORM**); provisional diagnoses (**Dx**); and treatment plan (**Tx**), which includes differential (**DDx**) and procedures/labs/testing to clarify diagnoses (**Test**), biologic treatments (**Rx**), psychotherapies (e.g., individual [**IT**], family [**FT**]) and psychosocial interventions (**PS**) for work, school, or individual quality of life improvement. This is illustrated in Figure 1-2.
2. **Simulate the interview.** People who practice for the Boards should take turns being the patient and the psy-

Interview Style

1. Opening and closing	Uses appropriate strategies
2. Informational cues	Follows vs. ignores leads
3. Affect cues	Explores appropriately vs. ignores
4. Communication	Uses adequate language and cultural sensitivity vs. a lack which interferes with obtaining data
5. Questioning technique	Uses open-ended but appropriately structured vs. abrupt forced choice questions
6. Control and direction of interview	Develops a cohesive interview vs. scattered fragmented series of questions

Substance of Interview

7. Presenting problem and history of present illness	Obtains adequate data vs. leaves vague or ambiguous
8. Past history—Family, social, medical, and developmental history	Gathers relevant data at least in a brief form vs. ignores major issues (e.g., child abuse)
9. History of drug and alcohol abuse	Sensitively gathers vs. ignores
10. Assessment of suicidal, homicidal risk	Sensitively explores vs. ignores

Presentation and Discussion

11. Summary	Presents important data concisely and coherently vs. disorganized
12. Mental status examination	Organizes and accurately presents vs. incomplete
13. Emergency issues	Considers suicide, violence, drug and alcohol abuse vs. ignores
14. Work-up—additional history, collateral information, test to be ordered	Considers appropriate diagnostic work-up vs. demonstrates a lack of rationale
15. Differential diagnosis	Presents pros and cons of pertinent Axis I, II, or III, and chooses an appropriate working diagnoses vs. too narrow or broad a differential
16. Biopsychosocial formulation	Includes all three dimensions of a formulation vs. a unidimensional view
17. Treatment plan	Provides a comprehensive and specific plan for this patient including appropriate use of medication, psychotherapy (justification for type of therapy used), criteria for hospitalization; knows milieu principles and family systems
18. Prognosis	Discusses positive and negative prognostic indicators, including anticipated transference/countertransference

Figure 1-1. Part II psychiatry grading criteria. Scoring: 1 = dangerous or grossly inadequate, 2 = fail, 3 = conditional, 4 = pass, 5 = high pass. (From McDermott et al., 1996.)

ID (Identifying information)

HPI (History of present illness)
SA (Substance abuse)

P (Psychiatric history)
PMHx (Past medical history)
D/S (Development/social history)
FHx (Family history)

MSE: (Mental status examination)
- **A** (Appearance)
- **M** (Mood)
- **S** (Sensorium)
- **I** (Intellect)
- **T** (Thought)

FORM (Formulation)

DX (Diagnoses)

TX (Treatment plan)
DDx (Differential diagnoses)

Labs/Tests (Labs/tests/procedures to clarify diagnoses)

Rx (Medications, somatic therapies)
IT (Individual therapies)
FT (Family/couples/group therapies)
PS (Psychosocial recommendations)

Figure 1-2. Sample presentation format. Only the abbreviations (bold) should be written down on the left side of the paper, and then clinical information is added in as it emerges during the interview.

chiatrist and have someone (*preferably, a Board examiner or someone who has passed the Boards*) question them about the interview. The "patient" reads about a diagnosis and presents with a disorder(s). The candidate should interview this "patient" *for 30 minutes* with someone sitting next to them. The more you practice, the more comfortable you will be with your interview and with the presentation format, and the less likely you will be derailed by anxiety.

3. **Videotape practice interviews and presentations. A very helpful strategy is to videotape practice interviews and discussions of the case.** Candidates are invariably amazed at how their appearance on tape (similar to what the examiner sees) diverges from what they thought transpired. This also helps a candidate recognize any idiosyncrasies or "quirks" that might alienate an examiner.
4. **Address cross-cultural factors.** Candidates with impressive ability must be able to communicate that in the current cultural context. **International students who have *integrated social assistance* into their learning have been more successful.** Specifically, foreign candidates have found it helpful to consider cultural differences that might impede forming a relationship with a patient, and to talk with someone who has passed the exam about any mannerisms that might disadvantage them while interviewing an American patient.
5. **Attire. Conservative, classic fashion is appropriate for Part II.** Women should wear a business suit or conservative dress. Men should wear shirt and tie, slacks, and a sports coat, or a suit. Consulting with a senior clothing store representative about appropriate apparel for a business interview may be helpful.

C. Test-Taking Skills for Part II

1. **The videotape interview**
   a. Successful candidates tend to **sit in the middle of the room where the monitors are easily viewable.**
   b. **Candidates may bring *blank* paper and writing instruments, but no audiovisual equipment** (e.g., tape recorder, camcorder) is allowed, and indeed would be cause for invalidation of Part II (Section I [H] 5). **Once seated, candidates may write down a psychiatric interview outline** (see Figure 1-2) to most easily organize the information from the videotape.
   c. **During the videotape, candidates may fill in information in the appropriate category,** including appearance and mannerisms which fit in the mental status examination.
   d. **At the conclusion of the videotape, candidates will be escorted to individual examining rooms where they should expect to begin with the summary** (see section C.2.e).
   e. After the examination, examiners will take any candidate notes/outlines. These are not "graded" but are discarded to preserve patient confidentiality.
2. **The live patient interview**
   a. **Meeting the examiners.** One or two examiners will meet the candidate in a waiting area. They may not appear friendly, and candidates should not initiate small talk with them. **Examiners are attempting to remain impartial,** so it is appropriate to simply shake hands, smile, and follow them to the examination room. They may review the time parameters with you before you meet the patient.
   b. **Greeting the patient.** The patient is often already in the room when the candidate arrives with the examiners. Patients have been prepared for the interview and should know

their role, and past research indicates most patients view this as a positive experience, so candidates should not feel guilty or apologize for interviewing them. Still, patients may forget the purpose of the interview, they may be psychotic or despondent, or they may act inappropriately. **Candidates should be prepared to be sensitive to their needs;** indeed, if the patient refuses to speak or "goes on a tirade," as has most likely occurred to every candidate during their four years of training, candidates should be respectful to the patient rather than attempt to force the patient to answer questions. As in real psychiatric practice, empathizing with the patient's difficulty or frustration may help such patients begin talking about their discomfort or frustration. **Examiners want to know that candidates can *contend* with whatever the patient presents.**

c. **The interview**

i. It is *not* appropriate for candidates to be familiar (e.g., talk about the weather or comment about clothing), but **it is appropriate for candidates to *clarify* to patients that this interview is to allow the examiners to watch candidates conduct an interview.**

ii. **After clarifying the purpose of the interview, candidates should follow the format of the psychiatric interview (Chapter 2) by beginning with an open-ended question** (e.g., "Can you help me understand what's led to you getting treatment?") that allows the patient the opportunity to describe, in their own words, their condition. **Examiners want candidates to be able to listen to a patient's story and fit the patient's descriptions into psychiatric categories, rather than observe the candidate ask a list of yes-no questions about diagnoses.** Candidates are expected to clarify whether this is a new problem or an exacerbation of a previous difficulty. Lists of diagnostic symptoms can be appropriately interjected during the history of present illness once a patient describes a major symptom, its onset, duration, and intensity. For example, once the patient indicates that depression (e.g., anxiety or mood swings) is the primary complaint, assessment of diagnostic criteria helps the examiner recognize that the candidate knows how to follow up on presenting symptoms to arrive at a diagnosis. When psychiatric history reveals, for example, substance abuse issues, follow-up with full diagnostic criteria questions again becomes appropriate.

iii. **While note-taking is allowed** (brief phrases or even single words may help candidates later remember specific details), **candidates will want to demonstrate *listening* to the patient** by exhibiting eye contact (to the patient, not the examiner), by nodding at appropriate intervals, by rephrasing patient descriptions in the patient's own words to show understanding (e.g., "It felt 'horrible' when your neighbor Lynn started moving things in your house."), and by gently interrupting, if necessary, to obtain clarification or more details about a symptom (e.g., "I'm sorry, help me understand your trouble sleeping.").

iv. **It is critically important for the candidate to follow the patient's cues, both informationally and affectively.** If the patient shows affect, such as tearfulness, **the candidate's capacity to empathize with the patient** (and not avoid the affect) **is as important as any question the candidate will ask during the interview.**

v. **Candidates should ultimately identify the constellation of patient symptoms so that a working diagnosis might evolve.** This usually requires that the candidate ask some structured but sensitive questions about the symptoms of specific psychiatric disorders.

- Some candidates find it helpful to devise or employ mnemonics for the most common diagnoses so that they might more easily recall specific criteria. Several of these mnemonics have been published (e.g., Reeves and Bullen, 1995; Short et al., 1992).
- Examiners are *explicitly* directed to check to see whether candidates **sensitively obtain** (vs. ignore) **psychiatric history** (including family, social, medical, and developmental history), **substance abuse history, HIV risk, and, particularly, suicide/homicide risks.** In addition, **candidates must attempt a mini-mental status examination,** and pursue any parts that appear significant (e.g., the patient appears disoriented, so ensure that orientation is specifically evaluated).

d. **Saying good-bye to the patient**

i. If at all possible, candidates should **ask questions until stopped by examiners** (examiners alert candidates when five minutes remain). Otherwise, it will not be possible for candidates to indicate that if they had had more time, they would have further investigated a topic in greater detail. "Disregarding time limits" is specifically identified as "irregular behavior" and could be cause for invalidation of the Part II. Thus, when time is "called," it would be dangerously inappropriate to question the patient any further.

ii. **Candidates should acknowledge that the interview is almost over, and ask if there is anything else that would be particularly important to know that has not been talked about.**

iii. **Patients should be thanked for participating.** *Only if* the patient asks a candidate about the patient's treatment (or can talk *more* with the candidate later), should the candidate clarify that they will discuss this case with these other doctors now. If the patient asks if the candidate will talk with their doctor, candidates should be honest and indicate that will not occur, empathize with the patient's need for understanding, and reiterate that this interview was to examine the candidate.

e. **Summarizing the case**

i. The examiners may allow the candidate "a moment to collect thoughts." This time is best used to **organize information to present in a coherent format. It is usually no longer than 1–2 minutes.**

ii. After the examiner takes the patient out of the room, the candidate will be asked to provide impressions. **The candidate's objective is to succinctly summarize the case in an organized presentation.** The case presentation ordinarily begins with identification ("Ms. Jones is a 34-year-old married black female who resides alone in an apartment and now complains of . . ."). The candidate should proceed *succinctly* through the history of present illness, psychiatric history, medical history, developmental/social history, family history, and mental status examination.

iii. The candidate should ***expect to be interrupted*** **during the summary, but be prepared to proceed on to the formulation.** If interrupted, candidates should not try to return to the presentation, but rather answer *concisely* whatever question the examiner poses. Examiners will either ask additional questions, or ask the candidate to resume presenting. If the candidate is unclear, asking the examiners if they want the candidate to resume with the presentation is appropriate. Some candidates find it helpful to leave their pen marking where they were in the presentation to make it easier to find where they left off.

iv. **If the patient evades an answer in an area (or if the candidate forgot to ask), the candidate should indicate that if more time had been available, further clarification in that area would have occurred and the importance of that information,** so that examiners know the candidate *knew* what should be covered in an evaluation.

f. **Formulating the case.** For candidates failing both the live patient and audiovisual components of Part II, an inadequate formulation is the most likely problem.

i. **Integrating the available information and presenting it with a biopsychosocial formulation is essential for all candidates.** This requires description of biological factors (e.g., family history of affective disorders, physical illnesses contributing to symptoms), psychological factors (e.g., how the patient perceives his/her predicament and understands the world), *and* social factors (e.g., work, family, spousal events that impact the illness). All three pieces should be described.

ii. **The formulation should conclude with *provisional diagnoses on axes I, II, III, IV, and V.***

iii. **Differential diagnoses *must* be entertained.** While it may seem obvious that a patient has major depressive disorder, it is *essential* candidates discuss this patient could also have bipolar disorder, depression secondary to medical illness/another psychiatric disorder/substance abuse, dysthymia, and/or "double depression." If any indication of a psychotic or anxiety disorder (e.g., obsessive-compulsive disorder [OCD]) were present, the candidate should discuss how they would monitor for the emergence of those symptoms. The candidate should briefly outline the necessary diagnostic criteria for each disorder in going through the differential, and evidence for and against each diagnosis based on the history obtained.

iv. Many patients have *co-morbid* disorders, so secondary or less severe disorders also warrant consideration.

g. **Planning treatment**

i. **Treatment planning should first include efforts to further clarify the diagnoses, by appropriate testing and by monitoring for additional or more persistent symptoms.** The patient may have taken great pains to conceal a disorder, e.g., OCD or substance abuse, so candidates should clarify that this first interview warrants treatment for the elicited disorder whereas a treatment alliance may reveal additional diagnoses in need of further intervention.

ii. Candidates should **describe treatment interventions with *both* medication and with psychotherapy.**

iii. **Organizing the treatment plan according to Bio, Psycho, and Social categories can be helpful when presenting a comprehensive approach.**

- Candidates should **be prepared to defend medication and psychotherapy choices;** it is never helpful to indicate convictions of not prescribing medications or not believing in psychotherapy.
- Candidates often find it helpful to **prepare (before the examination) single-sentence descriptions of treatment modalities** (e.g., couples therapy, electroconvulsive therapy, tricyclic antidepressants) and another sentence describing appropriate clinical indications for each of these modalities so that these are more easily described and defended during the actual interviews.
- This is *not* the circumstance to demonstrate creativity by recommending unconventional, unproven, or risky treatments.

iv. **Candidates should clarify the appropriate *treatment setting* for the patient.** Whether these treatments could be initiated as an outpatient or require hospitalization is important, and criteria for hospitalization and preferred milieu treatment (e.g., hospital, day programs) should be discussed.

v. **Family/support system interventions should be described,** particularly emphasizing how resources *in vivo* can be used to enhance the patient's care.

D. Test Anxiety (Part II)

Over 80% of candidates who pass Part II after failing it previously attribute their initial failure to their

"high level of anxiety that interfered with performance." When they pass Part II, candidates indicate that familiarity with the format of the examination and "knowing what to expect" were more important than remediating knowledge deficiencies. **Practicing the oral examination with someone who has passed or is familiar with Part II is encouraged.**

1. **Light exercise and adherence to normal routines** as in Part I remain appropriate.
2. **Medications.** Candidates should discuss these with their physician, and, if determined appropriate, a trial *prior to the exam* is recommended. Candidates should never try any medication *for the first time* at the Board exam.
   a. Low doses of beta-blockers, such as propranolol, nadolol, and atenolol, appear effective in "performance anxiety" situations (e.g., test-taking).
   b. Buspirone has not appeared effective in this situation.
   c. Deteriorations in performance have been reported with benzodiazepines, such as diazepam and lorazepam.
   d. Alcohol should never be used before or during any part of the Board exam.
   e. Alternative, over-the-counter agents, such as Bach-flowers (Germany) have not proven effective in controlled trials.

E. Handling Adversity

1. **When the candidate does not know the answer to a question.** This *usually* occurs. Examiners often want to know how a candidate contends with ambiguity. It is appropriate for candidates to indicate they are unsure of the answer, and then indicate how they would find the answer to something they don't know (e.g., refer to a book to find side effects, talk to a specialist regarding unusual drug interactions). Indicating that one would seek consultation in one's actual practice is reassuring to examiners. Even if the examiner probes the candidate to guess, the guess is made in the context of demonstrating appropriate caution. **Examiners *know* candidates don't know everything; candidates who try to prove otherwise can be perceived as arrogant or dangerous.**
2. **Ambiguous questions.** An examiner may ask a question that is unclear to the candidate. It is appropriate for the candidate to clarify the question before answering it ("I think you are asking X—is this correct?").
3. **The disastrous patient.** Sometimes patients will leave early in the examination. Although this experience is unusual, it is not unusual for another patient to be brought in. Candidates should *not request a different patient* if difficulties emerge, but **candidates should not feel disadvantaged if a patient leaves and a substitute patient is provided.**
4. **Failing the exam.** Unfortunately, a number of candidates do not pass the Board on their first try. Candidates fare best who remediate any areas of weakness, practice to regain confidence, and retake the exam at the next available opportunity. In order of importance, **candidates who initially failed Part II listed the following factors as most important in their subsequent successful passing of Part II: having taken the exam previously, having different examiners, having decreased anxiety, having studied more, getting feedback from others, having a more appropriate patient, being tested in different areas, having additional clinical experience, having a better examination environment, having additional colleague support, attending a Board review course, getting additional tutoring, and having easier and better travel/hotel arrangements.**

F. Testing Accommodations

1. Applicants with disabilities (including learning disabilities, attention deficit hyperactivity disorder) may complete an Application for Testing Accommodations in the application materials provided by the Board. Generally, the disability must have been formally diagnosed by someone specialized to do thorough evaluations (including appropriate objective testing), present during the previous three years, and a rationale must be provided for any accommodation requested.
   a. Part I accommodations include (but are not limited to) assistance in completing answer sheets, extended testing time, large print examinations, separate examination rooms, a reader, and use of assistive devices.
   b. Part II accommodations include (but are not limited to) infrared headphones during videotaped interviews and the use of assistive devices.

Suggested Readings

Ball, S. (1995). Anxiety and test performance. In C.D. Spielberger, P.R. Vagg, et al. (Eds.), *Test anxiety: Theory, assessment, and treatment (series in clinical and community psychology)* (pp. 107–113). Washington, DC: Taylor and Francis.

Cassady, J.C., & Johnson, R.E. (2002). Cognitive test anxiety and academic performance. *Contemporary Educational Psychology, 27,* 270–295.

Hagtvet, K.A., Man, F., & Sharma, S. (2001). Generalizability of self-related cognitions in test anxiety. *Personality & Individual Differences, 31,* 1147–1171.

Hong, E., & Karstensson, L. (2002). Antecedents of state test anxiety. *Contemporary Educational Psychology, 27,* 348–367.

Johnson, S. (1997). *Taking the anxiety out of taking tests: A step-by-step guide.* Oakland, CA: New Harbinger.

Juul, D., Scully, J.H., Jr., & Scheiber, S.C. (2003). Achieving board certification in psychiatry: A cohort study. *American Journal of Psychiatry, 160,* 563–565.

Kaufman, D.M. (1996). *Clinical neurology for psychiatrists* (4th ed.). New York: WB Saunders.

Luckie, W.R., & Smethurst, W. (1998). *Study power: Study skills to improve your learning and your grades.* Cambridge, MA: Brookline Books.

McDermott, J.F., Streltzer, J., Yen Lum, K., et al. (1996). Pilot study of explicit grading criteria in the American Board of Psychiatry and Neurology. Part II examination. *American Journal of Psychiatry, 153,* 1097–1099.

Morrison, J., & Munoz, R.A. (1996). *Boarding time: A psychiatry candidate's guide to Part II of the ABPN Examination* (2nd ed.). Washington, DC: American Psychiatric Press.

Reeves, R.R., & Bullen, J.A. (1995). Mnemonics for ten DSM-IV disorders. *Journal of Nervous and Mental Disorders, 183,* 550–551.

Short, D.D., Workman, E.A., Morse, J.H., & Turner, R.L. (1992). Mnemonics for eight DSM-III-R disorders. *Hospital and Community Psychiatry, 43,* 642–644.

Zeidner, M. (1998). *Test anxiety: The state of the art.* New York: Plenum.

Chapter 2

The Psychiatric Interview Examination

EUGENE V. BERESIN

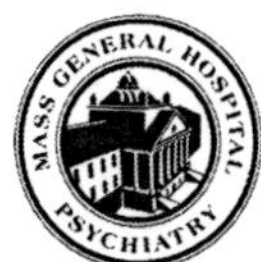

I. Introduction to the Oral Examination

A. Overview

The Oral Board Examination is the most anxiety-provoking part of the certification process. There are a number of reasons for the stress inherent in this component of the Boards. First, most clinicians are rarely observed doing psychiatric interviews, and certainly not by two examiners. The short time frame for examination and discussion is quite stressful. There is a great deal of uncertainty about what is expected of the examinee. And most clinicians, even recently graduating residents, have little opportunity to present a succinct history, mental status examination, formulation, differential diagnosis, and treatment plan on the spot. The purpose of this chapter is to help clarify the goals and objectives of the psychiatric interview examination and to provide a framework for preparing for a good performance.

There are two parts to the Oral Examination in General Psychiatry. One is **observation of a videotaped interview,** followed by the requirement to present a case history, differential diagnosis, and treatment plan based on what was seen. The second part is an **interview of a real adult patient** followed by a formal presentation. Both examinations are performed in front of two examiners, and the team leader may drop in to ask a question or two. This chapter focuses on the live interview. All of the principles of preparation and presentation are the same for both examinations.

B. Format

The psychiatric interview for the Oral Board Examination consists of a **30-minute interview of a live adult patient, followed by a 30-minute case presentation and discussion.** The examinee will be introduced to the patient by name. There will be no identifying data, such as whether the patient is an inpatient, partial hospital patient, or ambulatory patient. The examinee will not be given any directions as far as conducting the interview is concerned. **It is up to the examinee to watch the time.** The examiners will inform the candidate when there are 5 minutes left. Following the interview, there will be a few minutes to collect one's thoughts, and then the examinee will be asked to present the case. It must be kept in mind that this is quite a different interview from a typical office-based or inpatient diagnostic evaluation for psychiatric treatment. **It is similar to an emergency ward visit or a crisis intervention evaluation. It is imperative that one is very familiar with this format.**

C. General Principles

The Interview Examination has three broad areas of concern: skill in gathering information, skill in formulation and differential diagnosis, and skill in therapeutic planning.

1. **Skill in gathering information.** The examiners are looking to see whether the candidate can **establish rapport, follow the patient's lead, ask relevant questions, and focus on significant themes in the interview.** The data need to be collected by history-taking, performing a mental status examination, and determining what ancillary sources would be useful to fill in gaps in the history, such as talking with relatives and health care professionals, reviewing medical records, and determining the need for appropriate laboratory and psychological work-ups, as well as additional consultations.
2. **Skill in formulation and differential diagnosis.** A sound formulation must take into account the **biological, psychological, and sociocultural factors** that are intrinsic to the patient's life. There must be an **accurate interpretation of significant data and awareness of data that could be important but are missing.** The examiner should be able to integrate all significant findings and present a formulation that conveys reasonable clinical hypotheses based on supporting evidence. The formulation should include an assessment of the patient's strengths and maximal level of functioning, as well as the nature and degree of psychopathology.

   The differential diagnosis must be complete and include all pertinent symptoms and signs observed in the interview, as well as those that are reasonable to infer but were not elicited in the interview itself. The latter, of course, should be considered as hypothesis, since they were not obtained in the interview proper. **Consideration should be given to all possible diagnoses, and the examiner should be able to state the pros and cons of each.** Finally, the candidate would come to a reasonable number of working diagnoses for consideration in the treatment-planning presentation.
3. **Skill in treatment-planning.** The plan for treatment should be based on all data collected and those hypothesized from data missing in the interview. It would evolve from the differential diagnosis, and should consider ancillary means of data collection, such as laboratory tests, psychological tests, and professional consultations. It should include biological, psychological, and social approaches to treatment, and

be **framed in a multi-modal format. All possible treatment modalities should be considered, stating the relative priorities** for one modality compared with another. If there are contraindications for treatment, they should be proposed. The treatment plan should not at first be based on any particular health care delivery system, such as managed care, but should be an "ideal" treatment model regardless of constraints in the market. The interviewer, however, should be prepared to discuss later the feasibility of the proposed plan based on limitations in the health care delivery system. Above all, each treatment modality should be based on sound and specific therapeutic goals. Considerations of efficacy and prognosis should be discussed.

4. **Purpose and criteria for evaluation. The purpose of the clinical interview and presentation is to demonstrate that you are safe.** The age-old standard of care, "physician, do no harm," is the gold standard of the Boards. Now, what does safety entail in such an interview? The best way to think of this is to imagine that the patient you are examining comes into your emergency room or office, and you only have 30 minutes in which to make a reasonable assessment and plan for follow-up. Naturally, in such a short period of time with a complete stranger and without collateral sources of information, you need to be looking for the most serious problems, and understand that much important clinical and historical information will be lacking. What does such an interview require? First, one needs to **form an alliance** around the situation at hand. The relationship with the patient is the single most important element in an attempt to collect accurate historical and current symptoms. In a clinical setting, the alliance, of course, would be formed around the nature of the crisis. One would naturally attempt to develop rapport and comfort, respecting and listening to the patient. The clinician should elicit present and past data about the current illness, and make differential diagnostic hypotheses based on the data, leading on to a treatment plan. One would want to be sure that, once the patient leaves your presence, you are confident that you have a good idea of the nature of the clinical problems, that the patient is in no imminent danger, and that your prescription for treatment and follow-up are consistent with the data collected. This lets us all sleep at night. It also is exactly what the Board examiners are looking for.

   The examiners are not instructed to grill you, or to shake you up. They are, in fact, instructed to help you perform your best. This does not mean, however, that they will be warm and friendly, or nod their heads as some of your colleagues would were they to watch you perform an examination and hear your discussion. Nor will they prompt you. **They want to see that you are careful, thoughtful, and, most important, that your clinical reasoning is based on the data collected, and that it is logical and clinically sound.** The examiners are very interested in **the way you think—the way you organize your clinical approach, and base your clinical hypotheses on the data obtained.** They want to know that you have a logical, coherent, systematic way of organizing data, taking into account possible areas of concern that were not elicited in the interview.

5. **Focus.** Since the examiner only has 30 minutes and the most important issue is safety, the **primary concern is the present illness: its diagnosis, differential diagnosis, and management.** After you feel comfortable knowing the current clinical situation, then it is important to examine how it relates to the past psychiatric history, medical history, developmental, family, and social history.

6. **Preparation**

   a. **Books to review.** Although examiners are interested in your presentation being supported by a solid knowledge-base, they are not interested in psychiatric facts and figures from the literature. This was tested in the written exam, and, by virtue of passing it, you are qualified for the oral examination. The best study guide is to review the DSM-IV TR, and memorize the criteria from the Mini DSM-IV. In such a short interview, you will only have time to run though diagnostic criteria. Details (e.g., of epidemiology, course, and co-morbidity) are not necessary for review. It may be helpful to read the DSM-IV Casebook to see how data are put together from clinical vignettes. No other "book" study is needed.

   b. **Practice. One important reason for failing the Oral Boards is unfamiliarity with the format and too little practicing.** It is imperative to perform a number of these special interviews in front of one or two colleagues, so you can become comfortable with the time limitation of the interview, the stress of clinical presentation, and performing for an observer. It would be best to find colleagues you do not regularly work with in order to simulate the stress of evaluation by peers who are not your close professional friends. They should make the practice examinations as close to the real thing as possible: use patients unknown to you, and do not give you any feedback until after the interview and discussion.

   c. **Script.** It is essential to prepare and practice a systematic way of handling the interview and the data for discussion. This amounts to a **model for presenting the psychiatric history, mental status examination, differential diagnosis, and treatment plan.** A script is essential because it represents an outline of clinical categories. If one has this in mind, any gaps in the interview or discussion can be readily discerned, since they will be left out of the conceptual framework. I recommend the standard medical model for history and multiaxial DSM-IV axes for discussion of differential diagnosis. We all knew the medical history by heart. This was, indeed, essential for situations such as having been up all night as an intern and having to present a number of admissions to your attending on "auto-pilot." It was not that long ago that any one of us could rattle off data such as the following: "Chief complaint: This is a 64-year-old married Caucasian female presenting with shortness of breath, three-pillow orthopnea, four-plus pitting edema, and palpitations. History of present illness: #1 Cardiac: Mrs. Jones sustained her first myocardial infarction four years ago, having complained of progressive angina. She was brought to Country General. . . ." I am sure that any of us in those days could produce an entire medical history, physical examination, laboratory examination, differential diagnosis, and treatment plan with our eyes closed (and sometimes we were half-asleep!). **If some data were missing from the presentation, we knew exactly where they were, because we had a script memorized,** and had practiced it *ad nauseum*. And, we were all questioned by the attendings on our clinical reasoning. This is exactly the mind- and skill-set needed for excellent performance in the Oral Boards. All too rarely, however, do we continue to make such presentations in psychiatric practice. But this is what is needed for the Boards.

II. The Clinical Interview

A. Doctor-Patient Relationship

As noted earlier, **the alliance is critical for this examination.** You will be watched for how you make a relationship with the patient from the first encounter. Establishing rapport is a crucial part of safe, effective psychiatric history-taking and care.

1. **Introduce yourself, and explain the nature of the interview,** inviting cooperation. For example, "Hello, my name is Dr. Beresin. Has anyone told you about the nature of this interview? Let me explain. I am taking a clinical examination, and these two doctors watching us are going to see how effective I am in talking with you and understanding your problems. I want to thank you for coming here today. If there is anything you do not feel comfortable talking about, please feel free to tell me, and you do not have to talk about it. We will have 30 minutes to talk, and at the end I will offer you a chance to ask me any questions you have."
2. **Form an alliance around the task of exploring the current illness.**
3. **Help the patient feel comfortable.** Demonstrate politeness, empathy and concern, responsiveness, and respect. Respond honestly to the patient's questions/comments. **Thank the patient for cooperating.** Remember to be aware of cultural differences in beliefs and attitudes. It would be quite appropriate to ask how a symptom, problem, or its treatment is considered in the individual's culture. Demonstrating cultural competence is an important part of a sensitive and thoughtful examination.
4. **Maintain eye contact and avoid using medical/psychiatric jargon.** If you are used to taking notes, this is not a problem, so long as you keep good eye contact and do not look down too much.

B. Conducting the Interview

It is crucial to appreciate that no interview of this nature can be complete—some data will not be obtained. Moreover, the examiner needs to be flexible with different patients. **Remember, if questions are not asked, or data not collected, there is always an opportunity to make up for this in the presentation.**

1. **Begin, after your introduction, with open-ended questions for about five minutes.** It is valuable to see what is most important to the patient, and what his/her associations are. This may give you important clues about diagnosis and/or disposition. In addition, it gives you an opportunity to demonstrate empathic skill, respect, and concern for the patient's priorities. Furthermore, from a psychodynamic standpoint, which is still highly valued by examiners, it gives you a window into the mind-set and the cognitive and affective style of the patient. **After the initial five minutes, start to focus down on specific areas of concern and detailed questions.** For patients who ramble, or are tangential or circumstantial, gentle redirection will be needed.
2. **Focus on the primary concern, the present illness:** symptoms, precipitants, social setting and supports, current and past treatment, and complications.
3. **Listen to the patient.** Follow the patient's leads, be flexible, clarify the patient's use of terms (e.g., patient: "I was really nervous"; examiner: "What do you mean by 'nervous'?") and deal sensitively with the patient's affective responses.
4. **Collect relevant clinical data, if possible: past psychiatric history (previous disorders, therapies, hospitalizations), medications (their benefits and adverse effects), suicide, homicide, alcohol and drug use, medical history, family history (particularly psychiatric history), development, social history (including marital history, work, and interpersonal relationships).**
5. **Never forget: suicidal and homicidal potential (including access to firearms), alcohol and drug use, and current or past history of domestic violence.**
6. **Mental status examination.** A cornerstone of the psychiatric interview is the mental status examination. This should be a core part of the interview (but no more than five minutes), since much of the differential diagnosis will be based on history. The standard "textbook" examination is presented in III.A.1.

7. **Cognitive examination.** There is much controversy about whether to perform a formal cognitive examination. It is essential to perform an organized, brief assessment of cognition, such as one outlined below. A more formal, quantifiable examination, such as the **Mini-Mental State Examination,** is highly desirable. This type of highly structured examination **should be performed if there is suspicion of organicity or psychosis, with or without depression.** The Mini-Mental State Exam is outlined in Figure 2-1. It is brief, efficient, and quantifiable. If a formal cognitive examination is not performed, be able to say why it was not necessary; for example, "I did not perform a formal, quantifiable cognitive examination, such as the Mini-Mental State Exam, because the patient was lucid, well oriented, and in his/her normal discussion there was no evidence of a thought disorder, memory, attention, or concentration defect, or impaired judgment." When in doubt, perform the examination.

MINI-MENTAL STATE EXAM

Mean Scores	
Dementia	9.7
Depression with impaired cognition	19.0
Uncomplicated depression	25.1
Normals	27.6

Maximum Score	Score	
		Orientation
5	( )	What is the (year) (season) (date) (day) (month)?
5	( )	Where are we (state) (county) (town) (hospital) (floor)?
		Registration
3	( )	Name 3 objects: 1 second to say each. Then ask the patient all 3 after you have said them. Give 1 point for each correct answer. Then repeat them until he/she learns all 3. Count trials and record. TRIALS______
		Attention and Calculation
5	( )	Serial 7s: 1 point for each correct. Stop after 5 answers. Alternatively spell "world" backward.
		Recall
3	( )	Ask for 3 objects repeated above. Give 1 point for each correct answer.
		Language
2	( )	Name a pencil and watch. (2 points)
1	( )	Repeat the following: "no ifs, ands or buts." (1 point)
3	( )	Follow a 3-stage command: "Take a paper in your right hand, fold it in half, and put it on the floor." (3 points)
1	( )	Read and obey the following: "Close your eyes." (1 point)
1	( )	Write a sentence. Must contain a subject and a verb and be sensible. (1 point)
		Visual-Motor Integrity
1	( )	Copy design (2 intersecting pentagons. All 10 angles must be present and 2 must intersect). (1 point)

Total Score: ______

Assess level of consciousness along a continuum:

Alert Drowsy Stupor Coma

Figure 2-1. Mini-Mental State Exam. (Adapted from Folstein, M.F., Folstein, S.E., & McHugh, P.E. [1975]. Mini-mental method for grading the cognitive state of patients for the clinician. *Journal of Psychiatric Research, 12,* 189–198. Copyright 1975, Pergamon Press Ltd.)

8. **Always close by asking the patient if he/she has any questions and by thanking the patient.**

III. The Case Presentation

A. Format

Begin with a formal, concise, medical presentation, including the categories below. If you don't have data in a particular category, mention that fact and the material you would have obtained if you had had time. This gives the examiners the important information that you know what data you need in each relevant area.

1. **History and mental status examination**
   a. Chief complaint/identifying data
   b. History of present illness
   c. Past psychiatric history
   d. Past medical history
   e. Family history
   f. Developmental history
   g. Social history
   h. Mental status examination
      i. General appearance and behavior
      ii. Speech
      iii. Affect
      iv. Mood
      v. Perception
      vi. Cognition (or Mini-Mental State Examination; Figure 2-1)
         - Level of consciousness
         - Orientation
         - Attention and concentration
         - Memory: recent and remote
         - General information
         - Calculation
         - Abstraction
         - Judgment
         - Insight
2. **Formulation and differential diagnosis**
3. **Treatment plan**
4. **Prognosis**

B. Presenting the Differential Diagnosis

This is one of the most challenging parts of the presentation. The following are a few tips for a coherent, inclusive biopsychosocial case discussion.

1. **Begin with the descriptive signs and symptoms.** Build your diagnostic possibilities around constellations of specific symptoms. In other words, move from the specific to the generic. Begin with the most likely possibilities, and consider the pros and cons of all other possible psychiatric conditions. **It is crucial to mention all categories, even the very unlikely ones.** A core concept for this exam is the following: if you do not mention a diagnostic or treatment category, the examiners must assume that you do not know it exists. Thus, it is imperative to **be overinclusive.** I would mention ALL diagnostic categories in each of the DSM-IV Axes, even if some are clearly out of the question.
2. **Use the multiaxial framework as your script for the discussion.**
3. **Always run through the major Axis I diagnoses,** ruling in or out major illnesses, such as schizophrenia, mood disorders, substance-related disorders, anxiety disorders, including each of the subcategories of disorders within each of the major classes. This is best thought of as the "psychiatric biological axis."
4. **Use Axis II to discuss personality traits or disorders and include here a psychodynamic formulation.** Despite our reliance on DSM-IV for psychiatric nosology, good clinical care requires an understanding of the inner world of the patient. Surely, in a 30 minute interview, it may be difficult to make a personality disorder diagnosis, or fully understand the complexity of intrapsychic structure. However, this is a place to discuss your hypotheses on common defense mechanisms, personality trait disturbances, and possible intrapsychic conflicts, all of which may be important in treatment-planning and prognosis.
5. **Use Axis III to consider possible medical illness** that may be related as causes or complicating entities in the clinical picture. **Drug-drug interactions,** allergies, and other medical issues should also be raised here.
6. **Use Axis IV to discuss the social/environmental and cultural dimension,** such as nature of object relations, impact of ethnicity and cultural heritage, sources of precipitants, supports, and life stressors.
7. **Global assessment of functioning (GAF).** It is always useful to attempt to rate an approximate GAF currently and possible highest in the past.
8. **The key to the discussion.** Let the examiners know you have an organized way of **moving from the specific clinical data through the various diagnostic possibilities,** and that you take into account and integrate the biological, psychological, and social/environmental/cultural components of psychiatric health and illness.
9. **An important concept to keep in mind: making the "right" diagnosis is not as crucial as having a systematic approach to obtaining it.** It is always valuable to indicate your omissions; e.g., "I would have liked to explore this area further, if I had more time," or "I didn't ask about . . . , and this may have helped establish a . . . diagnosis."

C. Treatment Plan

Be sure the treatment plan includes multimodal components. Remember that each modality has multiple specific components, and each should be mentioned, even if not appropriate for the case at hand. Start with ancillary procedures that may be necessary either for clarifying the diagnosis or as helping in the treatment process:

1. **Laboratory and ancillary procedures**
   a. Clinical laboratory examination: e.g., CBC (complete blood count), LFTs (liver function tests), EKG (electrocardiogram), BUN (blood urea nitrogen), TFTs (thyroid function tests).
   b. Neuroimaging studies
   c. EEG (electroencephalogram)
   d. Psychological testing: cognitive and projective tests
2. **Biological therapies**
   a. Pharmacotherapy. Include all classes of drug treatment, even if certain agents are not appropriate for the clinical situation. State these as inappropriate and give reasons.
   b. ECT (electroconvulsive therapy)
3. **Psychotherapies.** These should include long- and short-term therapies, depending on the case. Possible categories to include are:
   a. Individual psychodynamic (specify type if possible: e.g., classical, ego psychological, object relations, self-psychology)
   b. Individual supportive
   c. Couples
   d. Family (specify type, if possible: e.g., structural, strategic, systemic, problem-solving)
   e. Cognitive and cognitive-behavioral therapy (specify type, as above: e.g., operant conditioning, dialectical behavior therapy)
   f. Group (homogeneous, heterogeneous, and specify model if possible)
   g. Interpersonal psychotherapy
   h. Relaxation techniques
   i. Hypnosis
   j. Biofeedback
   k. Other miscellaneous therapies as needed: e.g., 12-step programs, psychoeducational groups
4. **Hospital-based treatment**
   a. Inpatient: acute, subacute, chronic
   b. Partial hospital
   c. Residential: e.g., group homes, half-way houses

D. Helpful Tips on the Presentation and Discussion

1. **Interruptions and questions.** Remember to keep your scripts in mind for the history and differential diagnosis. Begin with your formal presentation, as indicated earlier. The examiners will, at times, interrupt you to ask questions. Do not assume that you have done anything wrong, or that they are questioning your reasoning. There are many reasons examiners ask questions. It is not up to you to figure them out. Try not to get rattled by interruptions. It is most useful to respond to an examiner's questions, then continue where you left off with your scripted presentation (again, a structured script is very reassuring in such situations, particularly if you are answering a difficult question). It is vital first to **demonstrate that you know the basics about psychiatric diagnosis and treatment.** Then, if time permits, and if you see from the nature of their questions that the examiners wish to go into greater depth, you can discuss the fine points, controversial issues, or current research data. For the most part, such detail is beyond the scope, goals, and objectives of this examination.

   If you do not know the answer to a question, do not attempt to guess. Such a response is an indicator that you are not safe. It is important to be comfortable saying: "**I don't know the answer to that question, but I would get assistance by** asking an expert colleague, looking up the topic in . . . journal or . . . textbook." Making references to specific journals, articles, or texts is useful here. Remember, the examiners do not expect you to know everything, and the hallmark of a safe physician is knowing where to get information and appropriate consultation quickly.
2. **Coping with anxiety.** It is useful in your practice exams to **know what makes you anxious,** e.g., which types of patients, which countertransference responses, and what kinds of questions from examiners. Once you discern the factors that heighten your anxiety, **practice a desensitization approach,** by making yourself face such situations before the Boards. For example, if you have problems with rambling, tangential patients, who give you vague, spotty clinical data, find as many as possible such patients to interview ahead of time. Beyond desensitization, there are other techniques to reduce anxiety. Deep breathing before the exam or talking to yourself to calm down are useful examples. For some, note-taking in a scripted format helps. For example, dividing your pad into three vertical sections—one for obtained clinical data, one for missing data, and one for diagnostic categories—may help. The most important form of self-reassurance is knowing that you have done many other exams successfully and that you know what works well for you.

   It is not usually a good idea to medicate yourself for such exams in advance unless this has been done repeatedly with success. There are individuals who do better with a tad of propranolol if they tend to develop a peripheral tremor when anxious, or those who use a small dose of lorazepam before testing. However, these methods are, for the most part, unnecessary, and could impair your cognition under stress.

   An important method of reducing anxiety is keeping good track of your time. Too often, under pressure, an examinee loses a sense of time and, on hearing there are only five minutes left, needs to do a cognitive examination, as well as cover a number of specific questions for one or more diagnostic categories.
3. **Monitor your style under stress.** Each of us has coping mechanisms under pressure. Be sure to appreciate

the ways you tend to react to stressful situations. Some examinees become **argumentative, flip or joking, or noncommittal and vague** under examination situations. Practice examinations are the best way to determine how you tend to respond under such conditions. There are rare situations when you disagree with an examiner, or when you know the literature on a particular topic in depth, and could get into a controversial discussion or argument with the examiner. This, of course, is not in your best interests, even if you know you are right. It is best to **avoid power struggles** and proceed with conventional clinical wisdom, avoiding the controversies. An excellent example comes from my own experience taking the Child Boards. I was discussing the treatment of a young adolescent with a tricyclic antidepressant, and the examiner asked me what I could do in the office, in the absence of a laboratory, to determine if the boy were toxic. I knew he was looking for taking the pulse and orthostatic blood pressure, but I knew there is not necessarily a correlation between anticholinergic adverse effects and blood levels of the drug. I answered that I would take the pulse and blood pressure. This, is, in fact, good clinical practice, and I would do it in my office. However, if I wanted to know if the child was in the toxic range, I would need a blood test and would like an EKG as well. I did not push the issue. It is typically the case that, when an examinee is asked about highly specific or controversial issues, it is a good indication of having passed.

Suggested Readings

Manley, M.R.S. (2000). Psychiatric interview, history, and mental status examination. In B.J. Sadock & V.A. Sadock (Eds.), *Comprehensive textbook of psychiatry* (7th ed., pp. 652–665). Philadelphia: Lippincott Williams & Wilkins.

Sadock, B.J. (2002). Psychiatric report and medical record. In B.J. Sadock & V.A. Sadock (Eds.), *Comprehensive textbook of psychiatry* (7th ed., pp. 677–689). Phildelphia: Lippincott Williams & Wilkins.

Silberman, S.E. (1997). Psychiatric interview: Settings and techniques. In A. Tasman, J. Kay, & J.A. Lieberman (Eds.), *Psychiatry* (pp. 19–34). Philadelphia: W.B. Saunders.

SECTION II

Approach to Psychiatric Diagnosis and Psychiatric Conditions

Chapter 3

The DSM-IV: A Multiaxial System for Psychiatric Diagnosis

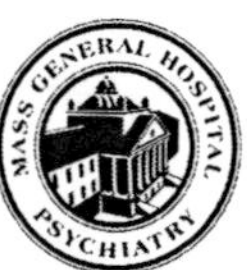

M. Elyce Kearns

I. Introduction

The *Diagnostic and Statistical Manual of Mental Disorders, Fourth Edition* (**DSM-IV**), published in 1994, is **the official classification system of psychiatric conditions currently in use in the United States.** All mental health professionals use this as a common means for communicating about the more than 300 specific disorders that have been characterized.

DSM-IV diagnostic criteria are used to facilitate communication among mental health and health care professionals, as a common standard for research criteria, and to communicate with third-party payors.

According to the DSM-IV, **a mental disorder is a disorder with significant behavioral or psychological symptoms** associated with present distress (e.g., pain), disability (i.e., impairment in one or more area of function), or with an increased risk of suffering death, pain, disability, or an important loss of freedom. The condition must not be merely an expectable and culturally sanctioned response to a particular event (e.g., the death of a loved one). Independent of its cause, it must be a manifestation of a behavioral, psychological, or biological dysfunction (American Psychiatric Association [APA], 1994, p. xxi).

II. Overview

The **DSM-IV is a descriptive classification system** that presents the clinical features that must be present for the diagnosis of a disorder. It does not address etiology or treatment related to disorders. Criteria have been made specific to increase the reliability of a diagnosis among clinicians (Sadock and Kaplan, 1995). **There are 16 major diagnostic classes and an additional section: "Other Conditions That May Be a Focus of Clinical Attention"** (Table 3-1). The diagnostic classes are listed in order of their priority in differential diagnosis, reflecting the hierarchical nature of the classification system.

The DSM-IV allows multiple diagnoses to be given to an individual who presents with symptoms that meet criteria for more than one disorder. In several situations the differential diagnosis is aided by exclusion criteria.

A. **When a mental disorder due to a general medical condition or a substance-induced disorder is responsible for the symptoms,** it pre-empts the diagnosis of the corresponding primary disorder with the same symptoms.

B. **When a more pervasive disorder** (e.g., schizophrenia) **has among its defining symptoms** (or associated symptoms) **the defining symptoms of a less pervasive disorder** (e.g., dysthymic disorder), **only the more pervasive disorder is diagnosed.**

C. **When there are particularly difficult differential diagnostic boundaries, the phrase "not better accounted for by . . ." is included, to indicate that clinical judgment is necessary to determine which diagnosis is most appropriate.** In some cases, both diagnoses may be appropriate (APA, 1994, p. 6).

III. The DSM Revision Process

The three-stage revision process from the *Diagnostic and Statistical Manual, Third Edition–Revised* (DSM-III-R) to DSM-IV included comprehensive and systematic reviews of the published literature, a re-analysis of already collected data, and extensive issue-focused field trials (APA, 1994, p. xviii).

The United States is under treaty obligation to maintain a terminology that is compatible with the disease classification, *International Classification of Disease* (ICD), that is used by the World Health Organization (WHO). ICD is in its tenth revision. Although ICD-9 remains in general use currently, the transition to ICD-10 is expected within the next several years. It includes a section of psychiatric diagnoses, "Mental and Behavioral Disorders," which correlate with those in the DSM-IV. Drafts of ICD-10 were reviewed by the DSM work-groups during the process of revision. The outcome was a diagnostic system in use in the United States that has terms and codes compatible with those accepted internationally.

Several other countries (including China, Japan, and Cuba) are adapting the ICD-10 classification system to their own independent psychiatric classifications (Mezzich, 1995). **DSM-IV also includes an appendix that addresses cultural formulations and culture-bound syndromes.**

In 2000, the *Diagnostic and Statistical Manual of Mental Disorders, Fourth Edition, Text Revision* (DSM-IV-TR), was published to update the descriptive text that accompanied the DSM-IV (American Psychiatric Association, 2000). The revision was made due to the length of time between the publication of DSM-IV and the expected publication of DSM-V. It includes correction of factual errors in DSM-IV; updated and new information based on reviews of recent literature, overseen by DSM-IV-TR work-groups; enhancement of the educational value of DSM-IV; and updated codes based on changes in ICD-9-CM codes since DSM-IV. Most changes were made in the associated features, prevalence, course of illness, risk factors, and co-mobidity sections. No changes were made in criteria sets. No new disorders or subtypes were considered. DSM-IV-TR includes expansion and clarification of procedures for rating Axis V, GAF. Descriptions

Table 3-1. Other Conditions That May Be a Focus of Clinical Attention

- Psychological factors affecting medical condition
- Medication-induced movement disorders
- Adverse effects of medication not otherwise specified
- Relational problems
- Problems related to abuse or neglect
- Additional conditions that may be a focus of clinical attention

of disorders containing significant text revision include Asperger's syndrome and dementia.

IV. Differences between the DSM and the ICD

Unlike the DSM, the ICD is a system used worldwide by clinicians in all medical disciplines and specialties to communicate about the characteristics of various disorders. This includes a common mode of diagnosis of mental disorders in which language, culture, and the approach to treatment may vary significantly from one area to another. The ICD system has some diagnoses that account for co-morbidity (e.g., depressive conduct disorder), unlike the DSM, in which all diagnoses are separate and co-morbidity is accounted for by listing co-occurring disorders separately on each axis (Schwab-Stone and Hart, 1996).

Some terminology has changed in the DSM-IV. The diagnosis of organic mental disorder and the terms "neurasthenia," "psychogenic," and "neurosis" have been eliminated from DSM-IV but remain in some form in the ICD-10. The ICD-10 does not use the term "bipolar II" (Sadock and Kaplan, 1995, p. 691).

ICD-10 uses a three-axis system: Axis I—Clinical Diagnoses; Axis II—Disablements; and Axis III—Contextual Factors. Appendix H in DSM-IV lists the ICD-10 codes that coincide with the DSM-IV diagnoses.

V. The Five Axes

Multiple diagnoses may be present on Axes I, II, and III.

A. **Axis I includes clinical disorders and "Other Conditions That May Be a Focus of Clinical Attention"** (see Table 3-2). There are codes that signify that there is either no diagnosis or that diagnosis is deferred on Axis I until further information is obtained.

B. **Axis II includes personality disorders and mental retardation.** If the principal diagnosis or reason for visit is a diagnosis coded on Axis II, the diagnosis should be labeled as such (see Table 3-3).

C. **Axis III includes general medical conditions** that are outside the "Mental and Behavioral Disorders" chapter of ICD. These diagnoses may have some bearing on the understanding and treatment of an individual's psychiatric condition. If a general medical condition is causing or is related to a psychiatric diagnosis, the diagnosis on Axis I may be "Mental Disorder NOS Due to . . ." for which the medical condition is listed on both Axis I and Axis III (see Table 3-4).

Table 3-2. Axis I: Clinical Disorders: Other Conditions That May Be a Focus of Clinical Attention

- Disorders usually first diagnosed in infancy, childhood, or adolescence (*excluding mental retardation, which is diagnosed on Axis II*)
- Delirium, dementia, amnestic, and other cognitive disorders
- Mental disorders due to a general medical condition
- Substance-related disorders
- Schizophrenia and other psychotic disorders
- Mood disorders
- Anxiety disorders
- Somatoform disorders
- Factitious disorders
- Dissociative disorders
- Sexual and gender identity disorders
- Eating disorders
- Sleep disorders
- Impulse-control disorders not elsewhere classified
- Adjustment disorders
- Other conditions that may be a focus of clinical attention

SOURCE: DSM-IV, p. 26.

D. **Axis IV describes the psychosocial and environmental problems experienced by the individual.** These may affect the diagnosis, treatment, and prognosis of mental disorders (APA, 1994, p. 29). Typically, factors have been present during the preceding year. Multiple factors may be recorded (see Table 3-5).

E. **Axis V involves the numerical assignment of a rank of global assessment of functioning of the individual considering only psychological, social, and occupational function** (APA, 1994, p. 30). It is based on a 100-point scale.

VI. Diagnostic Codes

Every diagnosis on Axes I, II, and III has its own distinct numerical code. The codes used in DSM-IV are compatible with those used in ICD-10. Codes are used for medical

Table 3-3. Axis II: Personality Disorders and Mental Retardation

- Paranoid personality disorder
- Schizoid personality disorder
- Schizotypal personality disorder
- Antisocial personality disorder
- Borderline personality disorder
- Histrionic personality disorder
- Narcissistic personality disorder
- Avoidant personality disorder
- Dependent personality disorder
- Obsessive-compulsive personality disorder
- Personality disorder not otherwise specified
- Mental retardation

SOURCE: DSM-IV, p. 27.

record-keeping, data collection, and reporting data and research activities.

In addition to the main code given to each diagnosis, **the subtypes of the diagnosis or specifiers as described in the narrative descriptions in DSM-IV are also coded, usually in the first two decimal positions.** This allows increased specificity of the diagnosis.

Subtypes are mutually exclusive. **Specifiers** do not designate mutually exclusive subgroupings. They provide an opportunity to define a more homogeneous subgrouping of individuals with the disorder (APA, 1994, p. 1).

VII. Specifiers

Specific criteria are noted for certain diagnoses in DSM-IV.

A. Severity. Level is based on the number of symptoms and functioning.

1. **Mild.** Few, if any, symptoms are present in excess of those required for diagnosis. There is no more than minor impairment in functioning.
2. **Moderate.** Intermediate between mild and severe in terms of symptom presence and impairment of function.
3. **Severe.** Many symptoms in excess of those required for diagnosis or several very severe symptoms are present, or there is marked impairment in functioning.

B. Course

1. **In partial remission.** The individual previously met full criteria for diagnosis and currently has some signs or symptoms.
2. **In full remission.** No signs or symptoms of the disorder remain, but the record should indicate that the disorder was present in the past.
3. **Prior history.** The person is considered to be recovered from the disorder.

Table 3-4. Axis III: General Medical Conditions (with ICD-9-CM Codes)

- Infectious and parasitic diseases (001–139)
- Neoplasms (140–239)
- Endocrine, nutritional, and metabolic diseases and immunity disorders (240–279)
- Diseases of the blood and blood-forming organs (280–289)
- Diseases of the nervous system and sense organs (320–389)
- Diseases of the circulatory system (390–459)
- Diseases of the respiratory system (460–519)
- Diseases of the digestive system (520–579)
- Diseases of the genitourinary system (580–629)
- Complications of pregnancy, childbirth, and the puerperium (630–676)
- Diseases of the skin and subcutaneous tissue (680–709)
- Diseases of the musculoskeletal system and connective tissue (710–739)
- Congenital abnormalities (740–759)
- Certain conditions originating in the perinatal period (760–779)
- Symptoms, signs, and ill-defined conditions (780–799)
- Injury and poisoning (800–999)

SOURCE: DSM-IV, p. 28.

C. Principal Diagnosis. The disorder was established, after evaluation, to be mainly responsible for the entrance into treatment.

D. Provisional Diagnosis. There is "strong presumption" that the person will meet the full criteria for a disorder, but information is currently inadequate.

E. Not Otherwise Specified (NOS). These terms are used to account for diversity in clinical presentation

Table 3-5. Axis IV: Psychosocial and Environmental Problems

- Problems with primary support group
- Problems related to the social environment
- Educational problems
- Occupational problems
- Housing problems
- Economic problems
- Problems with access to health care services
- Problems related to interaction with the legal system/crime
- Other psychosocial and environmental problems

when the more specific diagnoses do not fit. Each diagnostic category has designated at least one NOS diagnosis.

VIII. Exclusion Criteria and Differential Diagnosis

In addition to listing the criteria that must be met for the diagnosis of a certain disorder, DSM-IV specifies that other disorders should be considered during the diagnostic process. Due to the existence of co-morbid conditions and the desirability to establish a differential diagnosis and distinguish the boundaries of diagnoses when symptoms overlap, **the following qualifiers are used.** They serve to clarify when multiple diagnoses should be used.

A. **"Criteria have never been met for . . .":** defines a lifetime hierarchy.
B. **"Criteria are not met for . . .":** defines a cross-sectional hierarchy.
C. **"Does not occur exclusively during the course of . . .":** used to assure that the criteria for the disorder are not met only during the course of another disorder.
D. **"Not due to the direct physiological effects of a substance (e.g., a drug of abuse, a medication) or a general medical condition."** Any condition that is substance-induced or etiologically related to a general medical condition must be ruled out before the disorder can be diagnosed.
E. **"Not better accounted for by . . ."** The process of differential diagnosis should include the other disorders mentioned in the criteria, and clinical judgment should be used in differentiating diagnoses that occur on the border (APA, 1994, pp. 5–6).

IX. Areas Addressed in Descriptions of DSM-IV Diagnoses

Topics addressed include:

A. Diagnostic Features
B. Subtypes and/or Specifiers
C. Recording Procedures
D. Associated Features and Disorders
  1. Associated descriptive features and mental disorders
  2. Associated laboratory findings
  3. Associated physical examination findings and general medical conditions

E. Specific Culture, Age, and Gender Features
F. Prevalence
G. Course
  1. Age at onset
  2. Mode of onset
  3. Episodic versus continuous course
  4. Single episode versus recurrent
  5. Duration
  6. Progression

H. Familial Pattern
I. Differential Diagnosis

X. Algorithms

The DSM-IV has algorithms that were developed to assist clinicians in the process of identifying the presenting symptoms and considering how those symptoms may be reflective of a psychiatric diagnosis. **They aim to guide the clinician's thinking during the decision process for making a differential diagnosis.** The six areas for which they were developed are Mental Disorders Due to a General Medical Condition, Substance-Induced Disorders, Psychotic Disorders, Mood Disorders, Anxiety Disorders, and Somatoform Disorders.

XI. Conclusion

The purpose of the DSM-IV is to enhance communication among mental health clinicians and those who keep track of these disorders on an individual or population-wide basis. In addition, it is used to clarify the thought and decision-making processes about diagnosis when a clinician is faced with an individual presenting with any number of seemingly related or unrelated symptoms. **Keep in mind that symptoms and disorders are classified, not the individual. The DSM-IV does not minimize the importance of clinical judgment.**

Suggested Readings

American Psychiatric Association. (1994). *Diagnostic and statistical manual of mental disorders* (4th ed.). Washington, DC: American Psychiatric Press.

American Psychiatric Association. (2000). *Diagnostic and statistical manual of mental disorders* (4th ed., Text revision). Washington, DC: American Psychiatric Press.

Cooper, J. (1995). On the publication of the *Diagnostic and Statistical Manual of Mental Disorders*: Fourth Edition (DSM-IV). *British Journal of Psychiatry, 166,* 4–8.

First, M.N., & Pincus, H.A. (2002). The DSM-IV Text Revision: Rationale and potential impact on clinical practice. *Psychiatric Services, 53,* 288–292.

Frances, A.J., Widiger, T.A., & Pincus, H.A. (1989). The development of DSM-IV. *Archives of General Psychiatry, 46,* 373–375.

Mezzich, J.E. (1995). International perspectives on psychiatric diagnosis. In H.I. Kaplan & B.J. Sadock (Eds.), *Comprehensive textbook of psychiatry* (6th ed., pp. 692–703). Baltimore: Williams and Wilkins.

Sadock, B.J., & Kaplan, H.I. (1995). Classification of mental disorders. In H.I. Kaplan & B.J. Sadock (Eds.), *Comprehensive textbook of psychiatry* (6th ed., pp. 671–692). Baltimore: Williams and Wilkins.

Schwab-Stone, M.E., & Hart, E.L. (1996). Systems of psychiatric classification: DSM-IV and ICD-10. In M.L. Lewis (Ed.), *Child and adolescent psychiatry: A comprehensive textbook* (2nd ed., pp. 423–430). Baltimore: Williams and Wilkins.

Volkmar, F.R. Classification in child and adolescent psychiatry: Principles and issues. In M.L. Lewis (Ed.), *Child and adolescent psychiatry: A comprehensive textbook* (2nd ed., pp. 417–422). Baltimore: Williams and Wilkins.

Chapter 4

Child and Adolescent Development

ANNAH ABRAMS AND PAULA RAUCH

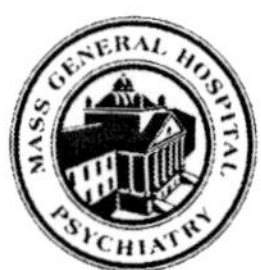

I. Introduction

This chapter outlines the normal development of a child, which occurs along a continuum. **Each age group is associated with physical, social, sexual, and cognitive changes.** Pediatricians and child psychiatrists use developmental screening tests to measure (monitor) the developmental tasks a child should achieve by a given age. **Developmental milestones as might appear in a screening test are outlined in Table 4-1.** Theories of child development describe and explain the social, sexual, and cognitive changes that occur for the child. The most often cited theorists in child development include Sigmund Freud, Erik Erikson, and Jean Piaget, who are discussed here. **Table 4-2 gives an overview of each theorist's approach to the development of the child.**

II. Infancy

Infancy begins at birth and lasts until the child is verbal (age 2+ years). During this phase the major emotional milestone is attachment. Attachment is the connection that develops between the infant and the primary caretaker. Bowlby and Mahler are key theorists who **describe the stages of attachment and separation.** Multiple developmental milestones in social, motor, and language skills are met (see Table 4-1).

III. Preschool (ages 2½–6 years)

Important aspects of the child's emotional and cognitive development during the preschool phase include egocentricity, magical thinking, and body image anxiety.

A. **Egocentricity** is the child's perception that all life events revolve around him.
B. **Magical thinking** is the creative weaving of reality and fantasy to explain how things occur in the world (**associative logic**).
C. **Body image anxiety** is a result of the child's immature sense of body integrity. The preschooler feels that his whole body is vulnerable when any body part is injured (e.g., my arm is broken, therefore I am broken).

IV. School Age/Latency (ages 6–12 years)

Latency is the **phase of development that is characterized by mastery of skills.** Children are gaining skills in many areas: academic, athletic, artistic, and social. **School and peer groups play a fundamental role** for the child. **Status within the peer group depends on a child's abilities** and how they compare with those of his/her peers. During this phase **children develop best friends.** Cognitively, the child is **able to use logical thinking (causal logic)** and appreciate another person's point of view. **The disorders that present during this phase are often related to school performance and peer relationships.**

V. Adolescence (ages 12–18 years)

The emphasis during adolescence **is on autonomy and sexuality.** The adolescent is **struggling to create a sense of identity that is separate from his or her parents.** His/her **emerging identity relies on the peer group** to determine what is "in" and what is "out." **Attractiveness is a key component of self-esteem.** There is tremendous self-consciousness, heightened by the range of maturation at any given age. Adolescents are reaching new levels both cognitively and emotionally. At this stage they are **capable of abstract thinking.**

VI. Theories of Development

A. Bowlby's Attachment Theory

1. **John Bowlby: attachment theory is a reciprocal process of bonding that is based on the care and the relationship that develop between the infant and his primary caregiver.** Attachment is the observable behavior of an infant responding to his caregiver. The infant at 6–8 weeks of age smiles in recognition of the mother and imprints the mother's face as the person to whom he will turn. A mutual connection and admiration has formed between the infant and the mother (caretaker). **The result of this attachment behavior is an infant who feels and is protected by his mother.** Bowlby asserts that attachment evolved to protect helpless infants from potential predators. **The three stages of mother-infant separation are:**
   a. Protest: the infant is separated from the caregiver and cries or calls out.
   b. Despair: the infant gives up hope that the mother will return.
   c. Detachment: the infant has emotionally separated himself from the mother.
2. **Mary Ainsworth created a model to determine the quality and strength of the attachment between the infant and the mother.** The **stranger situation was developed** to observe the infant in increasingly stressful situations. This **seven-step process** follows a sequence of the infant and the mother being together in a room → a stranger enters the room → the mother

Table 4-1. Developmental Milestones That Might Be Used in Screening Tests

Age	*Social*	*Gross Motor*	*Fine Motor*	*Language*
6 weeks	Social smile		Follows past midline	Responds to bell
2 months	Recognizes mother	Sits with head steady	Reaches for object	
4 months		Rolls over	Holds a rattle	Coos
6 months		Sits alone	Passes cube hand to hand	Laughs
8–10 months	Stranger anxiety	Stands	Thumb-finger grasp	Dada/mama non-specific
	Plays peek-a-boo	Creeps		
12 months	Drinks from a cup	Walks		Dada/mama specific
14–18 months	Imitates housework	Throws ball overhand	Four-cube tower	Combines two different words
24 months	Plays interactive games	Rides a tricycle	Eight-cube tower	Knows 50+ words
3 years			Copy a "0"	Gives first and last name
4 years	Dresses with supervision	Hops on one foot	Copy a "+"	Recognizes colors
			Draws man in three parts	
5 years	Dresses alone		Copies a square	

leaves the room → the infant is left alone with the stranger → the mother returns and the process is repeated. Through these observations, **Ainsworth concluded** that **more than 60% of infants have secure attachments by the age of 24 months.**

B. Mahler's Separation-Individuation Process

Margaret Mahler described the **separation-individuation process** that **occurs between a mother and a child.** This theory is based on behavioral observations. Mahler describes the **first phase as symbiosis** (birth to five months), during which the infant does not differentiate from the mother. The **separation-individuation process begins at approximately five months of age and follows four stages through the first three years of life.**

1. **Differentiation** (5–10 months)
   a. Physical movement away from the mother begins to occur.
   b. The infant begins to explore through play with his/her own body.
   c. Stranger anxiety develops.
2. **Practicing** (10–15 months)
   a. The infant gains physical distance through walking.
   b. Greater exploration occurs.
   c. Separation anxiety occurs.
3. **Rapprochement** (18–24 months)
   a. Self-awareness begins to develop. This increased self-awareness leads to anxiety and conflict.
   b. The child wants to stay close to the mother, but also wants to explore.
4. **Consolidation and object constancy** (24–36 months)
   a. The child is able to maintain an internal representation of the mother.
   b. The child tolerates separations from his mother, knowing that they will be reunited.

Table 4-2. Theorists' Approach to Child Development

	Cognitive Stages—Piaget	*Psychosocial Stages—Erikson*	*Psychosexual Stages—Freud*
Birth to 12 months	Sensorimotor stage	Trust vs. mistrust	Oral
1–2 years		Autonomy vs. shame Doubt	Anal
3–5 years	Pre-operational thought	Initiative vs. guilt	Phallic
6–10 years	Concrete operations	Industry vs. inferiority	Latency
11–18 years	Formal operations	Identity vs. role confusion	Adolescence

C. Freud's Psychosexual Model of Development

Sigmund Freud outlined the psychosexual development of the child from a psychoanalytic perspective. According to Freud, **the sexual goal of each stage is to derive pleasure and to relieve pain.** Accordingly, the infant is first soothed by the mother's breast and derives satisfaction orally; hence the first stage is the oral stage. **Freud's psychosexual stages are based on the child's development of sexual drives, body maturation, and nervous system development.**

1. **Oral phase** (birth to 1 year). The infant's urges are focused on feeding and sucking at the breast. This is the source of all the infant's satisfaction and frustration.
2. **Anal phase** (1–3 years). The child's urges are centered on bowel functioning. His/her ability to have control over his/her bodily functions becomes the main issue in the relationship between the child and the caregiver.
3. **Phallic (genital) phase** (3–5 years). The genitals become the child's focus for pleasure and satisfaction. Masturbation is used as a way of releasing tension and leads to anxiety and guilt.
   a. **Oedipal complex.** The child falls in love with the parent of the opposite sex. The child wants to have exclusive possession of the parent and wants to eliminate the other parent.
   b. **Castration anxiety.** The boy fears that his father will cut off his penis in retaliation for the boy's coveting his mother. This anxiety leads to repression of the sexual desire for the mother.
   c. **Penis envy.** A girl's curiosity and desire to have a penis.
   d. **Resolution of the Oedipal complex.** The child identifies with the same sex parent and begins to form relationships with same sex peers.
4. **Latency** (6–11 years). Sexual development during this phase is relatively stagnant.
5. **Adolescence** (12–18 years). Genital sexuality develops and proceeds into adulthood.

D. Erikson's Epigenetic Model of Development

Erik Erikson presents an **epigenetic model of development from birth to old age.** The epigenetic principle holds that the **eight stages of the life cycle are sequential, each stage relying on the next.** For successful development, a person must complete one stage before moving on to the next stage. If a stage is not completed, the unresolved issues continue to arise and create problems in the subsequent stages. **Each stage addresses cognitive, ego, sexual, social, and societal issues,** and offers positive and negative adaptations. Erikson also emphasizes the importance of adaptation to society.

1. **Basic trust vs. basic mistrust** (birth–1 year)
   a. A sense of basic trust is derived from the attachment that forms between the child and the parent who provides consistent care.
   b. Mistrust develops when the child is unable to rely on his or her parent for basic care, which leads to feelings of emptiness and despair.
2. **Autonomy vs. shame and doubt** (1–3 years)
   a. The child's sense of self is in part based on his or her ability to control his/her bodily functions (e.g., anal sphincter control).
   b. The child is able to explore and briefly separate from the parent without significant distress. The trust developed during the first stage gives the child the freedom to explore.
   c. Shame and doubt develop when the child is required to perform, but is unable.
3. **Initiative vs. guilt** (3–6 years)
   a. The child takes steps toward establishing a special relationship with the parent of the same sex.
   b. Fantasy allows the child to feel both the pleasure and the pride of being powerful and the guilt of having the imagined power to do harm to others.
4. **Industry vs. inferiority** (6–12 years)
   a. This stage corresponds to entering school. The main tasks for the child are ones of learning and doing.
   b. The child strives for a sense of accomplishment and develops a sense of mastery and control of his environment (i.e., school), avoiding failure at all costs.
   c. Feelings of inferiority develop when the child is unable to master all tasks.
   d. The child begins to understand that his family is a part of a larger society. Parents are no longer perceived as the only authorities.
5. **Identity vs. role confusion** (12–20 years)
   a. Adolescence is a phase of development that combines the potential for significant growth and crisis. Adolescents are at a fragile point of finding themselves at the same time as losing themselves.
   b. Multiple physical and social changes occur.
   c. Normative crises may evolve into disruptive and pathological behavior, but are not inherently maladaptive.
   d. Adolescents must identify within themselves and with the society at large.
6. **Intimacy vs. isolation** (20–40 years)
   a. The establishment of a stable love relationship requires that a person have a reasonable sense of self/personal identity.
   b. The fear of intimacy may lead one to choose isolation.
   c. The mature individual chooses the vulnerable position of intimacy over the loneliness of isolation.
   d. These adaptations also extend into one's career aspirations.
7. **Generativity vs. stagnation** (40–65 years)
   a. Adults can be generative through child rearing and mentoring in the community, passing along to the next generation what they have learned and achieved.
   b. Stagnation occurs when the adult is unable to give to others and remains isolated and self-involved.
8. **Ego integrity vs. despair** (65 years and older)
   a. Integrity develops for a person who feels that they have led a fulfilled life and are content with their place in the life cycle.
   b. Despair occurs for those who feel that life had no meaning. Death becomes a feared end to an unfulfilled life.

E. Piaget's Model of Cognitive Development

Jean Piaget focused on **the cognitive development of the child.** In this model the child follows a continuous pattern of behavior of adapting and responding to the various stimuli in the environment. Piaget describes this behavior as **a schema, a pattern or loop of behavior: stimulus-response-awareness.** The development of the child's cognitive abilities is categorized in **four stages:**

1. **Sensorimotor stage** (birth through 18–24 months)
   a. The senses receive a stimulus and the body reacts to it in a stereotyped way.
   b. **Object permanency** develops during the second year. The child is able to maintain a mental image of the object. The child will look for a toy where it disappeared.
2. **Pre-operational thought—prelogical** (2–6 years)
   a. **Symbolic functions develop.**
   b. Language development changes the child's ability to interact.
   c. **Egocentric thinking** (i.e., the perception that everything revolves around them) occurs. Minimal objectivity is involved.
   d. **Magical thinking,** in which reality and fantasy are interwoven to explain the world around them, arises. Unable to use a logical process to explain how and why they know what they know.
   e. Moral thought occurs, which is based on something being good or bad.
3. **Concrete operations** (7–11 years)
   a. Here, a rational and logical thought process is used.
   b. A more conceptual framework is applied to the world.
   c. An ability to understand someone else's point of view develops.
   d. The **concept of conservation.** The child is able to understand the combination of two variables (e.g., height and width). An example of a beaker experiment is often used: Water is placed in two identical beakers (A and B), then water from beaker B is transferred into a taller, narrower beaker C. The child is asked if the amount of water in beakers A and C is the same or different. A child at this stage of development will understand that the amount of water present in beakers A and C is the same even though the levels in the beakers are different.
4. **Formal operations** (12+ years)
   a. During this stage, **abstract thinking, deductive reasoning, and conceptual thinking develop.**
      i. **Abstract thinking** is the ability to manipulate ideas and theoretical constructs.
      ii. **Deductive reasoning** is the ability to go from the general to the particular.
      iii. **Conceptual thinking** is the ability to define concepts or ideas.

F. Chess and Thomas's Theory of Temperament

Stella Chess and Alexander Thomas described children as having individual styles that are shaped as the child and the family develop. The temperament of the child **takes into account nine observed behaviors** and **categorizes children as "easy," "difficult," and "slow to warm up."** These behaviors include activity level, rhythmicity, approach or withdrawal response, adaptability to change in the environment, threshold of responsiveness, intensity of any given reaction, mood, degree of distractibility, and persistence in the face of obstacles. They describe children as being active participants in their own development and experience.

G. Kohlberg's Model of Moral Development

Lawrence Kohlberg described **three major levels of development** of moral judgment. His theory has been criticized for being culture-bound, middle-class, and male oriented.

1. Level I: **Pre-morality (pre-conventional) morality.** Here, the child follows the rules set forth by his parents. Parents are the authority figures and they establish the standards of punishment and obedience.
2. Level II: **Morality of conventional role-conformity.** The child conforms to the norms of the group in order to gain acceptance and to maintain relationships.
3. Level III: **Morality of self-accepted principles.** The child voluntarily follows rules based on the concept of ethical principles and makes exceptions when they are determined to be appropriate.

H. Gilligan's Model of Morality

Carol Gilligan presented a view of the development of morality that includes **alternate pathways to the same moral pinnacle.** She proposed that **girls have a greater sense of connection and concern with relationships than with rules** and meet the highest level of moral development through other routes.

VII. Other Significant Issues during Childhood

A. Divorce

1. Over 1 million children each year are affected by divorce.
2. Marriages end in divorce after an average of 6–7 years.
3. The impact of divorce on children is significant and depends on multiple factors, including the parents' attention to the child and the age of the child. Half of children have difficulties during the first year after divorce. Factors that contribute to an adjustment period longer than 1 year include: parental discord, parental psychiatric illness, and poverty.
4. The impact on family is also significant:
   a. Relationships: the mother is the custodial parent 90% of the time.
   b. Psychiatric: higher rates of depression occur in parents after the divorce.
   c. Financial: women experience significant drops in their disposable income.

B. Child Abuse

1. **Physical abuse** (any inflicted rather than accidental injury) **and child neglect** (the major needs of the child, such as nutrition, shelter, protection, health care, education, and emotional needs, are not met) occur to more than 1 million children in the United States each

year. More than 3,000 deaths are caused by child abuse each year.

a. Risk factors include low birth weight, handicapped (e.g., mental retardation), and behaviorally-disordered children.

b. The abuser is most commonly a parent, often one who was abused in childhood himself or herself.

2. **Sexual abuse.** The engaging of the child in sexual activities that the child cannot comprehend, for which the child is developmentally unprepared to give consent for, and/or that violates the social and legal taboos of society.

a. In the majority of cases, the perpetrator is known to the victim, and most often is a father or stepfather/surrogate father.

b. The median age of victims is between 9 and 10 years.

c. Risk factors include physical or sexual abuse history of the perpetrator, substance abuse, impulsivity, sexual deviancy, and violent tendencies.

Suggested Readings

Abrams, A., & Rauch, P. (1998). Developmental considerations in critical care medicine. *New Horizons, 6,* 321–330.

Bowlby, J. (1969). *Attachment and loss: Vol. 1: Attachment.* New York: Basic Books.

Erikson, E. (1963). *Childhood and society* (2nd ed.). New York: W.W. Norton.

Gilligan, C. (1982). *In a different voice: Psychological theory and women's development.* Cambridge, MA: Harvard University Press.

Kohlberg, L. (1984). *The psychology of moral development: The nature and validity of moral stages.* San Francisco: Harper and Row.

Lewis, M. (1996). Normal growth and development: An overview. In M. Lewis (Ed.), *Child and adolescent psychiatry: A comprehensive textbook* (2nd ed.). Baltimore: Williams and Wilkins.

Mahler, M.S., Pine, F., & Bergman, A. (1975). *The psychological birth of the human infant: Symbiosis and individuation.* New York: Basic Books.

Thomas, A., Chess, S., & Birch, H.G. (1968). *Temperament and behavior disorders in children.* New York: New York University Press.

Vaughan, V.C., & Litt, I.F. (1992). Growth and development. In R.E. Behrman (Ed.), *Nelson textbook of pediatrics* (14th ed., pp. 13–104). Philadelphia: W.B. Saunders.

Wallerstein, J.S., & Kelly, J.B. (1980). *Surviving the breakup: How children and parents cope with divorce.* New York: Basic Books.

Chapter 5

Child and Adolescent Disorders

Annah Abrams and Jean Frazier

I. Overview

Approximately 10% of the child and adolescent population suffers from psychiatric disorders (Wilens et al., 1998). **When psychiatric illnesses present in childhood, they tend to be more familial and chronic, and to be associated with greater morbidity.** This chapter outlines the disorders of infancy, childhood, and adolescence, and presents them in the diagnostic categories as outlined in the *Diagnostic and Statistical Manual, Fourth Edition* (DSM-IV). In addition, treatment for these childhood-onset psychiatric disorders is addressed.

II. Disruptive Behavioral Disorders

A. Attention Deficit Hyperactivity Disorder (ADHD)

1. **Diagnosis. Attention deficit hyperactivity disorder (ADHD) is the most common psychiatric disorder in children; its prevalence is 3–5% in school-age children (DSM-IV).** It often **presents as a classic triad of inattention, hyperactivity, and impulsivity.** However, some children may be primarily hyperactive and others primarily inattentive.
2. **Symptoms** must include at least six signs of inattention and six signs of hyperactivity-impulsivity for 6 months.
   a. **Symptoms of inattention include** failure to pay close attention to details, difficulty sustaining attention in tasks or activities, failure to listen when spoken to directly, difficulty organizing tasks, avoidance of activities that require mental effort, losing things necessary for tasks or activities, distractibility, and forgetfulness in daily activities.
   b. **Symptoms of hyperactivity include** fidgeting with the hands or feet, inability to sit still, running around when it is not appropriate, difficulty engaging in leisure activities quietly, feeling "on the go" or "driven by a motor," and talking excessively.
   c. **Symptoms of impulsivity include** blurting out answers before questions are completed, having trouble waiting one's turn, and interrupting others.
3. The diagnosis is specified as either combined type, predominately inattentive type, or predominately hyperactive-impulsive type. The pattern of behavior must be more frequent and severe than that observed in other children of the same developmental level. The symptoms of the disorder must be present before the age of 7 years. Many children are diagnosed after this age, but the symptoms often have been present for years prior to the diagnosis. **Impairment must cross situations and must be noted in at least two settings (e.g., school and home).** The symptoms are not exclusively present when another disorder, such as depression, is present.
4. **Prevalence is 3–5% among school-age children.** The disorder is **reported to persist into adolescence and adulthood for approximately 50% of those affected. The male to female ratio is 4–9:1,** depending on the type and setting.
5. **Medication is the first line of treatment for ADHD. There is a 70–80% response rate to psychostimulants** (Wilens et al., 1998). The psychostimulants include methylphenidate, dextroamphetamine, magnesium pemoline, and amphetamine sulfate.
   a. **Psychostimulants**
      i. **Methylphenidate (Ritalin)** should be started at 2.5–5 mg/day, and increased if necessary by 2.5–5 mg/day (reaching an optimal dose of 0.3–2 mg/kg/day). **Side effects** include insomnia, decreased appetite, mood disturbance, tics (rare), headache, gastrointestinal distress, and psychosis (rare).
      ii. **Dextroamphetamine (Dexedrine)** is twice as potent as methylphenidate. It has a similar side-effect profile to methylphenidate.
      iii. **Magnesium pemoline (Cylert)** has a longer half-life and is dosed differently than methylphenidate and dextroamphetamine. The initial dose is 18.75 mg/day, which is increased by 18.75 mg every few days. The dose range is 1–3 mg/kg/day. Its side-effect profile is similar to that of methylphenidate; however, liver toxicity is a concern, and, as a result, pemoline is not a first-line treatment. Liver function tests (LFTs) should be checked at baseline and every 3–6 months.
      iv. **Amphetamine sulfate (Adderall)** is a long-acting amphetamine compound.
      v. **Long-acting methylphenidate preparations (Concerta, Metadate CD, and Ritalin LA)** release methylphenidate immediately followed by a sustained/second release with resulting plasma levels of methylphenidate lasting approximately 12 hours.
   b. **Antihypertensive** medications (which are alpha-agonists) may also be used to treat ADHD, especially if a tic disorder or aggression is present.
      i. **Clonidine** should be initiated at 0.025 mg b.i.d., and may be dosed up to 4–5 μcg/kg/day total. Side effects include sedation, depression, and rebound hypertension.
      ii. **Guanfacine (Tenex)** is similar to clonidine, but less potent and less sedating. It is dosed up to 1–2 mg t.i.d.

c. **Antidepressants.** Tricyclic antidepressants (TCAs) and bupropion (Wellbutrin) may also be used for the treatment of ADHD. TCAs have been shown to be 60–70% effective (Wilens et al., 1998).

B. Conduct Disorder (CD)

1. **Diagnosis. A child with conduct disorder (CD) has a pattern of behavior in which the rights of others or societal norms/rules are violated. Four categories of behavior are described:**
   a. Aggression toward people and animals
   b. Destruction of property
   c. Deceitfulness or theft
   d. Serious violation of rules
2. **The child must have the symptoms of the disorder in the past year and at least one symptom in the past 6 months. Affected children have impairment in social, academic, and occupational functioning.** If the person is over the age of 18 years, he or she may be diagnosed with conduct disorder if the criteria for antisocial personality disorder are not met.
3. **Subclassification:** There are **two subtypes** of the disorder:
   a. **Childhood onset:** at least one criterion must be present prior to the age of 10 years.
   b. **Adolescent onset:** no criteria are present prior to age 10 years.
4. **Prevalence.** There is an **earlier average age of onset for boys** than for girls: ages 10–12 years for boys and 16 years for girls. Prognosis is worse with an earlier onset of the disorder. Prevalence depends on the population sampled; ranges of 6–16% in males and 2–9% in females have been reported.
5. **Treatment. The mainstay of treatment for CD is behavioral therapy.** There are no specific medications for the core symptoms of this disorder. The symptoms of **aggression and agitation may be treated with medications,** including alpha-agonists, beta-blockers, mood stabilizers, and antipsychotics. It is important to assess and treat co-morbid conditions.

C. Oppositional Defiant Disorder (ODD)

1. **Diagnosis.** These children have **a pattern of negative, hostile, and defiant behavior** of at least 6 months' duration. The behavior is usually directed at an authority figure (e.g., a parent or teacher). The behavior causes significant distress in social or academic settings. Oppositional defiant disorder (ODD) is not diagnosed in the context of a mood or psychotic disorder. ODD cannot be diagnosed if conduct disorder (CD) is present.
2. **Prevalence.** Prevalence is reported to be **between 2–16%.** Males with the disorder are more prevalent than females prior to puberty; however, after puberty, the male to female ratio equals out. There is a gradual onset of symptoms, usually appearing before the age of 8 years. Approximately 25% of children diagnosed with ODD no longer meet the criteria after several years; others worsen and many are eventually diagnosed with CD.
3. **Treatment.** Treatment for ODD is **behavioral therapy.**

III. Mood Disorders

Mood disorders in children are classified as unipolar or bipolar, with major and minor levels of severity. Juvenile mood disorders tend to be more chronic and more refractory to pharmacologic interventions than adult-onset mood disorders. **The prevalence of these disorders increases with age.** Mood disorders are not classified as childhood disorders in the DSM-IV. For treatment of mood disorders in children, see Table 5-1.

Table 5-1. Characteristics and Treatment of Child and Adolescent Disorders

Disorder	*Main Characteristics*	*Treatment*	
Disruptive Behavior Disorders		*Therapy*	*Medication*
Attention Deficit Hyperactivity Disorder	Inattention, hyperactivity, impulsivity		Stimulants, TCAs, alpha-agonists, atypical antidepressants
Conduct Disorder	Patterns of aggressive and antisocial behavior	Behavioral therapy	No specific medications for core symptoms; assess and treat co-morbid conditions; may treat aggression and agitation with alpha-agonists, beta-blockers, mood stabilizers, and antipsychotics

Table 5-1. (*Continued*)

Disorder	*Main Characteristics*	*Treatment*	
Oppositional Defiant Disorder	Pattern of negative, hostile, and defiant behavior	As for Conduct Disorder	As for Conduct Disorder
Mood Disorders			
Depression	Sad or irritable mood and/or loss of interest in usual activities; neuro-vegetative symptoms; age-specific associated features (e.g., school refusal)	Psychotherapy, cognitive-behavioral therapy	SSRIs, TCAs, atypical antidepressants
Bipolar Disorder	Extreme irritability or explosive mood; neurovegetative symptoms as seen in adults	Supportive psychotherapy	Mood stabilizers, anti-psychotics (typical and atypical)
Anxiety Disorders			
Separation Anxiety Disorder	Excessive anxiety when a child is separated from caretaker	Cognitive-behavioral therapy	BZDs, buspirone, SSRIs
Obsessive-compulsive Disorder	Recurrent obsessions and compulsions, severe and distressing	Cognitive-behavioral therapy, psychotherapy	Clomipramine, SSRIs
Post-Traumatic Stress Disorder	Trauma followed by hypervigilance, autonomic reactivity, and avoidance	Psychotherapy, dialectical behavioral therapy	alpha-agonists, SSRIs, BZDs, occasionally antipsychotics
Social Phobia	Fear of embarrassment in social situations	Cognitive-behavioral therapy	
Generalized Anxiety Disorder	Excessive anxiety and worry	Cognitive-behavioral therapy	BZDs, buspirone, SSRIs
Psychotic Disorders	Delusions, hallucinations, bizarre behavior, thought disorder, and negative symptoms (inattention and anhedonia, avolition, apathy, and alogia)		Antipsychotics (typical and atypical)
Developmental Disorders			
Pervasive Developmental Disorders	Impairment in multiple areas: motor, language, social, and academic	Behavioral therapy; treat co-morbid disorder. Important interventions include appropriate school placement, OT/PT, and speech and language therapy	
Autistic Disorder	Same as above	Same as above	
Learning Disorders	Reading, mathematics, written expression	Appropriate school accommodation for the learning disability; tutoring	
Communication Disorders	Expressive and/or receptive language deficits	Appropriate school accommodation; tutoring; speech therapy	
Motor Skills Disorders	Coordination impairment	OT/PT	
Elimination Disorders			
Encopresis	Fecal incontinence	Behavioral therapy	Medical management of constipation and diarrhea
Enuresis	Urinary incontinence	Behavioral therapy (bell and pad conditioning)	TCAs (imipramine), ddAVP

(continued)

Table 5-1. (*Continued*)

Disorder	*Main Characteristics*	*Treatment*	
Feeding Disorders			
Pica	Eating of non-nutritional substances	Behavioral therapy	
Rumination Disorder	Rechewing or regurgitation of food		Treatment of medical consequences of disorder
Feeding Disorder of Infancy and Early Childhood	Failure to eat leading to weight loss or failure to gain weight	Infant–parent work, behavorial therapy	
Tic Disorders			
Complex Motor or Vocal Tics	Either motor or vocal tics		alpha-agonists, antipsychotics
Tourette's	Multiple motor and one or more vocal tics; co-morbid with OCD and ADHD		alpha-agonists, antipsychotics
Other Disorders of Childhood			
Selective Mutism	Does not speak in some social situations, but fluent in others	Psychotherapy, cognitive-behavioral therapy	SSRIs
Reactive Attachment Disorder	Disturbed ability to relate socially	Consistent placement/caregivers, infant–parent work	

ADHD, Attention Deficit Hyperactivity Disorder; BZD, benzodiazepine; ddAVP, imipramine and vasopressin; OCD, Obsessive-Compulsive Disorder; OT/PT, occupational/physical therapy; SSRI, selective serotonin reuptake inhibitor; TCA, tricyclic antidepressant.

A. Major Depression

1. **Diagnosis.** In children, major depression may present with **a sad or irritable mood and/or a loss of interest or pleasure in the child's usual activities.** Child-specific symptoms include **school difficulties, school refusal, somatic complaints, and aggressive/antisocial behavior patterns.** Physiologic changes, such as **weight change or sleep pattern disruption,** also may be present. Psychotic symptoms may be present in a depressed child.
2. **Prevalence. The prevalence is 0.3% in preschoolers, 1–2% in school-age children, and 5% in adolescents.** There is an equal male to female ratio until adolescence, when the adult pattern of 3:2 female to male emerges.

B. Bipolar Disorder

Mania in children often presents as an extremely irritable or explosive mood with poor psychosocial functioning. Children may exhibit unrestrained high energy, over-talkativeness, racing thoughts, decreased sleep, and increased goal-directed activity. Poor judgment, as manifested by reckless thrill-seeking behavior, may also be present. It is important to differentiate juvenile mania from ADHD, conduct disorder, depression, and psychotic disorders that commonly occur with mania (Wozniak et al., 1995). See Table 5-1 and chapter 14 for the treatment of bipolar disorder.

IV. Anxiety Disorders

Multiple anxiety disorders can be diagnosed during childhood; however, **according to the DSM-IV, only separation anxiety disorder is classified as a childhood-onset anxiety disorder.**

A. Separation Anxiety Disorder

1. **Diagnosis.** Separation anxiety is defined as **excessive anxiety that occurs when a child is separated from home or from significant attachment figures.** Such anxiety occurs as **part of normal development in children around the age of 2 years.** However, when the symptoms have an onset later during childhood and they become excessive to the point of impairing functioning, a disorder is diagnosed. Afflicted children have excessive anxiety when separated from parents (or other important figures) and excessive worry (about losing someone or about something untoward happening to their primary caretaker).
2. **Prevalence. Symptoms must last at least 4 weeks; the onset must occur before 18 years of age. The**

prevalence is 4% of school-age children and 1% of adolescents. It occurs equally in boys and girls.

3. **Treatment.** Treatment includes **cognitive-behavioral therapy** and **medications** (selective serotonin reuptake inhibitors [SSRIs], buspirone, and benzodiazepines).

B. Obsessive-Compulsive Disorder (OCD)

1. **Diagnosis. OCD is manifest by recurrent and distressing ideas (obsessions) that are intrusive in one's thoughts. These may lead to repetitive and purposeful behaviors (compulsions).** Children's thoughts may include fears of contamination, or feelings of self-doubt or guilt. The resulting compulsive behaviors that alleviate the obsessions include checking, counting, handwashing, and touching.
2. **Prevalence. The prevalence of the disorder is approximately 1–2%** in the adult population. The disorder often initially presents during childhood and adolescence. Treatment issues are the same as in adults; see Table 5-1 and chapter 15.

C. Post-Traumatic Stress Disorder (PTSD)

Children with PTSD **experience or witness a traumatic event and develop symptoms of the disorder subsequent to that trauma.** The symptoms of the disorder include **re-experiencing of the event** (e.g., recurrent intrusive recollections or recurrent distressing dreams of the event), **autonomic arousal** (e.g., increased heart rate or blood pressure), and **avoidance of any stimuli associated with the trauma.** For treatment, see Table 5-1 and chapter 16.

D. Social Phobia

Social phobia involves **a fear of embarrassment in social situations.** Children may exhibit their fears by crying or by staying close to familiar adults. They may appear to be very shy and often are on the periphery in social situations (e.g., not participating on the playground). Unlike adults, children often are unable to avoid the situations that cause the anxiety (e.g., school) and/or are unable to identify the source of the anxiety. The symptoms may interfere with class performance and social activities. The phobia must be present in same age peer group situations and not just with adults. The course depends on the age that it presents. If the onset is in childhood, it may lead to a failure to achieve, whereas adolescents may experience a decline in functioning. For treatment, see Table 5-1 and chapter 15.

E. Generalized Anxiety Disorder (GAD)

The main feature of this disorder **is excessive anxiety and worry present for at least 6 months.** Children tend to worry about their ability to perform. The worries may be focused on school or athletic performance, even when they are not being evaluated. The anxiety also may be focused on catastrophic events (e.g., a hurricane). Frequently, these children are perfectionistic, which causes them to re-do tasks and to seek constant reassurance that they have done well. For treatment, see Table 5-1 and chapter 15.

V. Psychotic Disorders

A. Psychotic Disorders of Childhood

1. **Diagnosis.** Psychosis may present in childhood (rarely); it refers to **abnormal behavior** that is accompanied by **impaired reality testing.** Psychosis is defined by the presence of positive symptoms, which include **delusions, hallucinations, bizarre behavior, thought disorder,** and negative symptoms of **inattention, anhedonia, avolition, apathy, and alogia** (poverty of speech). **Developmental issues complicate the diagnosis of a child with a psychotic disorder.** Normal children have rich fantasy lives in their preschool and latency years. Therefore, differentiating normal fantasies from delusions can be difficult. In addition, normal preschool and latency age children have speaking patterns that could be described as looseness of associations due to their language and cognitive development. However, if a child is psychotic he or she has extreme degrees of disordered thought. The diagnosis of a psychotic disorder in children should be reserved for those who are consumed with fantasy and who do not recognize how fantasy differs from reality. Children have visual hallucinations more commonly than do adults. These usually occur with auditory hallucinations. In addition, children may have delusions, but they are less fixed in nature than are the delusions in adults.
2. **Prevalence.** Childhood-onset schizophrenia **occurs rarely (in roughly 1/10,000 children)** and develops insidiously over more than 6 months. The male to female ratio ranges from 3:1 to 5:1 (Frazier et al., 1997). The majority of children who present with psychotic symptoms have a primary affective disorder. Afflicted children typically have an acute onset of symptoms (Frazier et al., 1997).
3. **Treatment.** The cornerstone of treatment for psychotic disorders in children is antipsychotic medication. Given the lower risk of tardive dyskinesia associated with atypical neuroleptics, they are now being used as first-line treatment. Adjunctive medications should be used according to the symptoms present (e.g., antidepressants for depression or mood stabilizers for bipolar disorder) and their side-effect profiles (e.g., benztropine for Parkinsonian symptoms).

VI. Pervasive Developmental Disorders (PPD)

Children with these disorders have **severe and pervasive impairment in multiple areas of development.** All these children require thorough evaluations. Treatment is multidisciplinary and includes behavioral, occupational, speech, and language therapy. These children also require individualized school programs to ensure appropriate placement and expectations. Recognition and treatment of co-morbid disorders is important. The identification of children with pervasive developmental disorders has increased over the past decade. Recent studies indicate a prevalence of autism spectrum disorders (autistic disorder, Asperger's disorder, and PDD NOS [not otherwise specified]) of 34/10,000.

A. Autistic Disorder

1. Children with autism have **impairment with social interaction, communications, and behavior.**
   a. **Impaired social interactions** may present as abnormal gaze, posture, and expression in social interactions. There is a relative lack of peer relationships, emotional reciprocity, and spontaneous seeking of enjoyment.
   b. **Impaired communication** (verbal and social play) may present as a delay or lack of speech, impaired ability to initiate or sustain conversations, repetitive use of language, and inability to play with others.
   c. **Impaired behavior** may present as restricted repetitive and stereotyped patterns of behavior, interests, and activities.
2. The **onset** of the disorder is **prior to age 3 years.** The **male to female ratio is 4:1. Approximately 75% of children with autism are mentally retarded.**

B. Asperger's Disorder

This disorder is similar to autism in terms of abnormal social interactions and restricted repetitive and stereotyped patterns of behavior, interests, and activities. In contrast to autism, Asperger's disorder has **no delay in language or in cognitive development.** These individuals also have **no delay in age-appropriate self-care, adaptive behavior (except in social interactions), or curiosity about the environment.** The prevalence is not known, but it appears to be more common in males.

C. Rett's Disorder

This disorder is similar to autism except that these individuals **function normally through the first five months of life.** Beginning between the ages of 5 and 48 months multiple deficits develop, including decreases in the following areas: head growth, hand skills, social engagement, gait and trunk movements, language, and motor skills. This disorder often is associated with severe or profound mental retardation. The prevalence is not known (uncommon) and **has only been reported in females.**

D. Childhood Disintegrative Disorder

This disorder is similar to autism except that these individuals **develop normally for the first 2 years of life and then experience significant regression in multiple areas.** The losses of previously acquired skills occur between the ages of 2 and 10 years and involve **language, behavior, bowel/bladder control, play, and/or motor skills. Abnormal** functioning in **social interactions, communication, and behavior** develop. **This disorder is usually associated with severe mental retardation.** The prevalence is **rare.**

E. Mental Retardation (MR)

1. **Subaverage general intellectual functioning** is based on a standardized intelligence test (IQ) **with** concurrent **impairment in adaptive functioning** in at least two of the following areas: communication, self-care, home living, and social/interpersonal skills. **Subaverage** is defined as a full-scale IQ of less than 70 (i.e., two standard deviations below the mean). **Four diagnostic severity levels of MR** are described:
   a. **Mild** (IQ range of 50–55 to 70). Children with mild MR can develop social and communication skills, and can function relatively normally as adults.
   b. **Moderate** (IQ range of 35–40 to 50–55). Children with moderate MR have limited social awareness. They can be trained to care for most personal needs and to work in sheltered job placements. Moderate supervision is usually required (e.g., as in a group home).
   c. **Severe** (IQ range of 20–25 to 35–40). Children with severe MR have slow and poor motor development. They have limited to no speech and require close supervision.
   d. **Profound** (IQ falls below 20–25). Children with profound MR have poor cognitive and social capacities. Speech is often absent. Constant supervision is needed (e.g., special care setting).
2. The **onset** of MR must occur **before age 18 years.** Prevalence is 2–3% of the school-aged population. See chapter 8 for a more complete review of MR.

VII. Learning Disorders

Learning disorders are **associated with below expected abilities in academic achievement in reading, mathematics, and/or writing,** based on the child's chronological age, measured intelligence, and age-appropriate education. **The difference between achievement and IQ must be at least two standard deviations below the mean.** Reading, mathematics, and writing disorders often are co-morbid. The disorder is usually diagnosed during or after first grade when reading, math, and writing are being taught in school. Children with learning disorders have a school dropout rate of 40% (approximately 1.5 times the average). The **prevalence of learning disorders ranges from 2–10%,** with approximately 5% of school children in the United States diagnosed as having a Learning Disorder. Treatment involves appropriate school accommodation for the learning disability and tutoring.

A. Reading Disorder

This condition is manifest by a below expected reading achievement accompanied by a decreased ability to recognize words, to comprehend, and/or to read accurately. This disorder was **previously known as dyslexia.** The

prevalence is 4% of school-age children, with **a male to female ratio of 4:1.**

B. Mathematics Disorder

This disorder involves a lower than expected mathematical ability as demonstrated by decreased skills in understanding, recognizing, copying, and following mathematical terms, symbols, figures, and steps. **The prevalence is 1% and occurs equally in males and females.**

C. Disorder of Written Expression

This condition is manifest by a below expected ability in spelling, punctuation, and grammar. The prevalence is not known. Children with this disorder are often grouped with other learning disorders.

VIII. Communication Disorders

The communication disorders interfere with academic achievement and social communication and usually present during or after first grade. Treatment includes tutoring and appropriate school accommodation, including speech therapy.

A. Expressive Language Disorder

In this condition, standardized test scores for expressive language are below those for non-verbal intellectual capacity and for receptive language development. The presentation of the disorder depends on the age of the child and may include a **limited amount of speech, a limited range of vocabulary, errors in tense, and an immature language sentence construction.** Two types are known: an **acquired type,** in which impairment occurs after a period of normal development as a result of an insult (e.g., neurological or medical), and a **developmental type,** in which impairment is not associated with a neurological or medical insult. The prevalence for the developmental type is about 3–5%, whereas the acquired type is less common.

B. Mixed Receptive-Expressive Language Disorder

This condition, an expressive language disorder with **receptive language deficit (difficulty understanding words and sentences),** has a prevalence that is less common than expressive language disorder (approximately 3%).

C. Phonological Disorder

Difficulties with phonological disorders occur in **speech production.** The prevalence of moderate to severe symptoms is 2–3% in 6- and 7-year-olds. This decreases to 0.5% by age 17 years.

D. Stuttering

Stuttering is a **disturbance in the normal fluency of speech.** Speech difficulties may include sound repetitions, prolongation, interjections, pauses within words, and word blocking. Stuttering is **often absent in singing.** The disorder begins between the ages of 2 and 7 years with a peak at age 5 years. Almost all cases present before the age of 10 years. The **prevalence is 1% in prepubertal children** with **a male to female ratio of 3:1.** The symptoms often remit in adolescence. There is a familial pattern for the disorder with the risk for a first-degree biological relative developing stuttering at three times the risk of the general population.

IX. Motor Skills Disorder

A. Developmental Coordination Disorder

This is a disorder with an impaired ability to perform daily activities due to a coordination difficulty not accounted for by a medical condition (e.g., cerebral palsy or hemiplegia). These children may be slow to crawl or walk and/or clumsy with fine and gross motor skills. Often this disorder is seen in premature infants. The **prevalence is 6%** in school-age children. The course is variable and may persist into adulthood. These children benefit from occupational and physical therapy.

X. Elimination Disorders

A. Encopresis

This condition is manifest by the repeated passage of feces into inappropriate places (intentional or involuntary); it is not due to a medical condition. This behavior occurs at least **one time per month for 3 months.** Encopresis may occur with or without constipation and overflow incontinence. There are two types of this disorder: **primary (i.e., never toilet-trained) and secondary (i.e., regressed after being toilet-trained). The child must be at least 4 years of age** (chronologically and developmentally). The prevalence is one % of 5-year-olds. It is more common in boys than in girls. The treatment of encopresis is behavioral therapy. Some children need medical intervention for constipation and diarrhea.

B. Enuresis

1. **Diagnosis. Enuresis is manifest by the repeated voiding of urine into bed or clothes (intentional or involuntary) that is not due to a medical condition.** This occurs at least **two times per week for 3 consecutive months** or causes significant distress or social impairment for the child. Enuresis may be **nocturnal, diurnal, or both.** Like encopresis there are two types of the disorder (primary and secondary). The child must be **at least 5 years of age** (chronologically and developmentally).
2. **Prevalence.** The prevalence varies with age ranging from 7% of 5-year-old boys and 3% of 5-year-old girls to 1% of 18-year-old boys and less than 1% of 18-year-old girls.
3. **Treatment.** Treatment should begin with behavioral therapies. Techniques include **star charts and the bell and pad technique** (i.e., a pad is placed on the bed, when the pad gets wet, the bell goes off). If these methods are not successful, medication is the next step. **Imipramine and vasopressin (ddAVP)** have

been shown to be effective. Enuresis may remit spontaneously; it is therefore important not to continue these medications indefinitely.

XI. Feeding and Eating Disorders of Infancy

A. Pica

Pica is the persistent eating of a non-nutritional substance for at least a 1-month period. This behavior is developmentally and culturally inappropriate and is often associated with mental retardation, poverty, and nutritional deficiencies. A medical etiology for the disorder must be ruled out. Behavioral techniques are used for treatment.

B. Rumination Disorder

Rumination disorder involves the repeated regurgitation and rechewing of food occurring for at least 1 month following a period of normal eating. This disorder may be associated with neglect and with developmental delay. The symptoms are not due to a gastrointestinal or medical condition. This disorder develops between the ages of 3 and 12 months. The prevalence is rare. Outcome ranges from spontaneous remission to death secondary to malnutrition (mortality rates as high as 25%). Treatment must address the medical consequences of the illness, such as dehydration and malnutrition, as well as the etiology of the illness, whether it is neglect or developmental delay.

C. Feeding Disorder of Infancy and Early Childhood

A failure to eat leading to an inability to gain weight or a significant loss of weight over a 1-month period characterizes the condition. The symptoms are not due to a medical condition. The disorder must present prior to the age of 6 years, but usually presents during the first year of life. This disorder may be associated with attachment issues, and treatment should involve work with the infant-caregiver dyad.

XII. Tic Disorders

A tic is a sudden rapid recurrent non-rhythmic stereotyped motor movement or vocalization. Tics are described as motor (e.g., eye blinking or neck jerking) or vocal (e.g., grunting or snorting) and as **simple or complex.** A complex tic has more purposeful movements or imitative behaviors. **Tics are involuntary movements, but may be voluntarily suppressed.** Anxiety and stress exacerbate tics. During sleep or while doing an absorbing activity (e.g., playing video games), tics are often decreased.

The disorders listed below **occur prior to the age of 18 years.** If the symptoms present after age 18 years, the diagnosis is tic disorder, not otherwise specified.

A. Tourette's Disorder

Tourette's disorder is a childhood-onset neuropsychiatric disorder with **multiple motor tics and at least one vocal tic** at some time during the illness, but the motor and vocal tics need not be concurrent. **The tics occur many times a day, usually daily, for at least 1 year,** and there is never a tic-free period of more than 3 consecutive months. Impairment occurs in social and/or academic functioning. The tics are not due to the effect of medications (e.g., stimulants) or a medical illness (e.g., chorea). The symptoms often diminish in intensity in adolescence. Tourette's disorder is commonly associated with OCD, ADHD, and anxiety disorders. There is a significant familial association of the disorder with evidence of genetic transmission for vulnerability. Onset occurs before the age of 18 years. The usual age of onset is 7 years with motor tics presenting prior to vocal tics. Prevalence is 4/10,000 to 5/10,000, and is about three times more common in males than females

B. Chronic Motor or Vocal Tic Disorder

This disorder is similar to Tourette's disorder except that children have either motor or vocal tics. This disorder is more common than Tourette's; it occurs in 1–2% of school-age children and is more common in boys. If a person has a history of Tourette's, they cannot be diagnosed with this disorder.

C. Transient Tic Disorder

The symptoms of this disorder are single or multiple motor and/or vocal tics. The symptoms occur for at least 4 weeks, but not greater than 12 months, and may remit without treatment.

XIII. Other Disorders of Childhood

A. Selective Mutism

The child with this disorder will not speak in specific social situations even though their speech is fluent in other settings (usually home). The child usually communicates non-verbally in these settings (e.g., eye contact or head nodding). The diagnosis should not be made if the child is not comfortable with the spoken language (e.g., an immigrant child). The symptoms must be present for at least 1 month. It is associated with anxiety and shyness. The disorder is uncommon and occurs in less than 1% of children. Treatments include psychotherapy, cognitive-behavioral therapy (CBT), and the use of SSRIs.

B. Reactive Attachment Disorder of Infancy and Early Childhood

The child with this condition has **a disturbed and developmentally inappropriate ability to relate socially.** There are two types: the **inhibited type** (in which the child fails to initiate or respond to most social interactions) and the **disinhibited type** (in which the child is indiscriminately social as manifested by diffuse attachments). **Pathological child care,** either emotional and/or physical disregard for the child's basic needs or repeated changes in the primary caregiver, often is the etiology of the disorder. The disorder is not accounted for by developmental delay. The symptoms present prior to age 5 years. It is an uncommon disorder. Treatment of reactive attachment disorder includes consistent placement and caregiver and infant dyad work.

C. **Other Significant Issues during Childhood**
   1. **Suicide** (see chapter 54). **Suicide is the third leading cause of death in adolescents behind accidents and homicide.** The death rate for adolescents from suicide is 13/100,000. As with adults, the ratio of males to females for completed suicide is 4:1, and the reverse is true for attempted suicide (i.e., 4:1 female to male). The most common successful means used is firearms for both males and females. Other means include hanging, suffocation, and poisoning/overdose (OD). Risk factors include a previous attempt (25%), substance abuse, chronic illness, depression, psychosis, gender identity issues (homosexuality), and family issues, including history of suicide, discord, and psychiatric illness/substance abuse.
   2. **Eating disorders. Anorexia** and **bulimia** are reviewed in chapter 21.

XIV. Child-Specific Pharmacologic Issues

A. Many of the disorders that present during childhood are responsive to medication. However, the use of medications in children is not as well established as it is in adults. The use of medications in children should occur only after completion of a thorough diagnostic evaluation. This process includes a full psychiatric assessment, structured psychiatric interviews and rating forms as indicated, and relevant laboratory studies to rule out underlying medical conditions.

B. **Children often benefit significantly from the initiation of medications for the treatment of psychiatric disorders.** Medication may decrease the symptoms of a disorder, effect a positive change in the social/emotional and behavioral presentation of the child, and optimize the developmental trajectory of the child.

C. **The following basic pharmacologic principles should be considered when medications are used in children.**
   1. **Children metabolize most medications more efficiently than adults** and may require two-fold greater weight-corrected doses of medications.
   2. **Children may have higher peak plasma concentrations.**
   3. **Children may have lower trough plasma concentrations.**

XV. Conclusion

This chapter underscores that psychopathology does occur in children and adolescents and that this inherently involves some degree of developmental deviance. It is important to be able to recognize the disorders and how they present in childhood in order to initiate appropriate therapeutic interventions. The aim of these interventions is to decrease the child's symptoms and to facilitate development.

Suggested Readings

American Psychiatric Association. (1994). *Diagnostic and statistical manual of mental disorders* (4th ed.). Washington, DC: American Psychiatric Press.

Frazier, J.A. (1999). The person with mental retardation. In A.M. Nicoli (Ed.), *The new Harvard guide to psychiatry* (pp. 660–671). Cambridge, MA: Harvard University Press.

Frazier, J.A., Spencer, T., Wilens, T., et al. (1997). Childhood onset schizophrenia: The prototypic psychotic disorder of childhood. In D.L. Dunner & J.F. Rosenbaum (Eds.), *The psychiatric clinics of North America: Annual of drug therapy* (vol. 4, pp. 167–193). Philadelphia: W.B. Saunders.

Pfeffer, C.R. (1996). Suicidal behavior in children and adolescents: Causes and management. In M. Lewis (Ed.), *Child and adolescent psychiatry: A comprehensive textbook* (2nd ed., pp. 666–673). Baltimore, MD: Williams and Wilkins.

Wilens, T., Spencer, T.J., Frazier, J.A., & Biederman, J. (1998). Child and adolescent psychopharmacology. In T. Ollendick & M. Hersen (Eds.), *Handbook of child psychopathology* (3rd ed., pp. 603–636). New York: Plenum Press.

Wozniak, J., Biederman, J., Kiely, K., Ablon, J.S., Faraone, S.V., Mundy, E., & Meninin, D. (1995). Mania-like symptoms suggestive of childhood-onset bipolar disorder in clinically referred children. *Journal of the American Academy of Child and Adolescent Psychiatry, 34,* 867–876.

Yeargin-Allsopp, M., Rice, C., Karapurkar, T., et al. (2003). Prevalence of autism in a US metropolitan area. *Journal of the American Medical Association, 289*(1), 49–55.

Chapter 6

Delirium

STEPHAN HECKERS

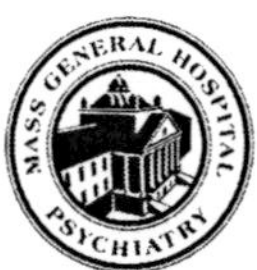

I. Overview

Delirium is a reversible organic mental disorder whose hallmarks are confusion and an altered level of consciousness. Most cases of delirium have an acute onset. It has, therefore, also been referred to as an *acute confusional state*. **Although delirium is usually reversible within a period of days to weeks, some cases progress to irreversible brain failure.**

II. Epidemiology

A. **The prevalence of delirium in medically and surgically ill patients is 11–16%; its incidence varies between 4% and 31%.** The highest incidence is found in the surgical intensive care unit (ICU), followed by the coronary care unit, and then on medical and surgical wards.

B. **Several risk factors for the development of delirium have been identified:**

1. **Being elderly.** Delirium tends to develop more frequently in the elderly than in younger patients, most likely as a result of pre-existing medical conditions (including impaired brain function and the frequent administration of numerous medications).
2. **Having a history of brain damage** (e.g., stroke, dementia), **drug dependency, and acquired immunodeficiency syndrome (AIDS).**
3. **Having cardiac surgery or being burned.** The prevalence of delirium after cardiac surgery is about 32%. The incidence of delirium in burn patients is approximately 18–30%; it increases with age and with the severity of burns.
4. Having certain psychosocial and environmental factors, especially sleep deprivation, has not been closely linked to an increased risk of delirium.

C. **Morbidity and Mortality**

1. **The majority of delirious patients recover without observable sequelae,** but the exact percentage is unknown. Patients undergoing drug withdrawal may develop seizures. **Some patients fail to recover from the acute confusional state, progress to stupor or coma, and die.**
2. **Delirium and agitation increase the risk for complications** (e.g., decubiti and aspiration pneumonia) **and tend to prolong the length of hospital stay.** A substantial number of elderly patients who develop delirium as inpatients (22–76% according to different studies) die during the hospitalization; **about 25% of delirious hospitalized patients die within 6 months of discharge.**

III. Clinical Features of Confusional States

Three domains (i.e., attention, orientation, and memory) are typically impaired in delirious patients; other features are more variable. Delirium can be diagnosed if the patient shows several features during parts of the evaluation process.

A. **Attention deficits are the *sine qua non* of confusional states.** The patient is easily distracted and cannot maintain his or her focus of attention during a task. Inattention and distractibility are often easily observed, or **can be assessed at the bedside by asking the patient to name the months of the year in reverse order or to repeat several numbers in sequence.**

B. **Memory is typically impaired.** Deficits are readily apparent when the patient is asked to encode new information (e.g., to recall three words) either immediately or after a delay of 5 minutes. Some patients will be partially or completely amnestic for the delirious episode.

C. **Impaired orientation is the third main feature** of confusional states. Except for lucid intervals, delirious patients are typically disoriented to time and to place, but rarely are to person.

D. **Thinking is often altered in acute confusional states.** Some patients are disorganized, irrational, and manifest impaired reasoning, whereas others are grossly impaired with delusions and paranoia.

E. **Poor insight and judgment** about medical treatment often make decision-making impossible.

F. **Altered perception** in the form of **illusions** or, less often, **hallucinations** are seen in some confusional states. **Visual hallucinations are more common than auditory or tactile hallucinations.** Confusional states secondary to sedative-hypnotic withdrawal are more likely to present with hallucinations.

G. **Neurological signs, such as tremor, myoclonus, or asterixis,** are seen in some types of delirium (e.g., hepatic encephalopathy). Other deficits, such as **impaired constructional ability, word-finding difficulties (dysnomia), or writing disturbances (dysgraphia),** are more generally found. The **clock-**

drawing test often provides a rapid screen for the presence and degree of delirium. **Dysgraphia,** easily tested by asking the patient to write a sentence, is a very sensitive, albeit non-specific, test for delirium.

IV. Differential Diagnosis of Delirium

A. Numerous **organic disturbances** have been **implicated in the etiology of delirium** and fall into **four major categories: primary intracranial disease, systemic diseases that secondarily affect the brain, exogenous toxic agents, and withdrawal from substances** on which the patient has become dependent.

B. **Three steps are important in the differential diagnosis** of delirium: rule out potentially life-threatening causes, rule out harmful effects of prescription or illicit drugs, and be aware of the complete list of conditions, illnesses, and medications that can lead to delirium.

1. **Rule out potentially life-threatening causes. The mnemonic WWHHHHIMP** can guide the clinician during the rapid assessment of serious and potentially life-threatening causes of delirium.
    a. **W**ernicke's encephalopathy is strongly suggested by the triad of confusion, ataxia, and ophthalmoplegia.
    b. **W**ithdrawal states occur after discontinuation of illicit or prescription drug use, even when small dosages are used for short periods of time.
    c. **H**ypertensive encephalopathy can be assessed with vital signs.
    d. **H**ypoxia can be assessed with arterial blood gases.
    e. **H**ypoglycemia can be assessed with a serum glucose level.
    f. **I**ntracranial bleed can be suggested by headache and confirmed by neuroimaging.
    g. **M**eningitis and encephalitis almost always produce focal neurological signs, as well as headache, loss of consciousness, and seizures.
    h. **P**oisons (including pesticides, solvents, or heavy metals) may lead to delirium.
2. **Rule out the impact of drugs.** Many prescription drugs and several illicitly used drugs cause delirium (Table 6-1). Drug overdose, either accidental or as a result of a suicide attempt, is a frequent cause of delirium in the medical intensive care unit.
3. **Continue the search. When life-threatening causes of delirium and the impact of several specific drugs have been excluded, the clinician will often proceed to empiric treatment of the delirious patient.** However, it is important to continue the search for an underlying cause, which can be found in more than 85% of cases. **Table 6-2 offers the mnemonic "I WATCH DEATH" to organize the differential diagnosis of delirium.** Considering the mortality associated with acute confusional states, the mnemonic is appropriate.

V. Treatment

Treatment of delirium includes specific treatment if the etiology is reasonably clear and empirical treatment to avoid immediate danger while awaiting clarification of the specific etiology.

A. Specific Treatment of Agitation and Confusion

1. **Maintenance of normal blood pressure, circulation, and blood oxygenation, correction of metabolic derangements, and treatment of local or systemic infections are essential to good medical care. Such treatment averts many mental status changes.**
2. **Treat drug toxicity and drug withdrawal.** Stop the offending drug and find an alternative compound without similar adverse effects. If necessary, antidotes can be administered.
    a. **Naloxone hydrochloride,** 0.4 mg subcutaneously or intravenously, is often used to reverse acute confusional states due to the use of narcotics.
    b. **Normeperidine** (the central nervous system [CNS]-stimulating metabolite of meperidine) **toxicity** leads to hallucinations, irritability, myoclonus, and seizures, and might require additional aggressive treatment with barbiturates or benzodiazepines.
    c. **Physostigmine,** 1–2 mg, infused slowly intravenously as a one-time dose or given as a continuous drip, can effectively treat anticholinergic delirium.
    d. Intravenous **verapamil** has been used for the treatment of phencyclidine intoxication.
    e. The benzodiazepine antagonist **flumazenil** has been used to reverse the effects of benzodiazepine excess.

B. Non-specific Treatment of Agitation and Confusion

Pharmacological intervention, mechanical restraints, and supportive measures (to re-orient and calm the patient) are central to the treatment of delirium.

1. **Pharmacological treatment. Neuroleptics and benzodiazepines are the primary drugs used to manage the agitated and/or confused patient.** If the patient's agitation cannot be controlled by these two classes of medications, narcotics, propofol, and paralyzing agents can also be used (Table 6-3).
    a. **Neuroleptics**
        i. **Haloperidol is most often used to treat the agitated, delirious patient.** Other typical neuroleptics (e.g., chlorpromazine, droperidol, thiothixene, and trifluoperazine) can also be used. Haloperidol is approved by the Food and Drug Administration (FDA) for intramuscular and oral use only, but it can be given intravenously. Typically the agitated patient will be given haloperidol at a starting dose of 0.5–5 mg. The elderly and those with known CNS dysfunction

Table 6-1. Drugs That Can Cause Delirium

Antibiotic	*Anti-inflammatory*	*Sedative-Hypnotic*
Acyclovir	Adrenocorticotropic hormone	Barbiturates
Amphotericin	Corticosteroids	Glutethimide
Cephalexin	Ibuprofen	Benzodiazepines
Chloroquine	Indomethacin	
Isoniazid	Naproxen	*Sympathomimetic*
Rifampin	Phenylbutazone	Amphetamine
		Phenylephrine
Anticholinergic	*Antineoplastic*	Phenylpropanolamine
Antihistamines	5-Fluorouracil	
Antispasmodics		*Miscellaneous*
Atropine	*Antiparkinson*	Aminophylline
Belladonna alkaloids	Amantadine	Bromides
Benztropine	Carbidopa	Chlorpropamide
Biperiden	Levodopa	Cimetidine
Chlorpheniramine		Disulfiram
Diphenhydramine	*Analgesics*	Drug withdrawal
Phenothiazines	Opiates	– Alcohol
Promethazine	Salicylates	– Barbiturates
Scopolamine	Synthetic narcotics	– Benzodiazepines
Tricyclic antidepressants		Lithium
Trihexyphenidyl	*Cardiac*	Metrizamide
	Beta-blockers	Metronidazole
Anticonvulsant	Propranolol	Podophyllin
Phenobarbital	Clonidine	Propylthiouracil
Phenytoin	Digitalis	Quinacrine
Valproic acid	Disopyramide	Theophylline
	Lidocaine	Timolol ophthalmic
	Mexiletine	
	Methyldopa	
	Quinidine	
	Procainamide	

SOURCE: Adapted from Wise, M.G., & Gray, K.F. (1994). Delirium, dementia, and amnestic disorders. In R.E. Hales, S.C. Yudofsky, & J.A. Talbott (Eds.), *The American Psychiatric Press textbook of psychiatry* (pp. 311–353). Washington, DC: American Psychiatric Press Inc.

(e.g., dementia, stroke) require doses as low as 0.5 mg two to three times per day; doses of 2–5 mg two to four times per day are not uncommon.

ii. **All neuroleptics predispose to extrapyramidal side effects.** Acute dystonia, especially the life-threatening **laryngeal dystonia, should be treated promptly** with benztropine mesylate 1–2 mg IV, or diphenhydramine 25–50 mg IV. **Akathisia responds well to reduction of the neuroleptic dose and concomitant administration of a beta-blocker** (e.g., propranolol 10–20 mg two to three times per day) or a benzodiazepine (e.g., diazepam or lorazepam 0.5–1 mg two to three times per day). Parkinsonian side effects occur more often in older individuals and respond to treatment with an anticholinergic agent, which unfortunately can aggravate the acute confusional state.

iii. **High doses of haloperidol have been associated with prolongation of cardiac conduction, leading to increases in the QTc (i.e., the QT interval corrected for heart rate).** In some patients, particularly

Table 6-2. Differential Diagnosis of Delirium ("I WATCH DEATH")

Infectious	Encephalitis, meningitis, syphilis
Withdrawal	Alcohol, barbiturates, sedative-hypnotics
Acute metabolic	Acidosis, alkalosis, electrolyte disturbance, hepatic failure, renal failure
Trauma	Heat stroke, severe burn, post-operative state
CNS pathology	Abscess, hemorrhage, normal pressure hydrocephalus, seizure, stroke, tumor, vasculitis
Hypoxia	Anemia, carbon monoxide poisoning, hypotension, pulmonary/cardiac failure
Deficiencies	Vitamin B_{12}, niacin, thiamine
Endocrinopathies	Hyper- or hypoadrenocortisolism, hyper- or hypoglycemia
Acute vascular	Hypertensive encephalopathy, shock
Toxins or drugs	Medications
Heavy metals	Lead, manganese, mercury

SOURCE: Adapted from Wise, M.G., & Gray, K.F. (1994). Delirium, dementia, and amnestic disorders. In R.E. Hales, S.C. Yudofsky, & J.A. Talbott (Eds.), *The American Psychiatric Press textbook of psychiatry* (pp. 311–353). Washington, DC: American Psychiatric Press Inc.

Table 6-3. Drugs Used to Treat Delirium and Agitation

Drug	*Route*	*Onset (min)*	*Peak Effect (min)*	*Starting Dose*	*Important Adverse Effects*
Neuroleptics					
Haloperidol	IV, IM	5–20	15–45	Degree of agitation:	
	PO	30–60	120–240	Mild: 0.5–2 mg	Cardiac arrhythmia (QTc increased,
				Moderate: 5–10 mg	torsades de pointes)
				Severe: >10 mg	Extrapyramidal side effects
Droperidol	IV, IM	3–10	15–45	2.5–10 mg	Hypotension; QTc prolongation
Chlorpromazine	IV, IM	5–40	10–30	25 mg	
Olanzapine	PO, SL	15–30	30–120	2.5–10 mg	
Quetiapine	PO	15–60	30–120	2.5–10 mg	Sedation
Benzodiazepines					
Diazepam	IV	2–5	5–30	2–5 mg	
	PO	10–60	30–180		
Lorazepam	IV, IM	2–20	60–120	1–2 mg	Respiratory depression
	SL	2–20	20–60	0.5–1 mg	May aggravate delirium
	PO	20–60	20–120	0.5–1 mg	
Midazolam	IV, IM	1–2	30–40	0.05–0.15 mg/kg	
Narcotics					Respiratory depression
Morphine sulfate	IV, IM	1–2	20	4–10 mg	May aggravate delirium
Paralytics					
Metocurine iodide	IV	1–4	2–10	0.2–0.4 mg/kg	Hypotension
Pancuronium bromide	IV	0.5–1	5	0.04–0.1 mg/kg	Tachycardia, hypertension

IV, intravenous; IM, intramuscular; PO, oral; SL, sublingual.

in those with pre-existing dilated ventricles and a history of alcohol abuse, ***torsades de pointes*** arrhythmia has developed.

iv. Atypical antipsychotics can be used instead of high-potency antipsychotics. Their use is associated with a very low incidence of extrapyramidal side effects.

b. **Benzodiazepines**

i. **Agitation due to panic attacks, generalized anxiety, or fear of being in the ICU** should be treated primarily with a benzodiazepine. Diazepam at a starting dose of 2–5 mg and lorazepam or clonazepam at a starting dose of 0.5–1 mg are effective in calming the anxious and agitated patient. In the case of panic attacks, maintenance treatment (e.g., with clonazepam 0.5 mg three times per day) is often recommended. Psychotic episodes and manic presentations have also been managed exclusively with clonazepam.

ii. **Midazolam, a benzodiazepine with a rapid onset of action and an elimination half-life of 1–4 hours, has been used successfully in the treatment of agitation.** Intramuscular administration of 2–3 mg of midazolam calms patients within 5–10 minutes. Continuous infusion of midazolam, with a mean infusion rate of approximately 0.6–6 μg/kg/minutes, is an effective treatment for severely agitated patients.

iii. **Many agitated patients benefit from the combined use of a neuroleptic and a benzodiazepine.** Benzodiazepines can cause respiratory depression if large doses are given. All benzodiazepines can lead to clouded consciousness, mimicking the mental status changes seen in acute confusional states.

iv. Increasingly, propfol has been used in ICUs to rapidly sedate agitated patients. However, when used as a continuous trip for extended periods, agitation and other signs and symptoms of sedative-hypnotic withdrawal may appear after its sudden discontinuation.

c. **Narcotics and nondepolarizing muscle relaxants**

i. **Morphine sulfate can be used for pain control and to sedate the agitated ICU patient.** Parenteral administration leads to a prompt effect that lasts 4–5 hours. Respiratory depression and aggravation of confusion are potential adverse effects.

ii. **Intubation, sedation, and paralysis using metocurine iodide or pancuronium bromide are the final treatment options when other measures fail to control severe agitation.** The cardiovascular effects of metocurine iodide and pancuronium bromide, pulmonary complications associated with intubation, and traction injuries that develop during paralysis are potential adverse effects of this treatment strategy.

2. **Mechanical restraints.** Even when optimally medicated with a neuroleptic and/or a benzodiazepine, the calm but confused patient might still perform dangerous maneuvers. In such situations it is recommended that the patient be placed in mechanical restraints. **The indication should be clearly documented in the medical record, and the need for restraints should be assessed continuously.**

3. **Supportive measures. The confused patient benefits from frequent reorientation to time and place. Adequate lighting can reduce the likelihood of illusionary misperceptions. The presence of calm and reassuring family member and nursing staff is helpful** for the patient. A "sitter" can also help reduce anxiety. **Education** of the staff, the patient's family, and the patient about the nature of confusion and/or agitation is **therapeutic for all of the parties involved.**

Suggested Readings

Crippen, D.W. (1990). The role of sedation in the ICU patient with pain and agitation. *Critical Care Clinics, 6,* 369–392.

Heckers, S., Tesar, G.E., & Stern, T.A. (1999). Diagnosis and treatment of agitation and delirium in the intensive care unit patient. In R.S. Irwin, F.B. Cerra, & J.M. Rippe (Eds.), *Irwin and Rippe's intensive care medicine* (pp. 2383–2393). Philadelphia: Lippincott-Raven.

Lipowski, Z.J. (1980). *Delirium: Acute brain failure in man.* Springfield, IL: Charles C. Thomas.

Lipowski, Z.J. (1988). Delirium (acute confusional states). *Journal of the American Medical Association, 258,* 1789–1792.

Tesar, G.E., Murray, G.B., & Cassem, N.H. (1985). Use of high-dose intravenous haloperidol in agitated cardiac patients. *Journal of Clinical Psychopharmacology, 5,* 344–347.

Thompson, T.L., & Thompson, W.L. (1983). Treating postoperative delirium. *Drug Therapy, 13,* 30–40.

Trzepacz, P.T., Baker, R.W., & Greenhouse, J. (1988). A symptom rating scale for delirium. *Psychiatry Research, 23,* 89–97.

Chapter 7

Dementia

Roy H. Perlis and William E. Falk

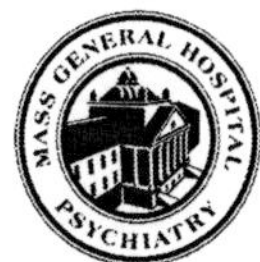

I. Definition

A. DSM-IV Criteria

The DSM-IV criteria for dementia require the demonstration of **a decline in memory, as well as impairment of at least one other domain of cognitive function:**

1. **Aphasia,** or difficulty with any aspect of language
2. **Apraxia,** or impaired ability to perform motor tasks despite intact motor function
3. **Agnosia,** or impaired object recognition despite intact sensory function
4. **Executive dysfunction,** or difficulty in planning, organizing, sequencing, or abstracting

B. Qualifiers to the Diagnosis

Several important qualifiers are included in the definition:

1. The condition must represent a **change from baseline** (i.e., patients with mental retardation would not meet the definition unless their cognition deteriorated further).
2. The deficits must be clinically significant in that they **interfere with social or occupational function.**
3. The deficits cannot occur exclusively during an episode of delirium.
4. The condition cannot be accounted for by another Axis I diagnosis, such as major depression.

C. Mild Cognitive Impairment

A decline in cognitive function compared with age-matched controls is seen in some individuals 65 and older. Although it may be a normal part of the aging process, mild cognitive impairment may be a precursor of Alzheimer's disease, particularly if symptoms progress over time and begin to cause impairment in social, avocational, or occupational function.

II. Epidemiology

Estimates of the prevalence of dementia vary widely, depending on which set of diagnostic criteria is utilized. Alzheimer's disease, which accounts for up to 70% of cases of dementia, affects some 4 million people in the United States. The cost of providing care for demented patients exceeds $113 billion each year.

A. Demographic Factors

The incidence of dementia increases with age: dementia affects 15–20% of individuals after the age of 65 years, and up to 45% after the age of 80 years. Whereas the etiology of dementia differs somewhat between genders (with higher rates of vascular dementia and lower rates of Alzheimer's disease in men), the overall incidence is equivalent in men and women.

B. Trends

As average life expectancies increase, the number of demented patients is expected to increase dramatically.

III. Differential Diagnosis

A. Confounding Disorders

As noted earlier, the diagnostic criteria for dementia require that a number of confounding disorders be ruled out. Chief among these is delirium, which requires a rapid medical and neurologic evaluation (see chapter 6). Other psychiatric illnesses, including major depression, may also resemble dementia. Differences in presentation may be useful in distinguishing delirium or depression from dementia.

Of note, **an underlying diagnosis of dementia may predispose a patient to delirium;** thus, further evaluation is required once the delirium has been treated successfully.

1. **Delirium generally differs from dementia in several important ways:**
   a. **The onset is acute or subacute** (hours to days).
   b. **The course often fluctuates.**
   c. **The level of consciousness, and attention in particular, may be impaired.**
2. **Depression may be difficult to distinguish from dementia, particularly as the two diagnoses are often co-morbid.** In addition, depression alone may cause cognitive impairment; in such cases, it may presage Alzheimer's disease by several years. **Certain features favor a diagnosis of depression:**
   a. A better pre-morbid level of function
   b. A more acute onset
   c. Poor motivation and/or prominent negativity on mental status testing. Depressed patients may state that they are unable to perform a particular task. At times, they can succeed at more difficult tasks and fail at easier ones.
   d. A family history that is positive for depression.

B. Reversible Conditions

Establishing a precise etiology (see Table 7-1) whenever possible allows more focused treatment and an accurate estimation of prognosis. Whereas **a reversible cause will be identified in fewer than 15% of cases,** a diagnosis may be comforting to patients and their families and useful in planning.

Table 7-1. Etiology of Dementia

Vascular:
Stroke, chronic subdural hemorrhages, post-anoxic injury, diffuse white matter disease
Infectious:
HIV infection, neurosyphilis, progressive multifocal leukoencephalopathy (PMLE), Creutzfeldt-Jakob disease, tuberculosis, sarcoidosis, Whipple's disease
Neoplastic:
Primary versus metastatic carcinoma, paraneoplastic syndrome
Degenerative:
Alzheimer's disease, frontotemporal dementia, dementia with Lewy bodies, Parkinson's disease, progressive supranuclear palsy, multisystem degeneration, amyotrophic lateral sclerosis (ALS), corticobasal degeneration, multiple sclerosis (MS)
Inflammatory:
Vasculitis
Endocrine:
Hypothyroidism, adrenal insufficiency, Cushing's syndrome, hypo/hyperparathyroidism, renal failure, liver failure
Metabolic:
Thiamine deficiency (Wernicke's encephalopathy), vitamin B_{12} deficiency, inherited enzyme defects
Toxins:
Chronic alcoholism, drugs/medication effects, heavy metals, dialysis dementia (aluminum)
Trauma:
Dementia pugilistica
Other:
Normal pressure hydrocephalus (NPH), obstructive hydrocephalus

IV. Evaluation of the Patient with Suspected Dementia

A. General Approach

History should be obtained from the patient, as well as family members or others who have observed the patient; family or other informants should be interviewed separately from the patient. Note that **patients themselves often fail to report deficits, usually because they are unaware of them.**

B. History

1. **Present illness**
   a. **Nature of presentation**
      i. An abrupt or precipitous onset favors a diagnosis of vascular dementia, whereas insidious onset suggests Alzheimer's disease.
      ii. Behavioral symptoms that precede cognitive ones suggest a frontotemporal dementia.
   b. **Course: a stepwise decline is more consistent with a vascular dementia,** whereas a gradual deterioration suggests a disorder such as Alzheimer's disease.
   c. **Associated symptoms** may favor a particular diagnosis; e.g., incontinence and gait apraxia are seen in normal pressure hydrocephalus (NPH).
   d. **Associated psychiatric symptoms,** such as hallucinations, paranoia, or personality change, may also implicate a particular diagnosis.
2. **Review of systems** should be completed and include incontinence, gait disturbance, and falls.
3. **A past medical history may reveal risk factors** for stroke (hypertension, obesity, hypercholesterolemia, cigarette smoking, diabetes mellitus, post-menopausal status) or other general medical or neurologic etiologies.
4. **A past psychiatric history may suggest co-morbid illness,** such as depression or alcohol abuse, particularly if prior episodes of psychiatric illness are elicited.
5. **Medications are implicated in up to 30% of cases of dementia. Common offenders include anticholinergics, antihypertensives, psychotropics, sedative-hypnotics, and narcotic analgesics.** Any drug is suspect if its first prescription and initiation of symptoms are temporally related.
6. **Family history is a significant risk factor for developing certain dementias, including Alzheimer's disease and frontal dementia.**
7. **A social and occupational history** is useful when assessing premorbid intelligence and education (both of which may confound cognitive screens for dementia), as well as a change in the level of function.

C. Physical Examination

1. A **general medical examination,** with a particular focus on the cardiovascular system, is an essential part of the evaluation of dementia. Endocrine, inflammatory, and infectious etiologies, for example, may also be suggested by physical findings.
2. A **complete neurologic examination,** including function of the cranial nerves, sensory and motor function, deep-tendon reflexes, and cerebellar function, can reveal focal findings that may suggest a vascular dementia or degenerative process (e.g., Parkinson's disease).
3. **Vision and hearing screening** may reveal losses that can masquerade as, or exacerbate, cognitive decline.

D. Psychiatric examination

D. Psychiatric examination may reveal evidence of delirium, depression, or psychosis. **On formal mental status testing, such as with the Folstein Mini-Mental State Examination** (MMSE; Table 7-2) **or other supplemental tests** (see Table 7-3), **documentation of particular findings, in addition**

Table 7-2. Folstein Mini-Mental State Examination

Task	*Instructions*	*Scoring*
Date: orientation	"Tell me the date"	One point each for year, season, date, day of the week, month
Place: orientation	"Where are you?"	One point each for state, county, town, building, floor/room
Register three objects	Name three objects, ask patient to repeat them	One point for each correctly repeated
Serial sevens	Ask the patient to count backward from 100 by 7. Stop after five answers. (Or ask the patient to spell "WORLD" backward)	One point for each correct answer or letter
Recall three objects	Ask the patient to recall the registered objects	One point for each correct object
Naming	Point to watch, ask "What is this?" Repeat with a pencil	One point for each correct answer
Repeating a phrase	Ask patient to say, "No ifs, ands, or buts"	One point if successful on first try
Verbal commands	Give the patient a piece of paper, and say, "Take this paper in your right hand, fold it in half, and put it on the floor"	One point for each correct action (out of three total)
Written commands	Show the patient a piece of paper with the words "CLOSE YOUR EYES"	One point if the patient's eyes close
Writing	Ask the patient to write a sentence	One point if the sentence has subject, verb, and makes sense
Drawing	Ask the patient to copy a pair of intersecting pentagons	One point if the figure has ten corners, two intersecting lines
		Total number of points: 30

Table 7-3. Supplemental Mental State Testing for Patients with Dementia

Area	*Test*
Memory	Recall name and address: "John Brown, 42 Market Street, Chicago"
	Recall three unusual words: "tulip, umbrella, fear"
Language	Naming parts: "lab coat: lapel, sleeve, cuff; watch: band, face, crystal"
	Complex commands: "Before pointing to the door, point to the ceiling"
	Word-list: "In one minute, name all the animals you can think of"
Praxis	"Show me how you would slice a loaf of bread"; "Show me how you brush your teeth"
Visuospatial	"Draw a clock face with numbers, and mark the hands to say 11:10"
Abstraction	"How is an apple like a banana?"; "How is a canal different from a river?"; proverb interpretation

to the overall score, allows cognitive function to be followed over time.

E. Laboratory Evaluation

1. **Guidelines established by the American Academy of Neurology for the evaluation of dementia include electrolytes, glucose, blood urea nitrogen (BUN) and creatinine, and liver function tests (which are often included in a comprehensive metabolic panel, or Chem-20), as well as a complete blood count, tests of thyroid function, a vitamin B_{12} level, and syphilis serology. The likelihood of detecting a reversible cause of dementia with this screen is generally less than 10%. A computed tomography (CT) scan of the brain,** without contrast, can also be useful to rule out a subdural hematoma, hydrocephalus, stroke, or tumor.
2. **Additional investigations are indicated if the initial work-up is uninformative, if a particular diagnosis is suspected, or if the presentation is atypical** (see Table 7-4). Such investigations are particularly important in young patients with rapid progression of dementia.
   a. **Neuropsychological testing may be useful,** and is essential in cases where a patient's deficits are mild or difficult to characterize. Briefer **screens, such as the Folstein**

Table 7-4. Supplemental Laboratory Investigations

What	*When*	*Why*
Neuropsychological testing	Patient's deficits are mild or difficult to characterize	The sensitivity of the MMSE for dementia is poor, particularly in highly educated or intelligent patients (who can compensate for deficits)
Lumbar puncture (including routine studies and cytology)	Known or suspected cancer, immunosuppression, suspected CNS infection or vasculitis, hydrocephalus by CT, rapid or atypical courses	Look for infection, elevated pressure, abnormal proteins
MRI with gadolinium	Any atypical findings on neurologic exam	More sensitive than CT for tumor, stroke
EEG	Suspected toxic-metabolic encephalopathy, partial complex seizures, Creutzfeldt-Jakob disease	Look for diffuse slowing (encephalopathy) vs. focal seizure activity
HIV testing	Risk factors or opportunistic infections	Up to 20% of patients with HIV infection develop dementia, although it is unusual for dementia to be the presenting sign
Heavy metal screening, screening for Wilson's disease or autoimmune disease	Suggested by history, physical exam, laboratory findings	May be reversible

Mini-Mental State Examination, have poor sensitivity and specificity for dementia, particularly in highly educated or intelligent patients. The MMSE also fails to assess executive function and praxis.

b. **Magnetic resonance imaging (MRI)** of the brain is more sensitive for recent stroke and should be considered when focal findings are detected on the neurologic examination.

c. An **electroencephalogram (EEG)** may be used to identify toxic-metabolic encephalopathy, partial complex seizures, or Creutzfeldt-Jakob disease.

d. A **lumbar puncture** may be informative when cancer, infection of the central nervous system (CNS), hydrocephalus, or vasculitis is suspected.

e. **Testing for human immunodeficiency virus (HIV)** is indicated in patients with appropriate risk factors as up to 20% of patients with HIV infection develop dementia. However, dementia is uncommon as a *presenting* sign of HIV infection.

f. **Heavy metal screening,** as well as tests for Wilson's disease or autoimmune diseases, should be reserved for patients in which these etiologies are suspected.

V. Alzheimer's Disease (Dementia of the Alzheimer's Type)

A. Diagnosis

A diagnosis of probable Alzheimer's disease (AD) is made when a patient meets the criteria for dementia as above and has **a gradual and progressive course,** once other etiologies have been ruled out. A definite diagnosis of Alzheimer's disease requires histopathologic confirmation and is generally made at postmortem examination.

In the early stages of Alzheimer's disease, a patient typically develops subtle **loss of short-term memory**. Subsequently, the individual becomes lost easily and develops **word-finding and naming difficulty**, which results in vague speech, circumlocution, and the use of clichés. At the same time, the individual may develop **apraxias** that affect such motor tasks as dressing and eating, and visual-spatial impairments that are apparent when driving or performing similar tasks. Finally, in the late stages, **judgment becomes impaired**, and the patient may develop personality changes, such as apathy, hostility, or social withdrawal. Disturbed sleep-wake patterns are also typical at this stage.

Psychiatric symptoms are often prominent in Alzheimer's disease (AD). Depression and anxiety may be presenting complaints; they are seen in up to 40% of cases. **Delusions** are also common, affecting up to 50% of patients; delusions often relate to theft or to other family members. **Hallucinations,** which are most often visual, affect up to 25% of patients with AD. **Agitation** is also a frequent symptom.

B. Risk Factors

Major risk factors for Alzheimer's disease include increasing age and positive family history; other risk factors include a history of head trauma and Down's syndrome. The genetic component of Alzheimer's disease is suggested by the fact that up to 50% of those with a first-degree relative with the disease will themselves be affected by the age of 90 years. **Three chromosomes have been linked to development of early-onset Alzheimer's disease:**

1. **Trisomy 21, or chromosome 21 mutations;** Down's syndrome patients older than age 30 years show Alzheimer's disease pathology in nearly all cases.
2. **Chromosome 14** contains the presenilin 1 gene; mutations here account for most cases of familial early-onset Alzheimer's disease.
3. **Chromosome 1** contains the presenilin 2 gene; mutations here have been associated with Alzheimer's disease in families from the Volga River area in Russia.

Nonetheless, **these mutations account for fewer than 5% of cases of Alzheimer's disease.** Additional **"vulnerability genes" have been identified for Alzheimer's disease; chief among them is the *ApoE-4* allele, which is associated with an increased risk for Alzheimer's disease and with an earlier age of onset.**

C. Histopathology

The typical histopathologic changes in Alzheimer's disease include senile plaques and neurofibrillary tangles. Plaques are extracellular and contain beta-amyloid; tangles are intracellular and contain cytoskeletal filaments. Other changes include synaptic degeneration and loss of cortical and subcortical neurons, particularly in the hippocampus, cortex, and nucleus basalis. **Neuron loss occurs first in the entorhinal cortex and the nucleus basalis.**

Neuron loss affects a number of neurotransmitter systems. However, **death of cholinergic neurons in the basal forebrain causes a particularly prominent decrease in levels of cortical acetylcholine.**

The role of imaging in the diagnosis of Alzheimer's disease is not yet clear. On positron-emission tomography (PET) scans, for example, parietal and temporal lobe hypometabolism is typically seen.

D. Course

The average **survival after the onset of symptoms in Alzheimer's disease is 8–10 years.** Predictors of more rapid institutionalization or death include the presence of extrapyramidal signs, the presence of psychotic symptoms, young age at onset, and current cognitive dysfunction.

VI. Other Selected Etiologies

A. Vascular dementia (formerly referred to as multi-infarct dementia) accounts for up to 20% of cases of dementia.

1. **Typical features include a step-wise progression of cognitive deficits and associated focal signs and symptoms** (e.g., deficits in sensory or motor function). Clinically, these features are often incorporated into an "ischemic score"; the diagnosis is confirmed by brain imaging.
2. **Risk factors** are those associated with vascular disease, vasculitis, or embolic disease (including atrial fibrillation).
3. A single strategically placed infarct, multiple infarcts, or white matter ischemia may all yield dementia; overall, **stroke yields a nine-fold increased risk of dementia.** The clinical significance of "periventricular white matter changes" or Binswanger's disease, commonly noted on imaging studies, is not yet well established.
4. **Treatment of vascular dementia focuses on secondary prevention by addressing underlying risk factors.** Anticoagulation, with coumadin or aspirin, is often utilized.

B. Dementia with Lewy bodies (DLB) may be more prevalent than previously recognized; postmortem studies reveal the presence of Lewy bodies in up to 25% of dementia cases.

1. Clinically, DLB shares features of both Alzheimer's disease and Parkinson's disease. A patient with DLB may suffer repeated falls and be unusually sensitive to adverse effects of typical neuroleptics. Common psychiatric symptoms include depression and systematized delusions. **In addition to progressive cognitive decline, the consensus criteria for clinical diagnosis require at least two of the following for a probable diagnosis:**
   a. **Recurrent visual hallucinations,** which are often well formed.
   b. **Parkinsonism.**
   c. **Fluctuating cognition,** with variation in attention and alertness.
2. **Risk factors** for DLB are not yet well understood, but some studies suggest a genetic predisposition may be important. The disease is more prevalent in males by a factor of 2:1; the age at onset varies from 50 to 80 years.
3. **The typical neuropathologic finding in DLB is the Lewy body, a round, eosinophilic intraneuronal inclusion.** Lewy bodies may be found in both cortical and subcortical structures. Of note, Lewy bodies are also detected in many cases of Alzheimer's and Parkinson's disease, as well as in a small number of otherwise well elderly individuals.
4. No specific treatment for DLB has yet emerged, although patients may respond to cholinergic agents (see below).

C. **Frontotemporal dementias** comprise a spectrum of disorders, including **Pick's disease.**

1. **Unlike most other dementias that present initially with cognitive change, frontal lobe dementia presents insidiously with behavioral changes. Common psychiatric symptoms include depression, anxiety, and delusions. Language impairments are also**

seen, including abundant speech and echolalia or repetition. Other typical changes include:

a. Decline in personal hygiene
b. Disinhibition and impaired social awareness
c. Impulsivity
d. Inflexibility and rigidity
e. Repetitive behaviors, particularly involving an obsessive focus on certain foods

2. Typically the age of onset is between 40 and 70 years; a family history of early-onset dementia is often present. In some familial cases, linkage has been shown to chromosome 17.
3. Neuropathologic changes typically include intraneuronal inclusions, known as Pick bodies, and loss of cortical neurons, particularly in the frontal and anterior temporal lobes. Structural neuroimaging demonstrates atrophy in these areas; SPECT (single photon emission computed tomography) studies often reveal frontal lobe hypoperfusion.
4. **Treatment** relies on management of behavior.

D. **Normal pressure hydrocephalus typically presents with a "magnetic gait" followed by urinary incontinence and then dementia.** Particular cognitive deficits include impaired concentration and mild memory deficits. On head CT, ventriculomegaly and diffuse cortical atrophy may be noted. Diagnosis relies on clinical improvement following serial lumbar punctures (LPs), known as the Miller Fisher test. If a patient benefits from LPs, ventriculoperitoneal shunting sometimes provides more persistent improvement.

E. **Parkinson's disease is associated with dementia in up to 70% of cases.** However, significant cognitive dysfunction usually occurs later in the disease course. A number of other dementias (including Huntington's disease, progressive supranuclear palsy, and corticobasal degeneration) manifest both neurologic and psychiatric features.

VII. Prevention

Prevention of dementia remains an active area of investigation. Some studies suggest that NSAIDs (non-steroidal anti-inflammatory drugs), but not acetaminophen or aspirin, and estrogen replacement may reduce the relative risk of developing Alzheimer's disease, or delay its onset.

VIII. Treatment

A. **Reversible etiologies should be addressed first.** Thus, any co-morbid medical problems identified in the initial evaluation must be treated, whether or not they contribute directly to the dementia. At the same time, drugs with cognitive side effects should be minimized and eliminated altogether whenever possible; as noted earlier, medications are implicated in 10–30% of cases of dementia.

B. **Psychosocial or behavioral interventions are essential in treating patients with dementia.**

1. **Educate the patient and the family** in a supportive and caring way, as presentation of an initial diagnosis may be extremely frightening. Seek the family's advice as to how to inform the patient.
2. **Ensure patient safety** by informing both the patient and the family that driving may become impossible.
3. **Address legal issues** (such as wills, health care proxies, and durable power of attorney) **early.**
4. **Suggest assistance with financial management,** such as bill paying.
5. **Continue routine health maintenance** visits every 3–6 months.
6. **When appropriate, raise the possibility of placement,** as nearly 75% of those with dementia will require a long-term care facility. Other options include adult day care, respite care, home health aides, outreach services, and homemakers.
7. **Address behavioral problems: wandering, agitation, screaming, incontinence, aggression, and psychosis. Most commonly these issues, rather than cognitive decline, precipitate nursing home placement.** Although pharmacotherapy may be beneficial in some cases, behavioral interventions remain a mainstay of treatment.
8. **Care for the caregivers** by providing referral to support groups or other sources of information and coping skills. **Over 50% of caregivers will develop clinically significant depression.**

C. **Pharmacologic treatment should target specific symptoms.** This strategy allows for more accurate assessment of treatment response and course over time. The Folstein Mini-Mental State Examination can be used to approximate cognitive status; similar scales exist for behavioral assessment. **Functional measures include the Activities of Daily Living** (see Table 7-5) **and the Instrumental Activities of Daily Living scales.** However, none of these measures is especially sensitive to change. Clinicians therefore need to attend to particular patient activities, such as hobbies, where treatment effects may be more pronounced.

In treating any geriatric patient, clinicians should in general start medications at low dosages and increase them slowly, paying careful attention to side effects.

1. Disease-**delaying and disease-modifying drugs** for Alzheimer's disease include estrogen, NSAIDs, and free radical inhibitors, such as vitamin E and selegeline.
   a. Estrogen replacement and NSAIDs are unlikely to be helpful once a diagnosis is established; however, both may

Table 7-5. Activities of Daily Living

Basic	*Instrumental*
Bathing	Shopping
Dressing	Cooking
Walking	Managing finances
Toileting	Housework
Feeding	Using telephone
Transfers (to/from bed, chair)	Taking medications
	Traveling outside of home

delay the clinically evident onset of symptoms in individuals at high risk for developing Alzheimer's disease.

b. Vitamine E, selegeline, or both may slow progression of Alzheimer's disease.

c. Ginkgo biloba does not appear to provide clinically significant benefit.

2. **Drugs that enhance cognition** in patients with Alzheimer's disease include four currently available cholinesterase inhibitors. While none stops the progression of cognitive decline, each agent may slow the rate of decline by 6 months to a year. All have cholinergic effects, such as nausea, vomiting, diarrhea, and bradycardia.
   a. **Tacrine** (Cognex) is the prototype of this class but its q.i.d. dosing, prolonged titration, frequent blood monitoring (for reversible elevation of liver enzymes), and high rate of attrition due to side effects limit its current use.
   b. **Donepezil** (Aricept), a reversible and specific inhibitor of acetylcholinesterase, has less gastrointestinal side effects and no hepatotoxicity. Once-daily dosing starts at 5 mg for 4–6 weeks, then settles at 10 mg per day thereafter.
   c. **Rivastigmine** (Exelon) is metabolized at its site of action rather than in the liver, thereby minimizing drug-drug interactions. Since it inhibits butyrylcholinesterase in addition to acetylcholinesterase, it may have a theoretical but unproven advantage in late-stage disease. This dual inhibition may also explain why patients often experience gastrointestinal side effects. Rivastigmine should be taken with meals, starting at 2 mg b.i.d. and increasing as tolerated to a maximum of 6 mg b.i.d.
   d. **Galantamine** (Reminyl) has, in addition to its inhibition of acetylcholine, a selective enhancement of nicotinic activity. This action may have a theoretical, unproven boosting effect on acetylcholine and other neurotransmitters. The initial dose of 4 mg b.i.d. is gradually increased to a maximum of 12 mg b.i.d.
   e. **Additional treatments**, such as agents that block amyloid production or modulate neurotransmitters other than acetylcholine, remain under study. A human study of an Alzheimer's vaccine was recently halted due to severe adverse events, but other potentially safer agents are being developed.
3. **Drugs which treat psychiatric or behavioral symptoms** are equally important.
   a. For depressive symptoms, SSRIs (selective serotonin reuptake inhibitors) are considered as first-line because of their relative safety.
   b. For hallucinations and psychosis, antipsychotic drugs at low doses may be helpful.
   c. Agitation and anxiety may respond to SSRIs or antipsychotics. **Benzodiazepines may cause disinhibition and can further impair cognition.**

D. **Referral** to a specialist in geriatric psychiatry or neuropsychiatry can be helpful in certain circumstances. **Patients with atypical presentations, with unusual symptoms or rapid progression, as well as those in whom no etiology can be identified, should be referred.** In some cases families may request a referral, particularly when they are interested in participating in a research protocol.

Suggested Readings

Cummings, J.L., Vinters, H.V., Cole, G.M., & Khachaturian, Z.S. (1998). Alzheimer's disease: Etiologies, pathophysiology, cognitive reserve, and treatment opportunities. *Neurology, 51*, S2–S17.

Daly, E.J., Falk, W.E., & Brown, P.A. (2001). Cholinesterase inhibitors for behavioral disturbance in dementia. *Current Psychiatry Reports, 3*, 251–258.

Falk, W.E., & Albert, M.A. (1997). Dementia. In N.H. Cassem, T.A. Stern, J.F. Rosenbaum, et al. (Eds.), *Massachusetts General Hospital handbook of general hospital psychiatry* (4th ed., pp. 123–147). St. Louis: Mosby.

Felician, O., & Sanderson, T.A. (1999). The neurobiology and pharmacotherapy of Alzheimer's disease. *Journal of Neuropsychiatry and Clinical Neuroscience, 11*, 19–31.

Helmuth, L. (2002). New Alzheimer's treatments that may ease the mind. *Science, 297*, 1260–1263.

Kaye, J.A. (1998). Diagnostic challenges in dementia. *Neurology, 51*, S45–S52.

Papka, M.P., Rubio, A., & Schiffer, R.B. (1998). A review of Lewy body disease, an emerging concept of cortical dementia. *Journal of Neuropsychiatry and Clinical Neuroscience, 10*, 267–279.

Peterson, R.C., Stevens, J.C., & Ganguli, M., et al. (2001). Practice parameter: Early detection of dementia: Mild cognitive impairment (an evidence-based review). *Neurology, 56*(9), 1133–1142.

Chapter 8

Mental Retardation

JOHN N. JULIAN

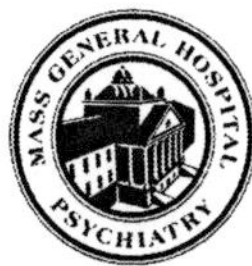

I. Overview

A. Historical Perspective on Mental Retardation

Mental retardation and psychiatric illness have had a shared ancestry. However, as the centuries have passed, they were often viewed quite differently. In the sixteenth century, the English Court of Wards and Liveries differentiated "idiots" from "lunatics." Later, in his initial diagnostic scheme Kraepelin listed mental retardation as a distinct form of psychiatric illness. It was not until the late nineteenth century that mental retardation and psychiatric illness were noted, at times, to co-exist. The phrase "imbecility with insanity" was noted in the *American Journal of Insanity* in 1888. Since then, mental retardation with co-morbid psychiatric illness has continued to be investigated, but at a slower than other areas of psychiatry.

B. Modern Investigations Regarding the Relationship between Mental Retardation and Psychiatric Illness

1. Several hypotheses have been formulated to explain why individuals with cognitive impairment seem to be at increased risk for psychiatric disorders.
2. With the occurrence of the "Decade of the Brain" and a shift in focus toward neurodevelopmental psychiatry, the relationship between mental retardation and psychiatric illness has generated more interest. Future investigation in this area is likely to shed light on complex issues; e.g., behavioral phenotypes and the relationship between coping abilities and the vulnerability to mental illness.

II. Epidemiology

A. Prevalence

1. **The prevalence of mental retardation is between 1% and 3%** depending on the criteria used, the methods used, and the populations sampled; most investigators believe the prevalence is probably closer to 1%.
2. Mental retardation is a condition with diverse etiologies; **more than 350 causes of mental retardation are known.** However, approximately 40% of cases have no clear etiology.
3. **The three most common causes of mental retardation account for about 30% of identified cases.** They include:
   a. **Down's syndrome** (chromosome 21), which is the most common genetic cause of mental retardation.
   b. **The fragile X syndrome** (X-linked gene *FMR-1*), which is the most common inherited cause of mental retardation.
   c. **The fetal alcohol syndrome** (with a triad of growth retardation, developmental delay, and classical facial features), which is the third most common known cause of mental retardation.

B. Co-morbid Psychopathology

1. **The mentally retarded population suffers from the full range of psychiatric illness,** and likely is afflicted at a higher rate than the general population.
   a. Some studies estimate that **the prevalence of psychiatric disorders is 4–6 times that of the general population.**
   b. In institutional settings upward of 10% of the mentally retarded population have some form of psychopathology; percentages are less clear in community samples. One must be cautious of methodological problems when interpreting data regarding this population.

C. Etiology of Psychopathology in the Mentally Retarded

1. Why there appears to be a higher prevalence of psychiatric illness in the mentally retarded population is unclear.
   a. One theory centers on the idea that mental retardation is a manifestation of damage to cortical and subcortical substrate, regardless of whether this damage can be identified with available technology. This damage confers a special vulnerability to psychiatric conditions.
   b. Another theory holds that individuals with mental retardation are chronically exposed to a confusing and stressful world; their decreased ability to cope with the demands of a complex society and an inadequate cognitive capacity to resolve emotional conflicts leads to increased psychiatric pathology.
   c. A third theory highlights the lack of psychiatric care in this population. It questions the psychiatric profession's unwillingness to treat psychiatric illness in the mentally retarded due to a prevailing view that behavioral disturbances and psychopathology are somehow more acceptable in individuals with mental retardation.

III. Diagnostic Features

A. Definition

1. The definition of mental retardation comes from work done by the American Association on Mental Retardation; it has basically been adopted by DSM-IV.
   a. **"Mental retardation refers to substantial limitations in present functioning. It is characterized by significantly subaverage intellectual functioning, existing concurrently with related limitations . . . [in several adaptive areas and] . . . manifests before age 18."**

b. In more objective terms, **mental retardation is defined by having a standardized IQ score at least two standard deviations below the mean and impairment in at least two out of eleven areas of adaptive functioning when compared to peers of the same age and culture.** The areas identified include communication, self-care, home living, social/interpersonal skills, use of community resources, self-direction, functional academic skills, work, leisure, health, and safety. However, it should be kept in mind that these domains were not empirically selected, and no single measure of adaptive function exists.

B. Classification of Mental Retardation

1. Mental retardation is classified into four levels of severity based on intellectual impairment (as measured by IQ scores). These categories do not reflect functional capabilities however, and IQ tests have a standard error of measurement of approximately 5 points. The levels of severity, their IQ ranges, and their prevalence within the mentally retarded population are as follows:
   a. **Mild** (IQ 55–70): 85%
   b. **Moderate** (IQ 40–55): 10%
   c. **Severe** (IQ 25–40): 3 to 4%
   d. **Profound** (IQ < 25): 1 to 2%
2. A proportion of individuals diagnosed with mild mental retardation as children lose this diagnosis in adulthood as their adaptive skills improve and with no psychologist around to test them. Those who retain this label into adulthood tend to be affected more severely.

IV. Evaluation and Differential Diagnosis

A. Evaluation

1. The evaluation for a diagnosis of mental retardation is relatively straightforward; it is based on the previously mentioned diagnostic criteria.
2. History of adaptive functioning from ancillary sources like school and primary caregivers and neuropsychiatric and adaptive behavior testing are the cornerstones of evaluation.
3. **A thorough medical and neurological examination is important to rule out correctable causes (including hearing impairment, vision impairment, and seizures) of observed dysfunction.**
4. These exams are also helpful to identify any physical features that may be associated with specific syndromes, as some syndromes have related psychiatric conditions.
5. There are no laboratory findings that are specifically associated with mental retardation.
6. However, some laboratory findings are associated with a variety of causes of mental retardation (e.g., metabolic disturbances and chromosomal abnormalities). It is helpful to identify these if not done previously, as this information can again lead to diagnosis of syndromes that may have associated psychiatric pathology.

B. Differential Diagnosis

1. The differential diagnosis for mental retardation also includes physical disabilities.
2. In addition, specific learning disorders, communication disorders, and borderline intellectual functioning must be considered.
3. Although pervasive developmental disorders (e.g., autism and autism spectrum disorders) are a separate diagnostic category, 70–80% of individuals with a pervasive developmental disorder also have co-morbid mental retardation.

V. Treatment Considerations

A. Overview

1. It is unlikely that a psychiatrist will be called upon to treat mental retardation per se, as specialized education and training in adaptive functioning is done in schools and vocational settings. It is more likely that a psychiatrist will be called upon to evaluate and treat a psychiatric or behavioral disorder that interferes with adaptive functioning.
2. The evaluation and differential diagnosis of psychiatric illness in this population is not as straightforward as the diagnosis of mental retardation itself. The full range of psychiatric disorders is found in people with mental retardation, at rates that are probably higher than they are in the general population.
3. **There are also certain behavioral disorders and syndrome-associated disorders that occur in people with mental retardation.**
   a. **Syndrome-associated disorders are specific disorders that have a high probability of being exhibited by people with a given syndrome.**
   b. The terms pathobehavorial syndrome and behavioral phenotype are concepts that have been used to try and conceptualize this phenomenon.
4. Finally, one must bear in mind that definitive diagnosis is both clinically and methodologically a challenge. This is often due to limited self-reporting by a substantial proportion of the population.

B. Traditional Psychiatric Disorders

What follows is a brief synopsis of traditional psychiatric disorders, behavioral disorders, and syndrome-associated disorders that present in the mentally retarded. In each category, differences in their presentation, if any, and any special treatment considerations will be highlighted.

1. **Affective disorders**
   a. **Depression and bipolar spectrum disorders may present differently in the mentally retarded population,**

with less subjective reporting and more reliance on change from baseline behavior, than they do in the general population. Observable mood changes, accompanied by quantifiable neurovegetative symptoms using sleep charts and calorie counts, are helpful. Behavioral difficulties may be primary in those with severe mental retardation.

b. Treatment can involve both medication and therapy, with the type of therapy chosen based on the individual's strengths. Medication with a high anticholinergic load should be avoided if possible, due to the potential of anticholinergic agents to cause cognitive blunting.

2. Anxiety disorders

a. The full spectrum of anxiety disorders has been reported in the mentally retarded population. **Somatic, more observable aspects of anxiety are often more helpful than is reliance on self-report.** The possibility of trauma must always be considered given the vulnerability of the population. Obsessive-compulsive disorder (OCD) is difficult to distinguish from stereotypy given the critical need for self-reported ego-dystonic feelings.

b. Treatment consists of behavior therapy and medication. Benzodiazepines may be used, but their potential for disinhibition should be considered.

3. Schizophrenia

a. The co-occurrence of schizophrenia with mental retardation has been noted since the days of Kraepelin and Bleuler. However, diagnostic clarity remains a problem. Observable behaviors related to psychosis must be present in addition to the chronic changes in baseline function associated with major mental illness.

b. Antipsychotics are the drugs of choice; newer, atypical agents cause fewer extrapyramidal symptoms. While the overuse of neuroleptics has been a problem in the past, it is not clear that extrapyramidal symptoms are worse or more prevalent in the mentally retarded population.

C. Behavioral Disorders

1. Aggression

a. **Aggression is one of the prime reasons for institutionalization and for consultation in the mentally retarded population.** Pain and discomfort, as well as environmental triggers and/or psychopathology, can precipitate aggression.

b. Behavioral treatment is usually a first-line intervention for aggression, followed by use of medication for any underlying psychiatric disorder or impulse control disorder.

2. Self-Injurious Behavior

a. Self-injurious behavior (SIB) either potentially causes or actually causes physical damage to an individual's body. It usually presents as idiosyncratic, repetitive acts that occur in an identical form.

b. Behavior therapy is the mainstay of treatment, but medications (e.g., selective serotonin reuptake inhibitors [SSRIs] and neuroleptics) that address compulsive acts have been reported as successful.

3. Stereotypy

a. **Stereotypies are invariant, pathologic, motor behaviors or action sequences without an obvious reinforcement pattern. They are often seen in circumstances of extreme stimulation or deprivation, and are noted in many institutionalized, mentally retarded adults.**

b. Behavior therapy is the primary treatment; SSRIs have been tried but have yet to be evaluated in a rigorous manner.

4. Copraxia

a. **Copraxia involves rectal digging, feces smearing, and coprophagia.** It is a rare phenomenon that is usually **only found in the profoundly retarded population.**

b. Behavior therapy is the first line of treatment after medical conditions are ruled out.

5. Pica

a. Pica involves eating inedibles (e.g., dirt, paper clips, and cigarette butts). It usually occurs in severely retarded individuals.

b. Behavior therapy is the mainstay of treatment. It is unclear that dietary supplements are helpful.

6. Rumination

a. Rumination involves repeated acts of vomiting, chewing, and re-ingestion of the vomitus. This condition occurs more often in the severely to profoundly retarded population.

b. Behavior therapy is the treatment of choice; overfeeding should be included in the differential.

D. Syndrome-Associated Disorders

1. Down's syndrome (trisomy 21)

a. Individuals with Down's syndrome have **a classical physical presentation of round face, a flat nasal bridge, and a short stature.**

b. **Psychiatric co-morbidities include Alzheimer's dementia,** which often begins after the age of 40 years, and depression.

2. Fragile X syndrome (q27, long arm of X chromosome)

a. Individuals with the fragile X syndrome present with **a triad of long face, prominent ears, and macroorchidism.**

b. The full range of psychiatric disorders has been reported but by far **the most prominent co-morbidity is attention-deficit/hyperactivity disorder (ADHD), which occurs in approximately 80% of affected individuals.**

c. One-third of female carriers may be mentally retarded.

3. Prader-Willi syndrome (chromosome 15 deletion, 70% of cases)

a. Individuals with Prader-Willi syndrome exhibit **a short stature, obesity, hypogonadism, and hyperphagia.**

b. Common co-morbidities include OCD and depression.

4. Williams syndrome (chromosome 7 deletion)

a. Individuals with Williams syndrome present with **elfin-like faces, a starburst iris, as well as supravalvular aortic stenosis and hypertension.**

b. There is also a loquacious communication style, known as cocktail party speech.
c. Co-morbidities include ADHD, anxiety, and depression.

VI. Conclusion

There are several important points to consider in the area of mental retardation and psychiatric illness.

A. Mental retardation is a prevalent condition with diverse etiologies that affects approximately 1% of the population.

B. Three of the most common causes of mental retardation are Down's syndrome, fragile X syndrome, and fetal alcohol syndrome.

C. People with mental retardation are susceptible to the full range of psychiatric illness and likely suffer psychiatric illness at a higher rate than do those in the general population.

D. Certain pathobehavioral syndromes are unique to the mentally retarded population.

E. Individuals with mental retardation are an incredibly underserved population when it comes to psychiatric services, both from a clinical and research perspective.

Suggested Readings

American Psychiatric Association. (1994). *Diagnostic and statistical manual of mental disorders* (4th ed.). Washington, DC: American Psychiatric Press.

Bergman, J.D., & Harris, J.C. (1995). Mental retardation. In H.I. Kaplan & B.J. Sadock (Eds.), *Comprehensive textbook of psychiatry* (6th ed.). Baltimore, MD: Williams and Wilkins.

Gualtieri, C.T. (1990). *Neuropsychiatry and behavioral pharmacology*. New York: Springer-Verlag.

King, B.H., State, M.W., Shah, B., et al. (1997). Mental retardation: A review of the past 10 years. Part I. *Journal of the American Academy of Child and Adolescent Psychiatry, 36,* 1656–1663.

Matlon, J.L., Bamburg, J.W., Mayville, E.A., et al. (2000). Psychopharmacology and mental retardation: A 10 year review (1990–1999). *Research in Developmental Disabilities, 21*(4), 263–296.

Russell, A.T., & Tanguay, P.E. (1996). Mental retardation. In M. Lewis (Ed.), *Child and adolescent psychiatry a comprehensive textbook* (2nd ed.). Baltimore, MD: Williams and Wilkins.

State, M.W., King, B.H., & Dykens, E. (1997). Mental retardation: A review of the past 10 years, Part II. *Journal of the American Academy of Child and Adolescent Psychiatry, 36,* 1664–1671.

Volkmar, F.R. (Ed.). (1996). Mental retardation. *Child and Adolescent Psychiatry Clinics of North America, 5*(4).

Chapter 9

Mental Disorders Due to a General Medical Condition

B.J. Beck

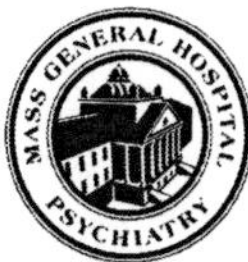

I. Introduction

A. Definition

1. **DSM-IV definition: Mental disorders due to a general medical condition (DTGMC) are psychiatric symptoms thought to be the direct, physiologic consequence of a non-psychiatric, medical condition.** The psychiatric symptoms themselves are severe enough to warrant recognition, and treatment, as a problem. This terminology is an attempt to replace the previously used functional versus organic dichotomy, and its unfortunate suggestion that the former has no biologic or physiologic basis, or that the latter is unaffected by psychosocial or environmental influences.
2. **General qualifiers. The mental disorder must:**
   a. **Be the direct pathophysiologic consequence of the medical condition.**
   b. **Not be better accounted for by another, primary mental disorder.**
   c. **Not occur solely during the course of delirium (i.e., a disturbance of consciousness in association with cognitive deficits).**
   d. **Not meet criteria for dementia (i.e., a syndrome with memory impairment and aphasia, apraxia, agnosia, or disturbances of executive function).**
   e. **Not be substance-induced.**

B. Disorders

1. **Mental disorder DTGMC should be part of the differential diagnosis for any psychiatric syndrome.** Alterations in cognition, behavior, or perception look much the same whether they derive from primary mental disorders, toxins, trauma, tumors, or seizures. For this reason, all but three of the individual disorders are listed in DSM-IV with disorders of similar symptomatology. These disorders are listed below, under the chapter titles in which they are located in DSM-IV:
   a. Delirium, dementia, amnestic, and other cognitive disorders
      i. **Delirium DTGMC**
      ii. **Dementia DTGMC**
      iii. **Amnestic disorder DTGMC**
   b. Schizophrenia and other psychotic disorders
      i. **Psychotic disorder DTGMC**
   c. Mood disorders
      i. **Mood disorder DTGMC**
   d. Anxiety disorders
      i. **Anxiety disorder DTGMC**
   e. Sexual disorders
      i. **Sexual dysfunction DTGMC**
   f. Sleep disorders
      i. **Sleep disorder DTGMC**
2. **Three diagnostic categories do not meet criteria for a psychiatric disorder,** and are listed separately in the chapter titled Mental disorders DTGMC:
   a. **Catatonic disorder DTGMC**
   b. **Personality change DTGMC** (coded on Axis I, not Axis II)
   c. **Mental disorder not otherwise specified (NOS) DTGMC**

II. Psychiatric Differential Diagnosis

A. Primary Mental Disorders

1. **It may be difficult to ascertain whether the mental disorder in question is the direct physiologic consequence of the medical condition, or whether the two merely co-exist. Correlation between the onset or severity of the medical and mental conditions is helpful, but inadequate, to establish a causal link.**

   Psychiatric symptoms may be the first symptoms of a medical condition (e.g., depression as the first manifestation of pancreatic carcinoma), or be out of proportion to the severity of the medical condition (e.g., depression or irritability in patients with early or minimal sensorimotor symptoms of multiple sclerosis). Alternatively, the psychiatric symptoms may occur late in the course of the medical condition (e.g., psychosis years after the onset of epilepsy), or may not resolve simultaneously with the medical condition (e.g., depression that continues after hypothyroidism is corrected).

   When treatment of the general medical condition does dissipate the psychiatric symptoms, an etiologic relationship is supported. However, some mental disorders DTGMC are amenable to, and require, treatment in their own right (e.g., interictal depression); this does not imply the diagnosis of a primary mental disorder.
2. **Atypical features of a primary mental disorder support an etiologic relationship to the medical condition:**
   a. **Age of onset:** e.g., the onset of panic attacks in a 65-year-old man
   b. **Course:** e.g., sudden onset of depression
   c. **Associated features:** e.g., cognitive deficits out of proportion to mildly depressed mood
3. **Typical features of the primary mental disorder** suggest that conditions may co-exist:
   a. **Recurrent past episodes** (in the absence of the medical condition)
   b. **Positive family history**
4. **The scientific literature supports the causal relationship between some medical conditions and the occurrence of certain psychiatric symptoms.** That

is, there is a greater than base-rate occurrence for a mental syndrome in patients with a particular medical condition, compared with an appropriate control group. Or, a mental syndrome may correlate with expected **deficits or symptoms based on the location of brain pathology** or pathophysiology (e.g., disinhibition or decreased executive function with frontal lobe damage). Although such studies may support the causal relationship between medical and mental disorders, the **diagnosis for a given patient must be considered individually.** Less stringent, but helpful, are individual **case studies** that suggest a link between a given medical condition and a mental disorder.

B. Substance-Induced Disorders

Prescription and over-the-counter medications, illicit drugs, or alcohol may be used, misused, or abused during the course of a general medical condition. **A careful history, and possibly the use of urine or blood tests, should alert the clinician to drug use and abuse and be part of every evaluation.** Use, intoxication, or withdrawal can cause mental symptoms that continue for up to a month after discontinuation of a substance. The therapeutic use of some medications causes psychiatric symptoms (e.g., steroids in a patient with systemic lupus erythematosus) that mimic the symptoms of the disease itself (e.g., mood lability).

C. If mental symptoms seem to be substance-induced *and* DTGMC, both conditions should be coded.

D. If one is not sure whether a mental disorder is due to a general medical condition, a primary mental disorder, or is substance-induced, the NOS code should be used.

III. General Medical Conditions

The mnemonic, GENeral MEDical CONDITions (Table 9-1), **should help the evaluating clinician recall the broad categories of medical conditions that can cause psychiatric syndromes.**

A. Infectious Diseases

Infection of the central nervous system (CNS), and especially the chronic meningitides, are increasingly prevalent as immune suppression is on the rise, either from acquired immunodeficiency syndrome (AIDS) or as a result of immune suppressant therapy for malignancy or organ transplantation.

1. **Herpes simplex virus (HSV) has a propensity for the temporal and inferomedial frontal lobes,** and is the most commonly encountered focal encephalopathy. Widely recognized to cause a loss of the sense of smell (anosmia), as well as olfactory or gustatory hallucinations, the limbic distribution of HSV may also result in psychosis, bizarre behavior, or personality change. These personality changes, along with affective lability and decreased cognitive function, may persist. Simple or complex partial seizures may also develop.

Table 9-1. Categories of General Medical Conditions

GENeral **MED**ical **CONDIT**ions
Germs (infectious diseases)
Epilepsy
Nutritional deficit
Metabolic encephalopathy
Endocrine disorders
Demyelination
Cerebrovascular disease
Offensive toxins
Neoplasm
Degeneration
Immune disease
Trauma

2. **Human immunodeficiency virus (HIV) infection is associated with neuropsychiatric symptoms of multiple etiologies, including, but not limited to, direct CNS infection** (e.g., HIV-related metabolic derangements, endocrinopathies, medication side effects, tumors, opportunistic infections). **Accepted terms for the neuropsychiatric syndromes of HIV CNS infection (e.g., HIV-1-associated cognitive/motor complex, AIDS dementia complex, dementia due to HIV disease)** are inadequate descriptors for the range of reported symptoms. The presence, severity, and location of HIV-related CNS pathology does not correlate particularly well with the reported symptoms. Besides the deficits suggested by the above terms (i.e., cognitive deficits: attention, concentration, and visuospatial performance; motor deficits: fine motor control and speed; and dementia: short-term memory loss, word-finding difficulties, and poor executive function), patients may experience depressed mood, apathy, social withdrawal, and a lack of energy, motivation, or spontaneity. Although much less common, mania and hypomania have also been reported. Psychosis is rarely reported as a new syndrome; when present, it generally occurs in the setting of advanced disease.
3. **Rabies, an acute viral disease of the mammalian CNS, is most often transmitted by exposure to infected saliva through an animal bite.** Rare in the United States, human rabies is more commonly seen following domestic animal bites received during foreign travel. The virus travels centripetally along

peripheral nerves to the CNS. The distance the virus travels, along with size of the innoculum and the degree of host defenses, is thought to be responsible for the extreme variability in incubation period, from 10 days to a year; the mean incubation period is 1–2 months.

The initial prodrome is similar to that of other viral illnesses, except for the distinct feature of local fasciculations or paresthesias at the inoculation site. Once rabies proceeds to acute encephalitis, brainstem dysfunction, coma, and death usually follow within 4–20 days. The encephalitis is heralded by agitation and motor excitation, followed by periods of confusion, psychosis, and combativeness which may initially be interspersed with lucid periods. Half of infected individuals experience painful, violent spasms of the diaphragm, laryngeal, pharyngeal, and accessory respiratory muscles when attempting to swallow liquids, which leads to classic hydrophobia. There is autonomic dysfunction, upper motor neuron weakness and paralysis, cranial nerve involvement, and often vocal cord paralysis.

4. **Lyme disease is a tick-borne spirochetal infection** most common in parts of Europe and the United States (especially the Northeast, upper Midwest, and Pacific Coastal states). **Because of the confusing array, and unreliable results, of serologic tests, as well as the prolonged, recurrent, and non-specific nature of the symptoms, the clinician must have a high level of awareness of the neuropsychiatric sequelae of Lyme disease.** Diagnosis may require both Lyme ELISA (enzyme-linked immunosorbent assay) and Lyme Western blot, as well as polymerase chain reaction assay (PCR) or culture.

   A flu-like syndrome and rash (erythema migrans) usually follow the initial tick (*Ixodes scapularis*) bite, with hematogenous spread taking place over days to weeks. Once lodged in the target organs (heart, eyes, joints, muscles, peripheral or CNS), the organism (*Borrelia burgdorferi*) may lie dormant for months to years, at which point memory of the initial event has often dimmed. Diagnostic delay is associated with a more chronic course, but **even with early, aggressive, antibiotic treatment, symptoms may recur or develop months to years later.**

   Lyme encephalitis may present with fatigue, mood lability, irritability, confusion, and sleep disturbance. Much less common, encephalomyelitis may mimic multiple sclerosis. **A more chronic encephalopathy may develop with a large range of disturbances in personality, cognition** (short-term memory, memory retrieval, verbal fluency, concentration and attention, orientation, processing speed), **behavior** (disorganization, distractibility, catatonia, mutism, violence), **mood** (depression, mania, lability), **thought processes** (paranoia), and **perception** (hallucinations, depersonalization, hyperacusis, photophobia). Strokes, seizures, and severe dementia are rare sequelae of neurologic Lyme disease.

5. **Neurosyphilis, of the symptomatic, parenchymal, general paretic type, is a form of late (tertiary) syphilis seen in less than 10% of untreated syphilitics, 20 years after primary infection.** Even more rare in the post-penicillin era, **general paresis may be on the rise among individuals with AIDS.** Antibiotics have also changed the classical picture, and patients may have mixed, more subtle, symptoms of late syphilis. With diffuse, but particularly frontal lobe involvement, signs and symptoms of general paresis (Table 9-2) include personality change, irritability, poor judgment and insight, difficulty with calculations and recent memory, apathy, and decreased personal grooming. **If untreated, mood lability, delusions of grandeur, hallucinations, disorientation, and dementia may follow, along with the classical neurological signs of tremor, dysarthria, hyperreflexia, hypotonia, ataxia, and Argyll Robertson pupils (small, irregular, unequal pupils that accommodate, but do not react to light).** Cerebral spinal fluid with elevated protein and lymphocyte count, and positive Venereal Disease Research Laboratories (VDRL) (a flocculation test that uses cardiolipin with cholesterol and lecithin), confirms the diagnosis.

6. **Chronic meningitis is a potentially treatable condition that sadly presents with minimal and subtle physical signs and symptoms (e.g., low-grade fever, headache), which, especially in the immunocompromised patient, may be overlooked or attributed to an underlying condition (e.g., AIDS).** Likewise, the common psychiatric concomitants (confusion, cognitive dysfunction, memory, and behavioral problems) are non-specific. **The most com-**

Table 9-2. Manifestations of General Paresis

PARESIS
Personality
Affect
Reflexes (hyperactive)
Eye (Argyll Robertson pupils)
Sensorium (illusions, delusions, hallucinations)
Intellect (decreased recent memory, orientation, calculation, judgment, and insight)
Speech

SOURCE: Lukehart, S.A., & Holmes, K.K. (1998). Syphilis. In A.S. Fauci, E. Braunwald, K.J. Isselbacher, et al. (Eds.), *Harrison's principles of internal medicine* (14th ed., p. 1027). New York: McGraw-Hill.

mon cause of chronic meningitis is *Mycobacterium tuberculosis;* common fungal agents are cryptococcus and coccidioides.

7. **Chronic and persistent viral or prion diseases of the CNS** are included here more for historic, rather than practical, significance. These tend to be increasingly rare disorders that, once manifest, lead unalterably to death in a matter of months to a few years. The neurologic signs may lag behind the psychiatric symptoms, but are so extreme and rapidly debilitating that they are unlikely to be attributed to primary mental disorders.
   a. **Subacute sclerosing panencephalitis (SSPE) occurs in children and adolescents (usually before age 11 years) following previous measles (rubeola) infection or, rarely, measles vaccination.** SSPE has steadily declined since the advent of widespread measles vaccination. With a predilection for males (3:1, male/female), the first signs are often deterioration in school work, distractibility, behavioral change (opposition and temper tantrums), sleepiness, and hallucinations. **Neurological signs, which appear within a few months, include myoclonic jerks, ataxia, seizures, and further intellectual deterioration.** Patients are generally bedridden within 6–9 months, and dead within 1–3 years.
   b. **Creutzfeldt-Jakob Disease (CJD) is a rare, rapidly progressive, and fatal illness of primarily 50–70-year-olds.** Most cases of this prion disease are sporadic, though **5–15% may be familial.** There is also evidence of person-to-person transmission through corneal transplantation, as well as transmission through cadaveric human growth hormone or cadaveric gonadotropins. The hallmarks of the disease, dementia and myoclonus, may be preceded by intellectual decline (memory difficulties, mood instability, poor judgment), sensorimotor disturbance (dizziness, vertigo, gait problems), and perceptual abnormalities (visual illusions or distortions). Hallucinations, delusions, and confusion may follow. Patients become spastic, mute, and stuporous, and usually die in less than a year. Characteristic electroencephalographic (EEG) changes late in the course, along with cortical and cerebellar atrophy seen on head computed tomography (CT) scan, are suggestive of the diagnosis.
   c. **Kuru, or "trembling with fear," is a fatal disorder of progressive dementia and extrapyramidal signs, which was endemic among a particular tribal group of New Guinea highlanders who ate the brains of their dead.** As this ritual cannibalism declined, so did the incidence of Kuru.

B. Epilepsy is a common (1% lifetime prevalence) neurologic disorder characterized by episodic, disorganized firing of electrical impulses in the cortex of the brain. The location of these impulses dictates the seizure phenomena, which may include altered consciousness, as well as motor, cognitive, behavioral, affective, perceptual, and/or memory disturbances. Seizures were often considered to be emotional problems prior to the use of the EEG which demonstrated a correlation between behavioral and objective findings. It is not surprising that psychiatric and neurologic syndromes were confused; the CNS has only certain, non-specific modes of response to stimulation, regardless of the source of the input. However, **seizures remain a clinical diagnosis, which may be supported, but not ruled out, by EEG.**

1. **Complex partial seizures,** often of temporal lobe or other limbic origin, are of particular interest to the psychiatrist. It is estimated that 60% of the roughly 2 million epileptics in the United States have nonconvulsive seizures, which are most commonly partial seizures. Of those with partial seizures, 40% do not show the classic, focal findings on EEG. A high level of suspicion must be maintained by the psychiatrist not to uncritically accept the neurologist's dismissal of the diagnosis based on a "normal" EEG.
   a. **Depression occurs in slightly more than half of patients with epilepsy, as compared with 30% of matched (medical and neurologic outpatient) controls.** The incidence is thought to be even higher in patients with partial complex seizures and left hemispheric foci, which suggests that depression may be caused by seizure-induced limbic dysfunction. **The suicide rate in patients with epilepsy is 5 times that of the general public; in patients with temporal lobe epilepsy, the risk may be 25-fold higher than in the general population.**
   b. **Anxiety** symptoms are also more closely associated with partial seizures than with other types of seizures. **It may be particularly difficult to differentiate partial seizures from panic attacks.** Both may occur "out of the blue," with hyperarousal, intense fear, perceptual distortion, and dissociative symptoms, such as depersonalization or derealization. Both may be responsive to benzodiazepines. Both may appear to begin with hyperventilation, a common symptom of panic that can also lower the seizure threshold in susceptible individuals. However, in panic disorder, the fear of passing out is common, while the actual loss (or alteration) of consciousness is rare; auditory or visual distortions may occur, but usually not olfactory or gustatory hallucinations; automatisms (chewing or lip-smacking movements) are not common; and there is usually no period of confusion following the episode. Panic attacks generally last 10–20 minutes, with memory of the event intact. It is precisely this memory that leads to the fear of the next attack and promotes the development of agoraphobia. In contrast, **complex partial seizures often start with cognitive (*déjà vu, jamais vu,* forced thinking), affective (fear, depression, pleasure) or perceptual (illusions, olfactory or gustatory hallucinations) auras, followed by a brief cessation of activity, then a minute or less of automatismic behavior and unresponsive-**

ness, concluding with a brief period (less than a minute to a half an hour) of lack of, or decreased, awareness. There is often incomplete memory of the episode, and agoraphobia is rare.

c. **Psychosis** is also more prevalent in patients with complex partial seizures. **The risk of psychosis in patients with epilepsy may be as much as 6–12 times that of the general public. Besides the psychotic symptoms experienced as auras or post-ictal delirium, there are brief episodic, as well as unremitting, chronic psychoses that are thought to result from sub-ictal, temporal lobe dysrhythmias.** The most common symptoms are hallucinations, paranoia, and thought disorders (e.g., circumstantiality, as opposed to the more common schizophrenic symptoms of thought blocking, derailment, and tangentiality). Psychosis often appears after many years of epilepsy, and may be preceded by personality changes. A notable difference in psychotic presentation is that the epileptic's affect is generally intact and warm, as compared with the affective flattening of the schizophrenic.

d. **Personality symptoms** associated with temporal lobe epilepsy are commonly described, but controversial, and not supported by controlled studies using structured, diagnostic tools. Nonetheless, **the inter-ictal traits reported include hyperreligiosity, hypergraphia, hyposexuality, dependence, obsessionality, and a marked humorlessness.** There is better agreement about **a sticky, or viscous, conversational style that is difficult to disengage.**

e. **Violence should be considered a rare ictal event, which is never an organized, purposeful act.** Episodic dyscontrol is a controversial syndrome, described as recurrent outbursts of uncontrollable rage, in response to minor irritations, which may occur more frequently in patients with early onset of temporal or frontal lobe epilepsy. However, such outbursts are also associated with psychosis and multiple psychosocial, educational, intellectual, socioeconomic, and family deficits, as well as a history of abuse. The overwhelming probability is that such attacks are related to (inter-ictal or primary) psychopathology or brain injury (which might also be the cause of seizures), and should not be attributed to seizure activity per se.

2. **The significance of epilepsy in psychiatric practice goes beyond its neuropsychiatric manifestations, and includes the psychosocial ramifications of living with a seizure disorder, the cognitive and affective side effects of common antiepileptic medications, and the seizure threshold-lowering effect of certain neuroleptic and tricyclic antidepressant medications.** Thus the presence of, for instance, mood symptoms and a seizure disorder does not automatically make the diagnosis of mood disorder due to epilepsy. Yet, inter-ictal mood symptoms deserve to be treated, even when they are most likely caused by the seizure disorder. **Finally, the difficulty or inability of confirming the clinical diagnosis of a seizure disorder, in the setting of psychiatric symptoms resistant to the usual treatments, should prompt a trial of an appropriate antiepileptic medication.**

C. Nutritional Deficits

1. **Niacin (nicotinic acid) deficiency, and deficiency of its precursor, tryptophan, lead to pellagra, which, when untreated, leads to a chronic wasting, diarrheal, neurologic (encephalopathy and peripheral neuropathy), and dermatologic (sun-exposed skin rash, angular stomatitis, and glossitis) syndrome. The early symptoms are non-specific and may easily be mistaken for depression: insomnia, fatigue, irritability, anxiety, and depressed mood.** Untreated, this progresses to mental slowing, confusion, psychosis, and dementia, which may be accompanied by a spastic spinal syndrome with leg weakness, hyperreflexia, clonus, and extensor plantar responses. Pellagra is rare since the advent of niacin fortification of cereals, but still occurs in alcoholics, refugee populations, and vegetarians in less developed nations. Most symptoms reverse quickly with niacin repletion. Dementia, however, a sign of severe and prolonged deficit, may clear slowly or incompletely.
2. **Thiamine (vitamin B_1) deficiency occurs in two forms: beriberi in areas of poverty or famine and Wernicke-Korsakoff syndrome in alcoholism.** There are cardiovascular, neuropathic, and cerebral signs and symptoms that generally occur in combination, but can less frequently present as isolated forms. Few alcoholics or malnourished individuals develop clinical deficiency, and other factors (e.g., activity and total calorie intake) affect the presentation. **The syndrome may be precipitated by the administration of glucose to asymptomatic, thiamine-deficient patients. The early symptoms may include decreased concentration, apathy, mild agitation, and depressed mood.** Confusion, amnesia, and confabulation are late signs of severe, prolonged deficit.
3. **Cobalamin (vitamin B_{12}) deficiency, from lack of absorption (e.g., from absence of intrinsic factor in pernicious anemia or after gastric surgery) or vegetarian diet, leads to megaloblastic macrocytic anemia and neurodegenerative changes in the peripheral and central nervous systems. Neuropsychiatric symptoms, which may precede hematologic findings, include apathy, irritability, depression, and mood lability.** Less common, and indicative of more severe disease, is **megaloblastic madness, a delirium with prominent hallucinations, paranoia, and intellectual decline.** Neurologic signs include peripheral numbness and paresthesias, sphincter dyscontrol, abnormal reflexes, and decreased position and vibratory sensation. Because the axonal demyelination and neurodegenerative changes lead ultimately to cell death, not all neurologic findings clear with treatment.

D. Metabolic encephalopathy should be considered whenever sudden or abrupt changes in mentation, orientation, behavior, or level of consciousness occur. Although the waxing and waning presentation of delirium may eventually be evident, early memory impairment, passivity, withdrawal, or anxiety, and agitation, may be wrongly attributed to a primary psychiatric disorder.

1. **Hepatic encephalopathy may result from acute, subacute, or chronic hepatocellular failure, with a range of neuropsychiatric symptoms from mild personality change to coma, many of which may precede the more classical neurologic or physical findings (e.g., asterixis or icterus, respectively).** Earliest signs, apparent only to close family and friends, are mild intellectual difficulties, often covered by intact verbal ability. **Objective mental slowing, mild confusion, decreased concentration, depressed or labile mood, irritability, sleep-wake reversal, and decreased personal grooming are common early signs.** There may be periods of intermittent disorientation, inappropriate behavior, and outbursts of rage before the progressive deterioration in consciousness, speech, cognition, and memory leave the patient somnolent, incoherent, disoriented, confused, and amnestic. The final stage is coma.
2. **Renal insufficiency, acute or chronic, is associated with neuropsychiatric symptoms.** Acute renal failure is most notable for delirium, often with bizarre visual hallucinations. **Chronic renal insufficiency is associated with a wide range of symptoms, from mild difficulties in concentration, problem-solving, or calculation to more severe cognitive impairment and lethargy.** While adequate dialysis may improve cognitive function, there are also problems of memory, concentration, and mental slowness associated with dialysis (even though the removal of aluminum has nearly eradicated the incidence of dialysis dementia). Depression also seems more prevalent in renal insufficiency, and in dialysis patients, although associated endocrine dysfunction (e.g., hyperparathyroidism) and disordered neurotransmission are thought to be contributing factors. Finally, uremia is associated with seizures, and complex partial seizures may be an occult cause of altered behavior, affect, perception, cognition, and consciousness.
3. **Hypoglycemic encephalopathy, whether from excess endogenous or exogenous insulin, can present with confusion, disorientation, or hallucinations and bizarre behavior.** Often, but not always, these symptoms are preceded by restlessness or apprehension. **Physical signs and symptoms include nausea, hunger, diaphoresis, and tachycardia.** Untreated, stupor and coma follow. **Repeated hypoglycemic episodes may cause permanent amnesia from hippocampal involvement.**
4. **Diabetic ketoacidosis can also present with non-specific symptoms of fatigue and lethargy, before the "three Ps" (polyphagia, polydipsia, polyuria), head-ache, nausea, and vomiting appear.** In a poorly controlled, elderly, diabetic patient, osmotic fluid shifts can cause a slowly resolving delirium that primarily affects cognitive function.
5. **Acute intermittent porphyria (AIP) is a rare, autosomal dominant enzyme deficiency that interferes with heme biosynthesis and causes the accumulation of porphyrins. More common in women than men, it is known for the classical triad of episodic, acute, colicky abdominal pain, motor polyneuropathy, and psychosis, usually with onset in those 20–50 years of age.** However, **AIP may present with only psychiatric symptoms:** insomnia, anxiety, mood lability, depression, and psychosis. A small percentage of chronic psychiatric patients have been found to have undiagnosed porphyria. Neurologic effects, hyponatremia, and other electrolyte imbalances from vomiting and diarrhea, can lead to seizures. **Attacks can be precipitated by drugs, alcohol, low calorie diets, or gonadal steroids (endogenous or exogenous). Porphyrinogenic drugs include most antiepileptic medications, meprobamate, sulfonamide antibiotics, and ergot derivatives.** Phenothiazines, bromides, narcotic analgesics, and glucocorticoids are among the safe medications.

E. Endocrine disorders are associated with psychiatric symptoms, most commonly depression and anxiety. In the past, when endocrinopathies were diagnosed later in their course, delirium and dementia were more common.

1. **Thyroid**
   a. **Hypothyroidism, which is at least 4 times more prevalent in women than in men, has an insidious onset of non-specific symptoms, such as fatigue, lethargy, weight gain, decreased appetite, depressed mood, cold intolerance, and slowed mental and motor activity.** Later in the course, the physical signs are dry skin, thin and dry hair, constipation, stiffness, a coarse voice, facial puffiness, carpal tunnel symptoms, loss of the outer third of the eyebrow, loss of hearing, and a delayed relaxation phase of deep tendon reflexes. Early symptoms may be attributed to aging, depression, dementia, or Parkinson's disease. Hallucinations and paranoia, the manifestations of the so-called "myxedema madness," are late findings. Roughly 10% of patients have residual psychiatric symptoms after hormone replacement.
   b. **Hyperthyroid patients appear restless, anxious, fidgety, or labile.** Symptoms may overlap with those of anxiety or panic, with palpitations, tachycardia, sweating, irritability, tremulousness, decreased sleep, weakness, and fatigue. Weight loss occurs despite increased appetite. **Elderly patients may manifest apathy, psychomotor retardation,**

and depression, rather than hyperactive symptoms; proximal muscle wasting and cardiovascular symptoms (failure and atrial arrhythmias) may predominate.

2. **Parathyroid** dysfunction is closely linked to perturbations in calcium, phosphate, and bone metabolism. However, attempts to correlate symptoms with absolute serum calcium levels have been inconclusive.
   a. **Hyperparathyroidism, and the resultant hypercalcemia, may be asymptomatic in as many as half of all patients, or present early on with non-specific signs of mental slowness, lethargy, apathy, decreased attention and memory, and depressed mood.** Delirium, disorientation, and psychosis are also reported.
   b. In **hypoparathyroidism, a gradual onset of hypocalcemia may cause personality change, or delirium, without the characteristic tetany of a more precipitous drop in serum calcium.**
3. **Adrenal dysfunction**
   a. **Adrenal insufficiency, whether from autoimmune Addison's disease (primary hypocortisolism) or the sudden withdrawal of prolonged glucocorticoid therapy (secondary hypocortisolism), presents with initially mild psychiatric symptoms that may be attributable to depression: apathy, negativism, social withdrawal, poverty of thought, fatigue, depressed mood, irritability, and loss of appetite, interest, and enjoyment.** Other signs and symptoms include nausea, vomiting, weakness, hypotension, and hypoglycemia. Psychosis, delirium, and eventually coma may develop. The treatment is glucocorticoid replacement, although psychiatric symptoms may not fully resolve and may require specific therapy, as well. Care should be taken to choose psychotropic medications that will not exacerbate hypotension. The relative roles of decreased glucocorticoids versus the increased levels of adrenocorticotropic hormone (ACTH) and corticotropin-releasing factor (CRF) versus the lack of normal diurnal and stress modulation in glucocorticoid replacement, in the development and continuation of psychiatric symptoms, are unclear.
   b. **Hypercortisolism may result from chronic hypersecretion of ACTH (ACTH-dependent) from a pituitary adenoma (Cushing's disease) or a non-pituitary neoplasm (Cushing's syndrome); or, less frequently, it may result from the direct, adrenal oversecretion of cortisol from a tumor or hyperplasia (ACTH-independent Cushing's syndrome).** The vast majority of patients will experience psychiatric symptoms, which may precede the (often partial) development of the classical, Cushingoid, stigmata: truncal obesity, peripheral wasting, hirsutism, moon facies, acne, and striae. **Psychiatric symptoms include anxiety (similar to general anxiety disorder [GAD] or panic disorder) and depression, with crying, extreme irritability, insomnia, decreased interest, energy, concentration, and memory.** Suicidal ideation may be prevalent. Although relatively rare, psychosis may develop. Prolonged administration of exogenous corticosteroids produces a similar syndrome and patients may be extremely responsive, psychiatrically, to small dose adjustments. High-dose, exogenous corticosteroids may also precipitate mania. In patients with a history of corticosteroid-induced mania and a need for episodic corticosteroid treatment, the prophylactic use of a mood stabilizer is indicated.
4. **Pituitary dysfunction** can disrupt the normal modulation of multiple systems in the body, and **thus can cause a wide range of psychiatric symptoms.** The post-partum, hemorrhagic destruction of the pituitary (**Sheehan's syndrome**), e.g., may cause depression, mental slowness, and mood lability. An overactive pituitary can lead to adrenal hyperplasia and all the symptoms of Cushing's syndrome, described earlier.

F. **Demyelinating disorders** are associated with neuropsychiatric symptoms, as well as motor and sensory changes. These disorders are relatively rare in the general public and may present initially with mild alterations in mood, behavior, cognition, or personality. **When the early physical complaints are intermittent, subjective, and variable, they may be attributed to depression, anxiety, somatization, or even malingering. Multiple sclerosis (MS) is by far the most prevalent of these disorders (50–60 cases per 100,000), with amyotrophic lateral sclerosis (ALS) a distant second (3–5 cases per 100,000).** Others include metachromatic leukodystrophy, adrenoleukodystrophy, gangliosidoses, and SSPE.

1. **Multiple sclerosis (MS), an episodic, inflammatory, multifocal, demyelinating disease of unknown etiology, affects the cerebral hemispheres, optic nerves, brain stem, cerebellum, and spinal cord. MS is more common in cold and temperate climates, with a predilection for women, and an onset between ages 20 and 40 years.**

   Studies suggest that psychiatric symptoms are prevalent throughout the course of MS, do not clear during remission of physical symptoms, and correlate poorly with magnetic resonance imaging (MRI) findings, severity of physical symptoms, or length of illness. In order of prevalence, **95% of MS patients experience some of the following alterations in mood, behavior, or personality: depressed mood, agitation, anxiety, irritability, apathy, euphoria, disinhibition, hallucinations, aberrant motor behavior, or delusions. Depressive symptoms may occur in over 75% of patients, and are associated with an increased rate of suicide.** Although the presence of depression does not vary by gender or age, the risk of suicide in MS is higher in men, the newly diagnosed, and those with onset prior to age 30 years. Despite the common wisdom that MS is associated with euphoria, only about a quarter of patients experience this mildly elevated mood at some point during their course of illness, and persistent euphoria probably occurs in less than 10% of patients. Euphoria should not be considered synonymous with mania, which is rarely seen. Rather, what passes for euphoria in MS is more of an upbeat nature that may seem incongruent with the patient's condition and pre-morbid personality style.

Mild to moderate cognitive deficits appear in more than half of MS patients, with more severe decline seen in 20–30%. Memory is most often affected, though severe dementia is not common.

2. **Amyotrophic lateral sclerosis (ALS), the most common degenerative motor neuron disease, is still relatively rare,** with an annual incidence of 1.6 per 100,000 population. It may begin with either upper or lower motor neuron involvement, but eventually both will be affected. It has a relentless course to death within 4 or 5 years, usually from diaphragmatic failure. The sporadic form is more common, although there are familial forms. Dementia may occur in familial ALS, but, even with advanced sporadic disease, cognitive function remains intact. **Uncontrollable laughing and crying (pseudobulbar affect) is the result of degenerative changes in the cortical bulbar projections to the brainstem.**
3. **Lipid storage disorders are a group of rare, inherited (autosomal recessive) enzyme deficiencies** that can present in adulthood with multiple psychiatric and neuromuscular signs and symptoms.
   a. **Metachromatic leukodystrophy** (MLD) is rapidly fatal when it presents in infancy. When it presents in adolescence or adulthood, however, it has an insidious, progressive course with cognitive decline, forgetfulness, deterioration of work or school performance, and personality changes. Mild cerebellar signs follow, with gait disturbances, masked facies, and strange postures. Patients become demented, and finally mute and bedridden.
   b. **Adrenoleukodystrophy** (ALD) also causes adrenal insufficiency (i.e., primary Addison's disease). It may present with aphasia, dementia, asymmetric myelopathic findings (e.g., homonymous hemianopsia, hemiparesis), or the psychiatric symptoms of Addison's disease. A progressive, more symmetric presentation follows, with spastic paraparesis or demyelinating polyneuropathy. Glucocorticoids treat the adrenal insufficiency, but there is no treatment for the overall disorder.
   c. **Gangliosidoses** are a group of lysosomal storage diseases that include the **adult form of Tay-Sach's disease.** Lower motor neuron and spinocerebellar symptoms may present in childhood or adolescence as clumsiness or weakness, with normal intelligence and vision. However, in some patients, psychosis or seizures develop, while the neuromuscular effects are mild.

G. **Cerebrovascular disease** is the third most common cause of death in the United States, behind heart disease and cancer. **The vast majority of strokes are ischemic (85%), and about a third of all strokes are the result of atherosclerotic thrombosis and cerebral embolism.** Essential hypertension is the most common cause of hemorrhagic stroke; spontaneous aneurysmal rupture, or arteriovenous malformation are much less frequent causes of parenchymal bleeding.

1. **Depression,** either major depression or dysthymia, is the most common post-stroke psychiatric syndrome, which occurs in over half of patients. Roughly two-thirds of these patients experience depressive symptoms in the immediate post-stroke period, while the rest become depressed after about 6 months. The natural course of untreated, post-stroke depression is about a year, while the course of dysthymia may be more protracted and variable. While the severity of deficits does not correlate with the onset of depression, depression is correlated with poor recovery and with a decreased ability to participate in rehabilitative therapies. Standard antidepressant therapies have been shown to shorten the course of post-stroke depression, underscoring the importance of timely recognition and initiation of treatment. There is suggestive, but questioned, evidence that stroke location (left hemisphere frontal, prefrontal, or basal ganglia) predisposes to depression; previous stroke, subcortical atrophy, and personal or family history of mood disorder may also increase the risk of post-stroke depression.
2. **Aprosodia,** the inability to affectively modulate speech and gestures (motor aprosodia), or the inability to interpret the emotional components of another's speech or gestures (sensory aprosodia), may follow right (nondominant) hemisphere insults. **The aprosodic patient often appears affectively blunted, or "flat," but this is a disorder of *expression,* not mood, and it should be carefully differentiated from depression.**
3. **Anxiety,** as an isolated syndrome, is relatively rare in the post-stroke period. However, almost half of patients with post-stroke depression have concomitant anxiety symptoms.
4. **Mania,** although rare, correlates with right-sided lesions of the orbitofrontal, basotemporal, basal ganglia, and thalamic areas. This secondary mania may be more common in those with pre-existing subcortical atrophy, or a personal or family history of mood disorder.
5. **Affective incontinence** may be seen, with **multiple lacunar infarcts** affecting the descending corticobulbar and frontopontine pathways. This release of cortical inhibition over lower brainstem centers results in uncontrollable outbursts of laughing or crying and loss of more moderate emotional expression, such as smiling. This affective dyscontrol occurs along with dysarthria,

dysphagia, and bifacial weakness, which together comprise the syndrome of **"pseudobulbar palsy."**

H. Toxins, of various types in miniscule amounts, are gaining notoriety as the putative cause of myriad non-specific symptoms in certain, sensitive individuals. While there are few data to support the existence of **multiple chemical sensitivity or environmental illness,** there are syndromes from common environmental toxins, such as carbon monoxide or low-level lead exposure, that may be overlooked because of their similarity to common medical or primary mental disorders.

1. **Carbon monoxide** (CO) poisoning, from faulty heating or exhaust systems, may cause a flu-like illness with cough, nausea, and general malaise. More chronic, low-level exposure can cause cognitive deterioration and depression. Severe, but sub-lethal poisoning can lead to memory dysfunction, visual problems, parkinsonism, confabulation, psychosis, and delirium.
2. **Lead,** a known toxin in young children, also poses a risk to adults who are exposed in a variety of occupational, recreational, and environmental settings. Potentially hazardous activities include home renovation, drinking from leaded crystal, and jogging in areas of heavy traffic. Stained glass, ceramic, and lead figure artisans, as well as artists who use lead-based oil paints, and even art conservators, are at risk. Firearm enthusiasts should also monitor their lead levels. The psychiatric symptoms of low-level lead exposure are non-descript, and easily dismissed as depression: after-work fatigue, sleepiness, depressed mood, and apathy. At higher levels, cognition and memory may be impaired, along with sensorimotor symptoms, restlessness, and gastrointestinal complaints. Organic lead exposure from gasoline, solvents, and cleaning fluids can cause psychosis, restlessness, nightmares, and, at very high levels, seizures and coma.
3. **Mercury exposure from organic mercury,** as well as from contaminated fish, **results in a primarily neurologic syndrome,** while **exposure to inorganic mercury presents initially with psychiatric symptoms.**
   a. In **organic mercury poisoning,** the prominent neurologic effects include motor-sensory neuropathy, cerebellar ataxia, slurred speech, paresthesias, and visual field defects. The primary psychiatric symptoms, depression, irritability, and mild dementia, may be less striking.
   b. With **inorganic mercury poisoning, the *Mad Hatter* syndrome,** the initial symptoms are depression, irritability, and psychosis, with less prominent headache, tremor, and weakness. Whereas exposure in the past was occupational or from broken thermometers, present-day sources may be less obvious. Mercury is found in readily purchased botanical preparations and folk medicines. It is also sold in easily broken capsules with instructions to sprinkle it in the home or car, a practice of certain cultural or religious sects.
4. **Drugs: overdose, herbal, non-prescription, prescribed, or recreational.** All should be considered potential toxins when evaluating changes in cognition, behavior, consciousness, or personality. (However, these would be substance-induced mental disorders, and are discussed elsewhere.)

I. Neoplasm, unregulated focal or diffuse growth within the cranial confines, can produce any of the symptomatic presentations available to the CNS. As compared with ischemic infarcts, tumors affecting similar brain volume are less symptomatic. The clinical presentation may suggest the type, location, and primary versus metastatic nature of the lesion. Metastatic brain lesions are more prevalent in adults than are primary brain tumors. In addition, paraneoplastic syndromes of non-brain tumors also cause psychiatric symptoms.

1. **Brain tumors,** such as **gliomas,** which account for 50–60% of primary brain tumors, **tend to produce diffuse symptoms** (e.g., cognitive decline), as they grow slowly and diffusely throughout the cortex. Multiple metastases or lymphoma can also present this non-focal pattern. **Meningiomas** (25% of primary brain tumors) grow extrinsically to the brain and **compress a limited area, causing progressive, more focal symptoms. Seizure is the third presentation of intracranial lesions,** which may be the result of abnormal excitation or interference of normal inhibitory mechanisms. Cortical invasion or compression, even from a relatively small meningioma, is more likely than sub-cortical tumors to cause seizures. Constitutional symptoms (fever, weight loss, fatigue) are more common with metastatic disease.

   Psychiatric symptoms occur in half of patients with brain tumors and, of those, over 80% have tumors in the frontal or limbic areas. Besides depression and personality changes, frontal tumors are associated with bowel and bladder incontinence. Temporal lobe tumors are especially likely to cause seizures, often with ictal or inter-ictal psychosis. Poor memory, or Korsakoff syndrome, aphasia, depression, and personality changes are also seen with temporal lobe tumors. Akinetic mutism, an alert but immobile state, occurs with upper brainstem tumors. Delirium is a sign of rapidly growing, large, or metastatic tumors.
2. **Paraneoplastic syndromes,** most common in small cell carcinoma of the lung, produce neuropsychiatric symptoms that may precede by many months the detection of the causative, non-CNS tumor. Tumors of the breast, stomach, uterus, kidney, testicle, thyroid, and colon may also cause paraneoplastic syndromes. These syndromes may arise from tumor production of hormones, with clinical manifestations of inappropriate

antidiuretic hormone secretion (SIADH), hypercortisolism, hypercalcemia, or hyperparathyroidism. Less well understood are the mechanisms responsible for encephalitic paraneoplastic syndromes, which involve non-reversible, often selective, inflammatory, and/or neurodegenerative destruction. **Paraneoplastic limbic encephalitis** has an insidious onset over weeks to months, with confusion and agitation. Depressed mood, anxiety, personality change, hallucinations, and catatonia are also reported, and may lead to psychiatric hospitalization. Initial memory loss progresses to dementia. Pathologically, there is neuronal loss in the medial temporal lobe and other limbic areas, along with meningeal and perivascular lymphocytic infiltration.

3. **Pancreatic cancer** is associated with a higher than expected incidence of depression, which may be its initial presentation.
4. **Colloid cysts,** non-malignant, space-occupying lesions of the third ventricle, exert pressure on diencephalic structures, and may increase intracranial pressure by ventricular obstruction. They have been associated with depression, mood lability, psychosis, personality change, and position-dependent, intermittent headache.

J. Degenerative disorders, especially of the basal ganglia, produce not only motor and sensory dysfunction, but also a spectrum of neuropsychiatric symptoms that include depression, psychosis, and dementia. In fact, the severity of the movement symptoms may vary with the level of emotional stress. This association between movement and emotion may be mediated by the largely limbic and cortical inputs to the basal ganglia and the shared neurotransmitter systems (dopamine, γ-aminobutyric acid [GABA], serotonin, norepinephrine).

1. **Parkinson's disease,** which affects 1% of the population over the age of 65 years, is known for its classical features of bradykinesia, rigidity, and tremor, and characteristic disturbances of gait and posture. The major degenerative loss is in the pars compacta of the substantia nigra, although other structures are also involved. Dopamine and to some extent norepinephrine and possibly other neurotransmitters are depleted, which may contribute to the depression experienced by over half of patients. Dementia is also more common in Parkinson's disease than in age-matched controls. Psychosis can develop, and is complicated by the dopaminergic and anticholinergic medications used to treat the disease.
2. **Huntington's chorea** is an autosomal dominant disorder of primarily striatal destruction and GABA depletion. Besides atrophy of the caudate and putamen, there is mild frontal and temporal wasting. Most common in the age range of 30–40 years, onset is extremely variable, and juvenile disease has a more rapidly progressive course (average duration of 8, as opposed to 15, years). The prevalence is 10 per 100,000 population. The classic choreiform movement disorder may present with, before, or after, prominent psychiatric symptoms. Early on, memory may be intact, but serious defects in attention, judgment, and executive function are evident. This may be followed by depression, apathy, social withdrawal, and a lack of attention to personal grooming. Irritability and impulsivity are common. The initial presentation may also mimic obsessive-compulsive disorder or schizophrenia. The depression is responsive to antidepressants and should be treated. The cognitive decline, like the movement disorder, is progressive, and leads to dementia.
3. **Wilson's disease** is an autosomal recessive defect in copper excretion that causes deposition of copper in the liver, brain, cornea, and kidney. This genetic deficiency of ceruloplasmin has a prevalence of 3.3 per 100,000 population. One person in 90 may be a heterozygous carrier. Symptoms are rare before age 6 years and commonly present in the teens. However, some patients remain asymptomatic well into adulthood. About half of patients present with liver manifestations: acute hepatitis, parenchymal liver disease, cirrhosis, or fulminant hepatitis. The vast majority of remaining patients present with neuropsychiatric symptoms, virtually always accompanied by gold or green-brown copper deposits around the cornea, the pathognomonic **Kayser-Fleischer rings.** Copper toxicity in the brain affects the lenticular nuclei and, to a lesser degree, the pons, medulla, thalamus, cerebellum, and cerebral cortex. Neurologic features include tremor, spasticity, rigidity, chorea, dysphagia, and dysarthria. Cognition is generally intact, although the dysarthria may be mistaken for mental retardation. About 10–25% of patients present with psychiatric symptoms, although those who present with neurologic findings also have psychiatric symptoms. Schizophreniform, bipolar, and more typical depressive symptoms may be seen, but bizarre, possibly frontal, behavior is more common. Psychiatric symptoms that respond incompletely to successful, excess copper removal require more specific treatment and psychopharmacotherapy.

K. Immune Diseases

1. **Acquired immunodeficiency syndrome** (AIDS) is caused by HIV infection, and is discussed earlier (see A.2) and elsewhere in this book.
2. **Systemic lupus erythematosus** (SLE) is an autoimmune, inflammatory disease of unknown etiology that affects women (9:1) more often than men, usually in the third to fifth decades. Tissue damage occurs in multiple systems, which gives the disorder an extremely variable presentation and course. Laboratory tests may be confirmatory, but are not totally specific

or reliable. When patients present with depression, sleep disturbance, mood lability, mild cognitive dysfunction, or psychosis, which up to one-half of patients do, the non-specific nature of their complaints may lead to the erroneous diagnosis of a primary mental disorder, such as major depression or somatization disorder. Correct diagnosis may lead to steroid therapy, which can worsen psychiatric symptoms.

L. **Trauma** to the head is extremely common in the United States, with roughly a million severe traumatic brain injuries each year. Young males are at highest risk. Motor vehicle accidents are responsible for about half of all closed head injuries, with falls, violence, and sports causing most of the rest.

1. **Penetrating head injury,** such as that received from a gunshot wound, is often dramatic; it tends to cause focal symptoms related to the size and location of directly involved brain tissue.
2. **Closed head injury** is far more common, and complicated, causing more diffuse symptoms and prolonged sequelae that do not correlate with the severity of the injury. The neurobehavioral dysfunction, including cognitive, somatic, and emotional symptoms, may clear in 3–6 months, or may persist for years after the injury. The mechanisms of injury in blunt trauma to the head may account for this variable course. Direct impact, acceleration/deceleration, and shearing forces, parenchymal stretching, and microscopic tears cause brain contusion and neuronal damage which may be followed by edema and bleeding. Limbic areas of the brain, the anterior temporal lobes and the inferior surface of the frontal lobes, are the major sites of damage. Cognitive slowing may occur with poor attention, increased distractibility, memory difficulties, perseveration, and poor planning. Personality changes, irritability, impulsivity, depression, anxiety, and mood lability are also common. Among the many somatic symptoms are headache, dizziness, fatigue, and sleep disturbance, which may be attributed to depression. Photophobia, noise sensitivity, tinnitus, and blurred vision also occur. Multiple head injuries, advanced age, and drug or alcohol use increase the risk of prolonged impairment. Patients with head injuries are often very sensitive to psychotropic medications, and may require "geriatric" doses.
3. **Post-concussive syndrome** (PCS) is the prolonged duration of cognitive, somatic, and emotional symptoms following "head trauma that caused significant cerebral concussion." DSM-IV has developed research criteria for PCS. A careful history for distant head trauma is necessary to recognize the syndrome.

IV. Evaluation of the Problem

Since mental disorder DTGMC should be part of the differential diagnosis for any psychiatric syndrome, the evaluation is the same as for any careful psychiatric evaluation. A high level of "medical suspicion" is required to gather the necessary information to make the diagnosis.

A. **History:** from records, the patient, other caregivers, and, when possible and appropriate (e.g., when the patient is a poor, or limited historian, or for medical or mental reasons), from family members or others close to the patient.

1. **Medical**
   a. A careful review of past and present illnesses, treatments, procedures, all medications, exposures, travel, head injury, seizure, habits (caffeine, tobacco), and recreational drug use.
   b. Correlation in time between medical events and psychiatric symptoms.
2. **Psychiatric:** close attention to the onset, course, treatment response, and past episodes, for typical and atypical features of primary mental disorders.
3. **Family:** the presence of similar symptoms, other psychiatric disorders, medical illnesses that "run" in the family; early or unexplained deaths.
4. **Social:** education, occupation, living situation, interpersonal relationships (fights, violence), recreational activities.

B. **Examination of the Patient**

1. **Laboratory examination** should be focused to support or rule out a suspected diagnosis.
2. **Imaging** should also be used to confirm a diagnosis, not to discover unsuspected pathology. Sudden onset, focal signs, rapid progression, infectious disease, or trauma are indications for appropriate brain imaging.
3. A **mental status examination** (MSE) is not specific for general medical conditions, but is comparable to the MSE in similar, primary mental disorders. Certain medical conditions, however, may present patterns of behavior or cognitive deficits that may be found on the MSE.
4. **Other tests** may be specific to a given medical condition (e.g., a sleep-deprived EEG in suspected complex partial seizures).

V. Treatment Considerations/ Strategies

A. **Some general medical conditions are chronic, stable, or unremitting,** and little can be done to change or treat them, or alter their course (e.g., previous stroke or toxic exposures, degenerative or demyelinating diseases). The mental disorder or **psychiatric symptoms should be treated** to the fullest extent possible, regardless of their medical etiology.

B. Whenever possible, **underlying medical conditions should be treated,** controlled, and/or stabilized. For example, infections should be treated with appropriate agents, metabolic perturbations should be normalized, and diabetic control and renal function should be optimized. **Some mental disorders will clear** when the underlying condition is treated, and thus long-term treatment of the mental disorder is unnecessary. Short-term comfort measures, however, may be necessary as the mental symptoms may lag behind the course of the medical condition. An example of this would be the judicious use of benzodiazepines in a patient being treated for hyperthyroidism.

C. **Often the medical condition and the psychiatric symptoms require ongoing treatment.** Maximal seizure control, for instance, may not be perfect, leaving the patient with inter-ictal symptoms, such as depression, that should also be treated. **The psychosocial stresses of chronic or acute medical conditions, as well as other primary mental or personality disorders, can exacerbate the psychiatric symptoms, interfere with treatment, and generally complicate the clinical picture.**

VI. Conclusions

Neuropsychiatric symptoms may precede, accompany, or follow the onset of a variety of general medical conditions. The psychiatrist must maintain a high level of suspicion, as well as a current knowledge of the broad categories and common features of these more prevalent conditions, to consider mental disorder due to a general medical condition in the differential diagnosis of every patient. Few, if any, general laboratory or imaging examinations are necessary, but the judicious use of specific examinations to support or confirm the suspected diagnosis is recommended. Although the underlying condition should be treated, when possible, psychiatric symptoms may also require specific treatment.

Suggested Readings

American Psychiatric Association. (1994). *Diagnostic and statistical manual of mental disorders* (4th ed.). Washington, DC: American Psychiatric Press.

Blumer, D., Wakhlu, S., Montouris, G., & Wyler, A.R. (2000). Treatment of interictal psychoses. *Journal of Clinical Psychiatry, 61,* 110–122.

Diaz-Olavarrieta, C., Cummings, J.L., Velazquez, J., & de la Cadena, C.G. (1999). Neuropsychiatric manifestations of multiple sclerosis. *Journal of Neuropsychiatry and Clinical Neuroscience, 11,* 51–57.

Geffken, G.R., Ward, H.E., Staab, J.P., et al. (1998). Psychiatric morbidity in endocrine disorders. *Psychiatry Clinics of North America, 21*(2), 473–489.

Hartman, D.E. (1998). Missed diagnoses and misdiagnoses of environmental toxicant exposure. *Psychiatry Clinics of North America, 21*(3), 659–670.

Hutto, B. (2001). Syphilis in clinical psychiatry: A review. *Psychosomatics, 42,* 453–460.

Lambert, M.V., Sierra, M., Phillips, M., & David, A.S. (2002). The spectrum of organic depersonalization: A review plus four new cases. *Journal of Neuropsychiatry and Clinical Neuroscience, 14,* 141–154.

Leroi, I., O'Hearn, E., Marsh, L., et al. (2002). Psychopathology on patients with degenerative cerebellar diseases: A comparison to Huntington's disease. *American Journal of Psychiatry, 159,* 1306–1314.

Racette, B.A., Hartlein, J.M., Hershey, T., et al. (2002). Clinical features and comorbidity of mood fluctuations in Parkinson's disease. *Journal of Neuropsychiatry and Clinical Neuroscience, 14,* 438–442.

Raymond, V., Gultekin, S.H., Rosenfeld, M.R., et al. (1999). A serologic marker of paraneoplastic limbic and brain-stem encephalitis in patients with testicular cancer. *New England Journal of Medicine, 340,* 1788–1795.

Skuster, D.Z., Digre, K.B., & Corbett, J.J. (1992). Neurologic conditions presenting as psychiatric disorders. *Psychiatry Clinics of North America, 15*(2), 311–333.

Tager, F.A., & Fallon, B.A. (2001). Psychiatric and cognitive features of Lyme disease. *Psychiatric Annals, 31,* 173–181.

Tucker, G.J. (1998). Seizure disorders presenting with psychiatric symptomatology. *Psychiatry Clinics of North America, 21*(3), 625–635.

Wilkie, F.L., Goodkin, K., van Zuilen, M.H., et al. (2000). Cognitive effects of HIV-1 infection. *CNS Spectrums, 5,* 33–51.

Wise M.G., & Rundell, J.R. (Eds.). (2002). *Textbook of consultation-liaison psychiatry: Psychiatry in the medically ill* (2nd ed.). Washington, DC: American Psychiatric Publishing.

Chapter 10

Alcoholism and Alcohol Abuse

JOHN A. RENNER

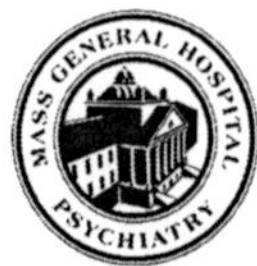

I. Introduction

A. Incidence

According to the National Co-morbidity Study (1990–1992), the lifetime prevalence for alcohol abuse is 6% in women and 12% in men; for alcohol dependence it is 8% for women and 20% for men. The 12-month prevalences for alcohol abuse (2% for women and 3% for men) and alcohol dependence (4% in women and 11% in men) are also high.

B. Alcohol abuse spans the continuum from brief episodes of excessive drinking to chronic patterns that produce significant problems, yet it never progresses to either psychological or physical dependence (Table 10-1).

C. Alcohol dependence (alcoholism) is defined as the excessive and recurrent use of alcohol despite medical, psychological, social, or economic problems (Table 10-1).

Table 10-1. DSM-IV Diagnostic Criteria

ALCOHOL ABUSE: One or more of the following present at any time during the same 12-month period.

1. Alcohol use results in failure to fulfill **major obligations.**
2. Recurrent use in **physically dangerous situations** (such as drunk driving).
3. Recurrent alcohol-related **legal problems.**
4. Continued use despite recurrent **social or interpersonal problems.**
5. Has never met criteria for Alcohol Dependence.

ALCOHOL DEPENDENCE: Three or more of the following present at any time during the same 12-month period.

1. **Tolerance.**
2. **Withdrawal.**
3. Use in **larger amounts,** or for **longer periods** than intended.
4. Unsuccessful **efforts to cut down** or control use.
5. A great deal of **time spent** obtaining alcohol, using or recovering from alcohol use.
6. **Important activities given up.**
7. **Continued use despite knowledge of problems.**

SOURCE: Adapted from DSM-IV Criteria for Substance Abuse and Substance Dependence, American Psychiatric Association, 1994.

D. Diagnostic criteria for alcohol dependence, as classified in DSM-IV, include tolerance and withdrawal symptoms. Although these signs of physical dependence are not required for the diagnosis, they are associated with more severe forms of the disorder. Specifiers can be added to the diagnostic criteria:

1. With physiological dependence: tolerance or withdrawal.
2. Without physiological dependence: no tolerance or withdrawal.
3. Early full remission: no criteria for dependence or abuse present for at least 1 month but less than 12 months of remission.
4. Early partial remission: one or more criteria for dependence or abuse present for at least 1 month but less than 12 months; full criteria not met.
5. Sustained full remission: no criteria for dependence or abuse present for 12 months or longer.
6. Sustained partial remission: one or more criteria for dependence or abuse present for 12 months or longer but full criteria not met.
7. In a controlled environment: no criteria for dependence or abuse present for at least the past month, but the individual is in an environment in which access to alcohol and controlled substances is restricted.

E. Co-morbid Conditions

1. **In 1994, the National Co-morbidity Survey (NCS) reported that the majority of patients in the United States with serious psychiatric disorders also abuse alcohol or other drugs.** Individuals in this group accounted for more than half of all lifetime psychiatric disorders in the United States; they usually had a history of three or more disorders, one of which was a substance abuse disorder.
   a. **The majority of individuals with an alcohol disorder have at least one other psychiatric disorder.**
   b. Co-morbid conditions (in rank order) associated with a substance abuse diagnosis are:
      i. Abuse of a second substance (most common)
      ii. Antisocial personality disorder
      iii. Phobias (and other anxiety disorders)
      iv. Major depressive disorder
      v. Dysthymic disorder (least common)
   c. Most lifetime co-occurring alcohol disorders begin at a later age than at least one other NCS/DSM-III-R disorder.
   d. Anxiety disorders and affective disorders co-occur more frequently with alcohol disorders in women.

e. Substance disorders, conduct disorder, and antisocial personality disorder co-occur more frequently with alcohol disorders in men.
f. 25–50% of suicides involve alcohol.

2. **Alcohol-related problems affect over 10% of drinkers and are the third leading cause of death in the United States. Alcoholism causes 80% of hepatic cirrhosis. Patients injured under the influence of alcohol fill 50% of trauma beds in the United States.**

II. Neurobiology of Alcohol

A. The positive reinforcement of alcohol appears to be mediated by:
1. Activation of γ-aminobutyric $acid_A$ receptors ($GABA_A$) which open chloride channels for a primary central nervous system (CNS) depressant effect.
2. Release of opioid peptides and dopamine.
3. Inhibition of glutamate NMDA (*N*-methyl-D-aspartate) receptors.
4. Interaction with serotonin systems.

B. Chronic alcohol use causes:
1. Upregulation of excitatory glutamate NMDA receptors
2. Downregulation of inhibitory neuronal GABA receptors
3. Increased central norepinephrine activity

C. The response to the termination of alcohol consumption involves CNS hyperactivity due to a lack of opposition to an alcohol-induced excitatory state.

III. Alcohol Metabolism

A. The primary metabolism of alcohol occurs through oxidation in the liver. Ethanol is metabolized via alcohol dehydrogenase to acetaldehyde, which is converted to acetate via aldehyde dehydrogenase; thereafter, carbon dioxide and water are produced.

B. Disulfiram (Antabuse) inhibits the action of aldehyde dehydrogenase and produces toxic blood levels of acetaldehyde.

C. A healthy liver oxidizes 0.75 ounces of 80-proof alcohol in 1 hour; in regular drinkers, the metabolic rate is even faster.

D. Elimination of alcohol: 90% is oxidized by the liver; 10% is excreted unchanged by the lungs and kidneys.

E. Asians have lower levels of both alcohol dehydrogenase and aldehyde dehydrogenase. Therefore, they metabolize alcohol more slowly and become intoxicated on lower amounts of alcohol than do Caucasians.

F. Blood alcohol concentration (BAC) helps determine alcohol intoxication (Table 10-2). (Note: A 160 pound man who drinks 5 ounces of whiskey in 1 hour develops a BAC of 0.10%.)

Table 10-2. Blood Alcohol Concentration and Associated Clinical Findings

BAC	*Clinical Findings*
0.05%	Exhilaration, loss of inhibitions
0.10%	Slurred speech, staggering gait
0.20%	Euphoria, marked motor impairment
0.30%	Confusion
0.40%	Stupor
0.50%	Coma
0.60%	Respiratory paralysis → death

A BAC over 150 mg% in an individual who does not appear very intoxicated, or over 300 mg% in any awake person, is evidence of physical addiction (tolerance) to alcohol.

G. The decreased gastric oxidation of alcohol by women causes a higher BAC in women than in men.

IV. Physiologic Effects of Alcohol

A. Cardiovascular Effects
1. Increased cardiac output (in alcoholics)
2. Elevated blood pressure
3. Increased heart rate and cardiac oxygen consumption (in non-alcoholics)
4. An increased risk of myocardial infarction

B. Increased incidence of cancer: esophageal, head, neck, liver, stomach, colon, and lung

C. Miscellaneous
1. Hypoglycemia occurs with acute intoxication.
2. Increased blood estradiol levels in women.
3. Dysregulation of triglycerides and lipoproteins.

V. Alcohol-Related Syndromes

A. Acute Alcoholic Hallucinosis (alcohol psychotic disorder, with hallucinations; 291.3) (see Table 10-3)
1. This condition occurs after cessation of drinking in an alcohol-dependent person (the onset of symptoms is during withdrawal).
2. It can also occur without a drop in BAC (with an onset during intoxication).
3. No delirium, tremor, or autonomic hyperactivity develops.
4. Hallucinations are usually auditory and paranoid.
   a. Symptoms can become chronic.
   b. Symptoms are not due to schizophrenia (it has a late onset, and no typical pre-morbid personality).

B. Alcohol Withdrawal Delirium/Delirium Tremens (DTs); 291.0 (see Table 10-3)

Table 10-3. Delirium Tremens vs. Acute Alcohol Hallucinosis

Condition	*Sensorium*	*Tremor*	*Hallucinations*	*Pupils*	*Vital signs*	*Onset*	*Duration*
Delirium tremens	Confused	Yes	Visual	Dilated, slow to react	↑	Gradual	3–10 days
Alcohol hallucinosis	Clear	Rare	Auditory	Normal	±	Rapid	5–30 days

1. **Minor (early) withdrawal symptoms include:**
   a. Onset 8–9 hours after the last drink
   b. Sweating, a flushed face, and insomnia
   c. Hallucinations in 25%
   d. Grand mal seizures (rum fits)
   e. Mild disorientation
2. **Major (late) withdrawal symptoms (DTs) include:**
   a. Onset 48–96 hours after the last drink
   b. Tremor and an increase in psychomotor activity
   c. Vivid hallucinations
   d. Seizures are absent
   e. Profound disorientation
   f. Increased autonomic activity and fever

C. Pathological Intoxication

Idiosyncratic alcohol intoxication is classified as alcohol use disorder not otherwise specified (291.9).

1. Intoxication develops after small amounts (4 ounces) of alcohol.
2. Automatic behaviors (usually combative or violent) are manifest.
3. Sleep or amnesia for the event often follows.

D. Alcohol Withdrawal Seizures

1. Involve generalized tonic-clonic seizures.
2. Occur within 24–48 hours after the last drink.
3. **Rarely involve more than one seizure, but a second seizure can occur within 3–6 hours of the first seizure.**
4. **Hypoglycemia, hyponatremia, and hypomagnesemia are often present in chronic alcoholics.**
5. **They are easily treated with benzodiazepines.**
6. Status epilepticus occurs in less than 3% of patients.

E. Fetal Alcohol Syndrome (FAS)

1. **Signs:**
   a. An affected infant may show signs of alcohol withdrawal.
   b. An early stage of liver disease may be evident.
   c. Mental retardation is common (44% had an IQ of 79 or below).
   d. A delayed weight and height curve may develop.
2. Congenital heart disease and other defects appear: wide-set eyes, short palpebral fissure, short and broad-bridged nose, hypoplastic philtrum, a thinned upper lip, and flattened midface.
3. **Incidence: six-fold increase between 1979 and 1993, to 6.7 per 10,000 births** (CDC, 1995).
   a. 17% are stillborn or die shortly after birth.
   b. 20% have birth defects (32% show full "fetal alcohol syndrome").
4. Maternal alcohol use while breastfeeding impairs a child's motor development, but not his/her mental development.
5. **Long-term effects of FAS:** Less than 6% able to function in school; most never hold a job. The average IQ in 61 subjects with FAS was 68 (Streissguth, 1991); 72% have major psychiatric disorders (Famy, 1998).

VI. Genetics and the Biologic Correlates of Alcoholism

The Virginia Twin Registry Study supports the findings of other current research that suggests that **genetic factors have a major influence on the development of both alcohol abuse and alcoholic dependence.** The specific biologic mechanisms affected by these genetic factors are less clearly understood. This large population-based twin study also demonstrated that environmental factors shared by family members had little influence on the development of alcoholism in males (Prescott and Kendler, 1999). The **social use of alcohol, however, is primarily influenced by environmental factors,** such as peer pressure, cultural attitudes, price, and availability.

A. Summary of Risk Data in the United States

Non-familial alcoholism accounts for 51% of all alcoholics; it is characterized by less severe alcoholism, later onset, better school and work histories, smaller families, higher socioeconomic status, and less psychopathologic or antisocial behavior (Frances, 1980).

1. **Any drinker** has a 5–10% risk of becoming an alcoholic.
2. If one parent is alcoholic, the risk doubles to 20%.
3. If both parents are alcoholic, the risk is between 20% and 50%.
4. The risk for fathers, sons, and brothers of alcoholics approaches 50%.
5. Risk for male and female twins is 28% for fraternal twins and 54% for identical twins.
6. If the father is severely alcoholic and criminal, the son's risk is 90%.

B. The Stockholm adoption study included 862 males and 913 females, adopted and raised by non-relatives; two types of alcoholism were identified (Cloninger et al., 1981).

1. **Type I or "milieu-limited" alcoholism**
   a. Affects both men and women.
   b. Reflects a congenital susceptibility (both parents can have mild, adult-onset alcohol abuse).
   c. Has a severity that is determined by post-natal stress.
   d. Estimates a risk in sons that is twice the normal incidence.
   e. Is associated with a risk in daughters with an alcoholic mother that is three times the normal incidence.
2. **Type II, or "male-limited" alcoholism**
   a. Is passed only from fathers to sons.
   b. Involves fathers who are both severely alcoholic and criminal.
   c. Sons of affected individuals have nine times the normal incidence.
   d. Has an early onset of alcohol abuse (before age 25 years).
   e. Post-natal environmental has no influence.
   f. Daughters of such fathers have no increased incidence.

Prospective personality "trait" studies (e.g., involving the Minnesota Multiphasic Personality Inventory [MMPI]) have failed to document a typical pre-alcoholic personality. However, certain constellations of personality traits, and biological findings, may be associated with specific alcoholic subtypes (Buydens-Branchey et al., 1989; Cloninger, 1987). Type II males are three times as likely to be depressed and four times as likely to have attempted suicide as type I males.

C. Brain Wave Studies

Event-related potential-evoked P300 brain waves studied in 6–13-year-old sons of alcoholic fathers showed a neurophysiological deficit, compared with controls, that was identical to that seen in chronic abstinent alcoholics (Begleiter et al., 1984).

D. Abnormal Response Patterns in Males at Risk for Alcoholism

1. An enhanced thyrotropin response was seen in sons of familial alcoholics. Daughters showed no abnormalities (Moss et al., 1986).
2. Schuckit (1994) demonstrated that a low level of response to alcohol at age 20 years predicts the likely development of alcoholism at age 30.

E. Neurobiologic Susceptibility to Alcoholism (Tarter et al., 1984, 1985)

1. **Temperamental deviations.** Biologic and psychologic characteristics associated with a vulnerability to alcoholism have been identified in pre-alcoholic males. They manifest cognitive and behavioral deficits and electrophysiologic abnormalities suggestive of dysfunction along the prefrontal-midbrain neuraxis.
2. **A pre-existing serotonin deficit has been identified in type II alcoholics** (Buydens-Branchey et al., 1989). Low serotonin metabolites in the cerebrospinal fluid (CSF) are associated with depression, impulsivity, and violence (Brown and Linnoila, 1990); early onset alcoholism (Linnoila and Virkhunen, 1992); and insomnia.
3. **A mutation on the D_2 dopamine receptor gene (D_2DR) associated with severe alcoholism, Tourette's syndrome, attention-deficit/hyperactivity disorder (ADHD), autism, and post-traumatic stress disorder (PTSD) has been investigated.** The mutant A-1 allele causes a reduced density of D_2 receptors. Although it does not cause alcoholism, it is a modifier gene that is associated with a more severe form of alcoholism (Blum, et al., 1990; Comings, et al., 1991; Noble, et al., 1991).

VII. Subtypes of Alcoholics

Research by Babor et al. (1992) using empirical clustering techniques has demonstrated two homogeneous subtypes among both male and female alcoholics. Both groups differ in the course of their illness and their response to treatment. These findings are consistent with the subtypes identified by Cloninger (1987).

A. Type A Alcoholics

1. **Later onset**
2. **Fewer childhood risk factors**
3. **Less severe dependence**
4. **Fewer alcohol-related problems**
5. **Less psychopathological dysfunction**

B. Type B Alcoholics

1. **Early onset of alcohol-related problems**
2. **Familial alcoholism**
3. **Childhood risk factors**
4. **Greater severity of dependence**
5. **Polydrug use**
6. **More chronic treatment history (despite younger age)**
7. **Greater psychopathological dysfunction**

VIII. Evaluation of the Patient

A. General Recommendations

Screening for alcohol-related problems should be routine for all mental health patients regardless of setting, and **is mandatory in patients examined for the Boards.** Individuals with alcohol problems are also at high risk for the abuse of other drugs; they should therefore be screened for the abuse of other legal and illegal substances.

B. Psychiatric and Social Problems Associated with Alcoholism

1. **Mental disorders commonly co-morbid with alcoholism** include other substance abuse, antisocial personality disorder, conduct disorder, mania, and schizophrenia.
2. **Mental disorders sometimes co-morbid with alcoholism** include major depressive disorder (especially in females), anxiety disorders, ADHD, and PTSD.
3. An erratic school or employment history.

4. Domestic violence.
5. Marital problems, especially multiple divorces.

C. Alcoholism Screening Instruments

In addition to questions regarding the quantity and frequency of drinking, several instruments are available for detecting less overt problems.

1. **The CAGE test has four simple questions** (Table 10-4) that can be easily inserted into the psychiatric interview. Two or more positive responses correlate with significant alcohol-related problems. This is a quick and reliable screening tool, even for those patients who try to hide their alcohol abuse; it is a more reliable indicator than elevated liver function tests.
2. **The Michigan Alcoholism Screening Test (MAST)** is a 25-question instrument (Table 10-5) that takes longer to administer, but is a more accurate screening tool than the CAGE, especially for women and the elderly.

D. Interviewing the Patient

Suspected substance abuse patients should be approached in a respectful and non-judgmental manner. A confrontational approach by the clinician does not facilitate the interview process, and has been shown to decrease the rate of successful referral to alcohol treatment. A moralistic approach is never helpful, and is also likely to alienate and to demoralize patients; it may also increase denial and diminish motivation for treatment.

E. Abnormal Blood Chemistries Commonly Seen in Alcoholics

No one test is considered diagnostic for alcohol dependence.

1. CDT (carbohydrate-deficient transferrin) is the most sensitive indicator of alcoholism.
2. GGTP (or GGT, γ-glutamyltranspeptidase): a blood level of > 30 units/L of this liver enzyme is induced with 4+ drinks per day for 2 weeks. It is the earliest indicator of an alcoholism relapse and will return to normal (< 30 units/L) if the patient stops drinking.
3. A MCV (mean corpuscular volume) > 95 μm^3 is found in males and > 100 in females in chronic alcoholism.
4. Liver function tests (LFTs): elevated aspartate transaminase (AST) (or serum glutamic-oxaloacetic transaminase [SGOT]), alanine aminotransferase (ALT) (or serum glutamic-pyruvic transaminase [SGPT]), and alkaline phosphatase.
5. cAMP (cyclic adenosine monophosphate) levels in white blood cells (WBC) of alcoholics are three times normal.

Table 10-4. The CAGE Questionnaire

"C"	Have you ever felt you should **C**ut down on your drinking?
"A"	Have people **A**nnoyed you by criticizing your drinking?
"G"	Have you ever felt bad or **G**uilty about your drinking?
"E"	Have you ever had a drink first thing in the morning to steady your nerves or to get rid of a hangover (**E**ye opener)?

SCORING: Item responses on the CAGE are scored 0 or 1, with a higher score indicative of alcohol problems. A score of 2 or more is considered clinically significant.

SOURCE: Published in the American Journal of Psychiatry, 1974, by the American Psychiatric Association.

IX. Differential Diagnosis

Many disorders may mimic alcoholism and complicate the diagnostic process.

A. Medical Problems

1. Mild alcohol intoxication is marked by disinhibition; more severe intoxication results in delirium, ataxia, or even coma. The clinician needs to rule out life-threatening conditions (e.g., head injuries) and other neurologic and metabolic problems (e.g., hypoglycemia).
2. Alcohol use disorders may mimic insomnia and can cause a variety of medical problems, including gastrointestinal bleeding, pancreatitis, cirrhosis, hepatitis, cardiomyopathy, labile hypertension, intracranial hemorrhage, sexual dysfunction, and peripheral neuropathy.

B. Psychiatric Problems

The presence of a non-alcohol-induced psychiatric disorder is suggested by psychiatric symptoms that precede alcohol use, are greater than what would be expected given the amount and duration of the drinking, and last longer than 4 weeks following detoxification. **Appropriate diagnostic assessment can not be accomplished while an individual is actively drinking.**

1. **Dysthymia and major depressive disorder,** with or without suicidality, can be difficult to distinguish from the depression induced by chronic alcohol consumption. **More than 60% of alcoholics are clinically depressed when admitted for detoxification, and many complain of dysthymia during the early months of sobriety.** Any alcoholic or intoxicated individual who expresses suicidal ideation should be considered a serious suicide risk, regardless of the presence or absence of major depressive disorder. In most cases, depressive symptoms should clear after 2 weeks of sobriety. If the patient remains depressed beyond 2 weeks, they should be assessed for a co-morbid depressive disorder.
2. **Anxiety** is a common symptom during alcohol withdrawal, but it usually clears within a few days. Some alcoholics also complain of generalized anxiety, and/or panic attacks lasting up to 12 months following detoxification. These symptoms are difficult to distinguish from a co-morbid anxiety disorder and require a

Table 10-5. Michigan Alcoholism Screening Test (MAST)

Clinical utility of instrument	To screen for alcoholism with a variety of populations
Research applicability	Useful in assessing extent of lifetime alcohol-related consequences
Copyright, cost, and source issues	No copyright Cost: $5 for copy, no fee for use Source: Melvin L. Selzer, M.D. 6967 Paseo Laredo La Jolla, CA 92037

Points		*YES*	*NO*
( )	0. Do you enjoy a drink now and then?	—	—
(2)	1. Do you feel you are a normal drinker? (By normal we mean you drink less than or as much as most other people.)[a]	—	—
(2)	2. Have you ever awakened the morning after some drinking the night before and found that you could not remember a part of the evening?	—	—
(1)	3. Does your wife, husband, a parent, or another near relative ever worry or complain about your drinking?	—	—
(2)	4. Can you stop drinking without a struggle after one or two drinks?[a]	—	—
(1)	5. Do you ever feel guilty about your drinking?	—	—
(2)	6. Do friends or relatives think you are a normal drinker?[a]	—	—
(2)	7. Are you able to stop drinking when you want to?[a]	—	—
(5)	8. Have you ever attended a meeting of Alcoholics Anonymous (AA)?	—	—
(1)	9. Have you gotten into physical fights when drinking?	—	—
(2)	10. Has your drinking ever created problems between you and your wife, husband, parent, or other relative?	—	—
(2)	11. Has your wife, husband (or other family members) ever gone to anyone for help about your drinking?	—	—
(2)	12. Have you ever lost friends because of your drinking?	—	—
(2)	13. Have you ever gotten into trouble at work or school because of drinking?	—	—
(2)	14. Have you ever lost a job because of drinking?	—	—
(2)	15. Have you ever neglected your obligations, your family, or your work for 2 or more days in a row because you were drinking?	—	—
(1)	16. Do you drink before noon fairly often?	—	—
(2)	17. Have you ever been told you have liver trouble? Cirrhosis?	—	—
(2)	18. After heavy drinking have you ever had delirium tremens (DTs) or severe shaking, or heard voices or seen things that really weren't there?[b]	—	—
(5)	19. Have you ever gone to anyone for help about your drinking?	—	—
(5)	20. Have you ever been in a hospital because of drinking?	—	—
(2)	21. Have you ever been a patient in a psychiatric hospital or on a psychiatric ward of a general hospital where drinking was part of the problem that resulted in hospitalization?	—	—
(2)	22. Have you ever been seen at a psychiatric or mental health clinic or gone to any doctor, social worker, or clergyperson for help with any emotional problem where drinking was part of the problem?	—	—

Table 10-5. (*Continued*)

Points		*YES*	*NO*
(2)	23. Have you ever been arrested for drunk driving, driving while intoxicated, or driving under the influence of alcoholic beverages?[c]	—	—
(2)	24. Have you ever been arrested, taken into custody, even for a few hours, because of other drunk behavior? (If YES, how many times? —)	—	—

[a]Alcoholic response is negative.
[b]5 points for each Delirium Tremens
[c]2 points for *each* arrest

SCORING SYSTEM: In general, five points or more would place the subject in an "alcoholic" category. Four points would be suggestive of alcoholism, and three points or less would indicate the subject was not alcoholic.

Programs using the above scoring system find it very sensitive at the five-point level, and it tends to find more people alcoholic than anticipated. However, it is a screening test and should be sensitive at its lower levels.

SOURCE: Selzer, M.L. (1971). The Michigan Alcoholism Screening Test: The quest for a new diagnostic instrument. *American Journal of Psychiatry, 127,* 1653–1658.

SUPPORTING REFERENCES:

Hedlund, J.L., & Vieweg, R.W. (1984). The Michigan Alcoholism Screening Test (MAST): A comprehensive review. *Journal of Operational Psychiatry, 15,* 55–64.

Skinner, H.A. (1979). A multivariate evaluation of the MAST. *Journal of Studies on Alcohol, 40,* 831–844.

Skinner, H.A., & Sheu, W.J. (1982). Reliability of alcohol use indices: The Lifetime Drinking History and the MAST. *Journal of Studies on Alcohol, 43,* 1157–1170.

Zung, B.J. (1980). Factor structure of the Michigan Alcoholism Screening Test in a psychiatric outpatient population. *Journal of Clinical Psychology, 36,* 1024–1030.

Zung, B.J., & Charalampous, K.D. (1975). Item analysis of the Michigan Alcoholism Screening Test. *Journal of Studies on Alcohol, 36,* 127–132.

comprehensive psychiatric evaluation after the patient has achieved sobriety.

3. **Schizophrenia** or other psychotic disorders may be confused with the hallucinations associated with delirium tremens or with alcohol hallucinosis.

X. Treatment Strategies

A. Overview

Effective treatment of drinking problems requires more than management of the medical aspects of detoxification. Psychiatrists must also understand:

1. The distinction between detoxification (the gradual elimination of alcohol from the body) and definitive treatment for alcohol dependence.
2. The stages of the recovery process and the way ambivalence impedes progress toward sobriety.
3. The types of psychiatric problems that complicate the management of these patients.

B. Chronic Disease Model

Although a brief office intervention may be sufficient for people with minor problems, long-term treatment is usually required for individuals who are alcohol dependent. Successful management of such patients can be a long-term process during which treatment interventions must be matched to the particular needs of each patient. Psychiatrists must understand the stages alcoholics usually pass through during the recovery process, the importance of using correct intervention skills, and the need to identify and treat co-morbid psychiatric conditions. The Project Match Study showed that "matching" patients to a specific type of alcoholism treatment did not improve outcome except in cases of psychiatric severity. Alcoholics Anonymous (AA), cognitive-behavioral therapy (CBT), and motivational enhancement are equally effective for other patients. The critical treatment question is, Which treatment for which patient at which time?

C. The Stages of Behavioral Change

The work of Prochaska, DiClemente, and Norcross has provided a paradigm for the process of behavioral change, including change in the addictive disorders. Individuals commonly move through a series of specific stages on the road from abusive drinking to stable sobriety. Successful treatment involves helping the alcoholic move from one stage to the next, through the use of those intervention techniques that are most effective for each stage. **Typically, patients cycle through this process several times before achieving stable sobriety.** This approach works best when the clinician recognizes the importance of a gradual stepwise progression through the stages of change, rather than demanding instant recovery (Table 10-6).

D. Motivational Interviewing Techniques

Based on the stages of change model, Miller and Rollnick have elaborated a counseling style designed to avoid patient resistance, to resolve ambivalence about drinking, and to induce change. The basic concepts of this approach are:

1. Therapist style is a powerful determinant of patient resistance and change.
2. **Confrontation of the problem is a goal, not an intervention style.**
3. Argumentation is a poor tool to induce change.
4. When resistance is evoked, patients tend not to change.
5. Motivation can be increased by specific treatment techniques.

Table 10-6. The Stages of Behavioral Change

1. **Precontemplation**	Drinker is unaware that alcohol use is a problem or has no interest in changing drinking pattern.
2. **Contemplation**	Drinker becomes aware of problems but is still drinking and is usually ambivalent about stopping.
3. **Preparation**	Previous pattern continues, but drinker now makes decision to change. May initiate small changes.
4. **Action**	Behavioral change begins; typically a trial and error process with several initial relapses.
5. **Maintenance**	New behavior pattern is consolidated; relapse prevention techniques help to maintain change.
6. **Relapse**	Efforts to change are abandoned; cycle may be repeated until permanent sobriety is established.

SOURCE: Adapted from Prochaska, DiClemente, and Norcross, 1992.

6. Motivation emerges from the interaction between patient and therapist.
7. Ambivalence is normal, not pathological.
8. **Helping patients resolve ambivalence is the key to change.**

This interviewing technique suggests the following approaches for use during each stage in the recovery process.

E. Moving Patients from Precontemplation to Contemplation

Many patients may be unaware that their drinking is problematic.

1. **Provide feedback** and explore the patient's perspective on alcohol and its effects, **but don't confront or argue.**
   a. Obtain a physical examination and laboratory data (e.g., LFTs, BAC, MCV).
   b. Administer an assessment instrument (CAGE or MAST).
   c. Review the quantity and frequency of a patient's drinking.
2. Summarize your findings and **connect drinking to identified problems.**
3. **Involve family** in this process whenever possible.
4. If the patient refuses to accept your conclusions, maintain medical follow-up, listen sympathetically to the patient's complaints, and encourage the patient to agree to an "evaluation" of his or her problems.
5. The goal is to help patients connect their problems to their drinking.

F. Moving Patients from Contemplation to Preparation

1. **Explore the patient's ambivalence about drinking;** start with the positives:
   a. Positive: "What do you like about your drinking?"
   b. Negative: "What problems does the drinking create?"
2. Help the patient internalize this conflict; don't become part of the conflict.
3. Help the patient discuss their anger, humiliation, guilt, and resentment.
4. **Search out their wish to control and/or stop their drinking.**
5. The goal is to help the patient resolve his or her ambivalence; do not recommend action until the patient has made the decision to stop.

G. Moving Patients from Preparation to Action

1. **Clarify the patient's goal:** to stop, to control drinking, or to explore problems?
2. Recommend treatment options if the patient wishes to stop drinking.
3. Recommend substance abuse counseling if the patient wishes to "control" use or remains highly ambivalent about his or her drinking.
4. Support the patient's self-efficacy: "You can do it!"
5. **The goal is to develop an action plan; let the patient choose from a menu of treatment options.**

H. Action: Active Quitting Begins

1. **Focus on directive behavior-based therapy** and other specific prescriptions for gaining and maintaining sobriety (e.g., go to AA, stop socializing with other drinkers, see a counselor).
2. Avoid passive, non-directive, forms of psychotherapy.
3. **Anticipate a trial and error process** to refine treatment needs.
4. Provide ongoing optimism and support.
5. **Work with self-help programs**
   a. **Alcoholics Anonymous (AA)** is the primary treatment resource for most alcoholics. It relies on group support to guide the alcoholic through a process of spiritual renewal and characterologic change. The emphasis on "one day at a time," reliance on one's "higher power," and spirituality are central to the AA philosophy.
   b. Psychiatrists rely on AA to complement other types of interventions. Its immediate accessibility, the connection to a strong social network of sober individuals, and the provision of free unlimited 24-hours-a-day support make it an invaluable resource.
   c. Schizoid individuals and persons with more severe psychopathology may be uncomfortable in any type of self-help group. Professionally run groups or individual counseling are the preferred options for such patients.
   d. Non-religious persons may find Rational Recovery or similar self-help programs an effective alternative to traditional AA.
   e. Psychiatrists may need to reassure patients that AA does not discourage psychotherapy or the use of appropriately

prescribed medication for the treatment of psychiatric conditions.

f. Successful referral to self-help programs requires familiarity with the resources available in the local community.

i. Try to match the program to the patient's age, race, social or professional status, and religious or sexual orientation, if the patient so desires.

ii. Insist that the patient initially attend four or five different groups, to "shop around."

iii. Most programs will provide a volunteer to escort a newcomer to his or her first meetings. This will greatly facilitate referral.

I. Maintenance

Relapse prevention is a specialized form of CBT developed by Marlatt to help maintain sobriety.

1. Alcoholics are taught to identify high-risk situations and predictors of relapse. Feelings, thoughts, and behaviors that trigger craving and relapse are explored, and the patient is taught to modify them.
2. Making the distinction between lapses (brief slips) and full relapses helps patients terminate drinking episodes promptly before they experience a complete loss of control. Redefining such events as opportunities for learning reduces guilt and demoralization and enhances the likelihood of successful outcome.
3. These techniques are most helpful after patients have achieved an initial period of sobriety.

XI. Medications in the Treatment of Alcoholism

In addition to the drugs used to treat alcohol withdrawal, medications are now available that significantly enhance the long-term management of alcoholism.

A. Detoxification

1. Benzodiazepines are the preferred medications for detoxification because of their excellent side-effect profile.

   a. **Long-acting benzodiazepines, such as chlordiazepoxide and diazepam,** are the standards for uncomplicated detoxification. When high enough initial doses (> 60 mg diazepam over 24–36 hours) are used, these drugs are self-tapering.

   b. **The short-acting benzodiazepine, lorazepam,** is recommended only for patients with significant liver disease, for those who are cognitively impaired, for patients over 65 years, and for any patient with unstable medical problems. This drug needs to be tapered over 4–8 days, but it is metabolized to the glucuronide form and is rapidly excreted by the kidney, giving the clinician more flexibility when managing unstable patients.

2. Symptom-triggered dosing based on withdrawal scales, such as the Clinical Institute Withdrawal Assessment (CIWA-Ar), works best, but requires frequent patient monitoring. This approach provides for adequate control of symptoms, avoids over-medication, and shortens the period of detoxification treatment.

B. Medications for Long-Term Treatment

1. **Naltrexone,** an opiate antagonist, has been found to reduce craving and relapse in alcoholics. Given in doses of 50 mg orally per day, it is well tolerated and seems to work best in motivated patients with a shorter history of alcoholism who describe intense craving. It is contraindicated for patients taking opiates or for those patients with acute hepatitis or liver failure. A positive response in terms of reduced craving and/or drinking is usually apparent within 7–10 days. If there is no response at 10 days, the medication should be discontinued.
2. **Disulfiram** inhibits the enzyme aldehyde dehydrogenase, leading to elevated levels of acetaldehyde. Doses of 250 mg orally per day can produce tachycardia, dyspnea, hypotension, facial flushing, nausea, and vomiting, if the patient drinks.

   a. In controlled trials disulfiram is no better than placebo in producing continuous abstinence, but it does reduce the number of days drinking and the severity of concurrent medical problems.

   b. Disulfiram works best in older, stable, motivated patients who are followed closely by their psychiatrist.

   c. Liver function tests (LFTs) need to be monitored periodically for signs of disulfiram-induced hepatitis.

   d. Disulfiram inhibits the metabolism of imipramine, desipramine, phenytoin, diazepam, and chlordiazepoxide. The doses of all of these medications need to be lowered when given in combination with disulfiram.

   e. Amitriptyline potentiates disulfiram. Lower doses may be used when prescribed with this antidepressant.

   f. Disulfiram also inhibits dopamine β-hydroxylase and may exacerbate psychosis in some schizophrenics. Reducing the daily dose to 125 mg and adding a high-potency dopamine-blocking agent, such as haloperidol, may resolve the problem.

3. **Serotonergic agents** have been shown to reduce craving and improve outcomes in specific alcoholic subtypes.

   a. **Ondansetron** (a selective 5-HT_3 antagonist) reduced alcohol consumption in early onset Type B alcoholics but not in Type A alcoholics (Johnson et al., 2000).

   b. **Sertraline** (a selective serotonin reuptake inhibitor) increased abstinence and reduced days drinking in Type A but not Type B Alcoholics (Pettinati et al., 2000). **Citalopram** had a similar effect, but only in male alcoholics (Naranjo et al., 2000). Fluoxetine did not improve drinking outcomes in either subtype (Kranzler et al., 1996)

C. Treating Associated Symptoms

Following detoxification, alcoholics may experience various distressing symptoms and may pressure the psychiatrist to provide medication for these complaints. After a careful evaluation to rule out co-morbid psychiatric disorders, patients should be reassured that these symptoms **are a normal part of early recovery** and will usually resolve with extended sobriety. Avoiding prescribed medications helps patients learn that they are moving beyond a dependency on exogenous chemicals.

1. **Anxiety.** Relaxation techniques and cognitive-behavioral interventions can be utilized. Avoid the prescription of benzodiazepines because of their abuse potential in this population.
2. **Depression.** The majority of alcoholics entering detoxification programs are clinically depressed. Following detoxification less than 3% of men and 12% of women meet DSM-IV criteria for a depressive disorder. These individuals should be considered for antidepressant therapy. Fluoxetine has been demonstrated to reduce both drinking and depression in severely depressed alcoholics. Paroxetine is well tolerated by this population, although efficacy data is less clear-cut. For individuals with less severe depressive symptoms, psychotherapy is often helpful in managing guilt and discouragement.
3. **Insomnia.** If appropriate sleep hygiene does not resolve the problem, use of the sedating antidepressant, trazodone (25–100 mg p.o. q.h.s.), may help. It has no significant abuse potential and is effective for long-term use. Sedative hypnotic drugs should be avoided because of their abuse potential.

XII. Managing Dual Diagnosis Patients

Psychiatric diagnoses made during periods of active drinking are highly unreliable. The patient should be observed following a minimum of 2 weeks of sobriety to confirm any diagnosis. Once it is clear that the symptoms are not secondary to the patient's alcoholism, any co-morbid psychiatric disorder must be treated. **Failure to adequately diagnose and treat co-morbid psychiatric disorders is the most common cause for the failure of alcoholism treatment.**

A. Anxiety Disorders

1. General considerations. If anxiety complaints are associated with alcohol craving or preoccupation, an initial response should be a 2-week trial of naltrexone. If there is no response, or if anxiety symptoms persist despite reduced craving, the patient should be evaluated for an independent anxiety disorder.
2. Specific treatment options for anxiety disorders comorbid with the substance use disorders are outlined in Table 10-7.
3. Use of benzodiazepines. Judicious use of the less abusable benzodiazepines, such as oxazepam or chlordiazepoxide, may be considered for patients with panic disorder or generalized anxiety disorder (GAD) who have failed to respond to the more conservative therapies recommended above. These patients should be monitored carefully for signs of abuse of these medications, and/or relapse to drinking.
   a. **Panic Disorder** may precede the development of alcoholism and usually becomes more severe following extended drinking. Behavioral psychotherapy and antidepressants, such as imipramine and paroxetine, have proved to be effective treatments.
   b. **Post-traumatic Stress Disorder (PTSD)** and co-morbid alcohol abuse are very difficult to treat. Such patients should be referred to specialized treatment programs. Improvement has been demonstrated in outpatient treatment utilizing the "seeking safety" cognitive-behavioral psychotherapy protocol (Najavits et al., 1998).

B. Major Depressive Disorder

Various tricyclic antidepressants (TCAs) and the selective serotonin reuptake inhibitors (SSRIs) have been used with some success in depressed alcoholics, though there are few adequately controlled clinical trials. Nefazodone appears to be effective in those alcoholics with a combination of anxiety and depressive symptoms, but it must be used with caution because of the risk of hepatotoxicity.

C. Bipolar Disorder

Mood-stabilizing drugs can have dramatic benefits in these cases. Adequate control of manic episodes often eliminates excessive drinking.

1. **Bipolar I:** lithium in the standard dose range is most effective.
2. **Bipolar II:** valproic acid may have some advantage in this group.

D. Schizophrenia

Intensive long-term substance abuse counseling must be provided in conjunction with comprehensive psychiatric management. Schizophrenic patients do poorly in most AA groups, and may be highly ambivalent about sobriety, since they often use alcohol to moderate psychotic symptoms or to reduce the side effects of their antipsychotic medications. There is evidence that clozapine and some other atypical antipsychotics may reduce alcohol craving and consumption.

E. Attention-Deficit/Hyperactivity Disorder (ADHD)

can be treated with methylphenidate 10–20 mg p.o. t.i.d., though these patients must be followed carefully for signs of stimulant abuse.

XIII. Criteria for Referral for Inpatient Detoxification

A. A history of failure in outpatient detoxification, or **multiple relapses.**

B. **Suicidal ideation or acute psychosis.**

C. A history of **delirium tremens.**

D. **Co-morbid medical problems** that require frequent daily monitoring during detoxification.

Table 10-7. Treatment of Specific Axis I Conditions in the Presence of an Alcohol-Related Disorder

Condition	*Primary Treatment*	*If No Response*
Panic Disorder	CBT + SSRI or nefazodone I	Alternative SSRI or venlafaxine
Social phobia		
1) Specific type	CBT + beta-blocker	
2) Generalized + depression	CBT + SSRI	
3) Generalized, no depression	SSRI or Nefazodone	
Post-traumatic Stress Disorder (PTSD)	Psychotherapy	Medications as needed
1) Plus depression	SSRI or Nefazodone	Alternative SSRI
2) With related psychosis	New generation antipsychotics	Alternative antipsychotic
3) With severe insomnia	Trazodone	Sedating TCA
Obsessive-Compulsive Disorder (OCD)	SSRI	Clomipramine, if no seizures or suicidal ideation
Generalized anxiety disorder (GAD)		
1) 90% are comorbid for panic disorder, PTSD, social phobia, or OCD	Treat any comorbid anxiety disorders, as above	
2) GAD + depression	SSRI or Nefazodone	
3) GAD, not depressed	CBT/relaxation therapy	Buspirone, up to 60 mg q.d.

XIV. Criteria for Referral for Specialized Long-Term Alcoholism Treatment

A. A history of **multiple treatment failures.**

B. **Serious co-morbid psychiatric conditions,** especially if they have failed to respond to initial efforts at psychiatric management.

C. Abuse of other drugs (**polysubstance abuse**).

D. **Living in very unstable environments,** e.g., the homeless.

Suggested Readings

American Psychiatric Association. (1994). *Diagnostic and statistical manual of mental disorders* (4th ed.). Washington, DC: American Psychiatric Press.

Babor, T.F., Hofmann, M., DelBoca, F.K., et al. (1992). Types of alcoholics, I. Evidence for an empirically derived typology based on indicators of vulnerability and severity. *Archives of General Psychiatry, 49*(8), 599–608.

Begleiter, H., Porjesz, B., Bihari B., et al. (1984). Event-related brain potentials in boys at risk for alcoholism. *Science, 255,* 1493–1496.

Bein, T.H., Miller, W.R., & Tonigan, J.S. (1993). Brief intervention for alcohol problems: A review. *Addiction, 88,* 315–335.

Blum, K., Noble, E.P., Sheridan, P.J., et al. (1990). Allelic association of human dopamine D_2 receptor gene in alcoholism. *Journal of the American Medical Association, 263,* 2055–2060.

Brown, G.L., & Linnoila M.I. (1990). CSF serotonin metabolite (5-HIAA) studies in depression, impulsivity, and violence. *Journal of Clinical Psychology, 51*(4, suppl), 31–41.

Buydens-Branchey, L., Branchy, M., Noumair, D., & Lieber, C. (1989). Age of alcoholism onset, I & II. *Archives of General Psychiatry, 46,* 225–236.

Center for Disease Control and Prevention, reported in *The Boston Globe*. (1995, April 7). More babies are found to suffer fetal alcohol syndrome.

Ciraulo, D.A., & Renner, J.A. (1991). Alcoholism. In D.A. Ciraulo & R.I. Shader (Eds.), *Clinical manual of chemical dependence.* Washington, DC: American Psychiatric Press.

Cloninger, C.R. (1987). Neurogenic adaptive mechanisms in alcoholism. *Science, 236,* 410–416.

Cloninger, C.R., Bohman, M., & Sigvardsson, S. (1981). Inheritance of alcohol abuse: Cross-fostering analysis of adopted men. *Archives of General Psychiatry, 38,* 861–868.

Comings, D.E., Comings, B.G., Muhleman, D., et al. (1991). The dopamine D_2 receptor locus as a modifying gene in neuropsychiatric disorders. *Journal of the American Medical Association, 266,* 1793–1800.

Famy, C., Streissguth, A.P., & Unis, A.S. (1998). Mental illness in adults with fetal alcohol syndrome or fetal alcohol effects. *American Journal of Psychiatry, 155,* 552–554.

Frances, R.J., Timm, S., & Bucky, S. (1980). Studies of familial and non-familial alcoholism. *Archives of General Psychiatry, 37,* 564–566.

Friedman, L., Fleming, N.F., Roberts, D.H., & Hyman, S.E. (Eds.). (1996). *Source book of substance abuse and addiction.* Baltimore, MD: Williams and Wilkins.

Johnson, B.A., Roache, J.D., Javors, M.A., et al. (2000). Ondansetron for reduction of drinking among biologically predisposed alcoholic patients: A randomized controlled trial. *Journal of the American Medical Association, 284*(8), 963–971.

Kessler, R.C., Crum, R.M., Warner, L.A., et al. (1997). Lifetime co-occurrence of DSM-III-R alcohol abuse and dependence with other psychiatric disorders in the National Comorbidity Survey. *Archives of General Psychiatry, 54,* 313–321.

Kessler, R.C., McGonagle, K.A., Zhao, S., et al. (1994). Lifetime and 12-month prevalence of DSM-III-R psychiatric disorders in the United States. *Archives of General Psychiatry, 51,* 8–19.

Koob, G.F., & Roberts, A.J. (1999). Brain reward circuits in alcoholism. *CNS Spectrums, 4,* 23–33.

Kranzler, H.R., Burleson, J.A., Brown, J., & Babor, T.F. (1996). Fluoxetine treatment seems to reduce the beneficial effects of cognitive-behavioral therapy in type B alcoholics. *Alcohol Clinical Experimental Research, 20*(9), 1534–1541.

Linnoila, M.I., & Virkhunen, M. (1992). Aggression, suicidality, and serotonin. *Journal of Clinical Psychology, 53,* 46–51.

Mayfield, D., McLeod, G., & Hall, P. (1974). The CAGE questionnaire: Validation of a new alcoholism instrument. *American Journal of Psychiatry, 131,* 1121–1123.

Miller, W.R., & Rollnick, S. (2002). *Motivational interviewing: Preparing people for change* (2nd ed.). New York: Guilford Press.

Moss, H.B., Guthrie, S., & Linnoila, M. (1986). Enhanced thyrotropin releasing hormone in boys at risk for development of alcoholism: Preliminary findings. *Archives of General Psychiatry, 43,* 1137–1142.

Najavits, L.M., Weiss, R.D., Shaw, S.R., & Muenz, L.R. (1998). "Seeking safety": Outcome of a new cognitive-behavioral psychotherapy for women with posttraumatic stress disorder and substance dependence. *Journal of Trauma Stress, 11*(3), 437–456.

Naranjo, C.A., Knoke, D.M., & Bremner, R.E. (2000). Variations in response to citalopram in men and women with alcohol dependence. *Journal of Psychiatry and Neuroscience, 25*(3), 269–275.

Noble, E.P., Blum, K., Ritchie, T., et al. (1991). Allelic association of the D_2 dopamine receptor gene with receptor-binding characteristics in alcoholism. *Archives of General Psychiatry, 48,* 648–654.

O'Malley, S.S., Jaffe, A.J., Chang, G., et al. (1992). Naltrexone and coping skills therapy for alcohol dependence. A controlled study. *Archives of General Psychiatry, 49,* 881–887.

Osser, D.N., Renner, J.A., & Bayog, R. (1999). Algorithms for the pharmacotherapy of anxiety disorders in patients with chemical abuse and dependence. *Psychiatric Annals, 29,* 285–301.

Pettinati, H.M., Volpicelli, J.R., Kranzler, H.R., et al. (2000). Sertraline treatment for alcohol dependence: interactive effects of medication and alcoholic subtype. *Alcohol Clinical Experimental Research, 24*(7), 1041–1049.

Prescott, C.A., & Kendler, K.S. (1999). Genetic and environmental contributions to alcohol abuse and dependence in a population-based sample of male twins. *American Journal of Psychiatry, 156,* 34–40.

Prochaska, J., DiClemente, C., & Norcross, J. (1992). In search of how people change. Applications to addictive behaviors. *American Psychology, 47,* 1102–1114.

Rollnick, N., Heather, N., & Bell, A. (1992). Negotiating behavior change in medical settings: the development of brief motivational interviewing. *Journal of Mental Health, 1,* 25.

Saitz, R., Mayo-Smith, M.F., Roberts, M.S., et al. (1994). Individualized treatment for alcohol withdrawal. *Journal of the American Medical Association, 272,* 519–523.

Sandberg, G.G., & Marlatt, G.A. (1991). Relapse prevention. In D.A. Ciraulo & R.I. Shader (Eds.), *Clinical manual of chemical dependence.* Washington DC: American Psychiatric Press.

Schuckit, M.A. (1994). Low level of response to alcohol as a predictor of future alcoholism. *American Journal of Psychiatry, 151,* 184–189.

Selzer, M.L. (1971). The Michigan Alcoholism Screening Test: The quest for a new diagnostic instrument. *American Journal of Psychiatry, 127,* 1653–1655.

Streissguth, A.P., Aase, J.M., Clarren, S.K., et al. (1991). Fetal alcohol syndrome in adolescents and adults. *Journal of the American Medical Association, 265,* 1961–1967.

Sullivan, J.T., Syhora, K., Schneiderman, J., et al. (1989). Assessment of alcohol withdrawal: The revised Clinical Institute Withdrawal Assessment for Alcohol Scale (CIWA-Ar). *British Journal of Addiction, 84,* 1353–1357.

Swift, R.M. (1999). Drug therapy for alcohol dependence. *New England Journal of Medicine, 340,* 1482–1490.

Tarter, R.E., Hegedus, A.M., Goldstein, G., et al. (1984). Adolescent sons of alcoholics: Neuropsychological personality characteristics. *Alcohol Clinical Experimental Research, 8,* 216–222.

Tarter, R.E., Alterman, A.I., & Edwards, K.L. (1985). Vulnerability to alcoholism in men: A behavioral-genetic perspective. *Journal of Studies on Alcohol, 46,* 329–356.

Chapter 11

Substance-Related Disorders: Cocaine and Narcotics

JOHN MATTHEWS AND ANNE E. MOYLAN

I. Cocaine-Related Disorders

A. **Cocaine abuse involves a pattern of use that is less intense and less frequent than cocaine dependence.** The use is maladaptive, leads to impairment, and is manifest by at least one of the following domains within a 12-month period:

1. A failure to meet obligations at home, work, or school.
2. Use of cocaine in situations that are considered physically hazardous.
3. The development of cocaine-related legal problems.
4. Continued use of cocaine despite social and interpersonal problems caused or worsened by cocaine use.

B. **Cocaine dependence involves a maladaptive pattern of use that leads to impairment and distress in at least three of the following areas within a 12-month period:**

1. The development of tolerance, defined by either a need for **a significant increase in the amount of cocaine to achieve the desired effect or a significant decrease in the effect of the usual cocaine dose.**
2. The **development of cocaine withdrawal symptoms** (see below) or the need to ingest cocaine to relieve or to prevent withdrawal symptoms.
3. The **use of cocaine in larger amounts** and for longer periods than was intended.
4. The **inability to cut down** or to control the use of cocaine.
5. An excessive amount of time spent obtaining cocaine and recovering from the effects of cocaine.
6. Stopping or reducing social, occupational, or recreational activities to maintain cocaine use.
7. **Ongoing use of cocaine despite persistent or recurrent physical or psychological problems** that are caused or exacerbated by its use. Dependence may be episodic or continuous.

It is important to note that a diagnosis of substance dependence does not necessarily require the development of tolerance to the substance or withdrawal symptoms.

C. **Cocaine intoxication involves clinically significant maladaptive behavioral or psychological changes** (e.g., euphoria, interpersonal sensitivity, anxiety, tension, anger, stereotypic behaviors, poor judgment, impaired social and occupational functioning, and hypervigilance) **that develop during or shortly after cocaine use. Two or more of the following symptoms develop during or immediately after the use of cocaine:**

1. Tachycardia or bradycardia
2. Pupillary dilation
3. Elevated or lowered blood pressure
4. Diaphoresis or chills
5. Nausea or vomiting
6. Weight loss
7. Agitation or psychomotor retardation
8. Muscle weakness
9. Chest pain
10. Arrhythmias
11. Respiratory depression
12. Confusion
13. Seizures
14. Dyskinesias
15. Dystonia
16. Coma

D. **Cocaine withdrawal involves dysphoric mood and two of the following physiological symptoms that develop within hours to several days following the cessation of, or a decrease in, cocaine use:**

1. Fatigue
2. Vivid and unpleasant dreams
3. Insomnia or hypersomnia
4. Increased appetite
5. Agitation or psychomotor retardation

E. **Other cocaine-induced disorders include:**

1. Cocaine intoxication delirium
2. Cocaine-induced psychotic disorder, with delusions
3. Cocaine-induced psychotic disorder, with hallucinations
4. Cocaine-induced mood disorder
5. Cocaine-induced anxiety disorder
6. Cocaine-induced sexual dysfunction
7. Cocaine-induced sleep disorder
8. Cocaine-related disorder not otherwise specified

II. Pharmacology of Cocaine

A. **Cocaine preparations include coca leaves, cocaine hydrochloride, coca paste, free base, and crack** (Gold, 1997).

1. **Coca leaves.** This form of cocaine is ingested orally and is the least potent of all of the preparations; its purity is 0.5–1.0%. The average acute dose is 20–50 mg, the onset of action is 5–10 minutes, and the duration of the high is 60–90 minutes. It is used primarily by natives of Central and South America.

2. **Cocaine hydrochloride (oral).** This form of cocaine is a powder; its purity ranges between 20% and 80%, and the bioavailability is 20–80%. The average acute dose is 100–200 mg, the onset of action is 10–20 minutes, and the duration of the high is about 45–90 minutes.
3. **Cocaine hydrochloride (intranasal).** The purity of this form is 20–80%, and the bioavailability is about 20–30%. The average acute dose is 30 mg per line, the onset of action is 2–3 minutes, and the duration of the high is about 30–45 minutes.
4. **Cocaine hydrochloride (intravenous).** Cocaine hydrochloride powder is dissolved in water to produce an intravenous form. This is a particularly potent form since it has a bioavailability of 100%. The average acute dose is 25–50 mg, the onset of action is 30–45 seconds, and the duration of the high is 10–20 minutes. It is on occasion combined with heroin, forming a mixture known as a "speedball."
5. **Cocaine alkaloid (free base).** Cocaine is separated from its hydrochloride base by heating it with ether, ammonia, or some other solvent. This is a procedure with risk since the solvent can ignite. The purity is 90–100%. The average acute dose is 250–1,000 mg, the onset of action is 10 seconds, and the duration of the high is 5–10 minutes.
6. **Cocaine alkaloid (crack).** Crack, a cocaine alkaloid, is extracted from cocaine hydrochloride by mixing it with sodium bicarbonate. The purity is 50–95%. The average acute dose is 250–1,000 mg, the onset of action is 10 seconds, and the duration of the high is 5–10 minutes.

B. Metabolism

Cocaine is **metabolized to benzoylecgonine,** which can be detected in the urine for up to 36 hours.

C. Impact on Neurotransmitters

1. **Cocaine blocks the uptake of dopamine (DA), serotonin (5-HT), and norepinephrine (NE)** from each of their neuron terminals by binding to the presynaptic transporter complexes. The reinforcing properties of cocaine are believed to be mediated by enhancing neurotransmission through the mesolimbic dopamine pathway (dopamine cells in the ventral tegmental area in the brainstem project to the nucleus accumbens). The nucleus accumbens and DA serve as the final common pathway for the rewarding experiences of most recreational drugs of abuse.
2. In animal studies, using microdialysis techniques to measure released DA concentrations in the nucleus accumbens, researchers found a dose-dependent relationship between self-administration of cocaine and DA concentrations.
3. In human studies using positron emission tomography (PET), researchers demonstrated cocaine binding to high-affinity receptor sites on DA transporters *in vivo.*

D. Physical and Psychological Effects of Cocaine

1. **The acute physical and psychological effects of cocaine include:**
   a. Vasoconstriction
   b. An increased heart rate
   c. An increased blood pressure
   d. Euphoria; increased energy
   e. A heightened alertness and sensory awareness (confirmed by desynchronization of brain waves on EEG recordings)
   f. Increased anxiety
   g. An increased risk of panic attacks (in predisposed individuals)
   h. An increased self-confidence
   i. A decreased appetite
   j. An increased sexual excitement and spontaneous ejaculation
   k. An increased **risk for psychosis** (including paranoid delusions).

   An individual's response to cocaine may be trait-dependent. Individuals who have a low level of arousal may have a positive experience from cocaine use, whereas individuals who have a high level of arousal may have a negative experience.
2. As a result of chronic use of cocaine, many individuals develop symptoms of depression, irritability, agitation, a lack of motivation, insomnia, panic attacks, hypervigilance, paranoia, and hallucinations. The long-term effects of cocaine may result from neurotransmitter depletion.

E. Co-morbid Substance Use

Sedating substances, such as alcohol, are frequently used to combat the stimulating effects of cocaine and to prolong the euphoria it produces. Alcohol combines with cocaine to produce cocaethylene which has similar neurochemical, pharmacological, and behavioral properties to cocaine. However, many believe that cocaethylene may have more cardiac toxicity.

III. Epidemiology of Cocaine-Related Disorders

A. Historical Trends

1. In the 1970s, cocaine was considered by professionals to be a safe and non-addictive drug. Reasons why cocaine use has declined include:
   a. Education about the detrimental effects of cocaine.
   b. Promotion of better health.
   c. The need to be competitive in today's society; much of the decline in use has been among the middle and upper classes.
2. **A community survey from 1991 demonstrated that 12% of the population had used cocaine at least once during their lifetime,** that 3% had used cocaine within the past year, and that less than 1% had used cocaine within the past month. It is not known how many of those individuals would have met criteria for a substance use disorder.

3. Data from the National Institute of Drug Abuse (1997) demonstrated that **55% of drug-abusing patients, mostly in outpatient treatment programs** (methadone, short-term inpatient, residential, and outpatient), are **dependent on cocaine.**

B. Social Impact

Cocaine use continues to be a serious problem among the disadvantaged, who have easy access to the drug and little hope of becoming a productive part of society. Crack has become very affordable; vials cost as little as $10. Cocaine use is more prevalent among African-Americans and is associated with violence and the transmission of acquired immunodeficiency syndrome (AIDS).

IV. Course of Cocaine-Related Disorders

A. Episodic use generally occurs during weekends or on one or two occasions during the week. Binges are a type of episodic use when large amounts of cocaine are consumed within a few hours or a few days. Binges end when cocaine supplies are depleted.

B. Daily use of cocaine generally progresses from small amounts to large amounts due to the development of tolerance to the euphoric effects of cocaine.

C. Progressive Use

The form and route of administration of cocaine also determine the course and progression of use. Intranasal use tends to show a more gradual progression from use to abuse or dependence over months to years, whereas IV use and smoking tend to show a rapid progression to eventual dependence over weeks to months.

V. Co-morbid Psychiatric and Cocaine-Related Disorders

A. Prevalence

1. **The rate for any psychiatric disorder (excluding other substance abuse) in cocaine abusers seeking treatment is 50%; the lifetime prevalence is 80%.** Among cocaine abusers the rate for a lifetime diagnosis of major depressive disorder is 50%, for dysthymic disorder it is 25–50%, and for bipolar spectrum disorders it is 25%.

B. Self-Medication

Many cocaine-dependent patients with co-morbid psychiatric disorders use cocaine as self-medication for their psychiatric symptoms:

1. Depressed patients use to elevate their mood.
2. Bipolar patients use to sustain their highs.
3. Patients with attention deficit disorder use to help their distractibility and their mood.
4. Patients with schizophrenia use to help relieve their negative symptoms.
5. Patients with borderline personality disorder use to help their mood.
6. Patients with antisocial personality disorder use to enhance stimulation and excitement.
7. Patients with narcissistic personality disorder use to further increase feelings of grandiosity.

C. Use of Other Substances

Other substances of abuse, such as alcohol, marijuana, benzodiazepines, and opiates, are associated with cocaine abuse and dependence. Alcohol, marijuana, and benzodiazepines are often used to treat the unpleasant stimulating effects of cocaine, whereas opiates are used to enhance the euphoric effect of cocaine.

D. Co-morbid Psychiatric Conditions

Patients with anxiety disorders, especially panic disorder, tend to avoid the use of cocaine since it heightens anxiety and may trigger panic attacks. Panic attacks often continue after stopping the drug in vulnerable individuals.

E. Differential Diagnosis

It can be difficult to distinguish cocaine-induced psychiatric disorders from primary psychiatric disorders. **Cocaine-induced psychiatric symptoms include depression, panic attacks, anxiety, psychosis, antisocial behaviors, and aggressive behaviors.** In contrast to primary psychiatric disorders, symptoms induced by cocaine resolve within a few hours to a few days.

VI. Medical Complications Associated with Cocaine Use

A. Cardiovascular

Cocaine causes adrenergic stimulation, which may result in **elevation of blood pressure, tachycardia, and arrhythmias. It may also cause vasospasm in coronary arteries.** Adrenergic stimulation, which increases oxygen demand of the heart, in combination with coronary artery vasospasm, may result in myocardial infarction.

B. Central Nervous System

Cocaine causes vasospasm in cerebral vasculature that results in cerebral vascular accidents. Single-photon emission computed tomography (SPECT) has demonstrated significant hypoperfusion in frontal and temporal-parietal areas among chronic users of cocaine. These findings correlate with cognitive impairment (e.g., diminished concentration, attention, and memory as measured by neuropsychological testing). Cocaine can also induce seizures, after either single or repeated use, by a phenomenon called "kindling."

C. Respiratory System

Cocaine-induced respiratory symptoms include **hemoptysis, fever, and productive cough, as well as chest pain due to the build-up of carbon monoxide.** Respiratory disorders secondary to cocaine include asthma, pneumonia, pneumothorax, pneumomediastinum, pneumopericardium, pulmonary edema, and sudden death from cocaine-induced respiratory depression. "Crack lung" is a recently identified condition that is manifest by fever, shortness of breath, chest pain, and pneumonia.

D. Other Systems

Chronic intranasal use of cocaine may cause **nasal septum necrosis** due to its vasoconstricting effects. Cocaine binges may result in **dehydration, malnutrition, and weight loss. IV cocaine use may lead to vasculitis, endocarditis, granulomas, hepatitis B and C infection, human immunodeficiency virus (HIV) infection, pulmonary emboli, and septicemia due to contaminants in the injection solution.**

E. Use in Pregnancy

Cocaine use **increases the risk of fetal hypoxia and placental abruption** due to its vasoconstrictive properties. Cocaine readily crosses the placenta and can have toxic effects on the fetus. Echocardiograms reveal left ventricular hypertrophy in the fetus. Cocaine can cause fetal growth retardation, reduced head circumference, decreased birth weight, congenital anomalies, malformations of the urogenital system, central nervous system (CNS) irritability ("jittery baby"), attentional problems, cerebral vascular accidents, and death. Cerebral vasoconstriction and hypoxia may interfere with brain development. Cocaine is found in breast milk up to 60 hours after use. Symptoms observed in babies who ingest cocaine from breast milk include rapid heart rate, increased blood pressure, apnea, diaphoresis, and mydriasis.

VII. Treatment of Cocaine Use

A. Treatment Settings

The goal is to use the least restrictive environment so that family, social, and occupational responsibilities are minimally disrupted. Most studies demonstrate that patients can be effectively treated in an outpatient setting. However, patients with complicated psychosocial, psychiatric, or medical problems may require a more structured environment. Criteria for inpatient treatment according to Washton (1990) and others include:

1. Lack of motivation to participate in an intensive outpatient program
2. Significant psychological, cognitive, or neurological deficits
3. Serious co-morbid psychiatric or medical problems
4. Several failed attempts at outpatient and partial hospital treatments
5. Lack of a support network
6. Use of highly addictive crack, freebase, or IV cocaine
7. Significant dependence on alcohol and/or other substances of abuse
8. The risk for aggressive behaviors towards self, others, or property

B. Intoxication

There is no specific antidote for cocaine intoxication. Treatment remains generally supportive. Benzodiazepines treat aggressive or agitated behavior in the acute setting. However, clinicians must recognize that many cocaine-users have personal or family histories of abusing other substances, and benzodiazepine use may convey an addictive liability for them. Patients with paranoia should not be treated initially with antipsychotic medications because of the risk of inducing a seizure. Their psychosis generally resolves within a few hours to 5 days. If the psychosis continues, the diagnosis should be reconsidered and antipsychotic medication started. Although cocaine increases the risk for seizures, prophylactic use of anticonvulsants has not been shown to be beneficial.

C. Withdrawal

There is no specific treatment for the typical withdrawal symptoms from cocaine dependence (see above for typical symptoms of withdrawal). Withdrawal from cocaine does not pose a medical threat. The symptoms begin within a few hours of discontinuing cocaine use and may persist for several days. Dopamine agonists, bromocriptine and amantadine, were initially used to treat cocaine withdrawal symptoms and cravings, but recent studies have failed to support their use.

D. Relapse Prevention

Cognitive-behavioral therapy (CBT) helps patients identify the internal (emotions) and external (situations) cues that activate addictive beliefs ("The only way I can have fun is to get high") which trigger cravings and urges to use. Once cravings and urges are activated, permissive beliefs ("I can stop after one smoke") and rationalizations to use are realized; permissive beliefs lead to strategies ("I'll drive to Bill's to buy crack") to use. The therapist helps the patient challenge the validity of his or her addictive and permissive beliefs. CBT relapse prevention strategies are particularly effective over a 12-week period with more severe cocaine abusers. Outcome studies at 6–12 months also demonstrate that cognitive-behavioral relapse prevention is significantly more effective than routine clinical management. **A behavioral approach using contingent vouchers has been particularly effective in keeping patients in treatment and maintaining abstinence.** In this approach, patients earn vouchers to purchase predetermined items (e.g., books or social events with their family) provided that they maintain "clean" urines.

In addition, results from a recent pilot study support the efficacy of group therapy to treat substance use disorders. In particular, for those with mood disorders, groups which integrate the treatment of substance use disorders and mood disorders proved the most helpful.

E. Self-Help Groups

Cocaine Anonymous (CA) is a 12-step program modeled after Alcoholics Anonymous. A recent study of day hospital cocaine-abusing patients showed that greater participation in self-help groups at three months post-treatment predicted less cocaine use at six months post-treatment.

F. Pharmacological Treatments

Pharmacological treatment is not indicated for cocaine dependence. Studies of pharmacological treatments that could reduce the subjective effects of cocaine and reduce symptoms of cocaine abstinence have been mixed and inconclusive. Multiple methodological problems (including differences in patient populations, absence of controls, differences in psychosocial interventions, differences in route of cocaine administration, and inconsistent outcome measures) have plagued clinical studies. Dopamine agonists (e.g., amantadine and bromocriptine) and tricyclic antidepressants (e.g., desipramine) initially showed promise in treating cocaine dependence, but more recent studies have failed to confirm earlier findings. In contrast, recent studies which examined the relationship between mood disorders and substance use disorders demonstrated that pharmacological treatment of the co-morbid mood disorder facilitated the treatment and control of the substance use disorder.

VIII. DSM-IV Opioid-Related Disorders

A. Opioid Abuse

A maladaptive pattern of opioid use leading to clinically significant impairment or distress, as manifested by one or more of the following, occurring within a 12-month period:

1. Recurrent opioid use resulting in a failure to fulfill major role obligations at work, school, or home.
2. Recurrent opioid use in situations in which it is physically hazardous.
3. Recurrent opioid-related legal problems.
4. Continued opioid use despite having persistent or recurrent social or interpersonal problems caused or exacerbated by the effects of the opioid.

B. Opioid Dependence

A maladaptive pattern of opioid use, leading to clinically significant impairment or distress, as manifested by three or more of the following, occurring at any time in the same 12-month period:

1. Tolerance, as defined by either of the following:
   a. A need for markedly increased amounts of an opioid to achieve intoxication or the desired effect.
   b. Markedly diminished effect with continued use of the same amount of the opioid.
2. Withdrawal, as manifested by either of the following:
   a. The characteristic withdrawal syndrome of opioids.
   b. The same or a closely related opioid is taken to relieve or avoid withdrawal symptoms.
3. The opioid is often taken in larger amounts or over a longer period than was intended.
4. There is a persistent desire or unsuccessful efforts to cut down or control opioid use.
5. A great deal of time is spent in activities necessary to obtain, use, or recover from the effects of the opioid.
6. Important social, occupational, or recreational activities are given up or reduced because of substance use.
7. The opioid use is continued despite knowledge of having a persistent or recurrent physical or psychological problem that is likely to have been caused or exacerbated by the opioid.

C. Opioid Intoxication

Clinically significant maladaptive behavioral or psychological changes (e.g., initial euphoria followed by apathy, dysphoria, psychomotor agitation or retardation, impaired judgment, or impaired social or occupational functioning) **that develop during, or shortly after, opioid use.** Physiological changes include pupillary constriction (or pupillary dilation with severe overdose) and one or more of the following signs developing in the context of opioid use:

1. Drowsiness or coma
2. Slurred speech
3. Impairment in attention or memory

D. Opioid Withdrawal

The development of at least three or more of the following symptoms with either reduction or cessation of opioid use or administration of an opioid antagonist may produce:

1. Dysphoric mood
2. Nausea or vomiting
3. Muscle aches
4. Lacrimation or rhinorrhea
5. Pupillary dilation
6. Piloerection or sweating
7. Diarrhea
8. Yawning
9. Fever
10. Insomnia

E. Other Opioid-Induced Disorders

According to DSM-IV, the following disorders are diagnosed instead of opioid intoxication or opioid withdrawal only when the symptoms are in excess of those usually associated with the opioid intoxication or withdrawal syndrome and when the symptoms are sufficiently severe to warrant independent clinical attention:

1. Opioid intoxication delirium
2. Opioid-induced psychotic disorder
3. Opioid-induced mood disorder
4. Opioid-induced sexual dysfunction
5. Opioid-induced sleep disorder

IX. Opiate Pharmacology

A. Opiates bind to three types of receptors in the brain, which are referred to as mu, delta, and kappa. Mu and delta receptors, when activated, influence mood, reinforcement, analgesia, respiration, blood pressure, gastrointestinal function, and endocrine functions. Kappa receptors, when

activated, **produce dysphoria and analgesia.** Receptor subtypes (mu 1, mu 2, kappa 1, and kappa 2) have been identified, but specifics as to what functions they mediate are yet to be determined.

B. Opiate drugs are categorized as to how they are able to bind and activate receptor types:

1. **Agonists readily bind to and activate receptors.**
2. **Antagonists readily bind to but do not activate receptors.**
3. **Partial agonists bind to receptors but only activate them to a limited extent; they may also block receptors from occupation by other agonists or antagonists.**

Morphine, methadone, fentanyl, and sufentanil are primarily mu receptor agonists, buprenorphine and pentazocine are partial agonists, and naloxone and naltrexone are pure antagonists. Opiate receptors are located throughout the CNS, parts of the autonomic nervous system, and the gastrointestinal system. The receptors most commonly targeted by prescribed medications are located in the CNS and gastrointestinal system. When CNS receptors are activated, individuals experience tranquillity, reduced apprehension, analgesia, cough suppression, respiratory depression, pupillary constriction, and changes in temperature. When gastrointestinal receptors are activated, individuals experience nausea, constipation, and vomiting.

C. The positive reinforcing effect of opiates is mediated through the ventral tegmental area (VTA) dopamine projections to the nucleus accumbens, and through direct effects of mu and delta agonists on neurons in the nucleus accumbens. Mu and delta agonists inhibit γ-aminobutyric acid_A ($GABA_A$) interneurons that normally tonically inhibit VTA dopamine cells. The net effect of mu and delta agonists is to increase VTA dopamine cells firing rates, resulting in an increased release of dopamine in the nucleus accumbens. Stimulants, such as cocaine and amphetamine, also increase dopamine release via different receptors. Stimulants combined with opiates significantly increase their euphoric effect without increasing their side effects. As mentioned earlier, the combination of opiates and cocaine given together intravenously is called a "speedball."

D. Urine Testing

Heroin is measured as morphine in urine. Most short-acting opioids are detected in the urine 12–36 hours after administration. Routine urine screens do not detect meperidine, fentanyl, and oxycodone. Poppy seeds contain small amounts of morphine and codeine, which can result in false positive urine tests for opioid abuse.

X. Epidemiology of Opiate Abuse

A. A United States **community survey** from 1991 **demonstrated that 6% of the population had used analgesics for non-medical reasons,** 2.5% used them within the past year, and 0.7% used them within the past month. Most opioid-dependent individuals are not receiving treatment.

B. Heroin abuse and dependence occur three times more frequently in males than in females. The non-medical use of opioids (excluding heroin) occurs at almost twice the rate in Caucasians than in African-Americans. Some studies suggest that heroin abuse is more frequent among minority groups; however, these data are based on surveys of public treatment facilities, which may exclude a significant number of white middle-class heroin addicts.

XI. Course of Opiate Abuse

A. Studies examining patterns of use in adolescents and young adults have discovered a progression of drug use beginning with cigarettes, alcohol, marijuana, and eventually opioids. **The onset of opioid abuse in general is in the teens and early twenties. Once opioid dependence develops, the course is generally longstanding for many years with frequent lapses and relapses.** Even after long periods of incarceration, relapse rates are high. According to some experts, the average duration of active opioid addiction is 9 years.

B. The death rate among opioid addicts is 20 times that in the general population, and the increased rate is due to overdose, infection, AIDS, suicide, homicide, and trauma.

XII. Etiological Factors Associated with Opiate Use

A. Not everyone who experiments with opioid use develops abuse or dependence. According to the National Co-morbidity Survey (1994), **7.5% of individuals who used opioids for non-medical purposes and 23% of individuals who used heroin eventually developed opioid dependence.** There are genetic, biological, and psychosocial factors that contribute to opioid dependence.

B. Genetic and Biological Factors

1. Animal studies demonstrate that various strains of rodents exhibit differences with regard to their ability to learn opioid self-administration behavior.
2. Family members of opiate addicts exhibit higher rates of addictive disorders and psychiatric disorders.
3. **Studies of twins have shown that monozygotic twins are more likely than dizygotic twins to be concordant for opioid dependence.**
4. Environmental stress can sensitize animals to self-administer opioids. Corticotropin-releasing factor (CRF), a peptide important in the brain's response to environmental stress, can stimulate opioid-seeking behavior in opioid-dependent animals, whereas CRF antagonists

can reduce stress-related opiate self-administration. There is evidence that corticosteroids can sensitize animals to self-administer opioids and that they also increase the sensitivity of the VTA dopamine neurons to excitatory input. In addition, addicts physically dependent on heroin have high serum levels of glucocorticoids during withdrawal, and there are increases in adrenocorticotropic hormone (ACTH) prior to the onset of withdrawal symptoms. This increase of hypothalamic-pituitary-adrenal axis (HPA axis) activity is thought by some researchers to trigger cravings to use opioids in opioid-dependent individuals via the VTA. Environmental stressors may influence drug-seeking behavior through increases in corticosteroids and through increases in VTA activity through excitatory input from prefrontal cortical areas.

C. Psychosocial Factors

1. **The self-medication hypothesis proposed by Khantzian argues that there is a strong relationship between type of dysphoric state and drug preference.** Khantzian emphasizes the "anti-rage" properties of opiates.
2. In adolescents, risk factors for the development of opioid dependence include marijuana abuse, symptoms of depression, lack of a close relationship with parents, and leaving school. In general, other risk factors include availability of opioids, alienation from social institutions, social deviancy, and impulsivity.
3. Opiate addicts tend to score low on sensation-seeking, and they tend to avoid excessive internal and external stimulation.

XIII. Co-morbid Psychiatric and Opiate Use Disorders

A. **Studies show that 80–90% of opiate-addicted individuals carry a lifetime diagnosis of a psychiatric disorder.** Major depressive disorder (25% current and 50% lifetime) and antisocial personality disorder (25–40%) are the two most common co-morbid psychiatric disorders in opioid-dependent individuals. There is also an increased risk of posttraumatic stress disorder (PTSD). Children and adolescents with conduct disorder are at greater risk of developing substance abuse problems, especially opiate dependence. Psychiatric treatment of Axis I disorders improves outcome. Those addicts who seek treatment have more depression and anxiety, lower levels of social functioning, and more drug-related legal problems than untreated opioid addicts. Biopsychosocial complications of opioid abuse appear to encourage addicts to seek treatment earlier.

B. **It can be difficult to distinguish the difference between a primary mood disorder from an opioid-induced mood disorder.** Chronic use of opioids may cause symptoms consistent with the diagnosis of major depressive disorder. Depression in opiate addicts could also be related to complications of psychosocial stressors from chronic opioid use.

C. **The diagnosis of antisocial personality disorder is questionable in the context of an addiction** unless antisocial behaviors predate the onset of the addiction; addictive disorders tend to promote antisocial behaviors.

D. **Alcohol, benzodiazepines, and cocaine are the most common co-morbid substances used by opioid addicts.**

XIV. Medical Complications of Opiate Use

A. Intravenous (IV) Opioid Use

1. **Complications from contamination.** The most common injectable opioids are heroin, dihydromorphine (Dilaudid), and meperidine (Demerol). Heroin is sold on the streets in "bags," and there is a wide variability of purity and potency. Contamination, both chemical and microbial, of the injectable opiate contributes to multiple medical complications. **Chemical contaminants include talc, starch, and quinine (used as adulterants), and cotton (used as a filter); the primary microbial contaminants include *Staphylococcus aureus*, β-hemolytic streptococci, and anaerobes. Some of the most common medical complications include:**
   a. Cellulitis
   b. Skin abscesses
   c. Endocarditis
   d. Septic arthritis
   e. Hepatitis A, B, C, and D infection
   f. Osteomyelitis
   g. Nephropathy
   h. Rhabdomyolysis
   i. Pulmonary emboli, pulmonary hypertension
   j. Pneumonia
   k. Meningitis
   l. Brain abscess
   m. Tuberculosis
   n. HIV infection
2. **Liver disease.** Studies using serological testing show that **two-thirds of IV drugs users have been exposed to hepatitis B and C.**
3. **Pulmonary disease. Talc and cotton can cause granulomatous pulmonary reactions.** Heroin is known to cause pulmonary edema, but the mechanism is unclear. The common causes of pneumonia include *Haemophilus influenzae* and *Streptococcus pneumoniae.* Tuberculosis (TB) has been on the increase in IV drug users over the past few years; thus, TB must be considered in the presence of pulmonary infiltrates.

One study showed that, in one population of IV drug users, one-fourth had latent TB. The antitussive property of opioids contributes to respiratory infection and pneumonia.

4. **Cardiac disease. Endocarditis occurs in 0.2% of addicts in a 12-month period.** Contaminated needles and opiates cause endothelial damage on heart valves followed by platelet fibrin deposition and bacterial infection. *Staphylococcus aureus* is the most common infectious agent followed by *Streptococcus.* Right-sided endocarditis may result in pulmonary emboli, which are generally not fatal, whereas left-sided endocarditis may result in systemic emboli, which are often fatal.
5. **Renal disease. Intravenous heroin use can lead to focal or diffuse glomerulosclerosis, which may progress to nephrotic syndrome and end-stage renal failure.** Hematuria and proteinuria are found on urinalysis. Frequently occurring skin abscesses and ulcerations may result in renal amyloidosis.
6. **HIV infection. Two-thirds of IV drug users in the Northeastern United States, according to one study, are HIV-positive.** 25% of individuals with AIDS use IV drugs. Infants born HIV-positive may have clinical features similar to those associated with fetal alcohol syndrome.
7. **Complications with pregnancy in the setting of opiate use. Results from several studies indicate that roughly 80% of infants born to mothers addicted to opioids experience opioid withdrawal.** The fetus is exposed to multiple episodes of going in and out of withdrawal as the mother continues to use short-acting opiates, and each episode of withdrawal places the fetus at risk of being aborted. It is now common practice to place pregnant opioid-dependent women on methadone maintenance. The dose of methadone needs to be high enough to block cravings and further opioid use and low enough to decrease withdrawal symptoms in the infant at the time of delivery. In general, the goal is to achieve methadone doses of 20 mg/day or less. Pregnant women already stable on methadone, at doses above 20 mg/day, should be tapered slowly at a rate of 1–2 mg per week to prevent miscarriage. The safest time for tapering methadone is during weeks 14–32 of the pregnancy. The most common withdrawal symptoms in neonates include hyperactivity, hyperactive reflexes, increased muscle tone, diaphoresis, a high-pitched cry, yawning, insomnia, decreased eating, tremor, and mottling of the skin. A few neonates will experience more severe withdrawal symptoms, including seizures, vomiting, diarrhea, and fever. In general, the mild withdrawal symptoms do not require treatment, but, for severe withdrawal, paregoric (for mu opioid withdrawal) and phenobarbital (for hyperactivity and seizures) are the most frequently used pharmacological treatments. The onset of withdrawal symptoms occurs as early as 12–24 hours after birth, depending on the half-life of the opioid used. However, since the neonate does not have the enzymes to metabolize and excrete opioids, the presence of withdrawal symptoms may be delayed and last many weeks. About 7% of neonatal deaths and 4% of stillbirths are accounted for by opiate exposure and withdrawal.

XV. Treatment of Opiate Use

A. Intoxication

Acute intoxication does not generally require any treatment. With ingestion of large amounts of opioids resulting in respiratory depression and coma, treatment in a hospital setting is required. Life supports, including a ventilator, are essential. **The respiratory depression can be reversed by use of IV naloxone (0.4 mg);** if there is no response within 2 minutes, naloxone 0.8 mg (IV) can be repeated twice more, 5 minutes apart. Signs of a response to naloxone include increased respirations, increased blood pressure, and reversal of constricted pupils. Depending on the half-life of the opiate used, naloxone may need to be repeatedly dosed until the effects of the opiate abate. For short-acting opioids like heroin, the crisis resolves in about 4 hours; however, for long-acting opioids, such as methadone or LAAM (L-α-acetylmethadol), hospitalization may be required up to 48 hours.

B. Detoxification

There are four commonly used strategies and two experimental strategies for opioid detoxification: **methadone substitution, clonidine, clonidine-naltrexone ultra-rapid detoxification, buprenorphine, lofexidine (experimental), and ultra-rapid opioid detoxification under anesthesia/sedation (experimental).**

1. **Methadone substitution.** Methadone has a long half-life, which provides for a smoother withdrawal from opioids. In general, some clinicians believe that it should only be used for detoxification from more addictive substances, such as heroin, morphine, meperidine, or hydromorphone. For less addictive opioids, such as codeine, oxycodone, propoxyphene, or pentazocine, simply tapering the dose or using clonidine is the best strategy. The starting dose of methadone can vary between 20 and 40 mg/day. Doses of methadone above 40 mg/day in a patient who is not opioid-dependent can be lethal. It may take a few days to determine the stabilizing dose of methadone (based on signs and symptoms of withdrawal) before starting the taper. For inpatients, the stabilizing dose may be decreased at a rate of 5–10% per day; however, for outpatients, the dose should be tapered at a rate of 10% per week until a dose of 20 mg/day is reached and then at a rate of

3% per week for the remainder of the detoxification. Outpatients are more likely to relapse during the detoxification due to the availability of opioids; thus, it is important to provide a more comfortable taper. Patients tend to tolerate the taper to 20 mg/day, but below 20 mg/day they express more sensitivity to withdrawal symptoms and significant fears of being off opioids. For the long-acting opioids (methadone and LAAM) that have been used for long periods of time in a methadone program, a gradual detoxification over a period up to 180 days (in a licensed facility) has been shown to put the patient at less risk for relapse.

2. **Clonidine. Clonidine is an alpha-2-adrenergic agonist which reduces symptoms of opioid withdrawal by inhibiting noradrenergic hyperactivity in the locus coeruleus.** Clonidine suppresses many symptoms of withdrawal, including rapid heart rate, increased blood pressure, sweating, nausea, vomiting, diarrhea, and cramps. Clonidine has no effect on craving, muscle aches, or insomnia, thus adjunctive medications need to be added, such as non-steroidal anti-inflammatory drugs for muscle aches and possibly benzodiazepines for symptomatic relief. The most common side effects of clonidine are sedation and hypotension. For short-acting opioids (Kleber, 1999), the starting dose is 0.1–0.3 mg every 4–6 hours up to a maximum of 1.0 mg the first day. During days 2–4, clonidine doses are increased based on the need to control withdrawal symptoms, up to a maximum daily dose of 1.3 mg. Beginning day 5, the dose of clonidine is reduced by 0.2 mg/day. For long-acting opioids (methadone, at a dose of 20–40 mg/day) (Kleber, 1999), the starting dose is 0.1 mg t.i.d. on day 1. On days 2–4 the dose of clonidine is increased to a maximum of 0.4 mg t.i.d. This dose is maintained until day 11 at which time the dose of clonidine is reduced by 0.2 mg/day, but not to exceed 0.4 mg/day. During detoxification with clonidine, blood pressure and pulse should be checked before each dose. The dose should be held and the daily dose reduced if the blood pressure is below 90/60 mmHg.
3. **Clonidine patch. The clonidine patch is a transdermal delivery system designed to provide a constant daily dose of clonidine over a 7-day period,** which provides for a smoother withdrawal from opioids. It is available in three strengths that are equivalent to oral clonidine: 0.1 mg, 0.2 mg, and 0.3 mg. For the first 2 days of detoxification, oral clonidine has to be given because it takes 48 hours for the transdermal clonidine to reach steady state. On day 1, oral clonidine 0.2 mg t.i.d. or q.i.d. is given along with transdermal clonidine. The strength of the patch dose depends on weight: 0.2 mg if one weighs 100 pounds; 0.4 mg if one weighs 100–200 pounds; or 0.6 mg if one's weight is greater than 200 pounds. On day 2, the oral dose is reduced by half and it is discontinued on day 3. The clonidine patch or patches are removed after 7 days and replaced with half the original dose for an additional 7 days if withdrawal symptoms continue. In general, detoxification is complete in 7 days for short-acting opioids and about 10 days for long-acting opioids. The patch or patches are removed if the systolic blood pressure drops below 80 mmHg or the diastolic drops below 50 mmHg.
4. **Clonidine-naltrexone. The addition of naltrexone to clonidine can significantly shorten the time to complete detoxification.** Naltrexone accelerates the withdrawal process and clonidine reduces withdrawal symptoms. Completion rates range between 55% and 95%. During the first day, outpatients need to be monitored for 8 hours because of the risk for serious withdrawal due to the naltrexone and the need to monitor blood pressure while taking clonidine. According to a protocol by O'Connor et al. (1995) and Vining et al. (1988), on day 1, the patient is premedicated with clonidine 0.2–0.4 mg and oxazepam 30–60 mg. Two hours later naltrexone, 12.5 mg, is given orally and clonidine 0.1–0.2 mg every 4–6 hours (up to 1.2 mg), and oxazepam 30–60 mg is given every 4–6 hours for the remainder of the day. On day 2, naltrexone 25 mg orally is given 1 hour after the first doses of clonidine (0.1–0.2 mg) and oxazepam (30–60 mg). Clonidine 0.1–0.2 mg every 4–6 hours (up to 1.2 mg) and oxazepam 30–60 mg every 4–6 hours are continued throughout day 2. On day 3, the only change is an increase in naltrexone to 50 mg. After day 3, clonidine and oxazepam are continued for an additional 2–3 days. Medications to treat muscle cramps (non-steroidal anti-inflammatory drugs) and nausea (prochlorperazine or ondansetron) may also be required. An inpatient protocol using even higher doses of naltrexone can decrease the time to complete detoxification to within 2–3 days.
5. **Lofexidine. Lofexidine is an alpha-2-agonist currently used in England for opioid detoxification.** Its advantages over clonidine include reduced risks for sedation and hypotension. The National Institute on Drug Abuse (NIDA) is now studying lofexidine for possible FDA approval.
6. **Buprenorphine. Buprenorphine is a partial mu agonist analgesic that is very effective for detoxification from opiates.** The only form available to clinicians is parenteral; however, a sublingual form combined with naloxone is being developed. When given intramuscularly, the pharmacological effect has its onset within 15 minutes and lasts about 6 hours. With IV use, the onset of action is earlier. The equivalent parenteral dose of buprenorphine compared with 10 mg of morphine is 0.3 mg. Buprenorphine is very safe when taken in overdose due to the "ceiling effect"

of being a partial mu agonist; it exhibits very little respiratory depression. There are three strategies used for opioid detoxification with buprenorphine: abrupt discontinuation, gradual taper, and discontinuation with precipitation of withdrawal with naltrexone. The first step in all three methods is to stabilize patients on buprenorphine for at least 3 days. Studies now available demonstrate that, with abrupt discontinuation, withdrawal symptoms are minimal and abrupt discontinuation has higher success rates than gradual withdrawal.

7. **Ultra-rapid opioid detoxification under anesthesia.** The procedure involves the induction of anesthesia with propofol, tracheal intubation, and the precipitation of withdrawal with either an IV preparation of naloxone or naltrexone via intragastric tube. Patients are under anesthesia up to 8 hours, and they are discharged within 24–48 hours. Antiemetics, antidiarrheal medications, clonidine, and benzodiazepines are used to treat breakthrough withdrawal symptoms. Deaths have been reported within 24 hours of this procedure. There are no controlled or outcome studies to validate its use.

C. Pharmacological Treatments

1. **Methadone maintenance. Only a licensed facility can dispense methadone maintenance for the treatment of opioid dependence.** The criteria for initiating treatment include: a minimum of a 1-year history of physiological dependence on opioids (episodic or continuous); current signs and symptoms of withdrawal; needle tracks; and positive urines. For previously treated patients, reinstatement into a methadone maintenance program may occur within 2 years of discontinuation of methadone without the presence of current physical dependence and with documentation from a physician that relapse to opioid dependence is imminent. Individuals who are released from a penal institution and who met the criteria for methadone maintenance prior to incarceration may be admitted to a methadone program without the presence of physical dependence. Women who are pregnant are eligible for methadone maintenance if they are physically dependent on opioids or if they were dependent on opioids in the past and are now at imminent risk of relapse. Patients under the age of 18 years must have failed at least two opioid detoxifications in the past and have the consent of a parent, legal guardian, or an adult designated by state authority to enter a methadone maintenance program. Patient characteristics that predict a successful outcome in a methadone program include a brief history of drug abuse, age greater than 25 years, psychological stability, good social supports, good work history, minimal legal problems, and a low severity of opioid abuse.

   Methadone has a half-life of 24–36 hours; thus, it can be given orally once daily. The combination of its slow onset of subjective effects and its long half-life results in fewer euphoric peaks and distressing withdrawal symptoms that tend to reinforce opioid use. Methadone is well tolerated, and its main side effects include sedation, constipation, excessive sweating, ankle edema, decreased libido, and mild euphoria. The starting dose of methadone is determined by the intensity of the withdrawal signs and symptoms. For mild withdrawal, the initial dose is about 10 mg/day, whereas for severe withdrawal the initial dose is 20–40 mg/day. The patient should be monitored for 2 hours after the first dose to determine the effectiveness of the starting dose in reversing withdrawal signs and symptoms. The maintenance dose is determined by the reduction or elimination of opioid abuse as determined by negative urine screens, the lack of reinforcing properties (such as euphoria), and minimal side effects. Although there is a broad range of effective maintenance doses (10–100 mg/day), recent studies have shown that doses averaging 70–80 mg/day are needed to block opioid cravings and drug use. Methadone blood levels are helpful, and the goal is to achieve trough blood levels of 150–600 ng/mL. The maximum allowable dose according to federal regulations is 120 mg/day. About one-third of methadone maintenance patients do well, and about one-third show no benefit. With doses of methadone greater than 60 mg/day, retention rates in methadone programs reach 60% at 6 months and achieve up to a 90% reduction in opioid abuse. Unfortunately, the treatment only reaches 20–25% of opioid addicts. The benefits from methadone maintenance include decreases in opioid use, criminal behavior, unemployment, and risk for contracting AIDS.

2. **L-α-Acetylmethadol (LAAM). LAAM is a long-acting congener of methadone that has been approved for the use of opioid substitution in methadone programs.** LAAM has the same eligibility criteria as methadone but it is unavailable for pregnant females and individuals under 18 years of age. Its safety in pregnant women has not been determined. Women who are on LAAM must get monthly pregnancy tests.

   LAAM has two active metabolites, nor-LAAM and dinor-LAAM, both of which are mu agonists. These two metabolites account for LAAM's slow onset of action, its long half-life of 72–96 hours, and its long time to steady state, up to 20 days (time to steady state for methadone is 5–8 days). Because of its long half-life, LAAM is given three times per week: Monday, Wednesday, and Friday. The dose on Friday is 20–40% greater than on the other two days to adequately cover the potential for withdrawal over the weekend. The starting dose of LAAM is 20–40 mg, and the usual maintenance doses are 60 mg on Monday and Wednesday and 80 mg on Friday. When starting LAAM, methadone supplementation can be given in doses of 5–20 mg/day to help the patient during the stabilization period. To switch from methadone to LAAM, the methadone dosage should be multiplied by 1.2; to switch from LAAM to methadone, the LAAM dosage should be multiplied by 0.8. The effectiveness of LAAM compares well with methadone; however, it seems to benefit a different subgroup of opioid addicts.

3. **Buprenorphine. Buprenorphine clinically exhibits characteristics of both methadone and naltrexone. Its mu agonist properties satisfy cravings and prevent opioid withdrawal and its mu antagonist characteristics block the reinforcing effects from abused opioids.** These characteristics have led researchers to test buprenorphine's usefulness for opioid substitution in addicts. It has a half-life of 24–36 hours, which allows for once-a-day dosing. It is available to clinicians in an injectable form; however, a sublingual form is available to researchers. The sublingual form has the disadvantage that it has to be held in the mouth for 3 minutes. Subcutaneous buprenorphine at a dose range of 8–12 mg/day is comparable to methadone 60 mg/day for maintaining abstinence from opioid abuse.
4. **Naltrexone. As an opioid antagonist, naltrexone can help patients abstain from using opiates after detoxification. The most significant medical risk from this treatment is hepatotoxicity. Clinicians must remind patients that a higher dose of opiate will not counter the blockade of euphoria but it can lead to respiratory failure.** Prior to the onset of naltrexone use, a patient's liver function must fall within three times the upper limit of normal. Clinicians should monitor liver function tests every 2 weeks for the first month of treatment, then monthly for the next 6 months. Dosing should begin at 25 mg per day for 3 days, and if well tolerated it can be increased to 50 mg every other day or every day. Experimentally, some patients receive up to 100 mg per day. Common side effects include nausea, dyspepsia, and headache. Some patients do well with a Monday/Wednesday/Friday schedule of 100 mg/100 mg/150 mg, respectively. If a narcotic analgesia is needed, patients should discontinue the naltrexone at least 5 days prior to the anticipated need.

D. Psychosocial Treatment

1. **Psychosocial treatments include individual, group, and family psychotherapy; therapeutic communities; and self-help groups, such as Narcotics Anonymous.** Typical outcome measures are the frequency and amount of opioid used, employment status, the level of psychosocial functioning, and the severity of psychiatric symptoms.
2. **Psychotherapy.** The greater the degree of psychopathology in opioid addicts, the poorer the treatment outcome. However, for opioid addicts with psychiatric disorders, psychotherapy can significantly improve treatment outcome as compared to treatment without psychotherapy. Antisocial personality predicts poor response to psychotherapy. Positive predictors of psychotherapy outcome include: establishing a good alliance between therapist and patient; treating psychiatric symptoms, such as depression; assessing and addressing psychosocial problems; and monitoring treatment compliance.
   a. **Supportive-expressive therapy** is more effective than drug counseling alone for opioid addicts with prominent psychiatric symptoms.
   b. **Cognitive-behavioral therapy.** Studies in community-based methadone clinics showed that CBT plus drug counseling, and supportive-expressive therapy plus drug counseling, are each more effective than drug counseling alone at 7 and 12 months in methadone patients with high levels of psychiatric symptoms. All three treatment conditions were equally effective in methadone patients with low levels of psychiatric symptoms.
   c. **Behavioral therapy.** Cue extinction and contingency management are two effective behavioral approaches. There is good evidence that cravings can be classically conditioned; thus, through repeated exposures to internal or external cues, cravings are extinguished. With contingency management, the therapist and the patient establish a set of rewards for maintaining abstinence and a set of aversive consequences for opioid use; urine toxicology screens are randomly used to determine treatment compliance. In a recent study of patients in a methadone maintenance program, adding psychosocial services (on-site medical and psychiatric services, family therapy, and employment services) to contingency management and methadone substitution significantly improved outcome. Patients treated soley with methadone substitution had to be terminated from the study by week 12 due to a high percent of opiate-positive urine samples.
   d. **Family therapy.** Family members can be helpful in assisting the treatment team initiate and monitor contingency management protocols and facility compliance.
   e. **Group therapy.** Relapse prevention groups combined with self-help groups are more effective in reducing opioid use, legal problems, and unemployment than in detoxified opioid-dependent patients without treatment.
   f. **Therapeutic communities.** Patients reside in these facilities from 6 to 18 months. The environment is structured and consists of a hierarchy of privileges and responsibilities. The community confronts denial and emphasizes personal responsibility for achieving abstinence. Only highly motivated individuals are successful; 50% drop out by 6 months and only 15–25% graduate.

g. **Narcotics Anonymous (NA).** There are essentially no differences between NA and Alcoholics Anonymous (AA). NA includes patients with an addiction to any illicit drug. The main purpose of NA is to provide a support network, confront denial, and to help prevent relapse by addressing thinking and behaviors that often lead to use. Outcome studies are lacking with regard to the efficacy of NA.

Suggested Readings

American Psychiatric Association. (1994). Substance-related disorders. In *Diagnostic and statistical manual of mental disorders* (4th ed., pp. 175–272). Washington, DC: American Psychiatric Press.

American Psychiatric Association. (1995). *Practice guideline for the treatment of patients with substance use disorders: Alcohol, cocaine, opioids.* Washington, DC: American Psychiatric Press.

Franklin, J.E., & Frances, R.J. (1999). Alcohol and other psychoactive substance use disorders. In R.E. Hales, S.C. Yudofsky, & J.A. Talbott (Eds.), *The American Psychiatric Press textbook of psychiatry* (3rd ed., pp. 363–423). Washington, DC: American Psychiatric Press.

Gold, M. (1997). Cocaine (and crack): Clinical aspects. In J.H. Lowinson, P. Ruiz, R.B. Millman, & J.G. Langrod (Eds.), *Substance abuse: A comprehensive textbook* (3rd ed., pp. 181–199). Baltimore: Williams and Wilkins.

Gold, M., & Miller, N.S. (1997). Cocaine (and crack): Neurobiology. In J.H. Lowinson, P. Ruiz, R.B. Millman, & J.G. Langrod (Eds.), *Substance abuse: A comprehensive textbook* (3rd ed., pp. 166–181). Baltimore: Williams and Wilkins.

Jaffe, J.H., Knapp, C.M., & Ciraulo, D.A. (1997). Opiates: Clinical aspects. In J.H. Lowinson, P. Ruiz, R.B. Millman, & J.G. Langrod (Eds.), *Substance abuse: A comprehensive textbook* (3rd ed., pp. 158–166). Baltimore: Williams and Wilkins.

Jaffe, J.H., & Jaffe, A.B. (1999). Neurobiology of opiates/opioids. In M. Galanter & H.D. Kleber (Eds.), *Textbook of substance abuse treatment* (2nd ed., pp. 11–19). Washington, DC: American Psychiatric Press.

Kleber, H.D. (1999). Opioids: Detoxification. In M. Galanter & H.D. Kleber (Eds.), *Textbook of substance abuse treatment* (2nd ed., pp. 251–269). Washington, DC: American Psychiatric Press.

McLellan, T.A., Lewis, D.C., O'Brien, C.P., & Kleber, H.D. (2000). Drug dependence, a chronic medical illness; implications for treatment, insurance, and outcomes evaluation. *Journal of the American Medical Association, 284,* 1689–1695.

O'Brien, C.P., & Cornish, J.W. (1999). Opioids: Antagonists and partial agonists. In M. Galanter & H.D. Kleber (Eds.), *Textbook of substance abuse treatment* (2nd ed., pp. 281–294). Washington, DC: American Psychiatric Press.

O'Connor, P.G., Waugh, M.L., Carroll, K.M., et al. (1995). Primary care-based ambulatory opioid detoxification: The results of a clinical trial. *Journal of General Internal Medicine, 10,* 255–260.

Senay, E.C. (1999). Opioids: Methadone maintenance. In M. Galanter & H.D. Kleber (Eds.), *Textbook of substance abuse treatment* (2nd ed., pp. 271–279). Washington, DC: American Psychiatric Press.

Simon, E.J. (1997). Opiates: Neurobiology. In J.H. Lowinson, P. Ruiz, R.B. Millman, & J.G. Langrod (Eds.), *Substance abuse: A comprehensive textbook* (3rd ed., pp. 148–158). Baltimore: Williams and Wilkins.

Vining, E., Kosten, T.R., & Kleber, H.D. (1988). Clinical utility of rapid clonidine-naltrexone detoxification for opioid abuse. *British Journal of Addiction, 83,* 567–575.

Washton, A.M. (1990). Structured outpatient treatment of alcohol vs drug dependence. *Recent Developments in Alcohol, 8,* 285–304.

Weiss, R.D., Griffin, M.L., Greenfield, S.F., et al. (2000). Group therapy for patients with bipolar disorder and substance dependence: Results of a pilot study. *Journal of Clinical Psychiatry, 61,* 361–367.

Chapter 12

Psychosis and Schizophrenia

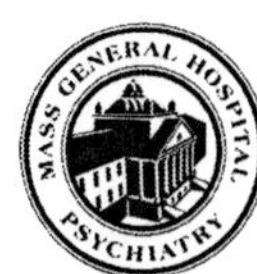

David C. Henderson, Laura Kunkel, and Donald C. Goff

I. Introduction

Psychosis is a gross impairment of reality testing which can result from a variety of psychiatric and medical problems. Psychotic symptoms generally fall into three categories:

A. Hallucinations

Hallucinations are sensory perceptions in the absence of external stimuli.

B. Delusions

Delusions are **firmly held false beliefs.** Delusions may be of persecution, of a somatic nature, of grandeur, of jealousy, or of the feeling that someone has been replaced by an impostor (Capgras' syndrome).

C. Thought Disorder

Formal thought disorder **refers to a disruption in the form or organization of thinking.** A patient may be incoherent and have difficulty communicating their thoughts to others, or have a loosening of associations, overinclusiveness, neologisms, thought blocking, clanging, echolalia, concreteness, or poverty of speech.

II. History of Diagnostic Classification of Schizophrenia

A. Kraepelin

In 1896, Kraepelin **distinguished "dementia praecox" from "manic depressive psychosis"** and **emphasized a chronic, deteriorating course.** (Major mental illnesses have different courses and outcomes.) The term "Kraepelinian schizophrenia" has been used by some investigators to refer to a condition in which a patient fails to achieve remission and to live independently for a 5-year period.

B. Bleuler

In **1911,** Bleuler described "schizophrenia" as a splitting of psychic functions. He **described specific fundamental symptoms of schizophrenia as the "Four As": autism, ambivalence, loosening of associations, and inappropriate affect.** He emphasized "negative symptoms" and described accessory symptoms which included delusions and hallucinations.

C. Schneider

In the 1970s, Schneider **described eleven "first-rank symptoms"** of schizophrenia, including hallucinations, delusions, thought withdrawal, thought insertion, imposed feelings, and impulses. He **emphasized the "positive symptoms" of schizophrenia** and believed that the diagnosis of schizophrenia can be made with second-rank symptoms, which include other disorders of perception (not first-rank), sudden delusional ideas, perplexity, emotional impoverishment, and depressive and euphoric mood changes.

III. DSM-IV Diagnosis of Schizophrenia

A. Features

The essential features of schizophrenia include:

1. **Active psychotic symptoms for at least 1 month (less if treated)**
2. **Functioning below the highest expected level**
3. **A duration of illness for at least 6 months (including prodromal or residual phases)**

B. Active Phase

The active phase requires either bizarre delusions or hallucinations (where two or more voices converse with each other, or a voice keeps a running commentary of the person's behaviors or thoughts), or two or more of the following symptoms: delusions, hallucinations, disorganized speech, grossly disorganized or catatonic behavior, or negative symptoms.

C. Prodromal or Residual Symptoms

Prodromal and residual phase symptoms include **social isolation or withdrawal, impairment of functioning, peculiar behavior, impaired personal hygiene, blunted or inappropriate affect, abnormal speech** (e.g., digressive, vague, overly elaborate), **odd beliefs** (e.g., superstitions, extrasensory perception [ESP]), **unusual perceptual experiences, and apathy.**

D. Subtypes of Schizophrenia

1. **Catatonic type:** catalepsy or stupor; negativism or mutism; excessive motor activity; peculiar voluntary movements (posturing, mannerisms, stereopathy, grimacing); echolalia or echopraxia.
2. **Disorganized type:** disorganized speech and behavior; flat or inappropriate affect, but not meeting the criteria for catatonic type.
3. **Paranoid type:** preoccupation with one or more delusions or frequent auditory hallucinations; the patient does not experience significant disorganization, catatonia, or inappropriate or flat affect.
4. **Undifferentiated type:** active psychotic symptoms, but not meeting criteria for other types.
5. **Residual type:** the absence of psychosis and not meeting criteria for other types.

IV. Differential Diagnosis of Psychotic Symptoms

A. **Mood disorders** (if present, they are of brief duration)
   1. Schizoaffective disorder: the mood disorder is prominent and the patient experiences psychotic symptoms for at least 2 weeks when euthymic.
   2. Bipolar disorder: psychosis is present only during manic or depressive episodes.
   3. Psychotic depression: psychosis occurs only during depressive episodes.

B. **Schizophreniform disorder:** involves a prodromal phase, an active phase, and has a residual duration of less than 6 months.

C. **Brief reactive psychosis:** the duration is less than 1 month.

D. **Schizotypal personality disorder:** acute discomfort with and reduced capacity for close relationships, cognitive or perceptual distortions, and eccentricities of behavior.

E. **Delusional disorder:** a persistent condition with non-bizarre delusions.

F. **Drug-induced psychosis**
   1. **Phencyclidine (PCP).** At high doses, PCP may cause illusions and hallucinations. PCP can cause effects that mimic the full range of symptoms of schizophrenia, such as delusions, paranoia, disordered thinking, a sensation of distance from one's environment, and catatonia. Speech is often sparse and garbled. People who use PCP for long periods report memory loss, difficulties with speech and thinking, depression, and weight loss. These symptoms can persist up to one year after cessation of PCP use.
   2. **Ketamine.** A dissociative anesthetic with a chemical structure and mechanism of action similar to PCP; it is a non-competitive antagonist of the NMDA receptor that produces psychosis, perceptual alterations, thought disorder, and mood changes in healthy subjects. Its effects are similar to those of PCP but they are of a shorter duration. Patients report sensations ranging from a pleasant feeling of floating to being separated from their bodies. Some experience a terrifying feeling of almost complete sensory detachment. PCP is odorless and tasteless, and therefore, it can be added to beverages without being detected. It induces amnesia and is used in the commission of sexual assaults.
   3. **Lysergic acid diethylamide (LSD).** The effects of LSD depend on the amount taken, the patient's personality and expectations, and the surroundings in which the drug is used. The patient may feel several different emotions at once or swing rapidly from one emotion to another. If taken in a large enough dose, the drug produces delusions and visual hallucinations. The patient's sense of time and self changes; patients may describe synesthesias (hearing colors and seeing sounds) which may lead to panic.
   4. **MDMA (Ecstasy):** MDMA (3,4-methylene dioxy-methamphetamine) has properties similar to both amphetamines and hallucinogens. Psychological effects can occur either during or weeks after use and include confusion, depression, sleep problems, drug craving, severe anxiety, and paranoia.

G. **Organic Etiologies**

These include (see Table 12-1) substance abuse, use of medications, seizure disorder, delirium, infectious diseases, endocrinopathies, nutritional deficiencies, neoplasms, heavy metal exposures, and neurologic disorders.

V. Evaluation of Psychosis

Most causes of psychosis (Table 12-1) can be ruled out by a good medical history, by a physical and neurological examination, and by screening laboratory examinations (see Table 12-2).

Table 12-1. Drugs and Medical/Neurological Conditions Associated with Psychosis

Drugs of abuse	**Infectious diseases**
Alcohol	Brain abscess
Amphetamines	Hepatic encephalopathy
Barbiturates	Infectious mononucleosis
Caffeine	Malaria
Cannabis (THC)	Meningitis
Cocaine	Syphilis
Hallucinogens (e.g., LSD, PCP, MDMA)	**Endocrine disorders**
Inhalants	Addison's disease
Opioids	Cushing's syndrome
Sedative-hypnotics	Hypo/hyperthyroidism
	Hypo/hyperparathyroidism
Neurological disorders	**Nutritional deficiencies**
Alzheimer's disease	Niacin deficiency (pellagra)
Complex partial seizures	Thiamine deficiency
Huntington's disease	(Korsakoff's psychosis, beriberi)
Hydrocephalus	Vitamin B_{12} (pernicious anemia)
Lupus cerebritis	**Other**
Parkinson's disease	Neoplasms
Pick's disease	Heavy metal exposures
Wilson's disease	Prescription medications-steroids

Table 12-2. Evaluation of Psychosis

1. Perform a complete physical and neurological exam
2. Conduct a mental status exam—ordering neuropsychological testing as indicated
3. Obtain a full laboratory screen: electrolytes, BUN, creatinine, calcium, glucose, CBC, thyroid panel, liver enzymes, VDRL, vitamin B_{12}, folate, HIV when indicated
4. Obtain a toxicological screen
5. Order brain imaging (CT or MRI)
6. Obtain an EEG if clinically indicated

A. **Important diagnostic questions** must be asked to distinguish medical from psychiatric disorders.
   1. Has a reversible, organic cause been ruled out?
   2. Are cognitive deficits (e.g., memory impairment) prominent? If so, consideration must be given to delirium or dementia.
   3. Is the psychiatric illness episodic or continuous?
   4. Have psychotic symptoms been present for at least 4 weeks?
   5. Are negative symptoms present?
   6. Has evidence of the illness been present for at least 6 months?
   7. Are mood episodes prominent?
   8. Have there been episodes of major depression or mania?
   9. Do psychotic features occur only during affective episodes?

B. **Neuropsychological testing** is frequently helpful to uncover underlying psychotic symptoms and cognitive impairments.

C. **Brain imaging** often yields little information in the absence of focal neurologic impairment. However, a brain scan (magnetic resonance imaging [MRI] or computed tomography [CT]) is generally recommended at least once in a patient with an atypical psychosis or with treatment-refractory psychotic symptoms.

D. An **electroencephalogram (EEG)** should be performed if clinically indicated.

VI. Epidemiology of Schizophrenia

A. Prevalence

1. The prevalence of schizophrenia is **1% worldwide.** The prevalence varies by region in the United States.
2. There appears to be a higher incidence of schizophrenia among the urban poor. In part, this may be related to economic drift and to the drift of chronically disabled patients toward urban areas.
3. The incidence of schizophrenia may be decreasing in Great Britain since 1950, but it is higher among British Afro-Caribbeans.
4. Substance abuse is seen in roughly 50% of individuals with schizophrenia.

B. Age of Onset

1. Psychotic symptoms associated with schizophrenia most often appear in adolescence or young adulthood. Males manifest the illness earlier (ages 18–25 years) than do females (ages 26–45 years).
2. 20% of cases occur after the age of 40 years; the majority of those are women (a second, smaller peak in women near menopause at ages 40–45 years).

C. Pre-morbid Deficits

1. Children at risk have lower scholastic test scores and poor social involvement.
2. Some evidence also suggests that children at risk experience a thought disorder and delayed developmental milestones as early as infancy.

D. Stress and Age of Onset

1. Stress appears to be a significant factor that impacts the age of onset of schizophrenia. In college, 44% of cases develop during the first semester.
2. Among army draftees, there is an eight-fold higher incidence of first-break psychosis during the first few months in the service as compared with episodes during the second year.
3. Child abuse victims have an earlier age of onset and a more problematic course.

E. Gender Differences

The lifetime risk of schizophrenia is approximately equal for males and females, with males experiencing an earlier age of onset and a more symptomatic course. Symptoms in females may worsen after menopause. 90% of males and 25% of females develop the illness before the age of 30 years. Gender differences have been reported for pre-morbid functioning (better in women), clinical course, and response to antipsychotic drugs.

F. Season of Birth

1. In a subset of patients, **there is a modest increase in the prevalence of schizophrenia among those born in the spring and early winter.** In the northern hemisphere, schizophrenic patients are more likely to have been born between January and April.
2. In the southern hemisphere, schizophrenic patients are more likely to have been born between July and September.
3. An increased incidence of schizophrenia exists among individuals exposed to influenza or to other viruses during the late second trimester (6 months). However, direct evidence of viral causation or contribution to disease development is lacking.

VII. Patterns of Inheritance

A. Both older and more recent studies consistently show higher rates of monozygotic concordance (45–50%) compared with rates of dizygotic concordance (10–15%).

B. Compared with a lifetime risk for schizophrenia in the general population of approximately 1%, the **risk for a sibling or child of a schizophrenic patient is approximately 10%.** The risk increases further with the number of affected relatives. For example, an individual has a 16% risk of developing schizophrenia when both a parent and a sibling are affected and a 46% risk when both parents are affected. Increased risk, although still present, decreases sharply for second- and third-degree relatives (5% and 2%, respectively). Estimates for the **overall heritability of the disease range from 63% to 85%.**

C. A genetic contribution to disease development is likely, but it is unlikely to be the result of a single gene. A number of chromosomal regions have been implicated consistently by linkage analysis (6p, 6q, and 8p). Regions for which data are suggestive include 1q, 5q, 10p, and 13q. Individuals with velo-cardio-facial syndrome, a disorder associated with a chromosome 22q11 microdeletion, have high rates of schizophrenia. There is new evidence that spontaneous mutations may play a role in the genesis of schizophrenia.

VIII. Biological Abnormalities

A. Structural Brain Abnormalities

1. **Reduced volume** of the prefrontal cortex, thalamus, hippocampus, and superior temporal gyri
2. **Increased volume** of the lateral and third ventricles, and basal ganglia (secondary to use of antipsychotic medications)

B. Functional Brain Imaging Abnormalities

1. Possible **"hypofrontality"** (decreased blood flow and metabolism of frontal lobes) at rest and during performance of the Wisconsin Card Sorting Test.
2. **Altered activation** observed in the prefrontal cortex (the dorsal lateral prefrontal cortex has been studied the most), hippocampus, amygdala, and thalamus during cognitive tasks.

C. Histopathological Changes

1. **Decreased size of the anteromedial temporal lobe,** along with cytoarchitectural abnormalities of the parahippocampal gyrus, may be found in some patients with schizophrenia.
2. **Reduced neuronal density** has been observed in the **prefrontal cortex, thalamus, and cingulate gyrus.**
3. **Absence of gliosis,** which suggests a developmental abnormality, and evidence of abnormal cell migration in the hippocampus and frontal cortex have also been observed.

D. Neuropsychological Functioning

1. An individual with schizophrenia generally exhibits **deficits in attention, memory, learning, and an inability to shift sets on neuropsychological testing. Problems with verbal memory and vigilance seem most predictive of poor functional outcome.**
2. **Cognitive deficits** appear pre-morbidly and worsen over the course of the illness.
3. **Smooth pursuit eye movements (SPEM) are abnormal in 50–85% of patients** with schizophrenia as well as in 45% of first-degree family members. This finding may represent an alternative expression of an autosomal dominant gene. The SPEM abnormality is non-specific and occurs in mania (state-dependent) and Parkinson's disease.
4. Evoked potentials P50 waveforms decrease after the first of paired stimuli in normal controls, but not in patients with schizophrenia. This may reflect an impairment of gating (filtering) auditory input; up to 50% of first-degree relatives have this defect. Finally, **impaired generation of P300 event-related potentials have been observed** in patients with schizophrenia.

E. Receptors and Neurotransmitters

1. **Dopamine D_2 receptor density may be increased in the striatum and the nucleus accumbens.**
2. **Norepinephrine receptor density may be increased in the nucleus accumbens.**
3. **Glutamate receptors are increased in the frontal cortex and hippocampus.**
4. Altered serotonin activity has also been suspected.
5. Integrative hypotheses suggest that schizophrenia is a disease of disordered neural circuitry involving multiple anatomical brain regions (i.e., cortex, thalamus, basal gangla, and medial temporal lobe) and their modulation by neurotransmitter-specific projection systems.

IX. Theories of Etiology

A. Dopamine Hyperactivity

1. **Schizophrenia and acute psychosis are associated with increased mesolimbic dopamine activity** (in the temporal lobes) which may be mediated, in part, by mesocortical hypoactivity (in the prefrontal cortex).
2. Supporting evidence for dopamine hyperactivity includes:
   a. The fact that dopamine agonists, such as amphetamine, produce psychosis.
   b. All conventional antipsychotic agents are dopamine antagonists and the affinity for dopamine D_2 receptors correlates with antipsychotic efficacy.

3. Evidence that complicates the dopamine model includes:
   a. Agents that act at other receptors also produce psychosis (lysergic acid diethylamide [LSD], and phencyclidine [PCP]).
   b. The antipsychotic effect may follow a delay of 2–10 weeks after dopamine blockade has occurred.
   c. Evidence of abnormalities in dopamine, its metabolites, or its receptor densities in patients with schizophrenia has been inconsistent.
   d. Negative symptoms are not clearly linked to dopamine.

B. Serotonin Dysfunction

1. LSD, a serotonin (5-HT) agonist, and 3,4-methylene dioxymethamphetamine ("ecstasy") (MDMA) toxicity, each produce chronic psychosis.
2. Clozapine, and other atypical antipsychotic agents, are active at the serotonin 5-HT_2 and 5-HT_{1c} receptors. Unfortunately, evidence of serotonin abnormalities has been inconsistent.

C. Phencyclidine (PCP) Model (Javitt, 1991)

1. PCP and ketamine produce delusions, hallucinations, thought disorder, negative symptoms, and catatonia in normal individuals. These drugs may also produce cognitive deficits and frontal lobe hypometabolism. In those with schizophrenia, ketamine can produce psychotic relapses.
2. Glutamate appears to mediate dopamine activity. The PCP receptor interacts with the *N*-methyl D-aspartate (NMDA)-type glutamate receptor complex by blocking ion channels.

D. Viral Hypothesis

Viral infection during the third trimester is suspected of compromising the development of the medial temporal lobe. This may account for the relationship between the season of birth and the decreasing incidence of schizophrenia in Great Britain.

E. Diathesis and Stress Model (Two-Hit Model)

1. In this model, the first factor (or hit) is an inherited vulnerability to schizophrenia, which may be manifested by neuropsychological deficits (e.g., impaired auditory gating).
2. The second factor is an environmental injury to the hippocampus (e.g., by an obstetrical injury, infection, trauma, or hypoxia).

F. The "two-hit" hypothesis has gained increasing attention. Genetic or environmental factors disrupt early CNS development which produce long-term vulnerability to a "second hit" that then leads to the onset of psychotic symptoms. Parallel disruption of cell-cell signaling in both the developing and the mature CNS provides a plausible way of integrating complex genetics, developmental biology, and environmental factors that contribute to schizophrenia.

X. Predictors of Outcome

Worse outcome is associated with insidious onset, younger age of onset, negative symptoms, poor pre-morbid function, substance abuse or other co-morbid disorder, disadvantaged minority status, and the absence of remissions. Better outcome is associated with affective symptoms and being female. The outcome most closely correlates with the initial response to medications. The outcome may be worse if pharmacotherapy is significantly delayed.

A. Course of Illness

1. Generally, the outcome is poor. **Approximately 10% recover and 20% have a good outcome.** With newer atypical antipsychotic agents, more patients are considered to have a good outcome. The outcome is generally better in under-developed countries
2. **While the suicide rate for patients with schizophrenia is 10–13%, 18–55% of patients with schizophrenia attempt suicide.** The incidence of suicide and attempts has decreased with the introduction of the atypical antipsychotic agent, clozapine.
3. For many patients, negative symptoms worsen over time. **Patients with schizophrenia, paranoid type, experience a later and a more rapid age of onset;** they have a better prognosis. **Those with a disorganized type, also called hebephrenia, and the undifferentiated type have an earlier age of onset and a more insidious onset;** they tend to experience a continuous but stable course.
4. Hallucinations and delusions may decrease, even without treatment, after the age of 50.
5. **Individuals with schizophrenia have an elevated rate of violence, particularly if they experience paranoia and disorganization.** Homicide rates are best studied in this group and may be increased by a factor of ten compared to the general population. Schizophrenics with the paranoid subtype or with delusions that promote violence are at greatest risk for violence. The presence of command auditory hallucinations is a risk factor in the context of a delusional system.

B. Awareness of Illness

1. **More than half of patients with schizophrenia have impaired insight into their illness.** This may reflect frontal-cortical dysfunction.
2. When evaluating a patient with denial or impaired insight into their illness, a focus on the developmental, education, employment, and social history may provide clues to the nature of the illness.

C. Negative Symptoms

1. **Negative symptoms of schizophrenia often receive less attention than do positive psychotic symptoms (e.g., hallucinations), but they can be just as disabling.**
2. Negative symptoms include anhedonia, asociality (social isolation), affective flattening, alogia (poverty of speech and thought), inattentiveness, and apathy.

3. Response of negative symptoms may occur independently of psychotic symptom response, and follow a different time course.

D. Differential Diagnosis of Negative Symptoms

The evaluation of a patient with negative symptoms should include consideration of other disorders or conditions with similar symptoms. **These disorders include neuroleptic-induced akinesia, depression, frontal lobe injury, idiopathic or neuroleptic-induced parkinsonism, substance abuse (particularly of stimulants), hypothyroidism, trauma, and post-traumatic stress disorder.**

XI. Psychosocial Treatment

It has been shown that antipsychotic medications are effective in the treatment of acute psychosis and in the prevention of relapse for patients with schizophrenia. However, 25–50% of individuals with schizophrenia will continue to have disabling residual symptoms and impaired social functioning, and many will experience a relapse.

A. **Cognitive-behavioral therapy** results in reduction of delusions and hallucinations in patients receiving optimal pharmacological treatment. Interventions focus on rationally exploring the subjective nature of the psychotic symptoms, challenging the evidence for these, and subjecting such beliefs and experiences to reality testing.

B. **Individual psychotherapy** can assist patients with managing life stressors, enhancing medication compliance, and improving self-esteem.

C. **Group psychotherapy** provides a supportive social network and a good setting for teaching coping and interpersonal skills. Advantages include lower cost, social interaction, and peer support.

D. **Assertive Community Treatment (ACT)** provides comprehensive integrated community services. Patients are assigned to one multidisciplnary team (with a case manager, a nurse, and an M.D.). The team has a fixed caseload and a high staff/patient ratio; it delivers all services needed by the patient 24 hours a day, 7 days a week. It is has been shown to reduce time spent in the hospital, but it is less effective for social adjustment or employment. High-quality case management with adequate service availability may be equally effective.

E. **Family therapy** is effective in the prevention of psychotic relapse and rehospitalization. **Expressed emotion (EE)** is a measure of the family environment that is based on an index of criticism, hostility, and overinvolvement with a psychiatric patient. **High EE has been demonstrated to be a predictor of relapse** in schizophrenia with a greater magnitude of association in chronically ill patients.

F. **Social skills training** uses learning theory principles to improve social functioning by working with patients to remediate problems in activities of daily living, employment, leisure, and relationships. There are three forms: the basic model, the social problem-solving model, and the cognitive remediation model. It improves social skills (although it is methodologically difficult to demonstrate) but has no clear effect on relapse prevention, psychopathology, or employment status.

G. **Supportive employment programs** that use the place-and-train model can significantly affect the ability to obtain competitive employment (e.g., a regular community job as opposed to being employed in a program overseen by a rehabilitation agency).

Suggested Readings

American Psychiatric Association. (1994). *Diagnostic and statistical manual of mental disorders* (4th ed.). Washington, DC: American Psychiatric Press.

Bustillo, J.R., Laurriello, J., Horwan, W.P., & Samuel, K. (2001). The psychosocial treatment of schizophrenia: An update. *American Journal of Psychiatry, 158*(2), 163–175.

Freudenreich, O., & Stern, T.A. (2003). Clinical experience with the managemnt of schizophrenia in the general hospital. *Psychosomatics, 44*(1), 12–23.

Goff, D.C., & Henderson, D.C. (1996). Treatment-resistant schizophrenia and psychotic disorders. In M.H. Pollack, M.W. Otto, & J.F. Rosenbaum (Eds.), *Challenges in clinical practice: Pharmacologic and psychosocial strategies* (pp. 311–328). New York: Guilford Press.

Goff, D.C., Henderson, D.C., & Manschreck, T.C. (1997). Psychotic patients. In N.H. Cassem, T.A. Stern, J.F. Rosenbaum, & M.S. Jellinek (Eds.), *Massachusetts General Hospital handbook of general hospital psychiatry* (4th ed., pp. 149–171). St. Louis: Mosby.

Meltzer, H.Y. (1987). Biological studies in schizophrenia. *Schizophrenia Bulletin, 13,* 77–110.

Chapter 13

Mood Disorders: Depression

JOHN MATTHEWS AND GEORGE PAPAKOSTAS

I. Overview

The *Diagnostic and Statistical Manual, Fourth Edition* (DSM-IV), denotes three categories of unipolar depressive disorders:

A. **Major depressive disorder (MDD)** is characterized by one or more episodes of persistent depressed mood, or a loss of interest or pleasure, for a minimum of 2 weeks, with four or more of the following symptoms of depression: weight disturbance, appetite disturbance, sleep disturbance, fatigue or loss of energy, feelings of guilt or worthlessness, poor concentration, psychomotor agitation or retardation, suicide attempts, or thoughts of death.

B. **Dysthymic disorder** is characterized by a depressed mood, experienced more days than not, over at least a 2-year period, as well as by two or more of the following symptoms of depression: poor appetite or hyperphagia, insomnia or hypersomnia, low energy or fatigue, low self-esteem, poor concentration and difficulty making decisions, or feelings of hopelessness.

C. **Depressive disorder not otherwise specified (NOS)** identifies those individuals who do not meet criteria for MDD, dysthymic disorder, adjustment disorder with depressed mood, or adjustment disorder with mixed anxiety and depressed mood.

II. Major Depressive Disorder (MDD)

A. DSM-IV Criteria

1. **To diagnose MDD, at least five of the following symptoms must be present during the same 2-week period;** symptoms must also result in a deterioration of function. At least one of the symptoms must be either depressed mood or a loss of interest or pleasure. Symptoms due to medical disorders or mood-incongruent delusions or hallucinations are not to be included.
   a. **Depressed mood** most of the day and nearly every day as expressed by either subjective account or by observations made by others.
   b. Markedly **diminished interest** or pleasure in all, or almost all, activities most of the day, nearly every day, as expressed by either subjective account or by observations made by others.
   c. Significant unintentional **weight loss or weight gain** (e.g., more than 5% of body weight in a month), or a decrease or increase in appetite nearly every day.
   d. **Insomnia or hypersomnia** nearly every day.
   e. **Psychomotor agitation or retardation** nearly every day (observable by others, not merely subjective feelings of restlessness or being slowed down).
   f. **Fatigue or loss of energy** nearly every day.
   g. **Feelings of worthlessness or excessive** or inappropriate **guilt** (which may be delusional) nearly every day (not merely self-reproach or guilt about being sick).
   h. **Diminished ability to think or concentrate,** or indecisiveness, nearly every day (either by subjective account or as observed by others).
   i. **Recurrent thoughts of death** (not just a fear of dying), **recurrent suicidal ideation** without a specific plan, or a **suicide attempt** or a specific plan for committing suicide.
2. The symptoms must cause disruption in social, occupational, or other important areas of functioning.
3. The symptoms are not secondary to a medical condition (e.g., Cushing's disease) or to the physical effects of a substance (e.g., alcohol, recreational drugs, or medications).
4. The symptoms are not secondary to bereavement. After the loss of a loved one, bereavement may be complicated by MDD if the symptoms persist for 2 months or longer, or are characterized by a marked functional impairment, by preoccupation with worthlessness, by suicidal ideations or behavior, or by psychotic symptoms.
5. The symptoms do not occur in the context of schizophrenia, schizophreniform disorder, delusional disorder, or psychotic disorder not otherwise specified.
6. There are several specifiers that may be used to describe MDD: mild severity, moderate severity, severe without psychotic features, severe with psychotic features, in partial remission, in full remission, chronic, with catatonic features, with melancholic features, with atypical features, with post-partum onset, with or without full inter-episode recovery, with seasonal pattern.

B. Specifiers for Major Depressive Disorder

1. **MDD with psychotic features.** In this condition, delusions and hallucinations are present in addition to the symptoms of major depression. The psychotic symptoms may be mood-congruent (i.e., the content is consistent with depressive themes, such as guilt, poor self-worth, death, hopelessness, or punishment) or mood-incongruent (i.e., where the content is not consistent with typical depressive themes, such as delusions of control, thought broadcasting, thought insertion, or persecutory delusions). Both mood-congruent and mood-incongruent psychotic symptoms can be present concurrently. Delusions occur without hallucinations in about

one-half to two-thirds of adults, whereas hallucinations occur without delusions in one-fourth or less of adults. Once psychotic symptoms appear, they tend to be present in each subsequent depressive episode.

2. **MDD with melancholic features.** During the most severe period of the episode, there is either loss of pleasure in all or almost all activities or there is lack of reactivity to usually pleasurable stimuli. In addition, three or more of the following must be present: a depressed mood that is experienced as qualitatively different from the feeling experienced after a loss, depression that is worse in the morning, awakening at least 2 hours before the usual time, marked psychomotor retardation or agitation, significant anorexia or weight loss, and excessive or inappropriate guilt.
3. **MDD with atypical features.** In this condition mood reactivity occurs in response to actual or potential positive events. Two of the following features must be present: significant weight gain or an increase in appetite, hypersomnia, leaden paralysis or a heavy feeling in the arms and legs, and a long-standing pattern of sensitivity to interpersonal rejection that results in social and occupational dysfunction.
4. **MDD with post-partum onset.** The onset of episodes in this condition must occur within 4 weeks of delivery.
5. **MDD with a seasonal pattern.** A temporal relationship exists between the onset of episodes and the season of the year. Episodes of depression generally occur in the fall or winter.
6. **MDD with catatonic features.** At least two of the following must be present: motor immobility (including waxy flexibility or stupor), excessive motor activity that is purposeless and not influenced by external stimuli, extreme negativism (manifested by maintenance of a rigid posture or resistance to commands), unusual voluntary movements (manifest by posturing, stereotyped movements, mannerisms, or grimacing), echolalia or echopraxia.

C. Differential Diagnosis

1. **Mood disorder due to a general medical condition with depressive or with major depressive-like episode.** The diagnosis is based on history, physical examination, and laboratory results. A temporal relationship must exist between the onset of depressive symptoms and the development of the abnormal physiological condition.
2. **Substance-induced mood disorder with depressive features.** The diagnosis is based on history, physical examination, and laboratory results. The symptoms of depression must develop during or within a month of substance intoxication or withdrawal; otherwise, the substance use is etiologically related to the depression.
3. **Dysthymic disorder.** This diagnosis differs from major depressive disorder based on its severity, chronicity, and persistence. In dysthymic disorder, the depressed mood needs to be present more days than not for a period of 2 years.
4. **Dementia.** In dementia, there is a pre-morbid period of cognitive decline; whereas, in depression, the cognitive decline is associated with onset of depression.
5. **Manic episodes with irritable mood or mixed states.** This diagnosis requires the presence of manic symptoms. The presence of symptoms that meet criteria for both a manic episode and a major depressive episode, every day for at least 1 week, would constitute a mixed manic episode.
6. **Attention-Deficit/Hyperactivity Disorder (ADHD).** Distractibility and low frustration tolerance are common to ADHD and to MDD. The disturbance in mood in ADHD is one of irritability rather than sadness or loss of interest.
7. **Adjustment disorder with depressed mood.** This diagnosis is made if the depressive episode occurs in the context of a psychosocial stressor; it is not due to bereavement, and it does not meet criteria for MDD.

D. Epidemiology

1. **The lifetime prevalence for MDD** in community samples for Americans 18 years and older **ranges from 10–25% for women and 5–12% for men.** The point prevalence for MDD in community samples for adults is 5–9% for women and 2–3% for men.
2. Since World War II, there has been a trend toward both an earlier age of onset of depression and an increased rate of depression.
3. In pre-pubertal children, the rate of depression for boys is greater than the rate for girls. Between the beginning of puberty and age 50 years, the rate for depression in women is twice the rate for depression in men. After the age of 50 years, the rates of depression in women and men are equal.

E. Course of MDD

1. **The average age of onset for unipolar depression is 29 years.**
2. **The onset of MDD may be sudden or gradual** and develop over several weeks or months. Early signs may include insomnia, poor appetite, decreased concentration, loss of interest, or any of the other symptoms of depression, but they occur at a subthreshold level. Other prodromal symptoms include anxiety and panic attacks. MDD with a sudden onset often occurs in the context of a severe psychosocial stressor, especially divorce or loss of a loved one. 80% of acute episodes of MDD are associated with a significant stressor in the previous 6-month period.
3. **MDD is a recurrent illness.** The probability of having a recurrence is influenced by the number of previous episodes. **The risk for relapse after one episode is about 50%, whereas the risk of relapse after three**

episodes is greater than 80%. The average lifetime number of episodes is four. The inter-episode interval shortens with increasing numbers of episodes from 6 years after two episodes to 2 years after three episodes. The rate of recurrence after a full recovery from an episode of major depression, in patients with recurring illness, ranges from 50% within 2 years and approximately 90% within 6 years.

4. **Full recovery from an episode of MDD occurs in 50% of cases by 6 months.** For individuals evaluated at one year post-diagnosis of MDD, 40% will still meet criteria for major depression, 20% will be in partial remission, and 40% will be in complete remission. 20% of individuals evaluated at the end of 2 years, and 12% at the end of 5 years, continue to be significantly depressed.
5. The course of recurrent major depressive episodes is variable. **Factors that contribute to relapse include a high number of previous episodes, inadequate antidepressant treatment, partial response to treatment, discontinuation of effective treatment, rapid discontinuation of antidepressants, a highly emotional environment, and co-morbid medical or nonaffective psychiatric disorders.**
6. **5–10% of individuals with a single episode of major depression will eventually develop bipolar disorder.** Young individuals with first episodes that are severe or that are associated with psychotic features may develop bipolar disorder. Women with postpartum depression are at greater risk of developing bipolar disorder.

F. Etiology

1. **Family studies**
   a. MDD is common in families. **It is found 2 to 3 times more frequently in the first-degree biological relatives of individuals with the disorder than in the general population.** However, more frequent occurrence in families does not prove that the disorder has a genetic etiology.
   b. Family studies of depressed patients demonstrate significantly higher rates of depression in first-degree relatives, who share 50% of the genome, than in second-degree relatives, who share 25% of the genome. These findings suggest a genetic contribution, but they are inconclusive.
2. **Twin studies and adoption studies**
   a. Studies conducted in Europe and in the United States have demonstrated that **the concordance rate for major depression is about 50% in monozygotic twins, compared with 20% in dizygotic twins.** These results argue for a genetic factor in the development of MDD. However, most of the twins in these studies were raised together, and it has been hypothesized that twins' behavior can influence each other and that identical twins tend to be treated more alike by their environment than fraternal twins or sibs.
   b. Adoption studies attempt to differentiate the influence of genetic and environmental factors on the expression of an illness. A common strategy is to examine differences in rates of the illness among biological relatives versus adoptive relatives. Recent studies of adoptees with MDD have shown that the rates for depression are higher in their biological parents as compared with the rates in their adoptive parents.
   c. Studies of identical twins raised apart have shown a concordance rate of about 70% for unipolar and bipolar disorder, which is similar for identical twins raised together. These results provide further support for a genetic contribution to the development of MDD.
   d. However, in both twin and adoption studies, between 20% and 30% of identical twin pairs are not concordant for depression, thus arguing for an interaction of the environment with a genetic vulnerability in order for major depressive disorder to be expressed. Reviews of recent twin studies have shown that between 20% and 45% of the variance in the risk for depressive disorders is attributed to genetic factors and the remainder to environmental factors.
3. **Biochemical theories**
   a. **Biogenic amine hypothesis**
      i. The biogenic amine hypothesis was the first biochemical theory to explain the biological basis of both depression and mania. The theory evolved out of observations by clinicians that certain medications had either a negative or positive effect on mood. Reserpine, which depletes the brain of norepinephrine, serotonin, and dopamine, had a tendency to make patients feel depressed, whereas iproniazid, which inhibits the metabolism of norepinephrine, serotonin, and dopamine, had a tendency to improve the mood of some tuberculosis patients. The hypothesis argued that depression is the result of too little catecholamine or indoleamine neurotransmitter and mania is the result of too much catecholamine or indoleamine transmitter. Further support for the theory emerged with the finding from animal studies that the tricyclic antidepressants (TCAs) block the uptake of norepinephrine and serotonin from presynaptic terminals.
      ii. Problems with the theory became evident with the observation that the uptake-blocking mechanism takes place within minutes, whereas the therapeutic effect of TCAs takes about two weeks. Other explanations for the effectiveness of antidepressants were pursued with the new technological advances in receptor biology. Subsequent animal research demonstrated that TCAs, monoamine oxidase inhibitors (MAOIs), and electroconvulsive therapy (ECT) downregulate beta-adrenergic receptors over a period of time consistent with the time course to achieve a therapeutic effect. The downregulation of beta-adrenergic receptors did not fully explain the biochemical basis of depression since most of the new antidepressants have no effect on these receptors.

iii. Recent studies have demonstrated that norepinephrine and serotonin are important to the therapeutic effect of TCAs and serotonin reuptake inhibitors (SSRIs), respectively. In one study, dietary depletion of L-tryptophan, which decreases the synthesis of serotonin, resulted in a relapse of depression in SSRI-responders. In another study, subjects given α-methylparatyrosine (AMPT), which inhibits the synthesis of norepinephrine, resulted in a relapse of depression in TCA (primarily norepinephrine uptake blockers)-responders.

iv. The SSRIs and atypical antidepressants, except bupropion, increase serotonin neurotransmission nonselectively. However, two atypical antidepressants, mirtazapine and nefazodone, selectively increase serotonin neurotransmission through the 5-HT_{1a} receptor subtype by blocking the 5-HT_2 receptor. An increase in 5-HT_{1a} receptor activity may be important for the therapeutic effect of many of the newer antidepressants.

G. Biological Markers

1. Sleep dysregulation

a. Electroencephalographic (EEG) studies in patients with MDD have identified several **architecture abnormalities during sleep, including shortened rapid eye movement (REM) latency (decreased time from sleep onset to the onset of the first REM cycle), decreased non-REM sleep, increased REM density (increased number of REMs per unit of time during REM sleep), reduced total sleep time, and decreased sleep continuity.** Sleep architecture abnormalities are most commonly associated with the melancholic subtype of unipolar depression.

b. No single sleep architecture abnormality is closely associated with MDD. However, **the combination of decreased REM latency, increased REM density, and decreased sleep efficiency discriminates patients with MDD from controls.** These measures, however, are not specific to MDD; thus, they are not appropriate for use as a diagnostic test.

2. Hypothalamic-pituitary-adrenal axis (HPA) dysregulation

a. Hypersecretion of cortisol over the 24-hour circadian cycle has been repeatedly observed in patients with MDD.

b. **The dexamethasone suppression test (DST) has been used to assess the finding of hypersecretion of cortisol in depressed patients. The test consists of giving a 1 mg dose of dexamethasone at 11 P.M. and measuring serum cortisol the following day (usually at 8 A.M. and 4 P.M.).** Normally cortisol is suppressed to levels below 5 μg/dL. Decreased or non-suppression of serum cortisol in response to a 1 mg dexamethasone challenge occurs in about 50% of patients with MDD and melancholia and in about 80% of patients with MDD and psychotic features. The incidence of dexamethasone non-suppression is much lower in atypical MDD than melancholic or psychotic MDD. Increased activity could occur at any point between the hypothalamus and the adrenal gland. There is evidence of increased release of corticotropin-releasing factor (CRF) from the hypothalamus. CRF is regulated at the level of the hypothalamus, in part, by norepinephrine and serotonin, the same neurotransmitters implicated in the pathophysiology of depression. Recent evidence suggests a link between a certain polymorphism for the angiotensin converting enzyme and cortisol hypersecretion in patients with MDD.

c. Consistent with the physiologic abnormalities noted earlier are the findings that the pituitary and adrenal glands are hypertrophied in patients with MDD.

3. Hypothalamic-pituitary-thyroid axis dysregulation

a. Thyroid abnormalities have been associated with mood disorders: about 10% of hospitalized depressed patients have a diagnosis of hypothyroidism; thyroiditis is more common in patients with mood disorders; patients with rapid-cycling bipolar disorder are more likely to exhibit hypothyroidism; and triiodothyronine (T_3) is used to augment antidepressants for treatment-resistant depression. Recent evidence suggests a link between a certain polymorphism for gene coding for a protein involved in thyroid hormone receptor signaling and major depressive disorder. The role of thyroid hormones in MDD may be related to their effect on the energy metabolism of brain cells.

b. **The thyrotropin-releasing hormone (TRH) stimulation test can be used to challenge the hypothalamic-pituitary axis.** Protirelin, 55 IU, is given intravenously as the standard dose and thyroid-stimulating hormone (TSH) serum levels are measured at 0.5 and 1.5 hours after the infusion. An increase in serum TSH of less than 5 IU/mL after TRH infusion is considered a blunted response. One-third of euthyroid patients with melancholia have blunted responses. Some studies show the blunted response as a trait marker while others identify it as a state marker. The underlying mechanism for this abnormal response has not been determined.

4. One carbon cycle metabolism abnormalities

a. S-adenosyl methionine (SAMe), folate, B_{12}, and homocysteine are linked in the "one-carbon cycle," as homocycteine and 5-methylene tetrahydrofolate (5-MTHF), a product of folate, are required for the formation of SAMe. Methylcobalamin, a product of vitamin B_{12}, is a catalyst involved in the production of SAMe. SAMe, in turn, is uniformly distributed throughout the brain where it serves as the major donor of methyl groups required in the synthesis of neuronal messengers and membranes. A number of studies report high homocysteine, low folate, low SAMe, and/or low vitamin B_{12} levels in MDD. Other studies report an abnormally low activity for the enzyme, methionine adenosyltransferase (MAT), which is involved in SAMe production in MDD. There are also reports of a connection between an increased risk of depression and the presence of a certain allele that codes for the

5-MTHF-reductase gene. Finally, low folate levels have been reported to have an adverse impact on both the short and long-term course of MDD.

b. The antidepressant efficacy of SAMe has been studied in over forty open and randomized, controlled trials involving more than 2,200 depressed adults in Europe and the United States. Several double-blind studies suggest that parenteral and/or oral SAMe, compared with a number of standard TCAs such as clomipramine, amitriptyline, and imipramine, were generally equally effective.

5. **Lipid homeostasis imbalance**

a. A number of studies have reported an association between low cholesterol levels and major depression. Low cholesterol levels have also been associated with an increased risk of death from suicide. In contrast, several studies have reported high cholesterol levels in patients with anxiety disorders, or with co-morbid depression and anxiety. Specifically, patients who suffer from panic disorder (PD), generalized anxiety disorder (GAD), obsessive-compulsive disorder (OCD), and post-traumatic stress disorder (PTSD) all have been found to have higher cholesterol levels than patients with anxiety disorders and co-morbid MDD or healthy subjects.

b. Humans cannot desaturate the naturally occurring omega-3 and omega-6 fatty acids (FAs) but must obtain them from the diet. For this reason they are referred to as essential polyunsaturated fatty acids. Studies have reported a connection between low omega-3 fatty acid levels and depression. A recent study reported a relationship between the severity of depression and lower levels of red blood cell membrane omega-3 FAs. In addition, examination of omega-3 levels in cases of depression have shown that serum total omega-3 FAs were decreased in depressed subjects, compared to healthy controls and to individuals with minor depression. Finally, in a separate study, depression severity was shown to correlate positively with omega-6 FA/omega-3 FA ratio in plasma and red blood cell phospholipids, suggesting that a lower level of omega-3 FAs and/or a high level of omega-6 FAs may result in depression. Despite these preliminary findings, the etiology and significance of lipid imbalances in MDD remain, for the most part, unknown.

6. **Brain imaging**

a. **Enlarged ventricles are more frequently found in elderly patients with late-onset MDD compared with those patients whose depression had an early-onset.** Magnetic resonance imaging (MRI) studies have demonstrated regional abnormalities, including decreased volumes of the frontal lobes, the hippocampus, and the basal ganglia. The volumes of connections among the basal ganglia, amygdala, and the hippocampus are important for the regulation of emotions.

b. Studies utilizing positron emission tomography (PET) have shown decreased metabolic activity in the frontal cortex of patients with unipolar depression. This hypofrontality is reversed by a positive response to antidepressant medications.

c. Single photon emission computed tomography (SPECT) studies have shown global reductions in cerebral blood flow in patients with unipolar depression as compared with controls. However, the prefrontal and parietal cortex, the anterior cingulate, the hippocampus, and the amygdala show greater perfusion deficits.

H. Pharmacological Treatment of MDD

Traditional antidepressants can be classified into several categories: TCAs and tetracyclic antidepressants, monoamine oxidase inhibitors (MAOIs), selective serotonin reuptake inhibitors (SSRIs), and atypical antide-

Table 13-1. Tricyclic Antidepressants (TCAs)

Name	*Mechanism: Uptake blocker*	*Alpha$_1$-adrenergic blockade*	*Muscarinic blockade*	*Histamine H_1 blockade*
Amitriptyline (Elavil)	NE and 5-HT	+++	+++	+++
Amoxapine (Asendin)	NE	+++	+	++
Clomipramine (Anafranil)	NE and 5-HT	+++	+++	+
Desipramine (Norpramin)	NE	++	+	+
Doxepin (Sinequan)	NE	+++	++	+++
Imipramine (Tofranil)	NE and 5-HT	+++	++	++
Nortriptyline (Pamelor)	NE	+++	+	+
Protriptyline (Vivactil)	NE	++	+++	++
Trimipramine (Surmontil)	None	+++	++	+++
Tetracyclic antidepressant				
Maprotiline (Ludiomil)	NE	+++	+	+++

+, weak; ++, moderate; +++, strong.

Table 13-2. Selective Serotonin Reuptake Inhibitors (SSRIs)

Name	*Alpha$_1$-adrenergic blockade*	*Muscarinic blockade*	*Histamine H_1 blockade*
Fluoxetine (Prozac)	+/0	+/0	+/0
Fluvoxamine (Luvox)	++	+/0	+/0
Paroxetine (Paxil)	+/0	+	+/0
Sertraline (Zoloft)	+/0	+/0	+/0
Citalopram (Celexa)	+/0	+/0	+/0
Escitalopram oxalate (Lexapro)	+/0	+/0	+/0

0, none; +, weak; ++, moderate.

pressants (see Tables 13-1 to 13-4). In addition, a number of natural remedies, including *hypericum perforatum* (St. John's wort), s-adenosyl methionine (SAMe), folate, and omega-3 fatty acids among others, have been found to possess antidepressant properties in preliminary open trials and/or double-blind placebo controlled trials. Larger, more definitive studies testing the antidepressant efficacy of these natural remedies are underway.

1. **Efficacy**
   a. Double-blind placebo-controlled studies have demonstrated that **all antidepressants are equally effective in treating MDD. Response rates range from 60% to 80% for drugs** and from 30% to 40% for placebo. Remission rates range from 40% to 50% for antidepressants. Response rates are generally defined as a 50% reduction in scores on depression rating scales. As many as 29% to 46% of patients with MDD may show only a partial or no response to an adequate course of an antidepressant (i.e., treatment-resistant depression).
   b. In view of the absence of a difference in response rates or remission rates among the antidepressants, decisions concerning which antidepressant to use are based on side effect profiles, history of response, family history of response, potential for drug interactions, risk of aggravating an existing medical condition (e.g., cardiac conduction defect), risk in overdose, depression subtypes (e.g., atypical depression), and cost.
   c. Once an antidepressant has been chosen, the dose must be titrated slowly to minimize the risk of inducing side effects. The SSRIs have a flat dose-response curve that enables the clinician to achieve a therapeutic dose more quickly. With elderly and medically ill patients on multiple medications, the dose should be increased more slowly, and the final maintenance dose may be one-half or one-third of the usual average dose. An adequate trial for antidepressants is 4–6 weeks at an adequate therapeutic dose. Definitive evidence suggesting that any one antidepressant may work faster than others is lacking.
   d. **Blood levels can be obtained for all of the antidepressants, but a correlation between blood level and therapeutic effect has only been shown for three TCAs (desipramine, nortriptyline, and imipramine).** Other reasons to obtain blood levels include monitoring compliance, risk for toxicity, and potential drug interactions.
   e. The strategies and practices used by clinicians when treating patients with treatment-resistant MDD vary, but include switching to another antidepressant, adding a second antidepressant or a non-antidepressant agent (e.g.,

Table 13-3. Atypical Antidepressants

Name	*Mechanism*	*Alpha$_1$-adrenergic blockade*	*Muscarinic blockade*	*Histamine H_1 blockade*
Bupropion (Wellbutrin)	Blocks NE and DA uptake	+/0	+/0	+/0
Mirtazapine (Remeron)	Releases NE and 5-HT by blocking D_2 receptors; Blocks 5-HT_2 and 5-HT_3 receptors	+	+	+++
Nefazodone (Serzone)	Blocks 5-HT_2 receptor; Blocks NE and 5-HT uptake	+	+/0	+/0
Trazodone (Desyrel)	Blocks 5-HT_2 receptors and blocks 5-HT uptake	+++	+/0	+
Venlafaxine (Effexor)	Blocks 5-HT and NE uptake	+/0	+/0	+/0

0, none; +, weak; ++, moderate; +++, strong.

Table 13-4. Monoamine Oxidase Inhibitors (MAOIs)

Name	*Reversible/ Irreversible*	*Inhibits MAO-A*	*Inhibits MAO-B*
L-Deprenyl (Eldepryl)	Irreversible	—[a]	+
Moclobemide	Reversible	+	—
Phenelzine (Nardil)	Irreversible	+	+
Tranylcypromine (Parnate)	Irreversible	+	+

[a]L-Deprenyl at doses above 10 mg/day inhibits both MAO-A and MAO-B.

lithium, thyroid hormone, an atypical antipsychotic), or electroconvulsive therapy.

2. **Treatment phases**
   a. Treatment is divided into three phases: **the acute phase, the continuation phase, and the maintenance phase. The duration of the acute phase is typically up to 12 weeks,** which is the time it often takes to achieve full remission once there is evidence of a response to an antidepressant.
   b. **The continuation phase** begins when full remission is achieved. This phase **lasts from 4 to 6 months** and is considered a high-risk period for relapse. It is highly recommended that antidepressant medication be continued throughout this period. When the antidepressant is discontinued, it should be tapered gradually over several weeks or months in order to prevent withdrawal (from SSRIs), anticholinergic rebound (from TCAs), or increased risk for relapse. Psychotherapeutic approaches that focus on reducing stress and maintaining compliance are often helpful in preventing relapse.
   c. **The maintenance phase represents the long-term commitment to prophylactic treatment with an antidepressant.** Research has demonstrated that all classes of antidepressants not only treat the acute symptoms of depression but also prevent recurrence of episodes. Longitudinal studies demonstrate that a history of three or more episodes places patients at greater than 80% risk for recurrence. **There is also evidence that maintenance doses of an antidepressant should be the same as those used to achieve full remission.** Other factors that contribute to the risk for relapse include co-morbid psychiatric disorders (e.g., panic disorder), co-morbid substance abuse, dysthymic disorder, and chronic medical illnesses.
3. **Side effects** (see Tables 13-1 to 13-3)
   a. The side effect profile of antidepressants depends on their unwanted receptor-blocking properties and their effect on increasing certain neurotransmitters.
   b. **Side effects are related to receptor-blocking properties:**
      i. **Muscarinic blockade:** dry mouth, constipation, blurred vision, and difficulty initiating urination
      ii. **Alpha$_1$-adrenergic blockade:** orthostatic hypotension
      iii. **Histaminic blockade:** weight gain and sedation
   c. **Side effects are related to receptor activation:**
      i. **Norepinephrine**: rapid heart rate, increased anxiety, insomnia, tremor, and diaphoresis
      ii. **Serotonin**: insomnia, sexual dysfunction, gastrointestinal disturbances (e.g., nausea, vomiting, diarrhea), restlessness (akathisia), headaches, and appetite loss
      iii. **Dopamine**: psychosis, agitation, and elevated blood pressure
4. **Antidepressant discontinuation syndromes**
   Recent reports describe adverse events upon abrupt cessation of SSRIs and venlafaxine, including dizziness, insomnia, nervousness, nausea, and agitation.

I. Electroconvulsive Therapy (ECT)

1. **The primary indications for ECT include failure of several antidepressant trials, severe depression with psychotic features, high risk of suicide, medical emergency due to severe weight loss, previous good response to ECT.**
2. **Contraindications. There are no absolute contraindications to ECT;** however, certain high-risk medical conditions must be reviewed with an appropriate consultant. Some high-risk conditions include hypertension, cardiac arrhythmias, presence of a cardiac pacemaker, myocardial infarction, intracardiac thrombi, anticoagulant therapy, pregnancy, dementia, vascular aneurysms, respiratory disorders (e.g., chronic obstructive pulmonary disease, asthma, emphysema), brain tumor or mass, epilepsy, orthopedic problems, a history or family history of problems with anesthesia.
3. **Efficacy. ECT is more effective than antidepressants in treating MDD,** both with and without psychotic features. Response rates for MDD are between 70% and 90%. The response rate for major depressives with inadequate pre-ECT pharmacotherapy is about 85%, whereas the response rate for major depressives who are medication-resistant pre-ECT is 50%.
4. **Procedure. ECT is given 3 times per week with the average number of treatments between eight and twelve.** Unilateral ECT is the preferred procedure since it is less likely to cause confusion and/or memory disturbances. Bilateral ECT is indicated if there is no response to at least six unilateral treatments.
5. **Side effects. The primary side effect is memory loss for events close to the time of the treatment (retrograde) and for events 3–6 months after completing ECT (anterograde).** Post-ECT confusion is also common and can take up to 7 days to clear. Factors that

contribute to memory loss and confusion include long seizures, older age, a high-intensity stimulus, bilateral electrode placement, inadequate oxygenation, a large number of treatments, and a short interval between treatments. Recent advancements that have reduced memory loss and confusion include brief pulse stimulus, unilateral electrode placement, and hyperventilation with 100% oxygen prior to applying the stimulus.

J. Treatment of Subtypes of MDD

1. **MDD with psychotic features.** The standard treatment of psychotic depression includes use of an antidepressant and an antipsychotic medication. The response rate for an antidepressant alone is 40% and for an antipsychotic alone is 20%, whereas the response rate for the combination of an antidepressant and an antipsychotic medication is 70%. Recent studies have suggested that SSRIs are as effective as TCAs in combination with an antipsychotic medication.
2. **MDD with melancholic features.** Preliminary evidence shows that patients with melancholic depression may preferentially respond to clomipramine, a TCA with a dual effect on both the noradrenergic as well as the serotonergic system. However, conclusive evidence supporting an advantage of clomipramine or dual-acting antidepressants over SSRIs in melancholic depression is lacking.
3. **MDD with atypical features.** The MAOIs and SSRIs have been shown to be more effective in treating atypical depression than TCAs. The response rates for MAOIs and SSRIs are 70%, whereas the response rate for TCAs is 50%. Thus SSRIs and MAOIs are considered first-line treatments for atypical depression.
4. **MDD with seasonal features.** Artificial light with an intensity of 2,500 lux placed 1 meter from the patient is very effective in treating seasonal affective disorder (SAD). The response rate is as high as 75%, which is similar to the use of antidepressant medications. Light therapy is more effective in treating patients with SAD than patients with non-seasonal MDD. Patients can be exposed to the light at any time of the day; however, some patients require the exposure to light in the morning. Response to light occurs within a week, and relapse may occur as soon as 3–4 days after discontinuation. Light therapy should begin in the fall and be continued through the spring. SSRIs, MAOIs, and bupropion have also been shown to be as effective as light therapy for the treatment of SAD.

K. Psychotherapy

1. **Cognitive-behavioral therapy (CBT) and interpersonal psychotherapy (IPT)** have been shown in research studies to be effective for the treatment of mild to moderate depression. Brief forms of psychodynamic psychotherapies and supportive psychotherapy have also been considered as helpful by many clinicians.
2. **Cognitive-behavioral therapy (CBT)**
   a. The cognitive-behavioral approach for the treatment of depression focuses on the impact of maladaptive belief systems on patients' views of themselves, their environment, and their future. Patients who are depressed tend to see themselves as defective, their environment as unsupportive and too demanding, and their future as unchanging and hopeless. The primary tasks are to identify distorted beliefs and then to challenge their validity by using a variety of cognitive-behavioral techniques.
   b. **Cognitive therapy has been shown to be as effective as antidepressants in outpatients with mild to moderate acute depression.** However, antidepressants appear to be more effective than CBT in the treatment of acute severe depression in psychiatric inpatients.
   c. In one study, cognitive therapy was as effective as antidepressants in preventing relapse. Another study demonstrated that, for responders to cognitive therapy and responders to antidepressants who had their treatment discontinued, cognitive therapy-treated patients had lower relapse rates compared with antidepressant-treated patients at 2-year follow-up (21% vs. 50%, respectively).
3. **Interpersonal psychotherapy (IPT)**
   a. IPT focuses on interpersonal losses, role disputes and transitions, social isolation, and deficits in social skills as contributing factors for the precipitation of depression. Techniques, such as role-playing, are used to develop social skills, and role expectations are clarified in conjoint sessions for role disputes. IPT is focused on the present, and it is conducted by the use of a manual. It is time-limited, usually lasting 16 weeks. It makes use of psychoeducation and teaches patients that depression is a medical illness.
   b. **Studies evaluating the efficacy of IPT in the acute treatment of depression have concluded that IPT is more effective than antidepressants in treating depressed mood, suicidal ideation, and lack of interest, whereas antidepressants are more effective for disturbances of appetite and sleep.** In comparison to IPT, antidepressants may offer more rapid treatment response.
   c. Studies evaluating the efficacy of IPT for the maintenance treatment of depression have shown that, in a 3-year follow-up study, IPT relapse-free survival rates were 30–40%, whereas supportive care relapse-free survival rates were 10%. Also, patients receiving high-quality IPT had 2-year survival rates similar to those achieved with antidepressants. Inconsistent use of IPT may account for some of the differences between survival rates for IPT and antidepressants.

L. Combination Psychotherapy and Antidepressant Treatment

1. Data from studies that combined psychodynamic psychotherapy, cognitive therapy, or IPT with antidepressants have not confirmed an advantage for combined treatment. For the treatment of mild to moderate depression, an antidepressant or one of the brief forms of

psychotherapy is recommended. For severe depression, initial treatment involves an antidepressant.

2. Combined therapy should be used if treatment with one modality fails to produce a complete response, if the depression is chronic, or if multiple symptoms, are present. Problems with assertiveness might be more amenable to psychotherapy, whereas an appetite disturbance would likely respond best to an antidepressant.

III. Dysthymic Disorder

A. DSM-IV Criteria

1. **Depressed mood** (or an irritable mood in children and adolescents that lasts for at least 1 year) **must be present for most of the day, more days than not, for at least 2 years.**
2. When depressed, the patient exhibits at least two of the following symptoms: poor appetite or overeating, insomnia or hypersomnia, low energy or fatigue, low self-esteem, poor concentration or difficulty making decisions, or feelings of hopelessness.
3. During a 2-year period (1 year in children or adolescents) of the disturbance, the person has never been symptom-free for more than 2 months.
4. A lack of evidence for a major depressive episode during the first 2 years of the disturbance.
5. No history of mania, hypomania, or cyclothymia.
6. Symptoms are not caused by a medical condition, drug of abuse, or a medication.
7. The symptoms do not occur exclusively during the course of psychotic disorders.
8. The symptoms cause clinically significant distress or impairment in psychosocial functioning.

B. The lifetime prevalence for dysthymic disorder is 6%, and the point prevalence is 3%.

C. Course

Dysthymic disorder generally exhibits a slow and insidious onset that begins in childhood, adolescence, or early adulthood. When dysthymic disorder is co-morbid with MDD, the condition is referred to as a "double depression." The presence of dysthymic disorder increases the risk for an episode of MDD in vulnerable individuals.

IV. Depressive Disorder Not Otherwise Specified

A. DSM-IV Criteria

1. This category includes depressive disorders that do not meet criteria for MDD, dysthymic disorder, adjustment disorder with depressed mood, or adjustment disorder with mixed anxiety and depressed mood.
2. Examples include the following:
   a. **Minor depressive disorder,** which is manifest by at least 2 weeks of depressive symptoms but fewer than five of the required symptoms for MDD.
   b. **Recurrent brief depressive disorder,** which is manifest by depressive episodes lasting from 2 days to 2 weeks, and which occurs at least once a month for 1 year.
   c. **Premenstrual dysphoric disorder,** which is manifest by markedly depressed mood, marked anxiety, marked affective lability, and a decreased interest in activities during the last week of the luteal phase of the menstrual period. Each of these symptoms resolves within a few days of the onset of menses. The symptoms must be present during most menstrual cycles during the past year, be totally absent for at least 1 week after the menstrual period, and be severe enough to interfere with work, school, or usual activities.
   d. **Post-psychotic depressive disorder,** which is a major depressive episode that occurs during the residual phase of schizophrenia.
   e. **Depressive disorder NOS,** which is also used in situations where the clinician has identified a depressive disorder but is unable to determine if it is primary or secondary to a medical condition or to use of a psychoactive substance.

Suggested Readings

Alpert, J.E., Mischoulon, D., Nierenberg, A.A., & Fava, M. (2000). Nutrition and depression: Focus on folate. *Nutrition, 16*(7–8), 544–546.

American Psychiatric Association. (1994). Mood disorders. In *Diagnostic and statistical manual of mental disorders* (4th ed., pp. 317–391). Washington, DC: American Psychiatric Press.

American Psychiatric Association. (1993). *Practice guideline for major depressive disorder in adults*. Washington, DC: American Psychiatric Press.

Baghai, T.C., Schule, C., Zwanzger, P., et al. (2002). Hypothalamic-pituitary-adrenocortical axis dysregulation in patients with major depression is influenced by the insertion/deletion polymorphism in the angiotensin I-converting enzyme gene. *Neuroscience Letter, 16,* 328(3), 299–303.

Bernstein, J.G. (1995). *Drug therapy in psychiatry* (3rd ed., pp. 112–194). St. Louis: Mosby.

Blackburn, I., Bishop, S., Glen, A., et al. (1981), The efficacy of cognitive therapy in depression: A treatment trial using cognitive therapy and pharmacotherapy, each alone and in combination. *British Journal of Psychiatry, 139,* 181–189.

Cassano, P., Fava, M. (2002). Depression and public health: An overview. *Journal of Psychosomatic Research, 53*(4), 849–857

Danish University Antidepressant Group. (1990). Paroxetine: A selective serotonin reuptake inhibitor showing better tolerance, but weaker antidepressant effect than clomipramine in a controlled multicenter study. *Journal of Affective Disorders, 18,* 289–299.

Dording, C.M. (2000). Antidepressant augmentation and combinations. *Psychiatric Clinics of North America, 23*(4), 743–755

Dubzovsky, S.L., & Buzan, R. (1999). Mood disorders. In R.E. Hales, S.C. Yudofsky, & J.A. Talbott (Eds.), *The American Psychiatric Press textbook of psychiatry* (3rd ed., pp. 479–565). Washington, DC: American Psychiatric Press.

Fava, M. (2000). Management of nonresponse and intolerance: Switching strategies. *Journal of Clinical Psychiatry, 61*(suppl 2), 10–12.

Fava, M., & Davidson, K.G. (1996). Definition and epidemiology of treatment-resistant depression. *Psychiatric Clinics of North America, 19*, 179–200.

Fava, M., & Kendler, K.S. (2000). Major depressive disorder. *Neuron, 28*(2), 335–341.

Frazer, A. (1997). Antidepressants. *Journal of Clinical Psychiatry, 58*(suppl 6), 9–23.

Iosifescu, D.V., & Renshaw, P.F. (2003). 31P-magnetic resonance spectroscopy and thyroid hormones in major depressive disorder: Towards a bioenergetic mechanism in depression? *Harvard Review of Psychiatry, 11*(2), 1–13.

Klerman, G., Weissman, M., Rounsaville, B., & Chevron, E. (1984). *Interpersonal psychotherapy of depression*. New York: Basic Books.

Mischoulon, D., & Rosenbaum, J. (Eds.). (2002). *Natural medications for psychiatric disorders: Considering the alternatives*. Philadelphia: Lippincott Williams & Wilkins.

Nierenberg, A.A., & DeCecco, L.M. (2001). Definitions of antidepressant treatment response, remission, nonresponse, partial response, and other relevant outcomes: A focus on treatment-resistant depression. *Journal of Clinical Psychiatry, 62*(suppl 16), 5–9.

Papakostas, G.I., & Fava, M. (In press). SAMe in the treatment of depression: A comprehensive review of the literature. *Current Psychiatry Reports*.

Parker, G., Hadzi-Pavlovic, D., & Pedic, F. (1992). Psychotic (delusional) depression: A meta-analysis of physical treatments. *Journal of Affective Disorders, 24*, 17–24.

Perlis, R.H., Iosifescu, D.V., & Renshaw, P. (2003). Biological response predictors in mood disorders. *Psychiatric Clinics of North America, 26*(2), 323–344.

Philibert, R., Caspers, K., Langbehn, D., Troughton, E.P., Yucuis, R., Sandhu, H.K., & Cadoret, R.J. (2002). The association of a HOPA polymorphism with major depression and phobia. *Comprehensive Psychiatry, 43*(5), 404–410.

Quitkin, F.M., Harrison, W., Stewart, J.W., et al. (1991). Response to phenelzine and imipramine in placebo nonresponders with atypical depression. *Archives of General Psychiatry, 48*, 319–323.

Rosenbaum, J.F., Fava, M. (1998). Approach to the patient with depression. In T.A. Stern, J.B., Herman, & P.L. Slavin (Eds.), *The MGH guide to psychiatry in primary care*, pp. 1–14. New York: McGraw-Hill.

Rosenbaum, J.F., Fava, M., Hoog, S.L., et al. (1998). Selective serotonin reuptake inhibitor discontinuation syndrome: A randomized clinical trial. *Biologic Psychiatry, 15*, 44(2), 77–87.

Rosenbaum, J.F., Fava, M., Nierenberg, A.A., & Sachs, G.S. (1995). Treatment-resistant mood disorders. In G.O. Gabbard (Ed.), *Treatments of psychiatric disorders* (2nd ed., pp. 1275–1328). Washington, DC: American Psychiatric Press.

Rothschild, A.J. (1996). Management of psychotic, treatment-resistant depression. *Psychiatric Clinics of North America, 19*(2), 237–252.

Wright, J., Thase, M., & Sensky, T. (1992). Cognitive and biological therapies: A combined approach. In J. Wright, M. Thaes, A. Beck, & J. Ludgate (Eds.), *Cognitive therapy with inpatients*, pp. 193–218. New York: Guilford Press.

Chapter 14

Bipolar Disorder

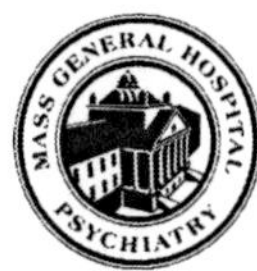

ROY H. PERLIS AND S. NASSIR GHAEMI

I. Overview

Mood disorders are among the most common psychiatric conditions. Although community studies suggest that around 5–10% of the general population in the United States experience a major depressive episode at least once in a lifetime, **bipolar disorder occurs in about 1–2% of the population.** Milder variations of bipolar disorder, such as cyclothymia, may account for another 2–5% of the population. Bipolar disorder may vary widely in its presentation, sharing features with both major depressive disorder (MDD) and schizophrenia. **An individual patient may look very different when manic or depressed; thus, bipolar disorder is frequently misdiagnosed.** Although effective treatment can result in almost complete recovery for many patients, this remains a potentially lethal illness, with a **lifetime risk of suicide among untreated patients as great as 15%.** Bipolar disorder is usually due to a primary mood disturbance, but it may be mimicked by medical conditions and by substance abuse.

II. Epidemiology

The lifetime prevalence of classical bipolar disorder is approximately 1%. Higher estimates are reported in studies that carefully assess milder symptoms of mood elevation and include cyclothymia and bipolar disorder, not otherwise specified (with a 2–5% lifetime prevalence). Of those identified as bipolar by epidemiologic studies, only one-third have already been diagnosed by a physician, and, of those, **only 27% have ever received treatment.** This rate of undertreatment is among the worst of any psychiatric illness.

A. Gender

The incidence of bipolar disorder is equivalent among males and females, unlike unipolar depression, which is more frequent in women. Some but not all studies suggest that a rapid-cycling bipolar course may be more common among females.

B. Age

According to recent studies, the average age of onset of bipolar disorder is around 19 years, with most cases presenting between 15 and 20. The reported age of onset of affective disorders has decreased in the last few decades, which likely reflects earlier diagnosis. The diagnosis of bipolar disorder in children is a subject of active research; in this age group accurate diagnosis may be complicated by developmental issues and co-morbidity, such as attention deficit hyperactivity disorder (ADHD). **New-onset bipolar disorder is rare after the fifth decade of life; when it occurs, it is usually secondary to a medical/neurological condition, or to the effects of medications, particularly antidepressants and steroids.**

C. Ethnicity

The prevalence of bipolar disorder is believed to be similar across ethnic groups. Some ethnic groups (African-Americans and Hispanics) with bipolar disorder may be more likely to be misdiagnosed with schizophrenia.

D. Socioeconomic Status

Unlike schizophrenia, bipolar disorder is not generally associated with a downward drift of socioeconomic class. Members of lower socioeconomic classes who have bipolar disorder may be more likely to be misdiagnosed as having schizophrenia.

E. Individual Factors

Bipolar disorder is associated with a lifetime rate of completed suicide of up to 15%. It is associated with extremely high rates of divorce, an occupational history of numerous jobs, often excellent academic achievement followed by a decline in occupational performance, and generally chaotic life histories (both personally and socially). Bipolar disorder is associated with elevated IQ in some studies. Women with bipolar disorder have a life expectancy that is diminished by 9 years.

F. Co-morbid Conditions

Co-morbidity may be the norm rather than the exception in bipolar disorder. **60% of individuals with bipolar disorder develop substance abuse at some point in their lifetimes.**

Anxiety disorders are also quite common, with a lifetime prevalence of anxiety disorders of approximately 50%. Among the most prevalent are social anxiety disorder, panic disorder, and post-traumatic stress disorder. Finally, attention deficit disorder may be an under-recognized co-morbidity in bipolar children and adults.

III. Differential Diagnosis

A. Differentiation from Other Axis I Disorders

Although depressive symptoms are common in all of the varieties of mood syndromes, technically the term "depression" is not a specific diagnosis but a symptom, like "fever." This can lead to confusion among patients and clinicians alike. Episodes of mood elevation (mania, hypomania, mixed states) and depression form the building blocks of mood disorders. The degree of severity of these episodes, and the presence or absence of mood elevation, determine the precise diagnosis.

1. **Major depressive episodes are identified using the standard DSM criteria (see chapter 13).** Some but not all studies suggest that atypical depressive symptoms (i.e., increased sleep, increased appetite, preserved reactivity of mood, leaden heaviness of the limbs, and oversensitivity to rejection) may be more common in bipolar depression than MDD.
2. **Manic episodes are associated with a period of irritable or euphoric mood, along with associated symptoms of mania as discussed below. Note it is *not* just euphoric mood.** While many persons with mania report "high" or "happy" mood, others have only an *irritable* mood. Manic episodes, while classically involving euphoria, can be characterized by an irritable mood. Either type can still be described as pure mania.
3. **Mixed states occur when depressed mood co-exists with manic symptoms;** during a mixed episode, patients meet mood and neurovegetative criteria for both depressive and manic episodes simultaneously. Mixed manic episodes are as common as are pure manic episodes.
4. **Bipolar disorder needs to be distinguished clearly from MDD, sometimes called unipolar depression.** In MDD, patients experience depressive episodes but never experience periods of mood elevation. Mood "swings"—rapid shifts in mood—may be seen in any mood disorder, or even among normal individuals, and are not by themselves indicative of bipolar disorder. **It takes *only one episode* of mood elevation for a diagnosis of bipolar disorder to be made, no matter how many times an individual becomes depressed.**
5. **Bipolar disorder must also be distinguished from schizophrenia. Psychotic features (most often delusions or auditory hallucinations) may be seen in 50% of bipolar patients during either manic/mixed or depressive episodes.** A key difference from schizophrenia is that, while schizophrenic patients exhibit depressive symptoms or agitation, they do not experience manic or mixed episodes.
6. **The presence of a single manic or hypomanic episode trumps all of the above diagnoses:** schizophrenia and unipolar depression are diagnosed only if bipolar disorder is absent. **Only schizoaffective disorder, bipolar type, remains a possible diagnosis once a manic/hypomanic episode is diagnosed:** When psychosis lasts for 2 weeks outside of a mood episode, schizoaffective disorder, but not bipolar disorder, may be present. In other words, schizoaffective disorder is distinguished from bipolar disorder by the persistence of psychotic symptoms in the absence of a manic, mixed or depressive episode.
7. **Distractibility and impulsivity are among DSM criteria for both bipolar disorder and attention deficit disorder; hence these two conditions can be confused, particularly in children. The key feature that distinguishes bipolar disorder from these other conditions is the manic or hypomanic episode; distractibility or impulsivity alone is insufficient for a mood episode.** Unlike bipolar patients, those with attention deficit disorder will continue to experience these symptoms in the absence of other mood symptoms. However, as the two diagnoses may co-exist, patients must often be reevalu-

Table 14-1. Distinguishing Criteria for DSM Mood Disorders

Diagnosis	*Manic/mixed symptom criteria*	*Depressive symptom criteria*
Major depressive disorder	Never	Yes (Major depressive episodes)
Dysthymic disorder	Never	Yes (but not major depressive episode) Depressed mood, more days than not, for 2+ years
Bipolar I	Yes At least one manic/mixed episode	Not necessary (usually major depressive episodes)
Bipolar II	Never manic/mixed episodes At least one hypomanic episode	Yes Major depressive episodes
Cyclothymic disorder	Numerous periods with hypomanic symptoms for 2+ years	Yes Never major depressive episode, but numerous periods with depressive symptoms
Bipolar, not otherwise specified	Yes (does not meet criteria for bipolar I, II or cyclothymia)	Not necessary

Adapted from Hirschfeld, R.M.A., et al. (2002). *Practice guideline for the treatment of patients with bipolar disorder (revision).* American Psychological Association.

ated for symptoms of attention deficit disorder once their mood episodes are adequately treated.

B. Subtypes of Bipolar Disorder (see Table 14-1)

In **bipolar disorder, type I,** at least one manic episode is identified, with or without major depression. In **bipolar disorder, type II,** not a single manic episode is identified, but at least one hypomanic episode, and at least one major depressive episode, is identified. In **cyclothymia,** symptoms of major depression do not reach the threshold for a diagnosis of a major depressive episode, and mood elevation, while present, does not reach threshold for diagnosis of a manic episode. Finally, in bipolar disorder not otherwise specified, mood elevation is present but patients do not meet full criteria for any of the above three diagnoses. **The key difference between mania and hypomania is that mania is associated with significant social or occupational dysfunction** (often involving spending sprees, sexual indiscretions, reckless driving, and impulsive traveling), **or with hospitalization, while hypomania is not.**

The diagnosis of a rapid-cycling bipolar disorder identifies an illness with a course of numerous (defined as four or more in a year) mood episodes.

IV. Theories on the Etiology and Neurobiology of Bipolar Disorder

The biological basis of bipolar disorder remains poorly understood. Recent investigations have focused on transmembrane and intracellular signaling, neurons and glial cells, and functional neuroimaging. These lines of evidence are beginning to identify brain abnormalities in bipolar patients and mechanisms of action of mood-stabilizing medications. Particular abnormalities may include:

A. Disruption of monoamine signaling and the hypothalamic-pituitary-adrenal axis
B. Changes in signal transduction involving protein kinase C and G-proteins
C. Abnormal regulation of factors involved in cell survival or neurotrophic pathways
D. Brain region-specific reduction in neurons or glial cells
E. Abnormalities in brain regions, including ventral and medial prefrontal cortex and amygdala

V. The Impact of Genetics and Environment

A. Genetics

Like other major mental illnesses, family and twin studies demonstrate that bipolar disorder has an important heritable component. Studies of twins indicate that the heritability of bipolar disorder may be approximately 60%, meaning that 60% of the risk is the result of heritable (though not necessarily entirely genetic) factors. The inheritance of bipolar disorder **is non-Mendelian, suggesting that multiple genes likely contribute to the risk of developing bipolar disorder.** Linkage studies and candidate gene studies are beginning to identify genes that may be associated with bipolar disorder.

B. Environment

Based on twin studies, the environmental influence is not likely to be familial or shared, but rather due to specific environmental effects that are unique to each individual. Obstetric complications, intrauterine viral infections, neurodevelopmental abnormalities in childhood, use of hallucinogenic drugs, and psychosocial trauma have been proposed as possible environmental influences. It is likely that the most potent environmental influences on the etiology of the illness occur early in life, before the illness's typical onset in adolescence and early adulthood.

Psychosocial stressors later in adulthood, such as the death of family and friends, the end of romantic relationships, and occupational stress, often serve as environmental triggers for mood episodes, acting on the underlying susceptibility to illness established earlier in life.

VI. Course of the Illness

A. Chronicity and Course

Bipolar disorder is generally both a chronic and a recurrent condition. A single manic episode heralds the near-certainty of future manic or depressive episodes and the need for long-term medication treatment. The interval between episodes is generally believed to decrease with time, then to plateau. Untreated, bipolar patients may experience episodes yearly, or even more frequently.

Even between DSM-defined mood episodes, some patients may continue to experience depressive symptoms which, while they do not meet criteria for a major depressive episode, continue to affect their functioning. Patients may spend a third or more of their time in either a full mood episode, or a subthreshold episode.

B. Seasonal Variation

Seasonal features are not uncommon in bipolar disorder; manic episodes occur more often in the summer, and depressive episodes in the winter or spring. This pattern should not be confused with that of seasonal affective disorder, a diagnosis made only when mood episodes almost always occur solely in certain seasons, and almost invariably fail to occur outside of those seasons for a number of years. Many patients who meet criteria for seasonal affective disorder are diagnosable with bipolar disorder, type II, based on the experience of major depression in the winter followed by hypomania in the spring.

C. Duration of Episodes

Depressive episodes (with a mean untreated duration of 6–12 months) tend to last longer than manic episodes (with a mean untreated duration of 3–6 months) in bipolar disorder.

VII. Evaluation

A. The Depressed Patient

Bipolar patients often present for treatment during a major depressive episode. In many cases, they do not recognize hypomanic episodes as indicative of illness. Indeed, all patients who meet criteria for major depression need to be screened for the presence of lifetime manic or hypomanic symptoms to rule out bipolar disorder. They must be screened for current symptoms of mania or hypomania to rule out a mixed episode. In fact, "I feel depressed" is a common complaint during mixed episodes.

Other than concurrent manic or hypomanic symptoms, there is no foolproof way to identify a bipolar depressed episode from current symptoms alone. While atypical depressive symptoms may be noted, they are also common among patients with MDD. Even a family history of bipolar disorder does not in and of itself make a diagnosis of bipolar depression. Ultimately, the best way to differentiate a currently depressed individual's diagnosis as bipolar depression is to screen carefully for past manic or hypomanic episodes.

B. The Manic Patient

A diagnosis of mania requires that a patient has experienced irritable or euphoric mood, with three (if euphoric) or four (if irritable) of the seven cardinal symptoms of mania, for at least 1 week. The cardinal symptoms of mania are easily remembered by a mnemonic (**"DIGFAST"**) that suggests the excessive activity of mania.

1. **Distractibility** is the most common manic symptom, but also the most subjective. It involves the inability to maintain one's focus on tasks for any extended duration.
2. **Injudiciousness,** or impulsivity (e.g., pleasure-seeking activities that do not display usual judgment, and, unlike increased goal-directed activities, are dysfunctional). Four common varieties are sexual indiscretions, reckless driving, spending sprees, and sudden traveling.
3. **Grandiosity** reflects inflated self-esteem. This can be delusional, or, in milder cases, it involves increased self-confidence out of proportion to one's circumstances.
4. **Flight of ideas,** or racing thoughts, indicates a rapid progression of one's thought processes.
5. **Activities** (i.e., an increase in goal-directed activities) that are functional and often appear useful fall into four categories:
   a. **Social:** increased socializing, calling friends, going out more than usual.
   b. **Sexual:** increased libido or hypersexuality.
   c. **Work:** increased productivity, cleaning the house more than usual.
   d. **School:** producing many projects, studying more than usual.

   In all cases, usual levels of activity need to be based on a comparison with activity levels during the euthymic state.
6. **Sleep** refers to **decreased *need* for sleep.** It differs from the insomnia of depression, which simply involves decreased sleep. An excellent way to differentiate the two is to ask about the patient's energy level. In mania, despite decreased sleep, the energy level is average or high. In depressive insomnia, it is low.
7. **Talkativeness** referes to speech that is pressured or a tendency to be more talkative, and perhaps more difficult to interrupt, than usual. Pressured speech may be present in the mental status examination. If not, one can ask the patient to compare their level of talkativeness with their speech during euthymic periods.

To qualify for a diagnosis of a manic episode, in addition to the above criteria, the patient must experience **significant social or occupational dysfunction** (which may include hospitalization) as a result of the above symptoms. If there is no social or occupational dysfunction, then a hypomanic episode is diagnosed. Also, for a diagnosis of a manic episode, the symptoms must last at least 1 week (or require hospitalization). If they last less than 1 week, but at least 4 days, then a diagnosis of hypomanic episode is made. An episode of hypomanic symptoms which lasts for more than 4 days is still considered hypomania if no dysfunction occurs; conversely, manic symptoms for fewer than 7 days constitute a manic episode if they result in hospitalization.

C. Ruling Out Secondary Mood Disorders

The medical causes of secondary mood disorders fall into several broad categories; these are discussed below in order of descending importance (see Table 14-2).

1. **Medications and drugs of abuse. Substance abuse** is the most common culprit; cocaine, in particular, may precipitate mania or induce manic-like symptoms. Drugs used to treat a variety of medical conditions can also precipitate mania or hypomania; among these, the most common classes are **antidepressants and steroids.**
2. **Neurological disorders.** These are the most common non-psychiatric illnesses that cause mood disorders. Probably the most common neurological disorder associated with mania is **multiple sclerosis. Frontal lobe syndromes,** whether due to head trauma, dementia, or stroke, can also simulate manic symptoms, especially impulsivity and hypersexuality. **Temporal lobe epilepsy,** particularly when the focus is in the non-dominant hemisphere, is associated with manic symptoms during the ictal period.
3. **Endocrine disorders.** These are less common, and mood disorders are unusual in the absence of other more characteristic physical symptoms. **Hyperthyroidism** and **Cushing's syndrome** may be associated with mania.

Table 14-2. Common Secondary Causes of Mania

Substance abuse/intoxication/withdrawal
Alcohol, cocaine, amphetamines, caffeine
Medications
Antidepressants, steroids, L-dopa, amphetamines, barbiturates, adrenocorticotropin (ACTH)
Neurological conditions
Multiple sclerosis, frontal lobe syndromes, temporal lobe epilepsy, stroke, head trauma, subcortical dementias, encephalitis, Huntington's disease, pseudobulbar palsy
Endocrine conditions
Hyperthyroidism, Cushing's syndrome
Other medical illnesses
Infections: herpes simplex encephalitis, HIV encephalitis, syphilis, other viral or parasitic encephalitides
Autoimmune disease: systemic lupus erythematosus
Metabolic states: hypoglycemia, hypoxia

4. **Other. Infectious diseases, metabolic states, and immunologic diseases** can produce mood disorders. Herpes simplex encephalitis and human immunodeficiency virus (HIV) infection, which may affect limbic areas of the brain, often simulates manic symptoms. Systemic lupus erythematosus is the most common autoimmune condition associated with mania. Hypoglycemia and hypoxia can each lead to mood instability.

In the treatment of secondary mood disorders, whenever possible the offending agent should be removed or the underlying medical condition treated. In the case of chronic medical conditions, long-term treatment with antidepressant or antimanic agents may be required to minimize mood symptoms.

VIII. Approach to the Bipolar Patient

A. General Strategies

1. **Establish a therapeutic alliance. Non-compliance with medications is a major problem** in bipolar disorder. Many medications utilized in the treatment of bipolar disorder carry substantial side-effect burdens and associated encumbrances, such as the need for blood draws. Some patients may exhibit a marked lack of insight into the nature of their condition, particularly regarding manic or hypomanic symptoms. They may be reluctant to take medications that they perceive as preventing mood elevation, misinterpreting the goal of mood stabilization as the absence of any positive or negative mood. Wherever possible, the treatment of bipolar disorder should represent a collaboration between patient and physician.
2. **Don't be fooled by depression or psychosis.** Clinicians make two common mistakes that lead to misdiagnosis. The first is to assume that, if patients experience psychotic symptoms, they must have schizophrenia. However, **one cannot make a diagnosis of schizophrenia based solely on the presence of psychotic symptoms.** Instead, the diagnosis of an affective disorder is based on affective symptoms; the diagnosis of schizophrenia is only made after having ruled out any affective disorder.

   The second, and more common, mistake is to assume that when patients experience depressive symptoms, MDD is present. However, as noted earlier, **depression is not just a diagnosis, it is a symptom.** Like "fever," depressive symptoms need further analysis to determine the underlying diseases. If present, one must ask, what type of depression is this? There are multiple possibilities: **It is either secondary (e.g., to substance abuse or a general medical condition) or primary.** If primary, it may be associated either with bipolar disorder or MDD. Secondary and bipolar depression need to be ruled out before MDD can be diagnosed.

   In summary, not all psychosis is schizophrenia, and not all depression is MDD.
3. **Obtain collateral history** from family, friends, or other treaters wherever possible. **As with numerous other psychiatric conditions, one cannot definitively rule out bipolar disorder based on an individual's self-report in a clinical interview,** even after inquiring about all possible manic symptoms. It appears that *part of the illness* is that the patient does not recognize possessing the illness. This *lack of insight* is more common in bipolar disorder than it is in those with unipolar depression. **Thus, the clinician cannot rely solely on an individual's self-report, which may be hindered by lack of awareness or denial of symptoms.** Diagnosis is based on the clinician's judgment, after searching all available sources of clinical information.
4. **Establish safety.** Assess for the possibility of suicide and violence. **Acutely manic patients usually require hospitalization. Depressed patients with an acute risk of suicide, or those whose depression is so severe that it impairs their ability to care for themselves, will also require hospitalization.** Not surprisingly, suicide risk is greatest during depressive episodes.

B. Goals of the Assessment

A major goal of an assessment for bipolar disorder is to determine if the patient has had at least one manic or hypomanic episode at any point in their lifetime. This will guide the diagnosis of a bipolar subtype and influence treatment.

C. Specific Elements of History

1. **Obtaining a medical history. Rule out possible secondary medical causes of bipolar disorder.** This requires that one take a careful medical history and obtain blood and urine samples to screen for the illnesses described previously.
2. **Obtaining a substance abuse history. Rule out secondary substance abuse-related mood disorders.** This requires taking a careful history as well as obtaining blood and urine screening samples. Remember that the presence of substance abuse does not establish a secondary mood disorder; 60% of individuals with bipolar disorder experience substance abuse at some point in their lives. Rather, **bipolar disorder would be secondary to substance abuse only if episodes of abnormal mood invariably occur during periods of substance abuse and not outside of those periods,** or (in those without a history of abstinence) if consistent substance abuse precedes the onset of a mood disorder.
3. **Assess manic symptoms. Use the DIGFAST mnemonic. Establish time-frames in which to use the mnemonic.** At least two time-frames are considered: current (the past 1–2 weeks), and past. When assessing for past manic symptoms, begin by assessing for mania, requiring that patients recall time-frames of 1 week or longer when they might have experienced elevated or irritable mood, decreased need for sleep, or other manic symptoms. If not volunteered, the stereotypic impulsive behaviors of mania (sexual indiscretions, reckless driving, spending sprees, impulsive traveling) should be assessed. One possible question is, "Have you ever had a period of time where you took more risks than usual, or made judgments that would be unusual for you?" If mania is not identified, then hypomania at any point must be assessed. Special attention should be given to establishing a patient's "normal" baseline in mood and energy. **Hypomania** represents any deviation above this baseline for 4 days or longer, associated with some manic symptoms but **without significant social or occupational dysfunction.** If significant dysfunction exists, mania should be diagnosed, even in the absence of the stereotypic behaviors described above. Conversely, because hypomania may not be experienced as illness, identifying these symptoms may require careful probing.
4. **Assess the family history.** Many but certainly not all patients with bipolar disorder have a family history of psychiatric illness. This history may include mood disorders, substance abuse, or schizophrenia. In part this variability may be the result of prior misdiagnosis of family members; however, family members of bipolar patients do not necessarily present with identical diagnoses, probably because bipolar disorder is a polygenic disease.
5. **Assess prior psychiatric treatment.** Frequently, individuals with bipolar disorder have been treated with antidepressants alone, which can worsen the course of the illness by precipitating mania or increasing the frequency of mood episodes (see below). Other than treatment-emergent mania or hypomania, or change in frequency of episodes during treatment, other hints of a bipolar diagnosis may include an initial rapid response to antidepressant agents followed by a loss of response, treatment resistance to multiple antidepressant trials, or a good response to the addition of a mood-stabilizing medication, such as lithium, to antidepressants.
6. **Assess for the presence of co-morbid psychiatric conditions.** Common co-morbid conditions include anxiety disorders (e.g., panic disorder and obsessive-compulsive disorder [OCD]), post-traumatic stress disorder, cluster B personality disorders (especially borderline personality), attention deficit disorder, and eating disorders. These co-morbid conditions may influence treatment decisions.
7. **Complete a mental status examination. Focus the examination on affect.** If a patient is currently manic, the **affect is either euphoric, irritable, or labile.** If a patient is currently in a mixed state or is depressed, the affect is usually depressed. Anxiety may or may not be present. Patients may express their mood as "down" or "sad" when depressed, but, when manic, mood may be reported as "fine." In some cases, euphoric mood may be described as "giddy," "high," or "up." Thought content is usually normal, although, in mild cases of mania, paranoid or grandiose ideas of reference may be present. Obsessions may occur with co-morbid OCD. In many cases of mania, thought process is characterized by **flight of ideas,** or a sense that one's thoughts are racing faster than one can speak them. Otherwise thoughts can be normal, circumstantial, or tangential. Looseness of associations tends to occur in patients with psychotic features. **Speech** in mania is often, but not always, characterized by a sense of **pressure.** Patients may be **overtalkative** and unduly prolong conversations. Patients may display psychomotor agitation, pacing or having difficulty sitting still in the chair, particularly during manic episodes. Psychomotor slowing may be observed during depression. Cognition is generally intact, with normal orientation to person, place, and time, and unimpaired immediate, short-term and long-term recall. (Disorientation should raise concern for delirium, which may be superficially similar to mania.) Concentration is often impaired in depression and mania; manic patients are often **distractible** and unable to maintain focus without jumping from topic to topic. Finally, suicidal and homicidal ideation should always be assessed.

8. **If current or past manic symptoms are identified, then the following features of the history should be determined:**
   a. Age of onset of first mania or hypomania
   b. Age of onset of first major depression
   c. Number of lifetime manic or hypomanic episodes
   d. Number of lifetime major depressive episodes
   e. Typical cycle of episodes (mania followed by depression followed by well interval, or depression followed by mania followed by well interval, or continuous cycling)
   f. Last and longest periods of euthymia
   g. Age of first psychiatric treatment
   h. Age of first bipolar diagnosis and previous psychiatric diagnoses, if present
   i. Presence of psychotic symptoms during any episode
   j. Sleep pattern
   k. Intentions to become pregnant, which may influence choice of pharmacotherapy
   l. Effect of illness on social and occupational functioning
   m. Last period of best occupational functioning

D. Management of the Bipolar Patient

1. **Assess and treat baseline medical and substance abuse conditions. Thyroid function, in particular, should be assessed in an individual with rapid-cycling bipolar disorder, since subclinical hypothyroidism may contribute to rapid-cycling. Substance abuse** should be assessed and treated aggressively while also treating the primary mood disorder.
2. **Maximize mood-stabilizing treatments.** The definition of mood stabilizers, which in the past referred primarily to lithium, valproic acid, and carbamazepine, has shifted somewhat with the addition of newer medications to the bipolar pharmacopeia. **A mood stabilizer is generally defined as a medication with efficacy in at least one phase of illness (depression, mania, or prophylaxis against depression or mania) and one that does not exacerbate any phase of illness.** By this definition, antidepressants would not be considered mood stabilizers, because while they are effective in treating depression, they may also precipitate or exacerbate mania.

   Although adjunctive medications may also be used during treatment, mood-stabilizing medications represent the foundation for treatment in bipolar disorder. Beyond lithium, valproic acid, and carbamazepine, newer medicines, which some studies suggest may also act as mood stabilizers, include lamotrigine and atypical antipsychotics.
3. **Eliminate and avoid mood-destabilizing agents.** The drugs most likely to destabilize mood are antidepressants, which can pose two kinds of risks. In the short-term, **they can cause mania;** in this regard, bupropion and paroxetine have been shown to carry a lower risk of "switching" a patient into mania than tricyclic antidepressants in bipolar depression. In the long-term, **antidepressants can lead to rapid-cycling or cycle acceleration, where patients suffer more manic and depressive episodes** than would have occurred if left untreated. While these agents have a role in the treatment of severe bipolar depression when used in combination with mood-stabilizing medications, they may be tapered if possible after the acute phase of treatment is over. Antidepressants are thus appropriate for acute depression in bipolar disorder, but not necessarily for prophylaxis of future depressive episodes in bipolar disorder. Table 14-3 provides a list of reasons for treatment resistance in bipolar disorder.
4. **Educate the patient and establish a therapeutic alliance.** Education is an important component of the long-term treatment of bipolar illness. Many patients have little knowledge or insight into their symptoms. If they improve, they need to understand and come to terms with the need to take medications most of their lives. Often, they must adjust to side effects, or work with their clinicians to adjust medication dosing to minimize the impact of side effects. To enhance compliance, a good therapeutic alliance is of the utmost importance. Psychological factors of the long-term treatment of bipolar disorder may be the missing link between the pharmacological efficacy of medications, such as lithium (i.e., how well they work in controlled trials) and their relative lack of effectiveness in some naturalistic long-term studies of real-world treatment. Adjunctive individual psychotherapy with a psychotherapist versed in bipolar disorder can be important, as can the use of cognitive-behavioral and interpersonal psychotherapies for the depressive phases of bipolar disorder. One particularly useful intervention can be mood charting, in which patients record their mood daily in a chart or mood diary. Self-help and family groups, such as the National Alliance for the Mentally Ill (NAMI) and the Depressive and Manic Depressive Association (DMDA), are also important resources for patients and family members.

Table 14-3. Causes of Treatment Resistance in Bipolar Disorder

- Mood-destabilizing effects of antidepressants
- Medication non-compliance
- Co-morbid substance abuse
- Misdiagnosis
- Specificity of response of diagnostic subtype
- Co-morbid psychosis
- Co-morbid medical conditions

Suggested Readings

Akiskal, H.S. (1996). The prevalent clinical spectrum of bipolar disorders: Beyond DSM-IV. *Journal of Clinical Psychopharmacology, 16*(suppl. 1), 4S–14S.

Ghaemi, S.N., Sachs, G.S., Chiora, A.M., et al. (1999). Is bipolar disorder still underdiagnosed? Are antidepressants overutilized? *Journal of Affective Disorders, 52,* 135–144.

Goodwin, F.K., & Ghaemi, S.N. (1998). Understanding manic-depressive illness. *Archives of General Psychiatry, 55,* 23–25.

Goodwin, F.K., & Jamison, K.R. (1990). *Manic depressive illness.* New York: Oxford University Press.

Harrow, M., Goldberg, J.F., Grossman, L.S., & Meltzer, H.Y. (1990). Outcome in manic disorders. *Archives of General Psychiatry, 47,* 665–671.

Hirschfeld, R.M.A., Bowden, C.L., Gitlin, M.J., et al. (2002). Practice guideline for the treatment of patients with bipolar disorder (revision). *American Journal of Psychiatry, 159*(4).

Kalin, N. (1996/1997). Management of the depressive component of bipolar disorder. *Depression Anxiety, 4,* 190–198.

Keller, M.B., Lavori, P.W., Coryell, W., et al. (1986). Differential outcome of pure manic, mixed/cycling, and pure depressive episodes in patients with bipolar illness. *Journal of the American Medical Association, 255*(22), 3138–3142.

Manji, H.K., & Lenox, R.H. (2000). Signaling: Cellular insights into the pathophysiology of bipolar disorder. *Biological Psychiatry, 48,* 518–530.

Pope, H.G., Jr., & Lipinski, J.F. (1978). Diagnosis in schizophrenia and manic-depressive illness. *Archives of General Psychiatry, 35,* 811–828.

Rajkowska, G. (2002). Cell pathology in bipolar disorder. *Bipolar Disorders, 4,* 105–116.

Sachs, G.S. (1996). Bipolar mood disorder: Practical strategies for acute and maintenance phase treatment. *Journal of Clinical Psychopharmacology, 16*(suppl. 1), 32S–47S.

Wehr, T.A., & Goodwin, F.K. (1987). Can antidepressants cause mania and worsen the course of affective illness? *American Journal of Psychiatry, 144*(11), 1403–1411.

Chapter 15

Anxiety Disorders

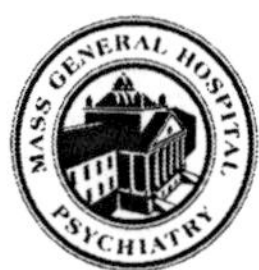

DAN V. IOSIFESCU AND MARK H. POLLACK

I. Introduction

A. Overview

Anxiety is an expected, normal, and transient response to stress; it may be a necessary cue for adaptation and coping. Pathologic anxiety is distinguished from a normal emotional response by four criteria:

1. **Autonomy:** it has no (or a minimal) recognizable environmental trigger.
2. **Intensity:** it exceeds the patient's capacity to bear discomfort.
3. **Duration:** the symptoms are persistent rather than transient.
4. **Behavior:** anxiety impairs coping, and results in disabling behavioral strategies, such as avoidance or withdrawal.

B. Definition of Anxiety

Anxiety results from an unknown internal stimulus, or is inappropriate or excessive when compared with the existing external stimulus. Anxiety differs from fear, which is a sense of dread and foreboding that occurs in response to an external threatening event.

C. Manifestations of Anxiety

1. **Physical symptoms** are related to autonomic arousal (e.g., tachycardia, tachypnea, diaphoresis, diarrhea, and light-headedness).
2. **Affective symptoms** that range in severity from mild (e.g., edginess) to severe (experienced as terror, the feeling that one is "going to die" or "lose control").
3. **Behavior** is characterized by avoidance (e.g., noncompliance with medical procedures) or compulsions.
4. **Cognitions** include worry, apprehension, obsessions, and thoughts about emotional or bodily damage.

II. Etiology

A. Neurophysiology

A burgeoning body of research points to the critical importance of several central nervous system (CNS) structures, including the amygdala, in the genesis of anxiety, as well as the involvement of a number of central neurotransmitter systems that generate and modulate anxiety symptoms.

1. **Central noradrenergic systems.** The **locus coeruleus (LC),** a small retropontine nucleus, is the major source of the brain's adrenergic innervation. LC stimulation generates panic attacks; LC blockade (e.g., by tricyclic antidepressants or alprazolam) decreases panic attacks.
2. The **γ-aminobutyric acid (GABA)** neurons from **the limbic system,** especially the septohippocampal areas, mediate generalized anxiety, worry, and vigilance. The highly concentrated GABA receptors in those structures bind benzodiazepines to reduce this heightened state of vigilance. Neuronal connections exist between the LC and limbic structures, including the amygdala.
3. **Serotonergic systems and neuropeptides** are important modulators of the two systems outlined above. The interconnections of these neuronal systems explain the efficacy of clinical interventions with diverse mechanisms of action (serotonergic and noradrenergic antidepressants, benzodiazepines, and cognitive-behavioral therapy [CBT]) on pathologic anxiety.

B. Cognitive-Behavioral Formulations

Cognitive-behavioral formulations of anxiety focus on the information-processing and behavioral reactions that characterize the anxiety experience. The emphasis is placed on the role of thoughts and beliefs (cognitions) in activating anxiety, as well as on the role of avoidance or other escape responses in the maintenance of both fear and dysfunctional patterns of thinking. Faulty cognitions are often characterized by overprediction of the likelihood, or impact, of negative events. Attempts to neutralize anxiety with avoidance or compulsive behavior serve to "lock in" anxiety reactions and contribute to the chronic arousal and anticipatory anxiety that mark anxiety disorders.

C. Developmental (Psychodynamic) Formulations

In Freud's later writing, anxiety was described as a signal of threat to the ego; signals are elicited because current events have similarities (symbolic or actual) to threatening developmental experiences (traumatic anxiety). Object relations theorists emphasize the use of internalized objects to maintain affective stability under stress.

III. Epidemiology

A. Prevalence

1. **Anxiety disorders are among the most prevalent psychiatric disorders in the general population.** Approximately one-fourth of the United States population experiences pathologic anxiety over the course of their lifetime (Table 15-1).
2. **First-degree relatives** of patients with anxiety disorders have a **significantly increased risk** for anxiety disorders compared with those in the general population. For first-degree relatives of patients with panic disorder the risk is increased four- to eight-fold. Limited data from twin studies are also consistent with a genetic contribution.

Table 15-1. Prevalence of Anxiety Disorders in the United States Population

Disorder	*Prevalence Lifetime (%)*	*12 months (%)*
Any anxiety disorder	24.9	17.2
Social phobia	13.3	7.9
Simple phobia	11.3	8.8
Agoraphobia	5.3	2.8
Generalized anxiety disorder	5.1	3.1
Panic disorder	3.5	2.3

IV. Course of Anxiety Disorders

A. Physical and Psychosocial Function

1. **Anxiety disorders are associated with marked impairments in physical and psychosocial function, as well as in quality of life.** Panic disorder is associated with increased rates of alcohol abuse, marital and vocational problems, and suicide attempts (in individuals with co-morbid depression and personality disorders). Panic and phobic anxiety are also associated with increased rates of premature cardiovascular mortality in men. Patients with panic disorder lose workdays twice as often as do those in the general population, with 25% of panic patients becoming chronically unemployed, and up to 30% receiving public assistance or disability. Patients with panic disorder are 5 to 7 times more likely to be high utilizers of medical services than are individuals without panic disorder.
2. **Most patients with anxiety disorders improve with treatment although the majority do not achieve full and sustained remission with current treatments.** High rates of relapse after discontinuation of pharmacotherapy support the need for maintenance therapy for many individuals.

V. Differential Diagnosis

Anxiety disorders should be differentiated from those medical and psychiatric conditions that are associated with anxiety. It is also important to recognize when anxiety symptoms mimic the symptoms of medical illness.

A. Organic Causes of Anxiety (medical illnesses that mimic anxiety disorders)

1. In a patient with a known medical illness, the condition, its complications, and its treatment should be suspected as potential causes of anxiety. For example, in a patient with chronic obstructive pulmonary disease (COPD), hypoxia, respiratory distress, and sympathomimetic bronchodilators can all cause symptoms of anxiety.
2. **Six factors associated with an organic anxiety syndrome** can help differentiate it from a primary anxiety disorder:
   a. Onset of symptoms after the age of 35 years
   b. Lack of personal or family history of an anxiety disorder
   c. Lack of a childhood history of significant anxiety, phobias, or separation anxiety
   d. Absence of significant life events generating or exacerbating the anxiety symptoms
   e. Lack of avoidance behavior
   f. A poor response to antipanic agents
3. A patient with an organic cause of anxiety may not otherwise meet criteria for panic disorder or generalized anxiety disorder; there is often a significant lack of **psychological** symptoms in the context of severe physical symptoms.
4. **Categories of medical conditions that are commonly associated with anxiety include:**
   a. **Endocrine dysfunction:** hyperadrenalism (pheochromocytoma), hypothyroidism, hyperparathyroidism
   b. **Drug-related:**
      i. **Intoxication:** e.g., use of caffeine, cocaine, sympathomimetics, theophylline, corticosteroids, and thyroid hormones
      ii. **Withdrawal reactions:** e.g., from alcohol, narcotics, or sedative-hypnotics
   c. **Hypoxia:** all causes of **cerebral anoxia,** including **cardiovascular** (e.g., arrhythmias, angina, congestive heart failure [CHF], anemia) and **respiratory** (e.g., COPD, pulmonary embolism)
   d. **Metabolic abnormalities:** e.g., acidosis, hyperthermia, electrolyte abnormalities (e.g., hypercalcemia)
   e. **Neurological disorders:** e.g., vestibular dysfunction, seizures (especially temporal lobe epilepsy)

B. Anxiety That Complicates Medical Illness

1. **Anxiety in the primary care setting.** Anxiety is particularly common in the general medical setting. The National Ambulatory Medical Care Survey (1980–1981) revealed that anxiety is the presenting problem for 11% of patients who visit primary care physicians (PCPs), and is the most common psychiatric problem seen by PCPs. More than 90% of the patients with anxiety present primarily with somatic complaints. Moreover, most patients with anxiety first seek help in primary care settings or in emergency rooms. The majority of heavy users of primary care services (including patients with chronic illness) have significantly higher rates of mood and anxiety disorders than do less frequent visitors to PCPs. High rates of anxiety disorders are found in patients presenting with chest pain, dizziness, dyspnea, and symptoms of irritable bowel syndrome.
2. **Work-up of the anxious patient.** The medical work-up of the anxious patient relies primarily on the medical and psychiatric history, the medication and drug history, and on an appropriate physical and neurologi-

cal examination. One should consider the anxiogenic effects of existing medications and medical conditions, as well as the effects of substance use and withdrawal (see above). A targeted physical examination, and laboratory and clinical tests are employed based on the clinical assessment, patient characteristics, and the focus of the patient's somatic complaints (e.g., cardiac, pulmonary, gastrointestinal, or neurologic).

C. Psychiatric Disorders, Other than Anxiety Disorders

Anxiety is also present in psychiatric disorders other than anxiety disorders. In **delusional disorders** there are persecutory fears which may mimic anxiety or phobias. Anxiety symptoms occur in the prodromal phase and during the course of **schizophrenia.** The presence of hallucinations, delusions, or disorganized speech associated with a marked decrease of social functioning over a long period differentiates schizophrenia from anxiety disorders.

More than half of all anxious patients also experience significant **depression.** Symptoms, such as dysphoria, hopelessness, anhedonia, early morning awakening, psychomotor retardation, and suicidal thoughts, are typically more indicative of depression than anxiety. Anxiety-disordered patients usually maintain their interest in their activities, but find it hard to negotiate them comfortably. Patients with anxiety should be evaluated for depression, given the frequency of their co-morbidity. When anxiety and depression co-exist, monotherapy with an antidepressant or the combination of an antidepressant and a benzodiazepine is indicated; treatment with a benzodiazepine alone is best avoided.

If anxiety develops in reaction to a stressful situation, and within 3 months of a stressor, but lasts less than 6 months after cessation of the stressor, a diagnosis of **adjustment disorder with anxious features** may be made. Treatment of this condition is typically aimed at reducing the impact of the known stressor. However, symptomatic relief with use of an anxiolytic or an antidepressant can markedly improve the patient's quality of life and prevent complications.

VI. Primary Psychiatric Disorders

A. Panic Disorder and Agoraphobia

1. **Definitions. Panic disorder is a syndrome characterized by recurrent unexpected panic attacks about which there is persistent concern. Panic attacks** are discrete episodes of intense anxiety, which develop abruptly and **peak within 10 minutes; they are associated with at least four other symptoms of autonomic arousal.** Associated features include:
   a. **Cardiac symptoms:** palpitations, tachycardia, chest pain, or discomfort
   b. **Pulmonary symptoms:** shortness of breath, or a feeling of choking
   c. **Gastrointestinal symptoms:** nausea or abdominal distress
   d. **Neurological symptoms:** trembling and shaking, dizziness, light-headedness, faintness, or paresthesias
   e. **Autonomic arousal:** sweating, chills, or hot flashes
   f. **Psychological symptoms:** derealization, depersonalization, a fear of losing control or going crazy, or a fear of dying

   Whereas the initial panic attack is usually spontaneous, subsequently, apprehension frequently develops about future attacks (anticipatory anxiety). **Agoraphobia,** a complication of panic disorder, involves anxiety about, or avoidance of, places or situations from which ready escape might be difficult, or from which escape might be embarrassing, or where help may be unavailable in the event of a panic attack. Agoraphobia can significantly restrict a patient's daily activities, to the point where he or she becomes dependent on companions to face situations outside the home; some individuals may become homebound.
2. **Epidemiology. Panic disorder has a lifetime prevalence of 1.5–3.5%;** it is more commonly diagnosed in women (2:1 female/male ratio). This difference may reflect a true gender difference or the observation that men tend to self-medicate with alcohol and are less likely to seek treatment. Many affected individuals recall a significant life event in the year before onset of the disease. The age of onset is typically between late adolescence and the third decade of life, but many affected individuals experience anxiety dating back from childhood, in the form of inhibited, anxious temperament or childhood anxiety disorders. Panic disorder tends to run in families; however, determining the relative contribution of genetic and environmental factors is an area of active research interest.
3. **Diagnostic features.** Based on the DSM-IV, the diagnosis requires:
   a. Recurrent, unexpected panic attacks.
   b. That at least one of the attacks is followed by more than a month of:
      i. Persistent concern about additional attacks
      ii. Worry about the implications of the attack and its consequences
      iii. A significant change in one's behavior related to the attacks
   c. That there is no organic factor (e.g., general medical condition or substance use) that generates these symptoms.
   d. That panic attacks are not accounted for by another mental disorder.
   e. That the presence or absence of agoraphobia be specified.

   A large number of patients have **limited-symptom attacks,** where only one or two of the panic symptoms are experienced. Limited-symptom panic attacks are also associated with significant morbidity.
4. **Disease course and treatment. Panic disorder is often a chronic disease,** with high rates of relapse

after discontinuation of treatment. Untreated panic disorder is often complicated by persistent anxiety and avoidant behavior, social dysfunction, marital problems, alcohol and drug abuse, as well as by increased utilization of medical services, and an increased mortality rate (from cardiovascular complications and suicide). Avoidant behavior can lead to progressive constriction of a patient's social interactions, and it prevents the individual from going to places where panic attacks have occurred or places where easy escape may be difficult or where assistance is unavailable. Affected patients may experience chronic distress and demoralization which can trigger depression. Although alcohol can temporarily alleviate symptoms of anxiety, patients who abuse alcohol may experience rebound anxiety, tolerance, and withdrawal, which may all exacerbate anxiety.

The established treatments of panic disorder include use of antidepressants, high-potency benzodiazepines, and cognitive-behavioral therapy (CBT) (see chap. 44).

B. Generalized Anxiety Disorder (GAD)

1. **Definition. Patients with GAD suffer from excessive anxiety or worry that is out of proportion to situational factors;** it occurs more days than not for longer than 6 months. These patients are often considered "worriers" or "nervous" by their families and friends. The anxiety is usually associated with muscle tension, restlessness, insomnia, difficulty concentrating, easy fatigability, and irritability. Affected patients typically experience persistent anxiety rather than discrete panic attacks, as in panic disorder.
2. **Epidemiology. The prevalence of GAD is about 5% in community samples;** it is more typically diagnosed in women (2:1 female:male ratio). The age of onset is frequently in childhood or adolescence, with some patients having an onset in their twenties. GAD is frequently co-morbid with other anxiety disorders (e.g., panic disorder or social phobia), depression, and with alcohol and drug abuse. The course of the disease is chronic but fluctuates in severity; it is frequently worsened by stress.
3. **Diagnostic criteria (DSM-IV)**
   a. Excessive anxiety and worry regarding a number of events or activities, that occurs more days than not for at least 6 months.
   b. The individual finds it difficult to control the worry.
   c. Three out of six symptoms (restlessness, easy fatigability, difficulty concentrating, irritability, muscle tension, and insomnia) are present.
   d. The worry is not related to features of other disorders.
   e. The anxiety causes significant distress or impairment in function.
   f. The anxiety is not attributed to an organic cause (e.g., substance use, medical condition).
4. **Treatment.** The treatment of GAD includes pharmacotherapy (antidepressants, benzodiazepines, buspirone) and CBT (see chap. 44).

C. Specific Phobia

1. **Definition. Patients with a specific phobia have marked and persistent fear of circumscribed situations or objects** (e.g., heights, closed spaces, animals, or the sight of blood). Exposure to the phobic stimulus results in intense anxiety and avoidance which interferes with the patient's life.
2. **Epidemiology. The lifetime prevalence of phobias is about 10% in the general population.** The age of onset varies depending on the subtype. Phobias to animals, natural environments (heights, storms, water), blood, and injections each have an onset in childhood. Situational phobias (e.g., triggered by airplanes, elevators, enclosed places) have a bimodal distribution with one peak in childhood and another peak in the mid-twenties.
3. **Diagnostic criteria (DSM-IV)**
   a. Persistent, excessive unreasonable fear of an object or situation.
   b. Exposure to a feared stimulus invariably provokes anxiety, including panic.
   c. Recognition that the fear is excessive or unreasonable.
   d. The phobic stimulus is avoided or endured with dread.
   e. The fear and the avoidant behavior interfere with the person's normal routine or cause marked distress.
   f. In a patient under the age of 18 years, symptoms last longer than 6 months.
   g. The symptoms are not better accounted by another disorder (e.g., obsessive-compulsive disorder [OCD], panic disorder).
   h. Specific subtypes (e.g., animal, natural environment, blood-injection-injury, situational) should be specified.
4. **Treatment.** Benzodiazepines are useful acutely to decrease phobic anxiety and to facilitate exposure (e.g., to take an airplane flight). However, CBT, involving exposure and desensitization to the feared stimulus, offers more comprehensive and persistent benefits.

D. Social Phobia

1. **Definition. Patients with a social phobia fear being exposed to public scrutiny; they fear that they will behave in a way which will be humiliating or embarrassing.** This perception leads to persistent fear and ultimately to avoidance or endurance with intense distress of the social situation. The anxiety can be limited to circumscribed performance situations, i.e., "performance anxiety" (e.g., speaking, eating, using a public bathroom, writing in public), or can affect more general social interactions. Although discomfort related to public speaking is a relatively frequent occurrence in the general population, a significant degree of distress or the presence of impairment is necessary to warrant the diagnosis of social phobia.

2. **Epidemiology. The prevalence of social phobia varies between 3% and 13% in different studies.** In epidemiological and community studies the prevalence is greater in females than in males; however, the prevalence is greater for males in clinical samples. This may be the result of males experiencing more pressure for social performance and thus becoming aware of existing pathology. The onset of social phobia is usually in adolescence, although most affected individuals have a history of anxiety that dates back to childhood.

   The symptoms of social phobia may overlap with those of panic disorder, avoidant personality, and shyness. Social phobia is frequently co-morbid with depression and with alcohol and drug abuse. The course of the disease is chronic but it fluctuates; it is frequently worsened by stress.

3. **Diagnostic criteria (DSM-IV)**
   a. Fear of showing anxiety symptoms or acting in a way that will be embarrassing or humiliating when scrutinized by others.
   b. The situation almost invariably provokes anxiety.
   c. The patient recognizes that the fear is excessive or unreasonable.
   d. The phobic stimulus is avoided or endured with intense anxiety.
   e. The fear and the avoidant behavior interfere with the person's normal routine or cause marked distress.
   f. In a patient under the age of 18 years, symptoms last longer than 6 months.
   g. The symptoms are not better accounted by an organic condition or by another mental disorder (e.g., trembling in Parkinson's disease, stuttering).
   h. The subtype ("performance anxiety" vs. generalized) should be specified.

4. **Treatment.** The treatment of social phobia includes pharmacotherapy (antidepressants, such as monoamine oxidase inhibitors [MAOIs] and selective serotonin reuptake inhibitors [SSRIs], as well as benzodiazepines and beta-blockers) and CBT (see chap. 44).

E. Obsessive-Compulsive Disorder

1. **Definitions. Obsessive-compulsive disorder (OCD) is characterized by recurrent, intrusive, unwanted thoughts (i.e., obsessions, such as fears of contamination), or compulsive behaviors or rituals (e.g., repetitive hand-washing).** The obsessions are recurrent, persistent thoughts, impulses or images, characterized by four criteria:
   a. They are experienced as intrusive and inappropriate and cause marked anxiety and distress.
   b. They are not simply worries about real-life problems.
   c. Attempts are made to ignore obsessions or neutralize them with some other thought or action.
   d. The person recognizes the obsession as a product of his/her own mind, rather than imposed from the outside as in thought insertion.

   The compulsive behaviors take place in response to obsessions or rigid rules. Compulsive behaviors are aimed at reducing distress or preventing a dreaded event; they are clearly excessive or unconnected in a realistic way with the event they are trying to neutralize.

2. **Epidemiology. The lifetime prevalence is 2–3% in the general population.** The mean age of onset is in the mid-twenties; less than 5% of patients develop the disease after the age of 35 years. The disease has a chronic course.

3. **Diagnostic criteria (DSM-IV)**
   a. The presence of obsessions or compulsions.
   b. The patient is or was able at some point to recognize that the obsessions or compulsions are excessive or unreasonable.
   c. The obsessions or compulsions cause marked distress, are time-consuming (more than 1 hour/day), or significantly interfere with the person's normal routine.
   d. The content of the obsessions or compulsions is not restricted to the features of any concomitant Axis I disorder.
   e. The obsessions or compulsions cannot be attributed to an organic cause (e.g., substance use, or a medical condition).

   The differential diagnosis includes obsessive-compulsive personality disorder, phobic disorders, depression, schizophrenia, and Tourette's disorder.

4. **Treatment.** The treatment of OCD includes pharmacotherapy (SSRIs and the tricyclic antidepressant, clomipramine) and CBT aimed at extinguishing intrusive thoughts and compulsive behavior (see chap. 44).

F. Post-traumatic Stress Disorder (PTSD)

1. **Definition. Patients with PTSD have experienced an event that involved the threat of death, injury, or severe harm to themselves or others; their response involved intense fear, helplessness, or horror.** Patients frequently re-experience the traumatic event in the form of nightmares, flashbacks, or by marked arousal when exposed to situations reminiscent of the event. PTSD patients avoid situations which remind them of the trauma; they may become emotionally numb, irritable, hypervigilant, or have difficulties with sleep and concentration.

2. **Epidemiology.** The syndrome was initially described long before the Vietnam War era; for those who were injured in combat the prevalence of PTSD is about 20%. PTSD can also occur in civilians who suffered life-threatening accidents or assaults; **the lifetime prevalence of PTSD in the general population is about 8%.** The syndrome may occur at any age. Symptoms usually begin within the first 3 months after trauma, although they can be delayed for months or years. The course is varied; complete recovery occurs within 3 months in half of those affected. Many

others experience symptoms for more than a year after the trauma.

The complications of PTSD include social withdrawal, depression, suicidality, as well as alcohol and drug abuse. Psychosocial risk factors for PTSD include a previous personality disorder, early trauma, a chaotic childhood, and previous mental illness. Protective factors include good self-esteem, external control, and social support.

3. **Diagnostic criteria (DSM-IV)**
   a. The patient must have experienced, witnessed, or confronted an event that involved actual or threatened death, serious injury, or threat to the physical integrity of self or others. The person's response involved intense fear, helplessness, or horror.
   b. Persistent re-experience of the trauma in the form of intrusive recollections, nightmares, flashbacks, psychological distress, and psychological reactivity occurs on cue exposure.
   c. Persistent avoidance of stimuli (thoughts and activities) associated with the trauma or numbing of general responsiveness (detachment or estrangement from others, or a sense of foreshortened future).
   d. Symptoms of increased arousal (e.g., sleep disturbance, irritability, anger, difficulty concentrating, hypervigilance, and a startle response).
   e. Symptoms last for more than 1 month.
   f. Symptoms cause significant distress and impairment. Subtypes: acute (symptoms for less than 3 months), chronic (symptoms for more than 3 months), and delayed onset (onset more than 6 months after trauma).

   The differential diagnosis includes **acute stress disorder,** in which symptoms occur within 4 weeks of the traumatic event and persist for less than 4 weeks.
4. **Treatment.** Pharmacological treatment (e.g., antidepressants for depression) targets reduction of prominent symptoms. A number of studies have demonstrated the efficacy of SSRIs for the treatment of PTSD. Exposure-based CBT is very effective for PTSD. Also important is psychotherapy aimed at survivor guilt, anger, and helplessness. Affected patients may benefit from family therapy and from vocational rehabilitation in the context of their significant impairment in social and professional functioning.

VII. Conclusions

Anxiety disorders are a group of psychiatric disorders associated with high morbidity and with mortality (through suicide, co-morbid substance abuse, and from cardiovascular problems). Given the similarities in presentations between certain medical conditions and anxiety disorders, a comprehensive medical, psychiatric, and substance use history is very important to the diagnostic process. Since most of the anxiety disorders tend to be chronic, many patients may benefit from ongoing pharmacotherapy and/or psychosocial interventions to optimize and to maintain improvement.

Suggested Readings

American Psychiatric Association. (2000). *Diagnostic and statistical manual of mental disorders (4th ed.), DSM-IV-TR (text revision).* Washington, DC: American Psychiatric Press.

Fyer, A.J., Gabbard, G.O., Pine, D.S., et al. (2000). Anxiety disorders. In H.I. Kaplan, & B.J. Sadock (Eds.), *Comprehensive textbook of psychiatry* (7th ed.). Baltimore, MD: Williams and Wilkins.

Pollack, M., Smoller, J., & Lee, D. (1998). Approach to the anxious patient. In T.A. Stern, J.B., Herman, & P.L. Slavin (Eds.), *The MGH guide to psychiatry in primary care.* New York: McGraw-Hill.

Rosenbaum, J., Pollack, M., Otto, M., & Bernstein, J. (1997). Anxious patients. In N.H. Cassem, T.A. Stern, J.F. Rosenbaum, & M.S. Jellinek (Eds.), *Massachusetts General Hospital handbook of general hospital psychiatry* (4th ed.). St Louis: Mosby.

Chapter 16

Trauma and Post-traumatic Stress Disorder

Rafael D. Ornstein and Roger K. Pitman

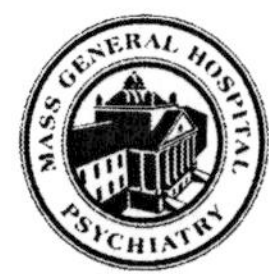

I. Overview

A. The puzzling, and disturbing effects of psychological trauma on human function have been described for generations, going back as far as Homer's *Iliad*. In more recent times, large numbers of American Civil War veterans complained of generalized weakness, palpitations, and chest pain, thought to result from the physical stress of war; it was referred to as **"soldier's heart."** In World War I, psychologically disabled veterans were thought to have suffered from brain damage or **"shell shock." Kardiner** described a syndrome in military veterans that foreshadowed the current diagnosis of **post-traumatic stress disorder (PTSD)**; he labeled it a **"traumatic neurosis of war,"** and made the point that the syndrome was physiological in nature. **Post-traumatic stress was virtually ignored until after the Vietnam War when both veterans groups and the feminist movement spoke out about psychological trauma. Later, Horowitz** helped to formulate the diagnosis that found its way into the DSM-III. Earlier in the century, **Freud** and **Janet** became interested in how psychological trauma led to psychopathology.

B. Since its inception in the DSM-III, **the diagnosis of PTSD has helped researchers study the connection between psychological trauma and psychiatric morbidity.** Initially, PTSD was described as a normal, expectable response to trauma. It was thought that the severity and chronicity of the syndrome might be related directly to the nature of the trauma. Subsequently, the diagnostic criteria for PTSD included several phenomena: an initial, expectable response to trauma, an initial pathological response, and a more prolonged, pathological state. **The onset of PTSD in any given person following a trauma is the exception rather than the rule. Current research suggests that individual vulnerabilities play a significant factor in the development of the syndrome.**

C. Acute and long-term responses to traumatic events are varied and multi-determined. Nearly every person can be expected to have some disruption in their mental function following a significantly traumatic event—a "normal" stress response. On average, most people are able to adapt following a traumatic event and return to their previous level of function, with or without some chronic symptoms. When the symptoms following a trauma impair functioning, they often appear as syndromes, labeled in the DSM-IV as **acute stress disorder and PTSD. Chronic exposure to trauma, and/or trauma occurring in childhood can produce long-lasting personality disturbances.** When the response to trauma reaches the level of PTSD, there are frequently a host of co-morbid psychiatric conditions. Exposure to trauma that does not result in a psychiatric diagnosis may still result in chronic symptoms that may have a significant impact on the individual.

II. Post-traumatic Stress Disorder

The DSM-IV criteria for PTSD define trauma and the three central groups of post-traumatic symptoms: **intrusive/re-experiencing, avoidance/numbing,** and **hyperarousal.** If these symptoms are pervasive, prolonged, and debilitating enough, they reach threshold for a diagnosis. **A typical post-traumatic response may involve any number of the above symptoms** as the person struggles to come to terms with the trauma and its consequences. **Common difficulties faced in integrating the traumatic experience include fear of repetition of the trauma, shame over helplessness, loss of a sense of invulnerability, feeling of personal failure, rage at the source of trauma and ensuing guilt, and guilt over having survived while others perished.**

A. The DSM-IV defines "trauma" in a specific way:

1. **"Trauma" involves a physical threat to life or bodily integrity;** examples include:
   a. **Exposure to military combat, violent assault, including rape and robbery, domestic violence, automobile accidents, childhood physical and sexual abuse or neglect, natural disasters, and sudden catastrophic medical illness.**
   b. **Witnessing a traumatic event.**
   c. **Being confronted with (e.g., being told about) a trauma** experienced by a loved one.
2. **A defining characteristic of a traumatic event, according to the DSM-IV, is that the person's response involves "intense fear, helplessness or horror."** Because of the intensity of the feelings associated with a trauma, **perception of the event may be distorted:** it may be experienced as fragments of sensations; time may be slowed or accelerated. **Feelings may be dissociated from events as they are occur.**

B. Intrusive, re-experiencing symptoms are a hallmark of PTSD. Traumatic memories are usually quite disruptive; they are often vivid sensory experiences, but also can be emotions or cognitions that intrude unbidden. **Nightmares** are common, often repetitive, life-like, and disruptive to sleep; a patient begins to dread sleep and will "fight it," to avoid the frightening nightmares. **Flashbacks, hallucinations,** and other experiences of **reliving the trauma** can occur. **Intense emotional distress** and **physiological reactivity,** such as palpitations, shortness of breath, chest tightening, and excessive sweating, occur in response to internal or external reminders of the trauma.

C. **Avoidance** of reminders of the trauma and **psychological numbing** can be the most disabling symptoms following a trauma. Following a trauma, persons may **avoid** anything that may remind them of the trauma, including thoughts or feelings, activities, places, or people that are associated with the event. There can be **amnesia** for aspects of the trauma itself. Numbing symptoms include an overall sense of **detachment, a diminished range of emotions,** and **withdrawal** from important activities.

D. **Hyperarousal** can create interpersonal problems. These symptoms include **disturbed sleep, irritability,** and **anger outbursts, difficulty with concentration, hypervigilance,** and an **exaggerated startle response.**

E. The duration of the disturbance is more than 1 month.

F. The disturbance causes clinically significant distress or impairment in social or occupational functioning.

G. The syndrome is **acute** if it has lasted less that 3 months and **chronic** if it lasts more than 3 months. PTSD has **delayed onset** if the onset of symptoms is greater than 6 months after the trauma.

III. Acute Stress Disorder

This disorder describes **an acute response to trauma.** It includes the criteria for PTSD but adds and **emphasizes dissociative symptoms.** An acute stress disorder may follow the same kind of traumatic event that can cause PTSD. A typical example includes a soldier responding to battle, becoming acutely disoriented, and being in a "daze." Acute stress disorder appears to be a good predictor of subsequent PTSD; the presence or absence of the diagnosis predicted PTSD at 6 months in 83% of cases in one study. The diagnostic criteria are listed below.

A. Diagnostic Criteria for Acute Stress Disorder

1. Exposure to a traumatic event in which both of the following were present:
   a. The person experienced, witnessed, or was confronted with an event that involved actual or threatened death or serious injury, or a threat to one's physical integrity or to the integrity of others.
   b. The person's response involved intense fear, helplessness, or horror.
2. Either during or after the distressing event, the individual had three or more of the following dissociative symptoms:
   a. A subjective sense of numbing
   b. A reduction of awareness of his or her surroundings (e.g., "being in a daze")
   c. Derealization
   d. Depersonalization
   e. Dissociative amnesia (inability to recall an important aspect of the trauma)
3. The traumatic event is persistently re-experienced with recurrent images, thoughts, dreams, illusions, flashback, or a reliving of the experience.
4. Marked avoidance of stimuli that arouse recollections of the trauma.
5. Marked symptoms of anxiety or increased arousal (e.g., difficulty sleeping, irritability, poor concentration, hypervigilance, exaggerated startle response, motor restlessness).
6. The disturbance causes clinically significant distress or impairment in social, occupational, or other important areas of function.
7. The disturbance lasts from 2 days to 4 weeks and occurs within 4 weeks of the traumatic event.
8. The disturbance is not due to the direct physiological effects of a substance (e.g., a drug of abuse, a medication) or a general medical condition.

IV. Epidemiology

A. Prevalence of PTSD in the General Population

1. The National Comorbidity Survey (NCS) found that approximately 50% of females and 60% of males experienced a traumatic event severe enough to cause PTSD. About 20% of those went on to develop the disorder.
2. The NCS found the overall lifetime prevalence to be about 8%, 10% for females and 5% for males. The most common cause of PTSD in men were combat and witnessing death or severe injury, and the most common cause in women was rape and sexual molestation.
3. A survey of 1,007 young adults in a Detroit HMO showed that 39% were exposed to a traumatic event and 24% of those exposed developed PTSD. The overall lifetime prevalence for PTSD was 9%, 11% for females and 6% for males.
4. The likelihood of developing PTSD is twice as high in females as in males. This is due to the vulnerability of women to developing PTSD following assaults. Although men more frequently experienced this trauma, women were 5 times more likely to develop PTSD following a violent assault.

B. Prevalence of PTSD Following Specific Traumas

1. The rates of PTSD following natural disasters vary. Following the Mt. St. Helens volcanic eruption, those exposed showed a lifetime prevalence of PTSD of 3.6%, compared with a rate of 2.6% in controls. Following a dam break and subsequent flood at Buffalo Creek, researchers found a 59% lifetime prevalence of PTSD; 25% still met criteria at 14-year follow-up.
2. For **war veterans,** rates can vary according to the traumatic exposure. Overall, the lifetime rate for PTSD for Vietnam veterans is 31%. Those exposed to median levels of combat showed rates of 28% compared with 65% among those exposed to the highest levels of combat. For political prisoners and prisoners of war, rates range from 30% to more than 70%. For torture victims, rates can be as high as 90%.
3. Among individuals who suffer a **violent assault,** there is a 20% rate of PTSD. Victims of rape have developed PTSD nearly half of the time in some studies. Witnessing a person being killed or seriously injured confers a risk of 7%.
4. Following a **traffic accident,** 10–30% still have PTSD 6–18 months after the accident.
5. In a group of individuals who experienced a sudden, unexpected death of a close friend or relative, 14% developed PTSD.

V. Longitudinal Course of PTSD

A. The clinical course of PTSD can vary considerably in any given individual. However, PTSD usually develops soon after a trauma. About 80% of those diagnosed still have the disorder at 3 months (chronic PTSD), and 75% have the diagnosis at 6 months. Recovery occurs most frequently in the first year; at 2 years, one-half of the cases have remitted. Over the next 5 years, another 20% or so recover. For about 30% of those initially diagnosed, PTSD can be a chronic and persistent illness. A study of survivors of the collapse of the dam at Buffalo Creek showed that 17% still had PTSD after 14 years. Similarly, another study found that 17% of women who were sexually assaulted had PTSD 17 years later. Among World War II prisoners of war, 50% manifest PTSD 40 years after their trauma.

B. Symptoms of PTSD can be **intermittent** and residual. It is common for PTSD to be reactivated, years after it has apparently resolved.

C. If the stressor involves interpersonal violence, victims are at greater risk for chronic PTSD.

VI. Risk Factors for Developing PTSD

A. The nature of the traumatic stressor remains the most important risk factor for developing PTSD. However, not every person will develop PTSD after exposure to a severe traumatic event. The stressors most likely to cause PTSD are (Tomb & Allen, 1994):

1. Stressors that are severe, unexpected, prolonged, intentional, and repetitive
2. Stressors that involve threat to one's physical integrity or to that of a loved one
3. Stressors that are isolating, demeaning, or in conflict with one's self-concept

B. Personal vulnerability is an important risk factor, especially in less severe trauma. Risk factors include:

1. A psychiatric history, including major depression, anxiety disorders, conduct disorder, neurotic personality, antisocial and narcissistic personality disorders
2. A history of previous trauma, including childhood sexual abuse
3. Low intelligence
4. Limited social supports
5. Childhood separation from parents, or divorce of parents in early childhood
6. A family history of major depression or anxiety disorders, which suggests a genetic component to PTSD
7. Genetic factors that appear to influence the risk of exposure to trauma as well as vulnerability to PTSD following that exposure

C. Dissociative symptoms experienced during or shortly after a traumatic event often predict future PTSD.

D. The presence of severe symptoms soon after a trauma appears to predict more severe symptoms later on.

VII. Associated Syndromes and Co-morbidity

A. Children exposed to physical or sexual abuse, or adults exposed to prolonged and repeated trauma may develop long-standing problems in psychological and interpersonal function. The younger the person the more vulnerable they may be to long-term difficulties. Although not yet recognized as a distinct diagnosis in the DSM, this syndrome is known in the literature as **complex PTSD** or **disorders of extreme stress not otherwise specified.** The syndrome describes a range of debilitating symptoms:

1. Difficulty with **affect regulation,** including problematic anger, self-destructive behavior, impulsive and risk-taking behavior
2. **Dissociation** and amnesia
3. **Somatization**
4. A range of **characterological difficulties,** including a damaged sense of self, chronic guilt and shame, a feeling of ineffectiveness, idealization of the perpetrator, difficulty in establishing and maintaining trusting relationships, a tendency to be re-victimized or to victimize others, and a chronic sense of despair and hopelessness

B. Although studies continue to show that PTSD is a distinct syndrome, co-morbidity is more frequently the rule rather than the exception; in the National Comorbidity Survey (NCS), 59% of men and 44% of women met criteria for three or more psychiatric diagnoses. Co-morbid conditions typical include major depression, other anxiety disorders, and substance abuse.

C. Major depressive disorder (MDD) is commonly co-morbid with PTSD. The NCS found that 48% of men and 49% of women with PTSD had MDD. MDD is a risk factor for PTSD, and PTSD is a risk factor for MDD. Often they can develop at the same time.

D. Anxiety disorders are also commonly co-morbid with PTSD. For example, simple phobias were co-morbid in 31% of men and 29% of women with PTSD, and social phobia was nearly as prevalent. Generalized anxiety disorder was found in about 15% of both men and women, and panic disorder was seen in 7% of men and 12% of women.

E. Substance abuse commonly co-occurs with PTSD; the NCS found that 52% of men with PTSD had alcohol abuse or dependence, and 35% had drug abuse or dependence. Of the women with PTSD in the survey, 28% had alcohol abuse or dependence, and 27% had drug abuse or dependence.

F. Clinical studies exploring the relationship between PTSD and eating disorders have found that childhood sexual abuse is a non-specific risk factor for bulimia nervosa but not anorexia nervosa. The National Women's Study (a large survey of U.S. women) found that women with bulimia had higher rates of PTSD than those without bulimia.

G. If a person develops PTSD following a trauma, he or she is at far greater risk of developing other psychiatric disorders, such as major depression, other anxiety disorders, or substance abuse, compared with a person who was exposed to a trauma, but who did not develop PTSD.

H. Exposure to trauma that does not result in PTSD *can* create long-standing symptoms, including depressed and anxious mood and damage to the victim's sense of self.

I. Suicide is a major concern in patients with PTSD. In one study 19% of those patients diagnosed with PTSD attempted suicide.

VIII. Neurobiology of PTSD

The neurobiology of PTSD is rapidly advancing. Although there is no single model that completely explains the pathophysiology of the disorder, data support the fact that PTSD is a discrete illness with biological correlates.

A. Review of the Neurobiology of the Normal Stress Response

1. **Norepinephrine** plays a role in orienting to new stimuli, in selective attention, and in autonomic arousal. The **locus coeruleus,** located in the pons, contains a large number of the brain's noradrenergic cell bodies that project throughout the brain.
2. **Cortisol** stimulates metabolic processes that prepare the body for fight or flight. Cortisol also modulates the stress response by counteracting catecholamines and restoring homeostasis; cortisol provides negative feedback for the stress response.
3. **Endogenous opiates** increase the pain threshold.
4. Neurotransmitters are linked in a **web of feedback loops.** For example, during stress, corticotropin releasing factor (CRF) increases the turnover of norepinephrine (NE), and NE increases concentrations of CRF in the locus coeruleus.
5. **Serotonin** appears to play a role in regulating the stress response.
6. In this theoretical scenario proposed by Rauch et al. (1998), the limbic system and the cerebral cortex process a stressful event. The **thalamus** relays information about threat to the **prefrontal cortex** and the **amygdala.** The **amygdala** is a limbic structure that is involved in threat assessment, emotional learning, and fear conditioning; it attaches emotional significance to incoming stimuli and facilitates the flight or fight response. The **amygdala** relays information to the **hippocampus,** the **paralimbic system,** the **sensory processing** systems, and other structures. The **hippocampus,** a limbic structure, is involved in learning and memory, especially of verbal information, events, places, and facts; it processes contextual information and provides feedback to the **amygdala** regarding one's experience and the current context. The **anterior cingulate cortex,** a part of the **paralimbic system,** sets priorities between emotional and cognitive processes and plays a role in inhibiting the **amygdala and** facilitating the extinction of conditioned fear responses.

B. The Neurobiology of PTSD

1. It has been hypothesized that **abnormalities in the sympathetic branch of the autonomic nervous system** play a role in the symptoms of intrusion and arousal.
   a. Animal models have shown that severe stress can cause dysregulation of the locus coeruleus, causing hypersensitivity to external stimuli.
   b. Combat veterans who suffer from PTSD have exaggerated heart rate responses during exposure to combat-related stimuli, as compared with combat veterans without PTSD and veterans with veterans with other anxiety disorders.
   c. Some studies have suggested that urinary excretion of norepinephrine is higher in patients with PTSD than in controls.

2. Abnormalities of the **hypothalamic-pituitary-adrenal** (HPA) **axis,** especially in regards to cortisol, are a principle finding in PTSD.
   a. **In PTSD, cortisol levels are chronically decreased,** there is increased glucocorticoid receptor sensitivity, stronger negative feedback, and sensitization of the HPA system. In sharp contrast, in **acute and chronic stress and major depression, cortisol levels are increased,** there is decreased glucocorticoid receptor responsiveness, a decrease in negative feedback, and desensitization of the HPA system (Yehuda, 2001).
   b. Patients with PTSD can show lower cortisol levels up to 50 years following the initial trauma.
   c. Lower cortisol levels immediately following a trauma can be a risk factor for developing PTSD at a later date. Studies have found that, following a rape, low cortisol was associated with prior rape or assault, which in turn was the strongest predictor of subsequent PTSD.
   d. In animal studies, high levels of cortisol are damaging to the hippocampus.
3. The **hippocampus tends to be smaller** in subjects with PTSD. MRI measurement of hippocampal volume in patients with PTSD detect slightly smaller hippocampal volumes, which are correlated with severity of traumatic exposure, cognitive deficits, and PTSD symptoms. The significance of these findings is unclear; lower volumes may represent a pre-morbid risk factor, a result of exogenous toxins, or the result of elevated cortisol. Magnetic resonance spectroscopy is able to quantify the amount of the amino acid *N*-acetyl aspartate (NAA) which reflects the density or viability of neurons; diminished hippocampal NAA has been found in PTSD.
4. A growing number of subjects have been studied with functional neuroimaging while stimulated with traumatic material. **A typical pattern of brain activation** in the face of traumatic stimuli in persons with PTSD is emerging. The studies show that the **amygdala is hyperreactive** to stimuli that are linked to a traumatic event. **Associated anterior paralimbic regions** of the brain are also activated in response to symptom provocation. Studies have also shown diminished activation of the **anterior cingulate cortex** in PTSD. As above, the anterior cingulate is thought to regulate emotion and play a role in extinction of conditioned fear responses. A study of women with PTSD showed decrease blood flow to the hippocampus during exposure to traumatic material. These findings support a model of PTSD where the **amygdala** and related structures (the "hot" and "emotional" memory system) are **overactive,** while the hippocampus (the "cool" and "cognitive" memory system) and anterior cingulate cortex is underactive. Current research is exploring and refining these models.

IX. Evaluation and Treatment Immediately Following a Traumatic Event

Immediately following a traumatic event, survivors rarely come to the attention of psychiatrists. Victims of trauma focus on practical concerns, such as re-establishing safety, obtaining information, responding to medical or legal concerns, securing food and shelter, and connection with family and other social supports. Most people adapt to traumatic events without professional help and often decline an offer of such help. There is a great deal of interest in determining whether or not acute psychological intervention can have an impact on the subsequent development of post-traumatic symptoms. A variety of debriefing strategies have been developed and research findings are mixed. Some studies suggest that well-trained clinicians, working in teams, can implement a highly structured debriefing process in a group setting that can diminish the development of PTSD symptoms. Other studies suggest that such interventions can actually worsen outcome, perhaps because of the expression of overwhelming feelings. Current research is evaluating whether such debriefings should be offered to all survivors or only those at high risk. Evaluation and treatment should include and be guided by the following principles.

A. **Help the individual regain a sense of mastery and control.** Communicate a sense of hope and expectation of recovery.
B. **Encourage the use of existing supports** and refer for psychological treatment only those at high risk; the option of follow-up should be made to all.
C. **Pay attention to the practical and immediate concerns** brought about by the traumatic event. Tell the patient any information available about the event.
D. **Assess the patient's mental status** to determine if he or she can manage safely with current available support. Dissociation can be pronounced and can be an important risk factor for the subsequent development of PTSD.
E. **Gently encourage the patient to review the trauma** and the surrounding events if he or she seems motivated to do so. If possible, identify the aspect of the trauma that was most distressing to the patient. However, the patient's capacity to tolerate the re-telling must be considered. It is not necessarily helpful and can be harmful for the patient to become overwhelmed by recounting the trauma. The need for the patient to face the "reality of the trauma" must be balanced with "denial," which may help the patient process the experience in a tolerable fashion. **Appreciate and respect the patient's coping style.**
F. **Assess the patient for risk factors for PTSD.** Those at highest risk may need ongoing treatment.

G. **Victims of rape,** for example, **need specialized follow-up.** They will need a medical work-up that evaluates their physical well-being, appropriately documents findings for any legal proceedings, and provides a sense of safety. Referral for specialized psychological services, such as those provided by a rape crisis center, can provide support, treatment, and assistance with legal issues.

H. **Assess whether the patient is at risk for ongoing trauma,** or is a victim of child or spousal abuse. Children need immediate protection (often with the help of social service agencies). Victims of domestic violence come from all socioeconomic groups; they will need encouragement to seek help; often they are reluctant to acknowledge the extent of their danger. Patients who face a persistent threat should be encouraged to write out a safety plan that details concrete steps they will take to avoid future trauma. These steps may include involving local law enforcement authorities. Although the clinician can encourage the patient to take steps to protect him- or herself, it is ultimately the patient who must make that decision.

I. **Tolerate the patient's feelings and help put them into context.** It can be very reassuring for a patient to know that feelings of fear, helplessness, guilt, shame, and anger are expected responses to a traumatic event. The patient may need to be reassured that he or she is not "going crazy."

J. **Educate the patients about the common responses to trauma,** which can help him or her feel more in control of their experiences. The patients should be told that he or she might experience insomnia, nightmares, intrusive memories, and irritability in the first few months or so after the trauma but that these symptoms should then begin to subside.

K. **Educate patients about possible maladaptive responses to trauma.** Alcohol abuse is common as patients attempt to manage hyperarousal and intrusive symptoms.

L. **Use medication sparingly.** There is no long-term benefit from heavily sedating a patient following a trauma. Severe anxiety, agitation, and insomnia may be treated with low-dose benzodiazepines. Supplies should be given for not more than a few days and are contraindicated in patients with alcohol or substance abuse.

X. Evaluation of Patients with PTSD

Patients are evaluated for PTSD in a variety of settings; the evaluation may be part of a general psychiatric evaluation in which the PTSD is not yet diagnosed, or part of a course of treatment specific for PTSD. The evaluation needs to be tailored to the needs of the current circumstances. An evaluation should include and be guided by the following principles:

A. **The time course of the patient's symptoms has important clinical implications.** Symptoms may cause clinically significant impairment in the first month (as in acute stress disorder), or after the first month (as PTSD). One group of patients will improve and return to an acceptable level of functioning, whereas another group will go on to have chronic PTSD. After 3 months, PTSD is a chronic psychiatric illness.

B. **PTSD, although prevalent, is notoriously difficult to diagnose.** In a general psychiatric evaluation, one should screen for exposure to traumatic events throughout the life cycle. **It may be more effective to ask about specific traumas than to ask about trauma in general, but questions should be introduced in a normalizing and non-judgmental manner.** For example, a clinician might say, "It is common for people to have been touched in ways they didn't want while they were growing up. Did you ever have the experience of being touched in a sexual or harsh way while you were a child?"

C. **Be aware of how the interview is affecting the patient.** Especially in regards to trauma, straightforward questions may evoke a sudden eruption of powerful and overwhelming feelings. Work with the patient to establish a tolerable level of distress appropriate for the circumstances of the interview. For example, a clinician might say, "I realize that some of these questions may bring up strong feelings, let me know if this is something that might be difficult to talk about." If the patient cannot tolerate talking about the trauma itself, it may be useful for the clinician to shift the focus to the effects of the traumatic event on various aspects of the individual's life.

D. **Offer the patient an opportunity to recount the traumatic event.** Note the patient's capacity to tell the story. Some patients will find it helpful to talk about the event, some will be so overwhelmed they think or speak of nothing else, others will not be able to speak of the trauma at all.

E. **Review the symptoms of PTSD and assess the intensity and the frequency of the patient's symptoms.** Patients will frequently report intrusive symptoms and be hyper-aroused, but rarely the symptoms of avoidance and numbing can be disabling. Ask the patient how he or she cope with symptoms. Are there ways he or she has learned to come out of a flashback or to manage the irritability of hyperarousal?

F. **Evaluate the patient's overall psychological, social, and occupational function.** Has the patient been able to resume his or her usual activities? Is there difficulty resuming activities which the patient associates to the trauma? How is the patient relating to family and friends? Is there an increase in social isolation or feelings of alienation? Assess the patient's pre-morbid functioning; has the trauma changed the patient's self-esteem, their capacity to tolerate loss, their ability to manage dependency, autonomy, and intimacy? Is the patient able to trust and to take risks?

G. **Assess how the trauma has affected the individual's "sense of themselves"** or self-schema and how the trauma may impact ongoing issues related to the individual's developmental stage. For instance, if a young man is assaulted, this may conflict with his idea of masculinity, which may be defined by his physical prowess. In another example, the effects of childhood sexual abuse may become evident as a young woman develops difficulties in a relationship with a man, or is flooded with memories as she cares for a young child.

H. **Formulate a differential diagnosis,** as several psychiatric illnesses share features of PTSD.
   1. **Psychotic disorders** and PTSD can each present with hallucinations. Hallucinations in a patient with PTSD typically involve a fragment of the traumatic event, or a voice of a perpetrator. At times a patients may hear their name called out. Patients with PTSD typically do not have delusions or a formal thought disorder.
   2. **Bipolar disorder** and PTSD can each present with irritable and labile mood, anger outbursts, a marked disturbance of sleep, and impulsive, risk-taking behavior. Patients with PTSD do not experience prolonged euphoria or expansive moods.
   3. **Major depressive disorder** and PTSD share a number of symptoms including emotional withdrawal, detachment, social isolation, helplessness, agitation, and sleep disturbance. It is common for PTSD patients to develop secondary depression. Weight loss or gain and generalized feelings of guilt are more typical of a primary depression.
   4. **Other anxiety disorders** and PTSD share a number of characteristics; patients with panic and agoraphobia are also avoidant, panic attacks manifest the same type of autonomic arousal that patients with PTSD experience when they have an intrusive memory, and the obsessive thought of a person with obsessive-compulsive disorder (OCD) can resemble the fixation with the trauma seen in PTSD.

I. **Screen the patient for frequently occurring comorbid conditions** that complicate treatment and recovery.
   1. Alcohol and other substance abuse
   2. Major depressive disorder
   3. Somatoform disorders
   4. Dissociative disorders
   5. Other anxiety disorders

J. **Evaluate the patient's strengths, and note the efforts made to successfully adapt to the trauma.** Patients may present for treatment due to a precipitant that disrupts previously successful adaptation to a traumatic event.

K. **Assess the patient's safety.** Is there a risk for ongoing trauma?

XI. Guidelines for the Treatment of PTSD

PTSD varies in its severity and its time course. Some patients use treatment to overcome overwhelming trauma, others appear to make little progress at all. For some, the passage of time and life events offer a chance for recovery; for others the trauma has made it impossible to move forward in life. The symptoms of PTSD can create a cycle that traps some patients within a world of the trauma. Traumatic memories, vivid, and timeless, threaten to overwhelm the survivor. Efforts are made to cope with such powerful and disorganized memories; the threat from within is that any intense feeling may trigger a traumatic memory, the threat from without is that many stimuli have become associated with the trauma. The person may withdraw into dissociative states or use alcohol to control intrusive memories and hyperarousal. People with PTSD may feel helpless in coping with the past and helpless in managing the present. The loss of control in the present stimulates traumatic memories and perpetuates the cycle. Psychiatric treatment for PTSD aims to address this cycle and is guided by the following general principles:

A. **Treatment generally involves an integration of several therapeutic approaches,** including **psychodynamic** and **cognitive-behavioral. Cognitive-behavioral approaches have been the most carefully studied and have been found to be the most effective. Medication** often plays an important role.

B. **Treatment is phase-oriented.** The initial goal is to **stabilize the patient** and address acute symptoms. The second phase involves **working through the trauma,** and the last phase focuses on **re-establishing social relationships.**

C. **Stabilization can be a prolonged phase**, and in some cases comprises the entire treatment. **Education** about post-traumatic experiences is the cornerstone of therapy. If patients can anticipate expectable post-traumatic responses, he or she can feel less helpless. **Identifying feelings** and putting words to bodily experiences begins to organize a chaotic emotional world. As a patient learns to notice how symptoms come and go, he or she can discover how to exercise more control over their emotional life. **Safety** is facilitated by the connection to the therapist in a treatment that has clear and predictable boundaries. Stabilization involves **addressing maladaptive behaviors,** such as substance abuse and self-destructive behavior. Ongoing exposure to trauma will undermine improvement, and patients may need to be taught to distinguish safe from unsafe behavior.

D. Treat co-morbid disorders.

E. Patients can **work through the trauma** in several different ways. They can learn to tolerate the traumatic memories and environmental triggers and become desensitized, thereby **diminishing avoidance.** Patients can also begin to create a narrative of the traumatic event and understand its personal meaning. The reality of the trauma and its impact becomes integrated into the survivor's sense of self.

F. Ultimately, the patient must return to daily life in the community. Facilitating the development of **social relationships** is an important part of recovery from trauma.

G. Treating a patient with PTSD can put the therapist under significant emotional strain. Hearing about the traumatic event and witnessing a patient's distress can be traumatic for the therapist. It can be difficult for the therapist to maintain the necessary balance between seeing the patient as a helpless victim *and* as a survivor capable of taking responsibility.

H. The therapist must balance the need for the patient to review the traumatic event with the danger that the patient will be traumatized by the re-telling.

I. Patients with a history of childhood sexual abuse or patients with **complex PTSD** are often challenging to treat. These patients often have significant **difficulties with affect regulation and trust.** It may take years for a patient to develop a relationship with the therapist sufficiently robust to manage the exploration of the trauma. For such a patient, learning **impulse control, affect regulation, boundary management, and basic positive self-regard** are prerequisites for exploration of the trauma itself.

XII. Psychosocial Treatment Modalities for PTSD

A. Cognitive-behavioral approaches include anxiety management, cognitive therapy, exposure therapy, and psychoeducation. Each have been found to be effective psychotherapy tools. They are often used in combination with each other.

1. **Exposure therapy** has been found to be the most effective treatment modality for those patients who can tolerate it. The goal of treatment is the **disruption of the link between trauma-related cues and the intense anxiety and avoidance that is typical for PTSD.** The technique often stimulates the patient to **experience a traumatic memory to modify the response to that memory.** Patients are taught to distinguish trauma memories and trauma-related emotions from current reality and thereby feel more in control of their world. Repeated exposure helps patients learn to master their fear. **Prolonged exposure** therapy, developed by Foa and colleagues (2000), has shown promising results. The treatment typically includes breathing training, psychoeducation, and discussions following the imaginal exposure to the traumatic memory. A course of treatment typically includes 10 twice-weekly sessions. On average, patients experience a 65% reduction in symptoms and its benefits appear to persist.
2. **Psychoeducation** involves teaching the patient about the range of responses to traumatic events. By explaining to the patient the nature of his or her symptoms, how they might arise and what function they may serve, it helps to organize a frightening experience. By outlining common maladaptive responses to traumatic events, patients can focus on behavioral interventions to address the maladaptive behaviors. For example, by understanding how avoidance commonly occurs following trauma, patients can begin to notice the behavior and try to alter it.
3. **Cognitive therapy** focuses on identifying underlying, **distorted, "all-or-nothing" beliefs** about the world following the trauma. For example, "I am a helpless person . . . the world is not a safe place . . . I am guilty for everything." These distorted thoughts can be addressed and altered.
4. **Anxiety management** teaches patients to handle anxiety. These techniques include relaxation training, breathing exercises, assertiveness training, and thought stopping.

B. Eye Movement Desensitization and Reprocessing (EMDR)

1. Shapiro (1995) found that negative responses to disturbing memories and thoughts were attenuated with rapid eye movements. She developed a treatment used for PTSD based on the following technique:
   a. An affect-laden image of the trauma is constructed along with a summary statement.
   b. Subjective distress is rated.
   c. An alternate, positive statement is formulated.
   d. Eye movements are initiated by the patient following an object moving across the visual field, while the patient holds in mind the traumatic image.
   e. After 12–24 repetitions, the patient notes his or her subjective distress.
   f. The cycle is repeated 3–15 times until there is significant reduction in distress.
2. The treatment is advocated as an adjunct to other modalities. Proponents suggest that several sessions can significantly reduce PTSD symptoms.
3. The psychiatric community and the scientific literature are divided over this technique. To date there is no

clearly documented method of action. Critics contend that, at best, EMDR is a non-intrusive exposure technique and that its benefits are non-specific. Advocates contend that, although its method of action is unclear, the benefits are impressive. Studies suggest that it is an effective treatment for PTSD.

C. **Psychodynamic approaches** are characterized by the following:
   1. This approach **emphasizes exploration of the personal meaning of the traumatic event** for the individual patient.
   2. **The impact of the trauma on the patient's self-concept is explored;** often feelings of shame, grief, and helplessness emerge. As the treatment progresses, feelings of guilt and anger and fantasies of omnipotent control are frequently encountered.
   3. **Unresolved conflicts from earlier in life may be exacerbated** by the trauma and dealt with in the treatment.
   4. **The patient's coping styles and defenses are noted.** Patients who are experiencing flooding of affects are helped to organize themselves, and those who are overcontrolled and detached are helped to gain access to feelings. Patients may need to explore their fears of losing control as they begin treatment.
   5. **The patient's relationship with the therapist is seen as an integral part of the treatment.** The connection helps contain affects and process transference reactions.

D. **Group treatment** can be an important component of an overall treatment plan, providing support and information. For some patients, group settings allow for a diffusion of the strong transference reactions that can impede treatment progress.

XIII. Pharmacotherapy of PTSD

Medication is an important part of the treatment for PTSD. Medication should be tailored to the stage of the illness and should target specific symptoms. Some level of anxiety may be necessary for the patient to make use of psychological treatment.

Until recently, there had been few controlled studies of medication for PTSD; recently sertraline and paroxetine have received FDA-approval as a treatment for PTSD. Medications that have been evaluated in open trials are now being subjected to more vigorous study.

A. **Selective serotonin reuptake inhibitors (SSRIs)** are first-line treatment and have been found to be most helpful in treating the intrusive, avoidant and hyperaroused symptoms of PTSD. **Sertraline** (Zoloft) 50–200 mg per day and **paroxetine** (Paxil) 20–60 mg per day have been FDA-approved for PTSD but **fluoxetine** (Prozac) 20–80 mg, **fluvoxamine** (Luvox) 100–300 mg, and **citalopram** (Celexa) 40 mg per day also appear to be helpful.

B. The data on **tricyclic antidepressants** are mixed, but they have been found to be somewhat helpful for intrusive symptoms and insomnia.

C. **Nefazodone** (Serzone), 300–500 mg, is frequently used and has been noted to be helpful, especially in veterans.

D. **Venlafaxine** (Effexor XR) 75–225 mg is popular with experts in the field, but it has not been well studied for PTSD.

E. **Monoamine oxidase inhibitors** have been shown to be effective in intrusive symptoms, but these medications are rarely used because of dietary restrictions and drug interactions.

F. **Antiadrenergics** are commonly used to treat **intrusive symptoms**, including nightmares. **Prazosin** was found to have benefit in a small placebo-controlled study. Data in open studies support the use of these medications: **propanolol** (Inderal) 20–60 mg per day or **clonidine** (Catapres) 0.1–0.2 mg b.i.d. or **guanfacine** (Tenex) 1–3 mg per day.

G. **Benzodiazepines** should be used with extreme caution, and some centers actively discourage their use. They can be helpful in acute situations. **Clonazapam** (Klonopin), **lorazapam** (Ativan), and other benzodiazepines can be used in low doses for symptoms of hyperarousal. Tolerance and abuse are common problems. The use of these medications in patients with a history of alcohol or substance abuse is contraindicated.

H. **Hypnotics.** Insomnia can be a persistent and distressing symptom in PTSD. **Trazodone** (Desyrel) 25–100 mg, **doxepin** (Sinequan) 25–50 mg, **amitryptyline** (Elavil) 25–50 mg and **mirtazapine** (Remeron) 15–45 mg may be useful as adjunctive treatments for insomnia.

I. **Mood stabilizers,** such as valproate (Depakote), carbamazapine (Tegretol), and lithium, have been studied in small, open studies. They can be used empirically for mood lability and anger outbursts. Newer anticonvulsants may also become useful. Anecdotal evidence has suggested some benefit from **topiramate** (topomax), with reduction of intrusive memories and improved mood

J. **Antipsychotic medication** is generally reserved for the most disorganized and psychotic patients. A recent study using olanzapine found some modest benefit in using the medication to augment SSRIs in non-responders. Improvement in sleep in particular was noted. Other atypical antipsychotics may find a role in the treatment of PTSD.

Suggested Readings

American Psychiatric Association. (2000). *Diagnostic and statistical manual of mental disorders (4th ed., Text Revised).* Washington, DC: American Psychiatric Press.

Breslau, N. (2001). The epidemiology of posttraumatic stress disorder. *Journal of Clinical Psychiatry, 62*(suppl 17), 16–22.

Foa, E.B., Davidson, J.R.T., & Frances, A. (Eds.). (1999). The expert consensus guideline series: Treatment of posttraumatic stress disorder. *Journal of Clinical Psychiatry, 60*(suppl 16).

Foa, E.B., Keane, T.C., & Friedman, M. (Eds.). (2000). *Effective treatments for PTSD: Practice guidelines from the International Society for Traumatic Stress Studies.* New York: Guilford Press.

Foa, E.B., Rothbaum, B.O., & Furr, J.M. (2003). Augmenting exposure therapy with other CBT procedures. *Psychiatry Annals, 33*(1), 47–53

Herman, J.L. (1993). Sequelae of prolonged and repeated trauma: Evidence for a complex posttraumatic syndrome (DESNOS). In J.R.T. Davidson & E.B. Foa (Eds.), *Posttraumatic stress disorder: DSM-IV and beyond* (pp. 213–228). Washington, DC: American Psychiatric Press.

Kessler, R., Sonnega, A., Bromet, E., Highes, M., & Nelson, C. (1995). Posttraumatic stress disorder in the National Comorbidity Survey. *Archives of General Psychiatry, 52*, 1048–1060.

Marshall, R.D., Beebe, K.L., Oldham, M., & Zaninelli, R. (2001). Efficacy and safety of paroxetine treatment for chronic PTSD: A fixed dose placebo-controlled study. *American Journal of Psychiatry, 158*(12), 1982–1988.

Ornstein, R. (1998). Approach to the patient following a traumatic event. In T.A. Stern, J.B. Herman, & P.L. Slavin (Eds.), *The MGH guide to psychiatry in primary care*. New York: McGraw-Hill.

Pitman, R., Shin, L., & Rauch, S. (2001). Investigating the pathogenesis of postraumatic stress disorder with neuroimaging. *Journal of Clinical Psychiatry, 62*(suppl 17), 47–54.

Raskin, M., Peskind, E.R., Kanter, E.D., et al. (2003). Reduction of nightmares and other PTSD symptoms in combat veterans by Prazosin: A placebo-controlled study. *American Journal of Psychiatry, 160*, 371–373.

Rauch, S., Shin, L., & Pitman, R. (1998). Evaluating the effects of psychological trauma using neuroimaging techniques. In R. Yehuda (Ed.), *Psychological trauma.* Washington, DC: American Psychiatric Press.

Saigh, P.A., & Bremner, D.J. (Eds.). (1999). *Posttraumatic stress disorder: A comprehensive text.* Boston: Allyn & Bacon.

Shalev, A.Y., Yehuda, R., & McFarlane, A. (1999). *International handbook of human response to trauma* (2nd ed.). Kluwer Academic Publishers.

Shapiro, F. (1995). *Eye movement desensitization and reprocessing.* New York: Guilford Press.

Stein, M.B., Jang, K.L., Taylor, S., et al. (2002). Genetic and environmental influences on trauma exposure and PTSD. *American Journal of Psychiatry, 159*(10), 1675–1681

Tomb, D.A., & Allen, S.N. (1994). Phenomenology of posttraumatic stress disorder. *Psychiatric Clinics of North America, 17*(2), 237–250.

Van der Kolk, B., McFarlane, A.C., & Weisaeth, L. (Eds.) (1996). *Traumatic stress.* New York: Guilford Press.

Wilson, J.P., Friedman, M.J., & Lindy, J. (Eds.). (2001). *Treating psychological trauma and PTSD.* New York: Guilford Press.

Yehuda, R. (2001). Biology of posttraumatic stress disorder. *Journal of Clinical Psychiatry, 62*(suppl 17), 41–45.

Chapter 17

Somatoform Disorders

CRISTINA BRUSCO AND EDYE GERINGER

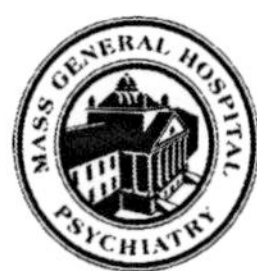

I. Introduction

A. Overview

Somatization can occur either as a symptom or as a psychiatric syndrome. All somatoform disorders share the feature of the over-importance of physical symptoms and illness in a patient's life, which may lead to the patient feeling misunderstood by health care professionals. This can lead to breakdown in the physician-patient relationship and to increased attempts to legitimize their quest for care.

1. **Definitions of somatization**
   a. Somatization is characterized by the tendency, in the absence of an organic etiology, to experience and communicate somatic distress in response to psychosocial stress, to attribute this distress to physical illness, and to seek medical help for these symptoms. This can range from normal complaints (e.g., headaches) to the belief that one has an illness (e.g., melanoma).
   b. Somatization also involves a disturbance in the way a person perceives, organizes, attributes, and/or expresses physical experiences.
2. **Impact of somatization.** Somatization accounts for a disproportionate number of users of medical care, laboratory tests, procedures, visits, hospital stays, and total health care costs (up to $30 billion per year). However, most individuals report numerous physical symptoms and do not seek medical attention.
3. **Etiologies of somatization.** Various physical, psychological, cultural, interpersonal, and biological theories have been proposed to explain somatization.
   a. The **"wandering womb"** refers to the ancient Egyptian belief that hysteria was caused by the uterus which migrated upward and displaced other organs to cause discomfort.
   b. Somatization can be used as an **intrapsychic defense,** whereby a patient can ward off unbearable impulses or affects, such as unacceptable bodily sensations, murderous rage, or forbidden sexuality. The pain and suffering are seen as "deserved" and used as atonement for hostile impulses.
   c. Somatization can be a means of **social communication** for some patients, allowing them to tell their doctor and the world that "I am a person deserving of care." A patient may attain the sick role and/or **secondary gain** by virtue of physical complaints.
   d. **"Abnormal illness behavior"** occurs when the provider and the patient have disparate assumptions about the nature of illness. This mismatch can lead to a failure to respond to treatment and to the excessive utilization of health care.
   e. **Learning theory** implicates a patient's ability to recall symptoms from either the patient's own or a role model's experiences as a means of expressing current distress.
   f. **Cultural stigma of psychiatric illness** can account for why patients express their symptoms physically. For example, it is easier for a Chinese patient to accept "neurasthenia" as a diagnosis rather than depression.
   g. The presence of lateralized defects on **structural and functional brain imaging studies,** alexithymia, and impaired selective attention on neuropsychological testing may help explain why some psychiatric states can only be expressed with physical symptoms.

B. DSM-IV Somatoform Disorders (see Table 17-1)

1. Somatization disorder
2. Undifferentiated somatoform disorder
3. Conversion disorder
4. Pain disorder
5. Hypochondriasis
6. Body dysmorphic disorder
7. Somatoform disorder not otherwise specified

II. Somatization Disorder (Hysteria, Multisymptomatic Hysteria, or Briquet's Disease)

A. Definition

Somatization disorder is a chronic disorder characterized by multiple, clinically significant somatic complaints that results in impairment of function and/or frequent use of medical services.

B. History

Thought of for thousands of years as a disorder of women, **Sydenham in 1679** linked the disorder in men and women to psychological stressors, referring to them as "antecedent sorrows." **Briquet, in 1859,** focused on a long course involving multisymptomatic complaints, and labeled the condition "multisymptomatic hysteria." In the 1950s, objective criteria were introduced; **in the 1970s the term "Briquet's disease" was coined.** Modern classification has moved away from use of eponyms. The current DSM-IV concept of somatization disorder has been criticized as being too narrow for clinical use. Instead, Kirmayer and Robbins proposed the idea of **presenting somatization**—"the predominantly or exclusively somatic presentation of psychiatric disorders, most commonly depression and anxiety" as distinct from **functional somatization**—"high levels of medically unexplained symptom reporting."

Table 17-1. Comparison of Somatoform Disorders

	Somatization Disorder	*Conversion*	*Pain Disorder*	*Hypochondriasis*	*Body Dysmorphic Disorder*
Main features	Recurrent, multiple, chronic, somatic complaints not accounted for by medical findings	Symptoms affecting voluntary motor or sensory systems, suggesting neurological disorder, preceded by stress	Pain is the predominant focus of treatment, psychological factors affect onset, severity, exacerbation, and maintenance	Fear of, or belief that one has a serious illness despite adequate medical evaluation and reassurance, NOT DELUSIONAL	Imagined ugliness, NOT DELUSIONAL INTENSITY
Age of onset	< 30	10–35	Any age	Early adulthood	Adolescence
Associated features	Repeated work-ups, multiple physicians, inconsistent history, chaotic lives	*La belle indifference,* suggestible symptoms do not conform to anatomical pathways	Disability, social isolation, search for the cure	Repeated work-ups, doctor shopping, childhood illness	Frequent checking, avoidance, feeling mocked by others; surgery makes it worse
Co-morbid medical illness	+/–	+/–	Common	Infrequent	No
Epidemiology	0.2–2% women, 0.2% men	25% of medical outpatients	?	4–9% medical outpatients	?
Gender	women > men	2:1–10:1 women > men	Equal	Equal	Equal
Course	Chronic	Usually self-limited, 25% recur in one year	Variable, often chronic	Chronic, waxes and wanes	Chronic
Secondary gain	+/–	+/–	+	+/–	–
Family history	Somatization disorder, antisocial, substance abuse	Conversion disorder	Depression alcohol abuse, pain disorder	Illness in family member when a child	
Co-morbid psychiatric illness	Major depression panic, substance abuse, personality disorder	Dissociative disorder, PTSD, depression	Substance abuse, depression anxiety	Anxiety, depression	Depression delusional disorder, social phobia, OCD, suicide
Treatment	Regular appointments, maintain vs. cure	Suggest cure, examine stress, no need to confront	Avoid iatrogenesis, multi-modal treatment, care not cure	? Selective serotonin reuptake inhibitors	Prevent iatrogenesis, SSRI, ? antipsychotics

C. DSM-IV Criteria

1. **A history of multiple and recurring physical complaints over several years, which begin before the age of 30. The physical complaints result in medical treatment or cause significant impairment in social, occupational, or other important areas of function.**
2. **To make the diagnosis all four of the following criteria have to be met at some time during the illness:**
   a. **Four pain symptoms,** each in a different area of the body or of a different function, such as headache, back pain, arthralgias, rectal and abdominal pain, dysmenorrhea, dysuria, and dyspareunia.
   b. **Two non-pain-related gastrointestinal symptoms,** such as bloating, nausea, vomiting, diarrhea, and food sensitivity.
   c. **One sexual symptom,** other than pain, such as decreased desire, erectile dysfunction, menorrhagia, or hyperemesis gravidum.
   d. **One pseudoneurological symptom,** including amnesia, fainting, blindness, double vision, aphasia, seizure, ataxia, and paralysis.

3. **The symptoms, after appropriate investigation, are not caused by a known medical condition or substance.** If a medical condition does exist, the complaints or impairment are deemed grossly in excess of expected.
4. **The symptoms are neither intentionally produced nor feigned.**

D. Clinical Features

1. **The patient's history**
   a. The major goal of the patient is apparently to communicate distress through a recitation of symptoms.
   b. The **history is often colorful and dramatic,** there is often little specific information, and it is often inconsistent from visit to visit. It may be presented as an unending laundry list of complaints with great detail. This means that a reliable diagnosis of this chronic illness can often be made only over time.
   c. A patient with this condition may not be able to distinguish between emotional and somatic feelings.
   d. **An afflicted patient is at risk for iatrogenic complications.**
   e. These patients may seek multiple treaters, including alternative health providers, and **doctor-shop** in search of a cure.
   f. **The relationship with treaters is often strained** and ends in mutual frustration and dissatisfaction.
2. **Clinical Course**
   a. The onset of symptoms can start in adolescence; the diagnostic criteria are usually met by age 25.
   b. The symptoms are chronic and fluctuate; rarely do the symptoms remit completely.

E. Epidemiology

1. Community surveys reveal that **women have a 0.2–2% lifetime prevalence of somatoform disorders.**
2. **In men the overall prevalence is 0.2%.** Greek and Puerto Rican men account for 5–20% of those with disorder.
3. Culture may also impact presenting symptoms. For example, burning in the hands and feet is more common in men from Southeast Asia, as compared with North American men. This may alter the review of systems.

F. Psychiatric Co-Morbidity

1. Axis I: 50% of patients with mood disorders. Anxiety disorders, substance abuse, and post-traumatic stress disorder are also common.
2. Axis II: 72% of patients with somatization disorder have personality disorders, most commonly histrionic, borderline, and antisocial personality disorders.
3. The co-morbidity of a history of childhood sexual abuse and neglect and somatoform disorder is high (30–70%).
4. **A family history of somatization disorder is quite common.**
   a. 10–20% of first-degree female relatives of female patients with somatization disorder develop it themselves.
   b. Male relatives of female patients with somatization disorder are more likely to have antisocial personality disorder and problems with substance abuse.
   c. Adoption studies have demonstrated that patients are five times more likely to present with somatoform disorders if either the biologic parents or the adoptive parents have had somatization disorder.

G. Differential Diagnosis

1. Since many medical conditions (e.g., acute intermittent porphyria, multiple sclerosis, systemic lupus erythematosus, endocrine disorders, chronic infections) present with variable and fluctuating courses, it is important to distinguish medical from psychiatric disorders.
2. **Somatization disorder is more likely than an underlying medical condition when there is:**
   a. Multiple organ involvement
   b. An early-onset of disease
   c. A chronic course
   d. An absence of any laboratory, radiographic, or physical abnormalities
3. **Other psychiatric disorders can mimic somatization disorder, and include:**
   a. Schizophrenia, when multiple somatic delusions are present
   b. Anxiety disorders, especially during a panic attack
   c. Depressive disorders, during a depressive episode
   d. Another somatoform disorder

H. Treatment

1. The goal of treatment is to **provide care for the patient but not to focus on curing the disease.**
2. The best **treatment occurs in the context of a long-term relationship** with an **empathic primary care provider** (PCP). The PCP should be encouraged to:
   a. Allow the patient to **maintain the sick role.**
   b. Schedule **regular follow-up appointments** of a **set length.**
   c. **Set the agenda** of the visit.
   d. **Prevent iatrogenesis** and limit work-ups to objective findings and not complaints.
   e. **Do no more and no less for the somatic patient than for any other patient.**
   f. **Set limits** on contacts outside of visit time.
   g. **Introduce psychosocial issues slowly,** using stress or mind-body language.
3. **Psychiatric referral** is useful to treat and manage co-morbid psychiatric disorders.
   a. Psychiatric **consultation decreases health care costs** and unnecessary utilization of services.

b. The goal of psychiatric consultation is to provide a **framework for treatment.** It should not be viewed as the end of the relationship with the PCP.
c. **Co-morbid psychiatric disorders should be treated** and managed by the PCP or psychiatric consultant.
d. **Individual or group psychotherapy** can be useful in either a dynamic or cognitive-behavioral model.
4. **Stress-reduction** education can be useful.
5. A small number of studies report symptom improvement with antidepressant use (independent of depression).

III. Undifferentiated Somatoform Disorder (Somatization Syndrome or Subthreshold Somatization Disorder)

A. Definition

This category includes subthreshold somatization disorders, such as chronic fatigue syndrome, ecological allergies, multiple chemical sensitivities, and fibromyalgia.

B. DSM-IV Criteria

1. **One or more physical complaints** (such as fatigue, loss of appetite, or a gastrointestinal complaint or urinary complaint) **must persist for 6 months or longer.**
2. Either:
   a. **The symptoms,** after appropriate evaluation, **cannot be fully explained** by a known medical condition or substance or
   b. **The complaints or impairments are grossly in excess of what would be expected** on the basis of the existing medical condition.
3. **The symptoms must cause significant distress or impairment** in social, occupational, or another important area of functioning.
4. **The symptoms are neither intentionally produced nor feigned.**

C. Clinical Features

1. The presentation is similar to that of somatization disorder, but it may be more culturally-based, as an idiom of distress, or as a manifestation of stigma avoidance.
2. The course is variable; an eventual diagnosis of a general medical disorder is more common than it is in somatization disorder.

D. Epidemiology

1. This disorder **occurs most commonly in young women of low socioeconomic status.** It is 30 times more frequent than is somatization disorder. **It's lifetime prevalence is 4–11%.**
2. **The diagnosis of multi-somatoform disorder, with three medically unexplained symptoms, has been proposed as clinically relevant as this threshold correlates significantly with increased disability.**

E. Differential Diagnosis

1. The differential diagnosis includes the same medical disorders that are found along with somatization disorder.
2. The psychiatric differential diagnosis includes somatization disorder, somatoform disorder NOS, major depression, anxiety, and malingering.

F. Treatment

The **treatment is similar to that of somatization disorder;** patients with this disorder may be more responsive to psychiatric referral.

IV. Conversion Disorder (Hysteria, Conversion Reaction, Hysterical Psychoneurosis, Conversion Type)

A. Definition

Conversion disorder involves the presence of symptoms or deficits that affect voluntary motor or sensory function in a fashion that suggests a neurologic condition but which is not explained by the medical findings.

B. History

1. Conversion disorders were described as early as **1900 B.C.** and labeled as hysteria, which led to the description of conversion and somatization disorders as indistinct until the 1850s. **Briquet** developed the first modern concept of conversion disorder as a central nervous system disorder. **Reynolds** introduced the idea of conversion as a loss of function secondary to ideas, and **Charcot** elaborated this by linking conversion symptoms and trauma. **Freud** used the concept to analyze the case of Dora. Currently, the importance of unconscious processes in diagnostic criteria has been reduced.

C. DSM-IV Criteria

1. **One or more symptoms or deficits affecting a voluntary motor or sensory function that suggests a neurological or general medical condition.**
   a. The sensory symptoms include double vision, blindness, deafness, and loss of touch or pain.
   b. The motor loss symptoms include paralysis, aphonia, difficulty swallowing, ataxia, tremor, and urinary retention.
2. **Symptom initiation or exacerbation is preceded by psychological conflict or stress.**
3. **The symptom, after appropriate investigation, cannot be fully explained by a general medical condition,** substance, or culturally-sanctioned experience, such as glossalia in religious rituals or hysterical epidemics.
4. **The symptom causes significant distress and is not feigned.**
5. **The symptom is not limited to pain or sexual dysfunction** and does not occur only in the course of somatization disorder.
6. Conversion disorder should be coded along with the type of deficit involved.

D. Clinical Features

1. **Patients**
   a. The more medically naive the patient, the greater the likelihood of implausible symptoms.

b. **Patients with this disorder tend to be suggestible.**
c. Conversion-disordered patients are more likely to have had **prior conversion symptoms** or symptoms or dissociation.
d. **One-third** of patients with conversion disorder **have concurrent neurological illness.** More than half of patients with pseudoseizures may have a neurologic illness.

2. **Symptoms**
   a. As opposed to the patient with somatization disorder or the patient with hypochondriasis who believes they are gravely ill, the patient with conversion disorder often presents with ***la belle indifference.***
   b. Symptoms are more likely to **occur following extreme stress.**
   c. Rather than following known anatomical pathways, the **symptoms tend to conform to a patient's own ideas** (e.g., a stocking-glove and a mid-line anesthesia).
   d. Symptoms are **inconsistent with the physical examination.** For example, a "paralyzed" arm doesn't fall on the patient's head, optokinetic nystagmus is maintained in hysterical blindness, and antagonistic muscle function is maintained in paralysis.
   e. The presentation may **resemble the patient's own symptoms** (e.g., epileptics who have pseudoseizures).
   f. The symptoms **rarely cause physical disability.**
   g. The symptoms **tend to recur.**
3. **Course**
   a. Conversion disorder is rarely reported in patients younger than 10 years, or older than 35 years of age; however, cases have been seen in people of all ages, including 90-year-olds.
   b. Patients with conversion disorder older than 35 years of age are more likely to have occult neurological disorders.
   c. The syndrome usually remits within 2 weeks after hospitalization, but it has a recurrence rate of 20–25% within the first year.
   d. Prior episodes increase the rate of recurrence.
   e. 20% of patients with conversion disorder develop somatization disorder within 4 years of their first episode.

E. Etiology

1. A **dynamic hypothesis** suggests that the conversion symptom is a solution to an unconscious conflict. Secondary gain is often an unconscious cause of conversion. For example, a woman whose husband had an affair may become paralyzed rather than walk away from the marriage.
2. **Altered structure and function** (especially of the right hemisphere) of both the dominant and nondominant **hemispheres,** as well as impaired cortical communication, seem to play a role in conversion symptoms.
3. **Hypercritical families** may create "unspeakable dilemmas" predisposing to conversion reactions.
4. Patients with conversion symptoms have higher levels of hypnotizability.

F. Epidemiology.

1. Conversion disorder is **the most common somatoform disorder.** Approximately 33% of female psychiatric outpatients report an episode of conversion. The annual incidence of conversion disorder in the general population is between 11 and 300/100,000. Conversion occurs in 25–30% of hospitalized veterans. Conversion is diagnosed in 5–16% psychiatric consultations and in 1–3% psychiatric outpatients.
2. The **rate of diagnosis is increasing** among rural populations, those with low socioeconomic status, and in developing regions.
3. A **gender bias exists,** with a ratio of 2–10:1, women to men. Left-handed women have a higher incidence.

G. Psychiatric Co-Morbidity

1. Conversion disorders can be a precursor to depression, somatization, and/or dissociative disorders.
2. Among Axis II–disordered patients (mostly with histrionic, dependent, antisocial personality disorders), conversion disorder can be an unconscious means to an end.
3. Patients with conversion disorder report more frequent and severe childhood trauma compared with patients with other psychiatric disorders.

H. Differential Diagnosis

1. Neurologic diseases are diagnosed in one-fifth to one-half of patients with conversion disorder. Early studies reported an even higher incidence.
2. The most common neurological disorders associated with conversion disorder are multiple sclerosis, myasthenia gravis, seizures, and dystonia.
3. Other somatoform disorders

I. Treatment

1. **A good prognosis is associated with an acute onset of disease, a clear stressor, a short interval between the onset of symptoms and initiation of treatment, rapid improvement in the hospital, an above-average intelligence, and a presenting symptom of paralysis, aphonia, or blindness.**
2. **A poor prognosis is associated with a presenting symptom of tremor and/or seizure, an increased interval between symptom onset and treatment, and a reduced intelligence level.**
3. The **use of suggestion** and **physical therapy** legitimizes the symptoms.
4. Confrontation of the patient is not helpful, as it results in a **"loss of face."**
5. **Indirect examination** of stressors can lead to relief.
6. **Behavioral techniques** should be instituted; referral to family therapy is often indicated.

V. Pain Disorder (Psychogenic Pain Disorder, Somatoform Pain Disorder)

A. Definition

Pain is the predominant focus of this clinical syndrome; it is associated with illness-affirming behavior.

B. History

In recent years there has been a movement away from etiology and towards a descriptive approach to this disorder. DSM-IV includes a subtype of pain associated with a medical disorder that is NOT a mental disorder.

C. DSM-IV Criteria

1. Pain occurs in one or more anatomical sites as the focus of attention.
2. Pain causes significant distress or impairment in social, occupational, or other areas of function. This includes disability, an increased use of health care facilities, an increased use of medications, and family problems.
3. Psychological factors have a role in the onset, severity, exacerbation, and maintenance of the pain.
4. The pain is not intentionally produced.
5. Pain disorder is not due to a mood, anxiety, or psychotic disorder, or to dyspareunia.
6. Subtypes and specifiers
   a. The 307.80 classification is used for a pain disorder that is associated with psychological factors.
   b. The 307.89 classification is a pain disorder associated with both psychological factors and a general medical condition.
   c. The last subtype is a pain disorder associated with a general medical condition (Axis III).
   d. Each subtype specifies an acute or chronic condition.

D. Clinical Features

1. Described as **severe and constant,** the pain may not be consistent with known anatomic pathways.
2. When the pain is consistent with a medical condition, the **severity is disproportionate to clinical findings.**
3. The most frequent sites of pain are the head, the face, the low back, and the pelvis.
4. **Pain is the main life focus** of a patient's energy; they frequently spend their life searching for a cure.
5. This behavior can lead to **disability** and **complications** that include iatrogenic substance abuse (opiates/benzodiazepines), fractured relationships, depression (which occurs in 30–50% of those with chronic pain), anxiety (with acute pain), and insomnia.
6. The **etiology is multi-factorial;** primary and secondary gain are often involved.

E. Epidemiology

The **prevalence** of these disorders is **unknown.** Pain disorder consumes a large amount of health resources with **$10 billion spent in 1980** on disability for chronic pain. The peak incidence occurs in the **third and fourth decade** of life. The **presenting symptoms** for male and females are different; **women** complain of more **headaches, men** complain more of **back pain.** A **family history** of increased depression, alcohol abuse, and pain disorders is often present. A **significant psychological stressor** is often the precipitating event.

F. Course

1. The **course is variable;** the syndrome can persist for years.
2. **A good prognosis is associated with continued work and the absence of pain as a focus of life.**
3. The differential psychiatric diagnosis includes malingering and factitious disorders.

G. Treatment

1. Emphasize **living with pain** and not removal of pain.
2. Employ a **multi-modal treatment** approach, combining physical, family, group and cognitive-behavioral therapy.
3. **Avoid iatrogenic** complications.
4. **Treat psychiatric illnesses** as they arise.

VI. Hypochondriasis

A. Definition

Hypochondriasis is a syndrome involving an excessive and pervasive preoccupation with fears of having, or the belief that one has, a serious illness that does not respond to reassurance after appropriate medical assessment.

B. History

Although it was described as a modern disease in the 1920s, hypochondrium before the nineteenth century meant abdomen. Therefore, hypochondriasis referred to disorders below the abdomen.

C. DSM-IV Criteria

1. **Hypochondriasis is a preoccupation with fears of having, or the idea that one has, a serious disease based on one's misinterpretation of bodily symptoms.**
2. **This preoccupation persists despite appropriate medical evaluation and reassurance;** the belief is not of delusional intensity (if so, a diagnosis of delusional disorder, somatic type is made).
3. This **preoccupation causes significant distress or impairment.**
4. **Hypochondriasis lasts at least 6 months** and is not accounted for by another mental disorder.

D. Clinical Features

1. **Symptoms**
   a. The **major presenting symptom** is a **fear of disease** and/or the **belief that one has a serious illness (disease conviction**). The symptoms are presented in excruciating detail as evidence of serious disease. The symptom reports can have a relentless quality.
   b. A patient's preoccupation can involve **any symptom or organ system** (e.g., heart rate, cough, headache). The complaints can be single or involve more than one system. It has been called **"medical student disease"** where

a patient reads about an illness and is convinced that he or she has it.

c. Hypochondriasis should be evaluated in a patient's **cultural context.**

2. **Doctor-patient relationship.** A patient with this problem frequently **doctor-shops,** which can be a source of frustration for both the doctor and patient. These patients are often **resistant to psychiatric referral.** Work-ups can become overzealous or inattentive.
3. **Clinical course**
   a. The **onset** is in **early adulthood.**
   b. **A chronic waxing and waning course is typical.**
   c. During a 5-year follow-up, two-thirds of patients still met criteria for hypochondriasis.
   d. Episodes may be **precipitated by stress,** especially the death of someone close.
4. **Etiology**
   a. **Amplification,** or misattribution hypothesis, refers to a patient that misinterprets a normal somatic sensation as an abnormal symptom.
   b. **Psychodynamic** hypotheses include the notion that hypochondriasis serves as an ego-defense against guilt, or as a vehicle for aggressive wishes toward others, or as a result of a transference to a physical complaint.
   c. **Learning theory** suggests that a patient may find that the sick role, reinforced by social interaction, can fulfill a need to be cared for.
   d. Variant theorists believe that **hypochondriasis is a form of another psychiatric disorder,** for example, OCD.

E. Epidemiology

1. **Hypochondriasis occurs in about 3–13%** of the general population in the United States. In Africa it occurs in 1% of the population (based on a survey of fourteen countries).
2. It can account for 4–9% of patients in general medical practice.
3. The incidence is equal in males and females.
4. The history often includes a childhood illness or illness of a significant family member when the patient was a child.

F. Differential Diagnosis

1. An underlying medical condition must be ruled out.
2. Hypochondriasis can occur as a transient response to medical illness.
3. Hypochondriasis can occur as a symptom of or co-morbidity with an Axis I disease, e.g., depression, anxiety disorders, specific disease phobia, OCD, somatoform disorders, psychotic disorders, or body dysmorphic disorder.

G. Treatment

1. A **good prognosis** for hypochondriasis **is associated with an acute onset** and **high levels of general medical co-morbidity.** It also includes an absence of a personality disorder, no secondary gain, high socioeconomic status, and less disease conviction.
2. Accompanying psychiatric conditions must be treated.
3. **Regular contact with a caring medical physician** should be maintained with palliation, and not cure, as the goal.
4. Patients may switch to **self-help** regimens.
5. The work-ups are based only on objective findings.
6. Cognitive-educational **group treatments** that include reattribution, distraction, and attentional tracking have been helpful.
7. Use of selective serotonin reuptake inhibitors **(SSRIs)** may have some benefit in these patients.

VII. Body Dysmorphic Disorder (BDD) (Dysmorphophobia)

A. Definition

BDD is a disease of imagined ugliness.

B. History

The disorder was described in European, Japanese, and Russian psychiatric literature over 100 years ago, yet not focused on in this country until the 1960s. Krapelin first described that as a compulsive neurosis, and Janet described it as an obsession of shame of the body.

C. DSM-IV Criteria

BDD is a preoccupation with an imagined defect in appearance, or a markedly excessive preoccupation if a slight anomaly is present. The preoccupation causes significant distress or impairment and is not accounted for by another mental disorder.

D. Clinical Features

1. Patients complain often of a **facial deformity** (e.g., asymmetry, size of nose), but it can be anything.
2. **Patients feel too ashamed to present for treatment** or to describe their anomaly.
3. Patients may frequently **check and groom** themselves (e.g., hair combing or skin-picking especially in mirrors or in other reflective surfaces).
4. **They may try to compensate for the imagined anomaly,** e.g., wearing a hat if hair loss is imagined or stuffing their shorts if a small penis is perceived.
5. **Complications** include social isolation (some only go out at night or are house-bound), imagined mockery, functioning below capacity, iatrogenic complications (7–9% of patients who undergo cosmetic surgery meet criteria for BDD), and suicide.

E. Clinical Course

The **onset occurs in adolescence;** 30 is the mean age for diagnosis. It can become **chronic.** The **presentation can be culture-specific,** e.g., in Southeastern Asia, there occurs a preoccupation that the penis is shrinking, which will disappear into the abdomen and cause death. Recently, males in the United States have presented with the belief that their musculature is abnormally small, despite intensive weight training.

F. Etiology

Psychodynamic features of the disease are thought to include displacement of a sexual or emotional conflict onto a body part.

G. Epidemiology

1. The frequency in males and females is equal. 2% of patients in a university plastic surgery clinic were diagnosed with this disorder.
2. Depression, delusional disorder, social phobia, and OCD can be co-morbid conditions. There is also a relationship between BDD and delusional disorder, somatic type.
3. There is a higher than expected family history of mood disorders and OCD.

H. Treatment

1. The **prevention of iatrogenesis** is optimal. After cosmetic surgery, for example, psychiatric pathology can re-emerge.
2. The use of **SSRIs can be helpful.** Relapse is common when the drug is discontinued.
3. **Antipsychotics** should be used for delusional disorder.

VIII. Somatoform Disorder Not Otherwise Specified

A. Definition

These disorders are residual categories for disorders where physical symptoms are the focus of treatment but which do not meet criteria for another somatoform disorder.

B. Examples

1. Pseudocyesis, or the belief that one is pregnant. Endocrine changes may be present and not explained by a general medical condition.
2. Non-psychotic hypochondriasis lasting less than 6 months.
3. Unexplained physical complaints lasting less than 6 months.

Suggested Readings

Barsky, A.J., Stern, T.A., & Greenberg, D. (1997). Functional somatic symptoms and somatoform disorders. In H. Cassem, T.A. Stern, J.F. Rosenbaum, & M.S. Jellinek (Eds.), *The MGH handbook of general hospital psychiatry,* pp. 305–336. St Louis, MO: Mosby.

Calabrese, L.V. (1998). Approach to the patient with multiple physical complaints. In T.A. Stern, J.B. Herman, & P.L. Slavin (Eds.), *The MGH guide to psychiatry in primary care,* pp. 89–98. New York: McGraw-Hill.

DeGucht, V., & Fischler, B. (2002). Somatization: A critical review of conceptual and methodological issues. *Psychosomatics, 43*(1), 1–9.

Ford, C.V. (1983). *The somatizing disorders.* New York: Elsevier.

Guggenheim, F.G., & Smith, G.R. (1995). Somatoform disorders. In H.I. Kaplan, & B.J. Sadock (Eds.), *Comprehensive textbook of psychiatry* (6th ed.). Baltimore, MD: Williams and Wilkins.

Kirmayer, L.J., & Robbins, J.M. (Eds.). (1991). *Current concepts of somatization: Research and clinical perspectives.* Washington, DC: American Psychiatric Press.

Martin, R.L., & Yutzy, S.H. (1994). Somatoform disorders. In R.E. Hales, S.C. Yudofsky, & J.A. Talbot (Eds.), *The American Psychiatric Press textbook of psychiatry* (2nd ed.). Washington, DC: American Psychiatric Press.

Phillips, K.A., McElroy, S.L., Keck, P.E., Jr., et al. (1993). Body dysmorphic disorder. 30 cases of imagined ugliness. *American Journal of Psychiatry, 150,* 302–308.

Simon, G.E., & Guerje, O. (1999). Stability of somatization disorder and somatization symptoms among primary care patients. *Archives of General Psychiatry, 56,* 90–95.

Smith, G.R. (1991). *Somatization disorder in the medical setting.* Washington, DC: American Psychiatric Press.

Stern, T.A. (1988). *Malingering, factitious illness and somatization.* In Hyman, S.E. (Ed.), *Manual of psychiatric emergencies* (2nd ed., pp. 217–225). Boston, MA: Little, Brown.

Chapter 18

Factitious Disorders

ADELE C. VIGUERA AND THEODORE A. STERN

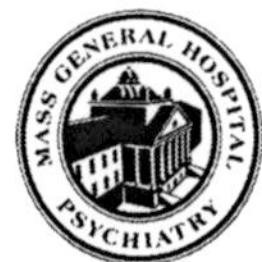

I. Overview

In factitious disorders, the individual's goal is to produce or feign signs of medical and mental disorders, and to assume the patient role. Factitious disorders are conditions that are, by definition, not real or natural. Although they tend to have a compulsive quality, the behaviors are considered voluntary even if they cannot be controlled. Obvious secondary gain, such as avoidance from work, revenue enhancement, or escape from legal authorities, is not a feature of factitious disorders; the search for secondary gain distinguishes these disorders from malingering. Factitious disorders can be incapacitating to the patient, who often produces severe trauma or develops untoward adverse effects from repeated surgical or medical interventions. Serial hospitalizations frequently make it impossible for these individuals to have meaningful sustained interpersonal or work relationships. **The prognosis in most cases is poor.** Although there are no adequate data about the long-term outcome of these individuals, a few of them die prematurely as a result of needless medications, instrumentations, or surgeries without the disorder ever being suspected.

II. Epidemiology

The prevalence of factitious disorders is unknown. Even when the diagnosis of factitious disorder is strongly suspected or confirmed, it is generally not recorded in hospital discharge summaries; determination of the prevalence is therefore difficult.

Although often described as a rare syndrome, **most clinicians have encountered at least one patient with this disorder.** These cases are often memorable because **patients with factitious disorders tend to wreak havoc on general medical and surgical units and induce strong countertransference feelings of hatred.** Conflicting data exist on whether factitious disorders are more common in males or females. It appears to occur most frequently among health care workers and those who have had extensive experience with illness, injury, or hospitalization during their early years.

III. Diagnosis

A. Diagnostic Features

There are three cardinal features of factitious disorder: an intentional production of physical or psychological signs or symptoms that are under voluntary control and that are not explained by any other underlying physical or mental disorder; a strong desire to assume the sick role; and a lack of incentives that reinforce behaviors, such as economic gain, and the avoidance of legal responsibility.

In the DSM-IV, factitious disorders are classified by their type: with predominately psychological signs and symptoms, with predominately physical signs and symptoms (also known as Munchausen syndrome), and with combined psychological and physical signs and symptoms. The DSM-IV also includes the category of factitious disorders not otherwise specified (NOS); the most notable example, factitious disorder by proxy (or Munchausen by proxy), is included in the appendix.

B. Subtypes

1. **Factitious disorder with predominately physical signs and symptoms (also known as Munchausen syndrome)** is a severe form of the disorder that may account for 10% of individuals with factitious disorders. Studies of fever of unknown origin have determined that 2.2–9.6% were factitious. One study reported a 9% rate of factitious disorders among all patients admitted to the hospital. Patients may present with a diverse array of physical complaints or signs, such as fever, hemoptysis, seizures, hypoglycemia, or abdominal pain. These patients characteristically travel from hospital to hospital trying to gain admission with a panoply of medical symptoms. **In factitious disorder by proxy (better known as Munchausen syndrome by proxy), someone intentionally produces physical signs or symptoms in another person who is under their care.** The most common scenario involves a mother who purposely deceives medical personnel by giving false information or by intentionally inducing illness or injury in the child. The motivation for the caretaker is to assume the patient role, albeit indirectly.
2. **Factitious disorder with predominately psychological signs and symptoms** is a difficult diagnosis to make; it is often made only after prolonged investigation. The feigned symptoms often include depression, hallucinations, dissociation, and bizarre behavior. Other symptoms include pseudologia fantastica and impostership. Pseudologia fantastica is characterized by extensive and colorful fantasies associated with the presentation of the patient's story. The listener's interest in the story pleases the patient and helps reinforce the behavior. The patient often gives false and conflicting accounts about their life, such as claiming the death of a parent or child to obtain sympathy. Impostership usually involves assuming the identity of a prestigious person. Men, e.g., may claim they are im-

portant war heroes who attribute their surgical scars to wounds received in battle.

3. Factitious disorders may present with **combined psychological and physical symptoms.**

IV. Clinical Features

A. **Factitious disorders typically begin in early adult life, although they may appear during childhood or adolescence.**

B. **Personality Disorders**
Many patients with factitious disorders fulfill the diagnostic criteria for borderline personality disorder, with a rigid defensive structure and a poor identity formation. They may have a masochistic personality in which pain serves as a punishment for imagined or real sins.

C. **Afflicted patients typically have a normal to above-average IQ, absence of a formal thought disorder, strong dependency needs, and confusion over their sexual identity.**

D. **A typical admission has several characteristics:**

1. **The patient often arrives in the emergency room late at night or on a weekend.** He or she is familiar with many of the diagnoses that usually require hospital admission or medication. **The patient uses convincing medical jargon and generally presents with an apparent acute illness or pain that is supported by a plausible and often dramatic case history.**
2. **The patient generally appeals to the qualities of nurturance and omnipotence in the physician** in an attempt to convince him or her to provide treatment.
3. Patients may insist on surgery. In about half the reported cases, the patient demands treatment with specific medications, usually analgesics.
4. **Once in the hospital, the patient's demands for attention increase;** irritation and anger develop when they are not met.
5. **Complaints of misdiagnosis and mistreatment arise and are directed toward staff.**
6. **The deception is often uncovered** by discovering, e.g., insulin-filled syringes in a patient's suitcase during his hospitalization for hypoglycemia.
7. **The staff become angry and lose interest in the patient's medical issues.** This results in either a swift discharge of the patient or elopement of the patient from the hospital.
8. **The patient arrives at a nearby hospital with a similar presentation** shortly after such a discharge.

V. Etiology

A. **Psychodynamic underpinnings of factitious disorders are poorly understood.** The patient may perceive one or both parents as rejecting figures who are unable to form close relationships. Feigning of an illness is carried out in an attempt to recreate the desired positive parent-child bond. The disorder may be considered as a form of repetition compulsion. The patient repeats the basic childhood conflict of needing and seeking acceptance and love while expecting that they will not be forthcoming. The physician and staff members are perceived by the patient as representing rejecting parents. Primitive defense mechanisms (including repression, regression, identification with the aggressor, and symbolization) are typically seen in those with factitious disorders.

B. **Many afflicted patients have suffered from childhood abuse or deprivation that resulted in frequent hospitalizations.** An inpatient stay may have been regarded as an escape from a traumatic home life, and the patient may have found a series of loving caretakers.

C. **Patients may identify with a close relative who was hospitalized for a particular illness.** They may feign the same illness in order to reunite with that particular relative in a magical way.

D. **Their behavior might represent an unconscious last-ditch effort to ward off further mental disintegration into psychosis.**

VI. Differential Diagnosis

A. **True Physical Disorders**
Factitious disorders must be distinguished from true physical disorders. Failure to diagnose and treat an underlying physical illness could lead to death of the patient.

B. **Somatization Disorders (Briquet's Syndrome)**
Somatization disorder and conversion disorder are distinguished from factitious disorders by the fact that the production of symptoms is not under voluntary control. The symptoms are a result of unconscious conflicts. Somatizing patients are typically not savvy about hospital procedures or medical diagnoses, nor is there any secondary gain from their complaints.

C. **Malingering**
Unlike patients with factitious disorders, malingerers have an obvious, recognizable secondary gain for the production of signs and symptoms. They generally seek admission to avoid the law, to receive financial compensation, or to avoid work.

VII. Approach to the Patient Who Presents with Factitious Disorder

A. **General Strategies**

1. **Gather information from collateral sources.** The psychiatric examination should emphasize corroboration of a patient's information with any available friend, relative, or other informant. Verification of all the facts presented by the patient concerning prior medical care is essential.

2. **Avoid confrontation.** When verifying facts initially, it is necessary to avoid pointed or accusatory questioning that may provoke evasiveness, defensiveness, or flight from the hospital. It may be nearly impossible to be certain of the diagnosis during the initial encounter.
3. **Be aware of negative countertransference.** Patients with factitious disorders usually evoke feelings of hostility and contempt among staff members. Try to embrace a non-judgmental approach to the patient. One appropriate intervention involves the realization that, even though the patient's illness is factitious, the patient is still ill.
4. **Be alert to specific elements of the history that typically suggest the presence of a factitious disorder. Such evidence includes:**
   a. Evidence of addiction or multiple hospital admissions
   b. Numerous forms of identification (e.g., hospital cards, insurance forms)
   c. Itinerant lives
   d. A facility for medical jargon
   e. A paucity of verifiable history
   f. An absence of close interpersonal relationships
   g. A history of having worked in a medically-related field
   h. An early history of sadistic or rejecting parents, chronic illness, or an important relationship with a physician
   i. History of personality disorder. Although a wide range of psychiatric diagnoses have been associated with this syndrome, these individuals are usually thought to have personality disorders.
   j. A multiplicity of scars.
5. **Recognize typical clinical presentations associated with factitious disorders.**
   a. **The acute abdominal type (laparotomaphilia migrans).** This type is the most common; many of these individuals have been operated on so frequently that abdominal symptoms may, in fact, be a consequence of intestinal obstruction from adhesions.
   b. **The hematologic type.** Profound anemia may have been produced by surreptitious bloodletting and by complications of self-administration of anticoagulants.
   c. **Neurologic type (neurologic diabolica),** often presenting with loss of consciousness, paroxysmal headaches, or seizure.
   d. **The dermatologic type (dermatitis autogenica),** frequently the result of self-inflicted wounds or chemical abrasions.
   e. **The febrile type (hyperpyrexia figmentatica).** These individuals often lose their fever when thermometers are placed, monitored, and removed under observation.
   f. **The endocrinologic type,** including those who present for evaluation of hyperinsulinemia, hyperthyroidism, and hypoglycemia.
   g. **The cardiac type,** including those individuals who complain of chest pain or arrhythmia.

VIII. Treatment

A. **No specific psychiatric therapy has been effective in treating factitious disorders.**

B. **Early identification of the disorder is perhaps the most important intervention** since determining the diagnosis can help prevent the patient from undergoing multiple, unnecessary, and potentially dangerous interventions.

C. **Focus on management, rather than on cure.** Reframe the patient's desire for medical attention as a cry for help. However, even the most empathic therapeutic confrontation may be met with profound denial, resistance, and anger. For this particular patient population, effective psychiatric care cannot be carried out in the absence of ongoing medical care. Good liaison between the psychiatrist and the medical/surgical staff is strongly advised.

D. **Legal intervention is sometimes needed,** particularly **in situations of Munchausen by proxy that involves children.** Child welfare services should be notified and arrangements made for ongoing monitoring of the child's health.

Suggested Readings

Asher, R. (1951). Munchausen's syndrome. *Lancet, 1,* 339–341.

Barsky, A.J., Stern, T.A., Greenberg, D.B., & Cassem, N.H. (1997). In N.H. Cassem, T.A. Stern, J.F. Rosenbaum, & M.S. Jellinek (Eds.), *Massachusetts General Hospital handbook of general hospital psychiatry* (4th ed., pp. 305–336). St Louis, MO: Mosby.

Ford, C.V., & Feldman, M.D. (2002). Factitious disorders and malingering. In M.G. Wise, & J.R. Rundell (Eds.), *Textbook of consultation-liaison psychiatry: Psychiatry in the medically ill* (2nd ed., pp. 519–531). Washington, DC: American Psychiatric Press.

Phillips, K.A. (Ed.). (2001). *Somatoform and factitious disorders.* Washington, DC: American Psychiatric Press.

Stern, T.A. (1980). Munchausen's syndrome revisited. *Psychosomatics, 21,* 329–336.

Stern, T.A. (1990). Factitious disorders. In S.E. Hyman, & M.A. Jenike (Eds.), *Manual of clinical problems in psychiatry,* pp. 190–194. Boston, MA: Little, Brown.

Chapter 19

Dissociative Disorders

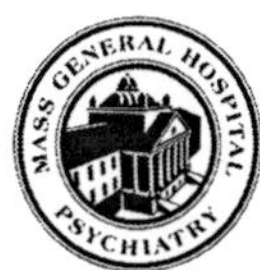

STEVEN C. SCHLOZMAN AND RAFAEL D. ORNSTEIN

I. Introduction

Dissociative disorders encompass a heterogeneous and sometimes controversial set of disorders. Although the concept of dissociation is more than 100 years old, dissociative phenomena are currently enjoying renewed interest. This increase is in part related to a burgeoning literature addressing the effects of trauma on memory and personality, as well as the apparent epidemic of dissociative disease during the 1980s. There is now a growing consensus that the increase in new cases deserves closer scrutiny and may represent an overdiagnosis of dissociative disorders. Nevertheless, dissociative phenomena have been consistently described throughout the history of psychiatry and when appropriate should be considered in the differential diagnosis.

Central to the conceptualization of dissociation is the understanding that a person's consciousness may not be fully integrated. Thus, a patient may experience a distinct alteration in personality or experience, in which thoughts, feelings, or actions are not logically integrated with other self-referential experiences. Traumatic experiences are often considered etiologic factors in the development of dissociation. Although the most well known of these disorders is dissociative identity disorder (previously called multiple personality disorder), it is important to note that current nosology also includes dissociative amnesia, dissociative fugue, depersonalization disorder, and dissociative disorder not otherwise specified. One must also be careful to consider factitious or malingered dissociative disorders when individuals present with symptoms of dissociation.

II. History of Dissociative Disorders

A number of historical figures have been instrumental in establishing the current conceptualization of dissociative phenomena.

A. **Franz Anton Mesmer** (1734–1815): **known for his theories of "animal magnetism,"** and today recognized as one of the first clinicians to explore the clinical utility of hypnosis in treating dissociation (see III, below).

B. **Pierre Janet** (1859–1947): with other clinicians, **he established hypnosis as a clinical intervention for dissociative states.** Most important, he was first to connect the etiologic nature of traumatic experiences.

C. **Sigmund Freud** differed from Janet by suggesting that dissociation results from the ego's vigorous defense against psychological pain. Thus, while Janet felt that the ego collapsed and fragmented under the weight of traumatic experiences, **Freud felt that trauma forced a powerful ego to wall off psychological pain, after which this pain manifests itself only in dissociative states.**

D. **Morton Prince** published *The Dissociation of a Personality* (1906), in which he described his patient, Sally Beauchamp, as "The Saint, the Devil, the Woman." His work was **likely the first clinical investigation into the notion of separate dissociative identities.**

III. Etiology of Dissociation

A. **Traumatic experience** is strongly correlated with dissociation. Multiple studies and case series document the relationship of trauma to dissociative states.

B. **Children appear more prone to dissociation than adults and may develop dissociative traits in response to trauma at a very young age.** Some researchers have theorized that these individuals remain more susceptible to dissociation than similarly traumatized older individuals.

C. Research suggests a potential clinical link between **dissociative states and hypnosis.** For example, patients with dissociative disorders are reportedly more hypnotizable than are control subjects. Moreover, hypnosis may represent a valuable clinical intervention for the treatment of dissociative disorders. Finally, some studies have found that subjects who have had traumatic experiences but who do not manifest a dissociative disorder appear more hypnotizable when compared to non-traumatized individuals.

D. **EMDR (eye movement desensitization and reprocessing therapy)** has also been implicated as a potentially useful treatment intervention for all forms of dissociation.

E. Recently, research has suggested that dissociative states (given the extent to which information about one's self is compartmentalized in those suffering from dissociative disorders) can be explored in terms of **state-dependent learning** (a broad concept meant to suggest that information stored in one "state" may only be retrieved in that specific state).

F. **Complex partial seizure** activity has been suggested as a cause of dissociation. However, a definitive link has not yet been revealed. Although some patients with dissociative disorders have concurrent seizure disorders, the seizures themselves do not necessarily cause their dissociative symptoms. **Electroencephalographic (EEG) studies** of patients with dissociative disorders have been contradictory; some studies suggest EEG differences within the same patient during different dissociative states.

G. **Neurochemical and pharmacologic agents** may be related to dissociative phenomena. Substances such as lysergic acid diethylamide (LSD), phencyclidine (PCP), and ketamine appear to provoke dissociative episodes, and some studies suggest a serotonin dysregulation as contributing to dissociative tendencies.

H. Dissociation has recently been hypothesized to involve **increased dorsal vagal tone,** similar to the autonomic changes postulated in the development of post-traumatic stress disorder (PTSD).

IV. Who Dissociates?

Dissociation can be measured clinically using the Dissociative Experience Scale (DES). This 28-item self-report questionnaire has achieved good reliability and validity. Higher scores represent more dissociative experiences. However, this scale has achieved only face validity, and can be purposefully misrepresented by the subject.

Other standardized assessments include the Structured Clinical Interview for Dissociative Disorders—Revised (SCID-D-R), as well as the Minnesota Multiphasic Personality Inventory (MMPI). Again, one must realize that the SCID-D-R has also achieved only face validity and that the MMPI has not been validated for dissociative disorders. Nevertheless, using these scales, as well as other means of assessment, several conclusions have been suggested regarding those who experience dissociative states.

A. **Gender**

Males and females (in both psychiatric and non-psychiatric samples) have similar DES scores. Thus, no gender differences are apparent in terms of the likelihood to dissociate. Similarly, there are no discernible differences on hypnotizability scores between males and females.

B. **Age**

There appears to be a negative correlation between age and the tendency to dissociate. Thus, younger individuals are more likely to dissociate. Similar findings have been documented for hypnotizability.

C. **Childhood Trauma**

Some studies have noted high DES scores in adults who suffered childhood trauma.

D. **Different dissociative disorders have epidemiological differences.** For example, while the tendency to dissociate is roughly equal in men and women, dissociative identity disorder is more common in women, while dissociative fugue might be more common in men (see below).

V. Dissociative Amnesia (Formerly Psychogenic Amnesia)

A. This condition is defined in DSM-IV as **"an inability to recall important personal information, usually of a traumatic nature, that is too extensive to be explained by normal forgetfulness."**

B. **Dissociative amnesia may be global, with total loss of autobiographic information, or it may be episodic, in which patients cannot recall specific episodes of behavior or traumatic experiences.** These experiences may include self-mutilation, criminal or sexual behaviors, traumatic events, or even marital or financial crises.

C. **Dissociative amnesia appears to be a common short-term reaction in both men and women to severe stress, such as civilian disasters.**

D. The **incidence** in both males and females appears roughly equal.

E. Dissociative amnesia may occur during any age, though its **peak incidence appears in the third and fourth decades.**

F. Three-fourths of cases last **between 24 hours and 5 days.**

G. **Differential diagnosis** includes organic syndromes (secondary to brain injuries, lesions, or seizures), as well as factitious disorders and malingering.

H. **Treatment** aims at restoring the missing memories, sometimes through psychotherapy and free association, but at times using hypnosis or an Amytal interview.

I. Generally speaking, patients with dissociative amnesia recover quickly and completely. However, many patients continue to display a propensity toward amnesia in the setting of trauma.

VI. Dissociative Fugue

A. Dissociative fugue is characterized in the DSM-IV as **"the sudden unexpected travel away from one's place of daily activities, with inability to recall some or all of one's past."** Often, patients suffering from dissociative fugue will **assume entirely new identities** during their fugue episode.

B. Note that dissociative fugue is essentially dissociative amnesia **plus** travel.

C. Dissociative fugue appears to be **more common during wartime or after natural disasters.**

D. Dissociative fugue may be the **rarest of the dissociative disorders.**

E. Patients suffering from dissociative fugue may appear normal, though they often become confused and distressed when asked questions about their personal history.

F. Although men appear to be affected as often as women, **the incidence of men suffering from dissociative fugue increases during war.**

G. Dissociative fugue occurs **primarily in adults, usually between the second and fourth decades.**

H. Although fugues may last from a few hours to several years, **most episodes last from a few days to a few months.**

I. **Alternative diagnoses** include brain pathology leading to fugue states, drug-induced fugues secondary to alcoholic or drug-related blackouts, and factitious disorders or malingering. In addition, some cultural syndromes (e.g., Amok and Latah) may mimic fugue states.

J. **Treatment** is similar to that for dissociative amnesia; the patient is helped to recall the events preceding the fugue, sometimes through hypnosis or Amytal interview.

K. **Prognosis varies.** When fugue states are of short duration, they tend to resolve spontaneously. Longer-lasting episodes may be intractable.

VII. Dissociative Identity Disorder (Formerly Multiple Personality Disorder)

Among the dissociative disorders, dissociative identity disorder (DID) has received the most attention over the last two decades. Thus, **the majority of research focusing on dissociative disorders has involved DID, and the diagnosis has endured considerable controversy.** The positive aspects of this controversy involve an ongoing debate about the interplay of society on psychiatric nosology, as well as a careful re-examination of all dissociative phenomena and their relationship to consciousness and pathology.

A. **DID is defined in the DSM-IV as "the presence of two or more distinct identities or personality states (each with its own relatively enduring pattern of perceiving, relating to, and thinking about the environment and the self)."** In addition, the DSM specifies that **"at least two of these identities" must periodically "take control of the person's behavior."** Finally, there must be a demonstrated **"inability to recall important personal information that is too extensive to be explained by ordinary forgetfulness."**

B. An important aspect of DID is the **amnestic quality for alternate personalities** displayed by the primary personality. However, in many instances different personality states have varying levels of awareness of other personalities (often called **"alters"**), and often a **dominant personality state** exists that is cognizant of all of the various personalities. **The term "co-consciousness" has been used to describe the simultaneous experience of multiple entities at one time.** Thus, one personality may be aware of another's feelings regarding an ongoing experience.

C. DID is characterized by **high rates of depression,** and often by affective symptoms that constitute the presenting complaint.

D. From **one-third to one-half of cases of DID experience auditory hallucinations.** Some researchers have suggested that these hallucinations are described as **"inner voices,"** helping to differentiate these symptoms from the external voices heard by those suffering from schizophrenia and other psychotic disorders. Furthermore, in contrast to individuals suffering from schizophrenia, patients with DID are **unusually hypnotizable and do not display evidence of a formal thought disorder.**

E. **The mean number of personality states in DID is approximately 13.** However, case series have shown that the number of alternate identities may vary from 1 to 50.

F. DID is reported more **commonly in women than in men.**

G. Prevalence estimates range from **rare to 1%.**

H. A number of **somatic symptoms may accompany DID,** including **headaches, gastrointestinal distress, and genitourinary disturbances.** In addition, there is an increased rate of **conversion disorders, pseudoseizures, and self-mutilation.** Finally, a number of **personality disorders**, including borderline personality disorder, are associated with DID.

I. **DID is usually diagnosed in the third or fourth decade, though those suffering from DID usually report symptoms during childhood and adolescence.** Most case series document a chronic, fluctuating course, characterized by relapse and remission. Making the diagnosis of DID in a particular patient is not without controversy. Some clinicians have proposed that the diagnosis must be persistently pursued if a patient's symptoms even subtly hint at the possibility of dissociation. These clinicians describe patients who are either unaware of, or who wish to hide their disorder, and need to be "educated" about DID. Critics contend that patients with DID are highly suggestible and that clinicians "create" such patients by "suggesting" symptoms. The critics emphasize that the symptoms are reinforced by clinicians who show interest and enthusiasm in the multiplicity of personalities.

J. **Extended psychotherapy remains the treatment of choice,** although approaches vary widely and remain controversial. Some clinicians describe specialized treatment for DID, including delineating and mapping the alters, inviting each to participate in the treatment, and facilitating communication between the various alters. Through careful exploration of all alternate identities, clinicians attempt to understand past episodes of trauma as experienced by each personality. Hypnosis is sometimes employed to reach dissociated states. Other clinicians focus on the function of the dissociative process in the here-and-now of the patient's life and the ongoing treatment. They help patients become aware of using dissociation to manage feelings and thoughts within themselves and to manage the closeness and distance within relationships. All approaches seek to increase affect tolerance and to integrate the dissociated states within the patient.

K. **Psychopharmacologic treatments,** such as **antidepressants and anxiolytics,** are often useful in treating the commonly accompanying complaints of depression and anxiety. However, no pharmacological treatment has been found to reduce dissociation per se. Benzodiazepines reduce anxiety but can also exacerbate dissociation. Although not routinely used for dissociative disorders, neuroleptics are sometimes employed in patients who are grossly disorganized; they should be used in the lowest possible doses and be discontinued if they are unhelpful.

VIII. Depersonalization Disorder

A. According to the DSM-IV, depersonalization disorder is characterized by **"persistent or recurrent episodes . . . of detachment or estrangement from one's self."** Often, patients with symptoms of depersonalization will **"feel like an automaton or like he or she is living in a movie."**

B. **Reality testing is intact** in those who suffer from depersonalization disorder. This represents an important distinction from other psychotic disorders.

C. **Transient depersonalization is common;** such events are not considered pathological. Studies have suggested that as many as 50% of people will at some point endorse transient symptoms.

D. **Transient depersonalization occurs equally in both men and women. However, depersonalization disorder is much rarer than is transient depersonalization; it occurs roughly twice as often in women.**

E. Depersonalization disorder usually **begins by late adolescence or early adulthood.**

F. Most **episodes last from hours to weeks.**

G. **Differential diagnosis** includes depression and psychosis, as well as illicit drug ingestion and iatrogenic drug effects. Brain pathology, such as seizures, migraines, or discrete lesions, may lead to depersonalization.

H. Treatment is difficult, and **patients are often refractory to intervention.** Treating accompanying psychiatric conditions, such as depression or anxiety, may help. As with other dissociative disorders, exploration of past traumatic events may prove useful.

IX. Dissociative Disorder Not Otherwise Specified

A. This category is reserved for presentations in which the predominant feature is dissociation without meeting clear criteria for any specific dissociative disorder.

B. Examples include patients who experience **derealization** (the quality of perceiving previously familiar objects in the external world as strange and unfamiliar) but not depersonalization, or patients with ill-defined alternate personalities. In addition, symptoms that result from torture or brainwashing may be classified in this category.

C. **Ganser's syndrome** (sometimes called **"prison psychosis"**) is classified as a dissociative disorder not otherwise specified. It is characterized by the provision of approximate answers, i.e., offering half-correct answers to simple inquiries, such as answering "5" to the question, "What is 2 plus 2?" The correct set of the response is given, but the answer is inaccurate. Ganser's syndrome is often reported in incarcerated populations.

D. **Culture-bound syndromes,** such as **Amok** in Indonesia or **Latah** in Malaysia, are often characterized by dissociation and sometimes by violence. These syndromes have been included in the DSM-IV as dissociative disorder not otherwise specified.

X. Factitious or Malingering Dissociative Disorders

A. Feigned dissociative symptoms may be more common than previously realized. A 1994 case series suggested that as many as 10% of patients with symptoms of DID in fact suffered from **factitious dissociative symptoms.** The motivation in this series appeared to be the **assumption of the sick role,** consistent with other presentations of factitious disorders.

B. Case reports detail dissociative symptoms expressed as a form of **malingering.** In these episodes, individuals feign dissociative symptoms for reasons other than assuming the sick role, such as **avoiding criminal or financial responsibilities.**

C. **Individuals attempting to feign dissociative symptoms are often extremely invested in the diagnosis of DID.** They may express their symptoms only when they feel they are being observed or heard, and they may refuse collateral interviews with other individuals in which the clinician attempts to gather additional information. One study suggested that approximately 50% of those with feigned DID admit their simulation of dissociation to a caretaker. Additionally, individuals who simulate these symptoms may have substantially more exposure to popular and scientific explorations of dissociation than do those with genuine dissociative disorders.

XI. Dissociative Trance Disorder

A. This is **not currently a formal classification,** but is listed in the DSM-IV as Criteria Sets and Axes Provided for Further Study.

B. Dissociative trance disorder might include apparent episodes of **demonic possession** or **religious ecstasy.** The feeling of being possessed is reported commonly in those who feel guilty about perceived transgressions. Examples might involve an individual who is unfaithful to his spouse and who becomes convinced that demonic possession is responsible for his infidelity.

C. It is important to rule out psychosis, malingering, and factitious disorder when considering this category.

Suggested Readings

Coons, P.M. (1998). The dissociative disorders. Rarely considered and underdiagnosed. *Psychiatric Clinics of North America, 21,* 637–648.

Dissociative disorders. (2000). In B.F. Saddock, & V.A. Sadock (Eds.), *Comprehensive textbook of psychiatry* (7th ed., pp. 1544–1576). Baltimore, MD: Lipincott, Williams and Wilkins.

Putnum, F.W. (1991). Dissociative phenomena. In A. Tasman, & S.M. Goldfinger (Eds.), *American Psychiatric Press review of psychiatry,* Vol. 10, pp. 145–160. Washington, DC: American Psychiatric Press.

Chapter 20

Sexual Disorders and Sexual Dysfunction

LINDA SHAFER

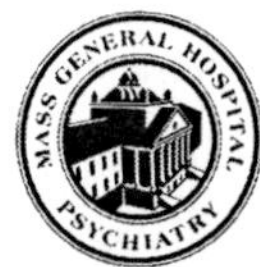

I. Introduction

A. Sexual Problems Occur Frequently and Cause Great Distress

1. 43% of women and 31% of men have experienced some form of sexual dysfunction.
2. 50% of American couples suffer from some type of sexual problem.
3. 24% of Americans will experience a sexual dysfunction at some time in their lives.
4. The primary care physician (PCP) is often the first to see the patient with sexual problems.

B. The *Diagnostic and Statistical Manual of Mental Disorders,* Fourth Edition (DSM-IV) divides sexual disorders into two groups:

1. **Sexual dysfunctions:** psychophysiologic impairment of sexual desire and/or of the sexual response cycle.
2. **Paraphilias:** recurrent, intense sexual urges or behaviors that cause marked distress and that involve unusual objects or activities.

II. Evaluation of the Problem: Sexual Dysfunction

A. General Recommendations

1. Sexual dysfunction is best understood by having knowledge of the stages of the normal sexual response, which vary with age and with physical status.
   a. **The four-step model (Masters and Johnson)**
      i. Excitement: arousal.
      ii. Plateau: the phase of maximum arousal prior to orgasm.
      iii. Orgasm: a stage that involves muscular contractions at 0.8-second intervals.
      iv. Resolution: a phase leading to a return to baseline.
      v. Refractory period: in men, a stage that increases with age; in women, there is no refractory period.
   b. **The triphasic model (Kaplan)**
      i. Desire.
      ii. Excitement (arousal): a vascular phenomenon, caused by innervation of the parasympathetic nervous system (2nd, 3rd, and 4th sacral segments of the spinal cord).
      iii. Orgasm: a muscular reaction, caused by innervation of the sympathetic nervous system, whose reflex center is in the lumbar cord.
   c. **Changes in the sexual response associated with aging**
      i. Males are slower to achieve an erection and need more direct stimulation to the penis to achieve an erection.
      ii. Females have decreased levels of estrogen which leads to less vaginal lubrication and to narrowing of the vagina.
   d. **Medications, diseases, injuries, and psychological conditions can affect the sexual response in any of its component phases and can lead to different dysfunctional syndromes** (Table 20-1).
      i. Several types of sexual dysfunction can co-exist.
      ii. One sexual dysfunction can be the cause of another.
      iii. A primary sexual dysfunction is one that has been present since the onset of sexual activity.
      iv. A secondary sexual dysfunction is one that occurs after a period of normal functioning.

B. Medical History

1. Although most sexual disorders were thought to have a psychological basis, newer diagnostic testing has identified more conditions having an organic etiology.
2. **Most sexual disorders are multi-causal and share a mixed etiology.**
3. Physical disorders, surgical disorders (Table 20-2), use of medications, and drug use or abuse (Table 20-3) can affect sexual functioning directly and/or cause secondary psychological reactions which can cause a sexual problem.
   a. **Sexual dysfunction is a common side effect, which occurs in more than 30% of patients taking a selective serotonin reuptake inhibitor (SSRI).**
      i. Treatment strategies include use of cyproheptadine, bupropion, yohimbine, amantadine, buspirone, sildenafil, ginkgo biloba, and/or a drug holiday.

Table 20-1. Classification of Sexual Dysfunctions

Impaired Sexual Response Phase	*Female*	*Male*
Desire	Hypoactive sexual desire Sexual aversion	Hypoactive sexual desire Sexual aversion
Excitement (arousal, vascular)	Sexual arousal disorder	Erectile disorder
Orgasm (muscular)	Orgasmic disorder	Orgasmic disorder Premature ejaculation
Sexual pain	Dyspareunia Vaginismus	Dyspareunia

Table 20-2. Medical and Surgical Conditions Causing Sexual Dysfunctions

Organic Disorders	*Sexual Impairment*
Endocrine	
Hypothyroidism, adrenal dysfunction, hypogonadism, diabetes mellitus	Low libido, impotence, decreased vaginal lubrication, early impotence
Vascular	
Hypertension, atherosclerosis, stroke, venous insufficiency, sickle cell disorder	Impotence, ejaculation and libido intact
Neurologic	
Spinal cord damage, diabetic neuropathy, herniated lumbar disc, alcoholic neuropathy, multiple sclerosis, temporal lobe epilepsy	Sexual disorder—early sign, low libido (or high libido), impotence, impaired orgasm
Local genital disease	
Male: Priapism, Peyronie's disease, urethritis, prostatitis, hydrocele	Low libido, impotence
Female: Imperforate hymen, vaginitis, pelvic inflammatory disease, endometriosis	Vaginismus, dyspareunia, low libido, decreased arousal
Systemic debilitating disease	
Renal, pulmonary, or hepatic diseases, advanced malignancies, infections	Low libido, impotence, decreased arousal
Surgical-postoperative states	
Male: Prostatectomy (radical perineal) abdominal-perineal bowel resection	Impotence, no loss of libido, ejaculatory impairment
Female: Episiotomy, vaginal repair of prolapse, oophorectomy	Dyspareunia, vaginismus, decreased lubrication
Male and female: Amputation (leg), colostomy and ileostomy	Mechanical difficulties in sex, low self-image, fear of odor

Table 20-3. Drugs and Medicines Causing Sexual Dysfunction

Drug	*Sexual Side Effect*
Cardiovascular	
Methyldopa	Low libido, impotence, anorgasmia
Thiazide diuretics	Low libido, impotence, decreased lubrication
Clonidine	Impotence, anorgasmia
Propranolol	Low libido
Digoxin	Gynecomastia, low libido, impotence
Clofibrate	Low libido, impotence
Psychotropics	
Sedatives	
Alcohol	Higher doses cause sexual problems
Barbiturates	Impotence
Anxiolytics	
Alprazolam; Diazepam	Low libido, delayed ejaculation
Antipsychotics	
Thioridazine	Retarded or retrograde ejaculation
Haloperidol	Low libido, impotence, anorgasmia
Antidepressants	
MAOIs (phenelzine)	Impotence, retarded ejaculation, anorgasmia
Tricyclics (imipramine)	Low libido, impotence, retarded ejaculation
SSRIs (fluoxetine, sertraline)	Low libido, impotence, retarded ejaculation
Atypical (trazodone)	Priapism, retarded or retrograde ejaculation
Lithium	Low libido, impotence
Hormones	
Estrogen	Low libido in men
Progesterone	Low libido, impotence
Gastrointestinal	
Cimetidine	Low libido, impotence
Methantheline bromide	Impotence
Opiates	Orgasmic dysfunction
Anticonvulsants	Low libido, impotence, priapism

4. Psychological causes of sexual disorders are complex; they range from superficial issues (e.g., fear of failure) to deep ones (e.g., profound depression).
   a. No direct correlation has been found between specific background factors and certain sexual dysfunctions.
   b. Predisposing, precipitating, and maintaining factors play a role in sexual problems (Table 20-4).

C. Taking a Sexual History

1. Be aware that patients are usually embarrassed to bring up and discuss sexual problems.
2. Remember that physicians, too, are often uncomfortable discussing sexual issues, in part because of fears of offending patients.
3. **Ask routine screening questions as part of the medical history to give the patient a chance to talk about sexual problems,** e.g.,
   a. Is there anything you would like to change about your sex life?
   b. Have there been any changes in your sex life?
   c. Are you satisfied with your present sex life?
4. **Additional routine questions to ask during the AIDS era include:**
   a. Are you sexually active?
   b. Do you practice safe(r) sex?
      i. Lack of knowledge of safe sex practices can contribute to the spread of AIDS.
      ii. Physicians should be prepared to discuss the benefits of safe sex techniques, including the use of condoms and spermicides that contain nonoxynol-9.
      iii. Failure to ask AIDS screening questions may result in complaints of inadequate treatment or a malpractice suit.
5. **Interview techniques**
   a. Attempt to be sensitive and non-judgmental.
   b. Move from the more general to more specific topics, in an appropriate context.
      i. Sexual issues can be integrated easily into the medical history during the review of systems, when discussing the initiation or introduction of a new medication, or when the chief complaint involves a gynecological or urological problem.
      ii. Physicians should be aware of covert presentations of sexual problems (e.g., headache, insomnia, and low back or generalized pelvic pain) that have no apparent medical basis.
   c. Vary questions depending on the patient's age, social class/occupation, and the nature of the patient's continuing relationship with you.
   d. Design the taking of the sexual history to fit the patient's needs and your time.
   e. If a sexual problem is uncovered, take a detailed history.
      i. Determine its onset.
      ii. Establish its progression. How often? With all partners? On masturbation? With fantasy?
      iii. Complete an assessment. Avoid use of "why" questions because this tends to make a patient feel defensive. Use "what" questions (e.g., What do you think caused your problems?).
      iv. Ask about attempts at resolution of the problem. Did they read or seek advice from books, friends, or clergy?
      v. Clarify the patient's expectations and goals. Do they wish to resolve the problem, save their marriage, or use the problem as an excuse for divorce?

Table 20-4. Psychological Causes of Sexual Dysfunction

Predisposing factors
Lack of information/experience
Unrealistic expectations
Negative family attitudes to sex
Sexual trauma: rape, incest
Precipitating factors
Childbirth
Infidelity
Dysfunction in the partner
Maintaining factors
Interpersonal issues
Family stress
Work stress
Financial problems
Depression
Performance anxiety
Gender identity conflicts

D. Examination of the Patient

1. **Physical examination**
   a. A thorough physical examination is indicated on every patient, with special attention paid to endocrine, vascular, neurological, urological, and gynecological systems.
2. **Laboratory examination**
   a. The extent of the laboratory examination depends on the nature of the problem.
   b. The extent of the laboratory examination depends on one's index of suspicion (i.e., is it organic or psychological?).
   c. The sexual history and physical examination together help determine the extent of the organic work-up, including what special laboratory studies and diagnostic procedures should be performed.
      i. Screening for unrecognized systemic disease should include a complete blood count (CBC), a urinalysis, a creatinine level, a lipid profile, thyroid function studies, and a fasting blood sugar (FBS).
      ii. Relevant endocrine studies for assessment of low libido and erectile dysfunction include levels of testos-

terone, prolactin, luteinizing hormone (LH), and follicular stimulating hormone (FSH).

iii. An estrogen level and microscopic examination of a vaginal smear for vaginal dryness should be obtained.

iv. A sedimentation rate, a cervical culture, and a Pap (Papanicolaou) smear should be obtained for evaluation of dyspareunia.

v. Diagnostic tests for erectile functioning include nocturnal penile tumescence (NPT) studies, ultrasonography, and angiography.

d. Referral to a specialist in urology, gynecology, endocrinology, neurology, and/or psychiatry is made on a case-by-case basis.

III. Psychiatric Differential Diagnosis of Sexual Disorders

A. Depression (Major Depression or Dysthymic Disorder)

1. Consider low libido or erectile dysfunction.

B. Manic Phase (Bipolar Disorder)

1. Consider increased libido.

C. Generalized Anxiety Disorder, Panic Disorder, Post-Traumatic Stress Disorder

1. Consider low libido, erectile dysfunction, lack of vaginal lubrication, or anorgasmia.

D. Obsessive-Compulsive Disorder

1. Consider "anti-fantasies" that focus on the negative aspects of a partner.
2. Consider low libido, erectile dysfunction, lack of vaginal lubrication, or anorgasmia.

E. Schizophrenia

1. Consider low desire or bizarre sexual desires.

F. Paraphilias

1. Consider deviant sexual arousal.

G. Gender Identity Disorder

1. Consider dissatisfaction with one's own sexual preference or phenotype.

H. Personality Disorder (Passive-Aggressive, Obsessive-Compulsive, Histrionic)

1. Consider low libido, erectile dysfunction, premature ejaculation, or anorgasmia.

I. Marital Dysfunction/Interpersonal Problems

J. Fears of Intimacy/Commitment

1. Consider deep, intrapsychic issues.
2. Consider a range of sexual disorders, including a lack of vaginal lubrication and erectile dysfunction.

IV. Diagnostic Criteria

A. Sexual disorders not caused by organic factors (medical conditions, medications, or drugs of abuse) or by another (psychological) Axis I disorder, all of which cause marked individual distress and/or interpersonal difficulties.

1. **Desire phase disorders in males and females**

a. Hypoactive sexual desire disorder (302.71 DSM-IV)

i. Hypoactive sexual desire disorder is a condition with persistently deficient sexual fantasies and an infrequent desire for sexual activity.

ii. Its incidence has increased from 37% in the early 1970s to 55% in the early 1980s.

iii. The lifetime prevalence of this condition is 40% in women and 30% in men.

b. **Sexual aversion disorder** (302.79 DSM-IV)

i. Sexual aversion disorder is a condition with a persistent and extreme aversion to, and avoidance of, all or almost all genital sexual contact with the sexual partner.

ii. Its exact incidence is unknown, but it is common.

iii. Primary sexual aversion is higher in men, but secondary aversion is higher in women.

iv. The syndrome is associated with phobic avoidance of sexual activity and/or the thought of sexual activity.

v. One-fourth of those with this condition also meet criteria for panic disorder.

vi. Affected individuals engage in intercourse once or twice a year.

vii. Patients tend to respond naturally to sexual relations if they can get past their high anxiety and initial dread.

2. **Arousal phase disorders**

a. **Female sexual arousal disorder** (302.72 DSM-IV)

i. Female sexual arousal disorder is a condition with the persistent inability to attain or maintain the lubrication/swelling response of sexual excitement until completion of the sexual act.

ii. Its lifetime prevalence is 60%.

iii. The condition is linked to problems with sexual desire.

iv. A lack of vaginal lubrication may lead to dyspareunia.

b. **Male erectile disorder** (302.72 DSM-IV)

i. Male erectile disorder is a condition involving the inability to attain or maintain a satisfactory erection until completion of sexual activity.

ii. Twenty to 30 million American men suffer from erectile dysfunction, accounting for more than 500,000 ambulatory visits to healthcare professionals annually.

iii. Between 50% and 85% of cases of erectile dysfunction have an organic basis (see Table 20-5 for risk factors).

iv. Primary (life-long) erectile dysfunction occurs in 1% of men under the age of 35 years.

v. Secondary (acquired) erectile dysfunction is manifest by the inability to achieve successful intercourse in 25% of attempts; it occurs in 40% of men over the age of 60 years, and increases to 73% in men who are 80 years old.

vi. Erectile dysfunction may be generalized (i.e., it occurs in all circumstances).

vii. Erectile dysfunction may be situational (i.e., it is limited to certain types of stimulation, situations, and partners).

Table 20-5. Risk Factors Associated with Erectile Dysfunction

Hypertension
Diabetes mellitus
Smoking
Coronary artery disease
Peripheral vascular disorders
Blood lipid abnormalities
Peyronie's disease
Priapism
Pelvic trauma or surgery
Renal failure and dialysis
Hypogonadism
Alcoholism
Depression
Lack of sexual knowledge
Poor sexual technique
Interpersonal problems

3. **Orgasm phase disorders**
   a. **Female orgasmic disorder** (302.73 DSM-IV)
      i. Female orgasmic disorder is a condition involving a persistent delay in, or absence of, orgasm, following a normal excitement phase.
      ii. Female orgasmic disorder is the most common type of female sexual dysfunction; its lifetime prevalence is 35%.
      iii. 5–8% of afflicted individuals are totally anorgasmic.
      iv. 30–40% of afflicted individuals are unable to achieve orgasm without clitoral stimulation during intercourse.
      v. The ability to reach orgasm increases with sexual experience.
      vi. The diagnosis should *not* be made for women who can experience an orgasm with direct clitoral contact, but who find it difficult to reach orgasm during intercourse. This is a normal variant.
      vii. Claims that stimulation of the Grafenberg spot, or G spot, in a region in the anterior wall of the vagina will cause orgasm and female ejaculation have never been substantiated.
      viii. Consider that the male sexual partner with premature ejaculation is contributing to female orgasmic dysfunction.
   b. **Male orgasmic disorder** (302.74 DSM-IV)
      i. Male orgasmic disorder is a condition with a persistent delay in, or absence of, orgasm following a normal sexual excitement phase.
      ii. It is an infrequent disorder with a lifetime prevalence of 2%; it occurs in men who are usually under the age of 35 years and who are sexually inexperienced.
      iii. Retarded ejaculation is usually restricted to failure to reach orgasm in the vagina during intercourse.
      iv. Orgasm can usually occur with masturbation and/or from a partner's manual or oral stimulation.
      v. The condition must be differentiated from **retrograde ejaculation,** where the bladder neck does not close off properly during orgasm, causing semen to spurt backward into the bladder.
      vi. One must rule out retarded ejaculation in a couple presenting with infertility of unknown cause. The male may not have admitted his lack of ejaculation to his partner.
   c. **Premature ejaculation** (302.75 DSM-IV)
      i. Premature ejaculation is a condition involving persistent ejaculation with minimal stimulation before or after penetration and before the person wishes it.
      ii. The lifetime prevalence of premature ejaculation is 15%.
      iii. With the condition, ejaculation usually occurs in less than 2 minutes or with fewer than ten thrusts.
      iv. Premature ejaculation is the most common male sexual disorder, affecting 30% of men.
      v. Prolonged periods of no sexual activity make premature ejaculation worse.
      vi. If the problem is chronic and untreated, secondary impotence often occurs.
4. **Sexual pain disorders**
   a. **Dyspareunia** (302.76 DSM-IV)
      i. Dyspareunia involves persistent genital pain before, during, or after sexual intercourse in either the male or the female.
      ii. The prevalence of dyspareunia is 15% in females and 5% in males.
      iii. Patients with dyspareunia often seek out medical treatment, but the physical examination is often unremarkable, without genital abnormalities.
      iv. If pain is caused solely by vaginismus or a lack of lubrication, the diagnosis of dyspareunia is *not* made.
   b. **Vaginismus** (306.51 DSM-IV)
      i. Vaginismus is the persistent involuntary spasm of the musculature of the outer third of the vagina that interferes with sexual intercourse.
      ii. The frequency of vaginismus is unknown, but probably accounts for less than 10% of female sexual disorders.
      iii. The diagnosis of vaginismus is often made on routine gynecologic examination when contraction of the vaginal outlet occurs as either the examining finger or a speculum is introduced.
      iv. There is a high incidence of associated pelvic pathology with vaginismus.

v. Life-long vaginismus has an abrupt onset, at the first attempt at penetration, and has a chronic course.

vi. Acquired vaginismus may occur suddenly, following a sexual trauma or a medical condition.

5. **Sexual dysfunction not otherwise specified** (302.70 DSM-IV)
   a. Sexual dysfunction not otherwise specified is a condition without subjective erotic feelings despite otherwise normal arousal and orgasm (female analog of premature ejaculation).
   b. It is unclear whether the sexual dysfunction is primary, due to a medical condition, or is substance-induced.

V. Treatment Strategies

A. Organically-Based Sexual Disorders

1. **Medical-surgical treatments**
   a. Treat pre-existing illnesses (e.g., diabetes).
   b. Stop, or substitute for, offending medications.
   c. Reduce alcohol and/or smoking.
   d. Add medications for psychiatric conditions (e.g., depression).
   e. Correct hormone deficiencies (e.g., testosterone for hypogonadism, thyroid hormone for hypothyroidism, estrogen/testosterone [Estratest] for post-menopausal females, or bromocriptine for elevated prolactin after neuroimaging of the pituitary).
   f. Initiate a trial of fluoxetine, sertraline, paroxetine, or clomipramine for premature ejaculation.
   g. Prescribe an oral agent for erectile dysfunction (* not yet FDA-approved).
      i. Phosphodiesterase type 5 (PDE-5) inhibitor: sildenafil (Viagra), vardenafil (Levitra*), tadalafil (Cialis*). Note: Contraindicated with nitrates.
      ii. Dopamine agonist: sublingual apomorphine (Uprima*)
      iii. α-adrenergic inhibitor: yohimbine (Yocon), phentolamine (Vasomax*)
      iv. Nitric oxide (NO) precursor: L-Arginine
   h. Prescribe topical agent for erectile dysfunction (* not yet FDA-approved).
      i. Prostaglandins (PGE_1): alprostadil gel (Topiglan*)
      ii. Vasodilator: minoxidil cream*, nitroglycerine gel*
   i. Consider transurethral penile suppository of alprostadil (MUSE) for erectile dysfunction.
   j. Initiate a pharmacologic erection program (PEP): alprostadil intracavernosal injections (Caverject), trimix (papaverine, phentolamine, and alprostadil combined).
   k. Consider use of an external penile suction device for erectile disorders.
   l. Implant a penile prosthetic device.
   m. Perform surgery for vascular problems (e.g., endarterectomy).
   n. For female sexual dysfunction, use the medications listed in g. and h., none of which are FDA-approved yet for use in women.
   o. Consider use of EROS-CTD, an FDA-approved clitoral therapy suction device.

B. Psychologically-Based Sexual Disorders

1. **General principles**
   a. If time is limited, schedule another appointment to take a detailed sexual history and to initiate treatment.
   b. Conduct discussions about sex in the office, while the patient is fully clothed, *not* in the examining room.
   c. Use the pelvic exam to teach the female patient about sexual anatomy.
   d. **Use the PLISSIT model** to recall the levels of treatment.
      i. **P:** permission. Help reassure the patient regarding sexual activity. Alleviate guilt about activities that a patient feels are "bad" or "dirty." Use statistics to reinforce the range of normal activities.
      ii. **LI:** limited information. Provide information about anatomy and physiology. Correct myths and misconceptions.
      iii. **SS:** specific suggestions. Apply behavioral techniques used in sex therapy. There are general principles and specific techniques for each of the sexual dyfunctions.
      iv. **IT:** intensive therapy. Patients with chronic sexual problems and/or complex psychologic issues may not respond to the above and may benefit from consultation with a mental health professional skilled in dealing with sexual problems.
2. **Behavior therapy (sex therapy): general principles**
   a. Improve communication between partners verbally and physically.
   b. Encourage experimentation.
   c. Decrease the pressure of performance by changing the goal of sexual activity away from erection or orgasm to feeling good about oneself.
   d. Relieve the pressure of the moment by suggesting there is always another day to try.
3. **Behavior therapy (sex therapy): specific suggestions**
   a. **Hypoactive sexual disorder**
      i. Behavioral treatment for hypoactive sexual disorder may include initiation of sensate focus exercises (non-demand pleasuring techniques) to enhance enjoyment without pressure.
      ii. Use erotic material.
      iii. Consider masturbation training with fantasy to help individuals become aware of conditions necessary for a positive sexual experience.
   b. **Sexual aversion disorder**
      i. Behavioral treatments for sexual aversion disorder are the same as for hypoactive sexual desire.
      ii. When the phobic/panic-type symptoms are displayed, the addition of antipanic medication (antianxiety or antidepressant) may be helpful.
   c. **Female sexual arousal disorder**
      i. Female sexual arousal disorder usually requires referral to a specialist.

ii. It is helpful to suggest the use of lubrication, such as saliva or KY jelly, for vaginal dryness.
iii. Post-menopausal women may benefit from topical estrogen cream, given intermittently.

d. **Male erectile disorder**
i. Prescribe "sensate focus" exercises.
ii. Prohibit intercourse, even if erection occurs.
iii. Prescribe the female superior position (female on top of male) to attempt non-demanding intercourse (heterosexual couple). The female manually stimulates the penis and if erection is obtained she inserts the penis into her vagina and gradual movement is begun.
iv. Educate the patient about ways to satisfy his partner without penile-vaginal intercourse.
v. Drug therapy (medication, injection, suppository) can be beneficial to restore confidence while exploring psychological issues.

e. **Female orgasmic disorder**
i. For women who have never had an orgasm suggest self-stimulation, use of fantasy material, and Kegel vaginal exercises (contraction of pubococcygeus muscles).
ii. For the woman who is anorgastic with her partner, recommend sensate focus exercises (from non-genital stimulation to genital stimulation). Use a back-protected position (male in seated position with female between his legs with back against his chest). Use controlled intercourse in the female superior position.
iii. If the woman is anorgastic during intercourse, use the "bridge technique," in which male stimulates the female's clitoris manually after insertion of the penis into the vagina.

f. **Male orgasmic disorder (during intercourse)**
i. When male orgasmic disorder is present, have the female stimulate the male manually until orgasm becomes inevitable.
ii. Insert the penis into the vagina and begin thrusting.
iii. Manual stimulation is repeated if ejaculation does not occur.

g. **Premature ejaculation**
i. When premature ejaculation is present, suggest an increase in the frequency of sex.
ii. Teach the "squeeze" technique, in which the female manually stimulates the penis. When ejaculation is approaching, as indicated by the male, the female squeezes the penis with her thumb on the frenulum. The pressure is applied until the male no longer feels the urge to ejaculate (15–60 seconds). Use the female superior position with gradual thrusting and the "squeeze" technique as excitement intensifies.
iii. "Stop-start" method is an alternative to the "squeeze" technique. The female stimulates the male to the point of ejaculation then stops the stimulation. She resumes the stimulation for several stop-start procedures, until ejaculation is allowed to occur.

h. **Dyspareunia**
i. Treat any underlying gynecologic problem first.
ii. Treat insufficient lubrication as described above.
iii. Treat accompanying vaginismus as described below.

i. **Vaginismus**
i. When vaginismus is present, the female is encouraged to accept larger and larger objects into her vagina (e.g., her fingers, her partner's fingers, Hegar graduated vaginal dilators, syringe containers of different sizes).
ii. Recommend the use of the female superior position, allowing the female to gradually insert the erect penis into the vagina.
iii. Use extra lubricant (KY jelly).
iv. Practice Kegel vaginal exercises to develop a sense of control.

VI. Evaluation of the Problem: Paraphilias

A. General Recommendations

1. Definition. Paraphilias are manifest by recurrent, intense sexually arousing fantasies, sexual urges, or behaviors, involving non-human objects, or the suffering or humiliation of oneself or one's partner, children, or other non-consenting persons that occur over a period of at least 6 months (see Table 20-6).
2. The diagnosis should only be made if the individual has acted on the urges or is markedly distressed by them.
3. Some individuals may always need paraphiliac fantasies for erotic arousal.
4. Some individuals have paraphiliac preferences only during periods of stress.
5. Paraphilias almost always occur in males.
6. Paraphilia replaces the older terms "perversion" and "sexual deviation."
7. Paraphilias may have legal and societal significance, as they may involve non-consenting partners.
8. A strong association exists between paraphilia and childhood attention deficit hyperactivity disorder (ADHD).
9. A strong association exists between paraphilia and substance abuse (64%), major depression or dysthymia (39%), and phobic disorder (42%).

B. Medical History

1. **Most paraphilias are thought to have a psychological basis.**
   a. Individuals with paraphilias have difficulty forming more socialized sexual relationships.
   b. Paraphilias may involve a conditioned response in which non-sexual objects become sexually arousing when paired with a pleasurable activity (masturbation).
2. **A medical evaluation should be completed to rule out endocrine and neurologic etiologies,** as well as reactions to medications, to drug use, or to drug abuse.

Table 20-6. Diagnostic Criteria of Specific Paraphilias

Disorder (DSM-IV Code)	*Definition*	*Features*
Exhibitionism (302.4)	Exposure of genitals to unsuspecting strangers in public.	Primary intent is to evoke shock or fear in victims. Offenders are usually male.
Fetishism (302.81)	Sexual arousal using non-living objects (e.g., female lingerie).	Masturbation occurs while holding the fetish object. The sexual partner may wear the object.
Frotteurism (302.89)	Sexual arousal by touching and rubbing against a non-consenting person.	The behavior occurs in a crowded public place from which the offender can escape arrest.
Pedophilia (302.2)	Sexual activity with a prepubescent child. The patient must be at least 16 years of age and be 5 years older than the victim.	Pedophilia is the most common paraphilia. Most of the victims are girls. Victims are often relatives. Most pedophiles are heterosexual.
Sexual Masochism (302.83)	Sexual pleasure comes from physical or mental abuse or humiliation.	A dangerous form is hypoxyphilia, where oxygen deprivation enhances arousal, and accidental deaths can occur.
Sexual Sadism (302.84)	Sexual arousal is derived from causing mental or physical suffering to another person.	Sexual sadism is mostly seen in men. It can progress to rape. 50% of those afflicted are alcoholic.
Transvestic Fetishism (302.3)	Cross-dressing in heterosexual males for sexual arousal.	The wife (partner) may be aware of the activity and help in the selection of clothes or insist on treatment.
Voyeurism (302.82)	Sexual arousal by watching an unsuspecting person who is naked, disrobing, or engaging in sexual activity.	Most commonly occurs in men, but it can occur in women. Masturbation commonly occurs. A variant is telephone sex.
Paraphilia Not Otherwise Specified (302.9)	Paraphilias that do not meet criteria for any of the above categories.	Categories include necrophilia (corpses), zoophilia (animals), urophilia (urine), and coprophilia (feces).

3. **An organic diagnosis underlying a paraphilia should be suspected when:**
   a. The behavior begins in middle age or later.
   b. There is regression from a previously normal sexuality.
   c. There is excessive aggression.
   d. There are reports of auras or seizure-like symptoms prior to, or during, the sexual behavior.
   e. There is an abnormal body habitus.
   f. There is an abnormal neurologic examination.

C. Sexual History

1. Most people with paraphilias will not spontaneously reveal their behavior and are very secretive about their sexual activities.
2. Many people when questioned will not admit to a paraphilia because of the illegal nature of the behavior and the impact of the behavior on close relationships.
3. Individuals with paraphilias may first come to the attention of others after their arrest by police.
4. A variety of interview techniques exists.
   a. Use screening questions that will not sound judgmental.
      i. When you want to be sexual, do you engage in sexual activity that other people find unusual?
   b. Appreciate the patient's shame and embarrassment when discussing atypical sexual behavior.
   c. Alert the patient of legal reporting requirements if sexual behavior is harmful or illegal (children in need of protection).
   d. If the sexual behavior is not illegal or harmful, assure the patient of confidentiality.
   e. When one form of atypical sexual behavior is found, ask about others in the same individual.

D. Examination of the Patient

1. Perform an appropriate physical examination.
2. Perform an appropriate laboratory examination.
   a. Penile plethysmography is used to assess paraphilias by measuring an individual's sexual arousal in response to visual and auditory stimuli.

VII. Psychiatric Differential Diagnosis of Paraphilias

A. Mental Retardation
B. Dementia
C. Substance Intoxication
D. Manic Episode (Bipolar Disorder)

E. Schizophrenia
F. Obsessive-Compulsive Disorder
G. Gender Identity Disorder
H. Personality Disorder
I. Sexual Dysfunction
J. Non-paraphiliac Compulsive Sexual Behaviors

1. Compulsive use of erotic videos, magazines, or cybersex
2. Uncontrolled masturbation
3. Unrestrained use of prostitutes
4. Numerous brief, superficial sexual affairs

K. Hypersexuality/Sexual Addiction

VIII. Diagnostic Criteria

A. Disorders may begin in childhood or early adolescence and become better defined during adolescence or adulthood. The disorders are chronic and life-long, but fantasies and behaviors often diminish with advancing age. The behaviors increase in response to psychosocial stress, other mental disorders, and an increased opportunity to engage in the paraphilia (see Table 20-6).

IX. Treatment Strategies

A. General Considerations

1. **People with paraphilias rarely seek treatment, unless forced by their arrest or by their discovery by a family member.**
2. The paraphilia produces intense pleasure and is difficult to give up; it is like an addiction or compulsion.
3. Paraphiliacs in therapy often try to convince therapists that their behavior has stopped when actually it continues.
4. Treatment outcome for paraphilias is poor, and recidivism is high.
5. Treatment requires active monitoring.

B. Specific Techniques

1. **Psychotherapy:** insight oriented or supportive
   a. Psychotherapy is relatively ineffective for paraphilias.
2. **Behavior therapy**
   a. Aversive therapy is used to reduce the behavior by conditioning.
   b. Desensitization is used to neutralize anxiety of non-paraphiliac sexual situations by gradual exposure.
   c. Social skills training (individual or group) is used to help form better interpersonal relationships.
   d. Orgasmic reconditioning is used to teach the paraphiliac to become aroused by more acceptable mental imagery.
3. **Medications**
   a. Anti-androgen drugs
      i. Intramuscular injections of medroxyprogesterone acetate (MPA) and cyproterone (not FDA-approved) acetate lower testosterone levels by competitive inhibition of androgen receptors and thus decrease aberrant sexual tendencies.
      ii Intramuscular injections of leuprolide (approved for treatment of prostatic cancer) and triptorelin (although not FDA-approved), synthetic gonadotropin-releasing hormone analogs, decrease testosterone to castrate level (after an initial transient increase) and may completely abolish deviant sexual tendencies.
      iii. Use of oral estrogen (ethinyl estradiol) has a lower success rate.
   b. Antidepressant drugs
      i. Clomipramine and the selective serotonin reuptake inhibitors (SSRIs), including fluoxetine, setraline, and fluvoxamine, may lower aberrant sexual urges by decreasing compulsivity/impulsivity of the act.

Suggested Readings

American Psychiatric Association. (1995). *Diagnostic and statistical manual of mental disorders* (4th ed., Primary care version). Washington, DC: American Psychiatric Press.

Basson, R., McInnes, R., Smith, M.D., et. al. (2002). Efficacy and safety of sildenafil citrate in women with sexual dysfunction associated with female sexual arousal disorder. *Journal of Women's Health and Gender-Based Medicine, 11*(4), 367–377.

Berman, J.R., Berman, L.A., & Goldstein, I. (1999). Female sexual dysfunction: Incidence, pathophysiology, evaluation, and treatment options. *Urology, 54*(3), 385–391.

Crenshaw, T.L., & Goldberg, J.P. (1996). *Sexual pharmacology.* New York: W.W. Norton.

Fava, M., & Rankin, M. (2002). Sexual functioning and SSRIs. *Journal of Clinical Psychiatry, 63*(suppl 5), 13–16.

Feldman, H.A., Goldstein, I., Hatzichristou, D.G., et al. (1994). Impotence and its medical and psychosocial correlates: Results of the Massachusetts Male Aging Study. *Journal of Urology, 151,* 54–61.

Goldstein, I., Lue, T.F., Padma-Nathan, H., et al. (1998). Oral sildenafil in the treatment of erectile dysfunction. *New England Journal of Medicine, 338,* 1397–1404.

Herrmann, H.C., Change, G., Klugherz, B.D., & Mahoney, P.D. (2000). Hemodynamic effects of sildenafil in men with severe coronary artery disease. *New England Journal of Medicine, 342*(22), 1622–1626.

Kafka, M. (2000). Psychopharmacologic treatments for nonparaphiliac compulsive sexual behaviors. *CNS Spectrums, 5*(1), 49–59.

Kaplan, H.S. (1995). *The sexual desire disorders: Dysfunctional regulation of sexual motivation.* New York: Brunner/Mazel.

Laumann, E.O., Paik, A., Rosen, R.C. (1999). Sexual dysfunction in the United States: Prevalence and predictors. *Journal of the American Medical Association, 281,* 537–544.

Lue, T.F. (2000). Erectile dysfunction. *New England Journal of Medicine, 342*(24), 1802–1813.

Maurice, W. (1999). *Sexual medicine in primary care.* New York: Mosby.

McKinlay, J.B. (2000). The worldwide prevalence and epidemiology of erectile dysfunction. *International Journal of Impotence Research, 12*(suppl 4), S6–S11.

NIH Consensus Development Panel on Impotence. (1993). *Journal of the American Medical Association, 270*(1), 8390.

Rosler, A., & Witztum, E. (1998). Treatment of men with paraphilia with a long-acting analogue of gonadotropin-releasing hormone. *New England Journal of Medicine, 338,* 416–422.

Shafer, L. (1998). Approach to the patient with impotence. In T.A. Stern, J.B. Herman, & P.L. Slavin (Eds.), *The MGH guide to psychiatry in primary care,* pp. 281–287. New York: McGraw-Hill.

Shafer, L. (1998). Approach to the patient with sexual dysfunction. In T.A. Stern, J.B. Herman, & P.L. Slavin (Eds.), *The MGH guide to psychiatry in primary care,* pp. 271–280. New York: McGraw-Hill.

Shafer, L. (2000). Approach to the patient with sexual dysfunction. In A. Goroll, L. May, & A. Mulley (Eds.), *Primary care medicine,* pp. 1178–1183. Philadelphia: J.B. Lippincott.

Shafer, L. (2002). Sexual dysfunction. In K. Carlson, & S. Eisenstat (Eds.), *Primary care of women,* pp. 415–420. St. Louis, MO: Mosby.

Shifren, J.L., Baunstein, G.D., Simon, J.A., et al. (2000). Transdermal testosterone treatment in women with impaired sexual function after oophorectomy. *New England Journal of Medicine, 343,* 682–688.

Vickers, M.A., & Satyanarayana, R. (2002). Phosphodiesterase type 5 inhibitors for the treatment of erectile dysfunction in patients with diabetes mellitus. *International Journal of Impotence Research, 14*(6), 466–471.

Wincze, J., & Carey, M. (1991). *Sexual dysfunction.* New York: Guilford Press.

Chapter 21

Eating Disorders

ANNE E. BECKER

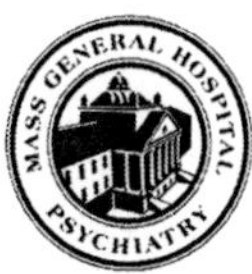

I. Overview

Eating disorders are characterized by disordered patterns of eating, accompanied by distress, disparagement, preoccupation, and/or distortion associated with one's eating, weight, or body shape. Both anorexia nervosa and bulimia nervosa are also associated with efforts made to lose weight or to prevent weight gain.

A. Etiology

The etiology of eating disorders appears to be multifactorial, with both genetic and environmental contributions to risk.

B. Course

Approximately 50% of individuals with anorexia nervosa and bulimia nervosa make a full recovery, whereas 30% partially recover, and 20% follow a chronic course. Individuals with binge-eating disorder (BED) appear to have a slightly more favorable outcome. The mortality rate for anorexia nervosa is 0.6% annually, nearly twice as high as the rate for female psychiatric inpatients of similar age.

II. Epidemiology of Eating Disorders

A. Prevalence

Anorexia nervosa is the least prevalent eating disorder, affecting approximately 0.3% of young adult females. Bulimia nervosa affects approximately 1% of young adult females. BED is the most prevalent eating disorder, affecting approximately 2.6% of young adults (and up to 29% of adults seeking weight treatment). In addition, clinically significant partial syndromes or atypical eating disorders (eating disorders, not otherwise specified), may occur in up to 5–13% of young adult females.

B. Demographics

Eating disorders typically affect young, adult females with 85–95% of cases of anorexia and bulimia nervosa and approximately 60% of cases of BED occurring among females.

C. Onset

The onset of anorexia is typically slightly earlier than the onset of bulimia, but both generally begin during adolescence; however, both disorders can occur at much older ages. Onset of BED tends to be slightly later, generally beginning in late adolescence or in the early twenties.

D. Sociocultural Factors

Although previously thought to be more common among affluent White women, eating disorders affect individuals of diverse ethnic and socioeconomic backgrounds. Eating disorders have been reported all over the globe, but they are more prevalent in industrialized and/or Westernized societies. Several epidemiologic studies have linked immigration, modernization, and urbanization to risk.

III. Diagnostic Features

Symptoms of eating disorders commonly overlap phenomenologically (e.g., binge-eating can occur in anorexia nervosa, bulimia nervosa, binge-eating disorder, and eating disorder, not otherwise specified (ED NOS), and patients often cross over into a different diagnostic category. Because treatment approaches differ among the disorders, it is essential to establish as clear a diagnosis as possible. Up to half of patients with clinically significant disordered eating present with atypical features or with partial syndrome disorders consistent with ED NOS (Figure 21-1).

A. Anorexia Nervosa

Anorexia nervosa is divided into two subtypes: restricting type (in which there is dieting, fasting, or excessive exercise, but no regular bingeing and/or purging), **and binge-eating/purging type** (in which there is regular bingeing and purging of calories). **Anorexia nervosa is characterized by the following diagnostic features:**

1. The refusal to maintain a minimally normal weight (often defined as 85% of the expected body weight for height and age).
2. A fear of gaining weight or becoming fat.
3. A disturbance in the way one's weight or body shape is experienced, a self-evaluation that is unduly influenced by weight or body shape, or the denial of the seriousness of low weight.
4. Amenorrhea (in post-menarcheal females).

B. Bulimia Nervosa

Bulimia nervosa includes two subtypes: purging type (in which there is regular use of self-induced vomiting or abuse of laxatives, enemas, or diuretics), **and non-purging type** (in which the inappropriate compensatory behaviors include excessive exercise or fasting but not the regular use of self-induced vomiting or abuse of laxatives, enemas, or diuretics). **Bulimia nervosa is characterized by the following diagnostic features:**

1. Recurrent, episodic binge-eating (at least twice weekly for at least 3 months). Binges are characterized by an unusually large amount of food eaten in a discrete period of time and associated with a sense of lack of control.
2. Recurrent, inappropriate compensatory behaviors to prevent weight gain (at least twice weekly for at least 3 months). These compensatory behaviors include

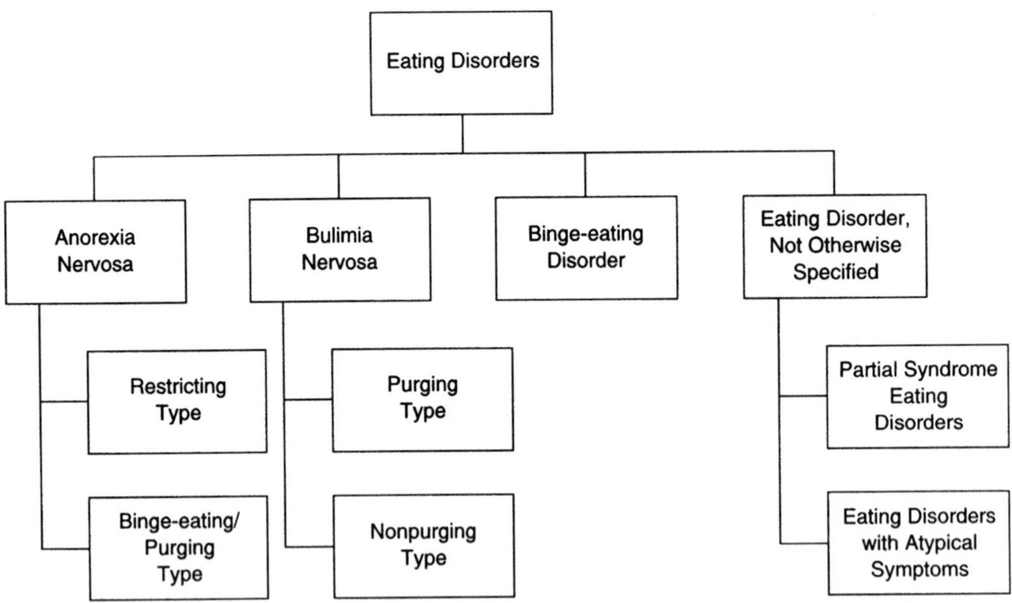

Figure 21-1. Types and subtypes of eating disorders. (Adapted from Becker, A.E., Hamburg, P., Herzog, D.B. (1998). The role of psychopharmacologic management in the treatment of eating disorders. In D.I. Dunner & J.F. Rosenbaum (Eds.), *Psychiatric Clinics of North America: Annual Drug Therapy.* Philadelphia: W.B. Saunders.)

self-induced vomiting, use of laxatives, enemas, diuretics, stimulants, as well as diet pill abuse, restrictive-pattern eating (e.g., meal-skipping), and exercise.
3. A self-evaluation that is excessively influenced by weight or body shape.
4. Symptoms that do not occur exclusively during episodes of anorexia nervosa.

C. Binge-Eating Disorder

Binge-eating disorder is characterized by the following diagnostic features:

1. Recurrent, episodic binge-eating (at least 2 days weekly for at least 6 months) without regular inappropriate compensatory measures to prevent weight gain.
2. The binge-eating episodes are associated with marked distress as well as with at least three of the following:
   a. Eating abnormally rapidly
   b. Eating until uncomfortably full
   c. Eating large amounts when not hungry
   d. Eating alone because of embarrassment
   e. Feeling disgusted, depressed, or guilty after bingeing
3. Symptoms that do not occur exclusively during the course of anorexia nervosa or bulimia nervosa.

IV. Evaluation and Differential Diagnosis

Because individuals with eating disorders are often reluctant to seek treatment or to disclose their symptoms, their illness may go undetected for years, even in clinical settings. It is also not unusual for some individuals to deny or actively conceal their symptoms, making the diagnostic process a challenge. **Evaluation of the eating-disordered patient should include medical, nutritional, and psychiatric assessments.**

A. Medical Evaluation

Medical evaluation of an eating-disordered patient centers on identification of any complications of undernutrition, obesity, excessive exercise, and/or purging behaviors, and exclusion of any organic causes of appetite or weight change (e.g., thyroid disease) by medical history, physical examination, and laboratory analysis.

1. **Medical history should include a thorough review of systems, a history of weight changes, and an inventory of dietary patterns, purging behaviors, and exercise patterns** (see below). **Current medications should be reviewed** for possible contributions to appetite or weight changes.
   a. **Assessment of individuals with suspected or known anorexia nervosa or bulimia nervosa** should include questions about fatigue, postural and non-postural lightheadedness, palpitations, cognitive changes, peripheral neuropathy, dental caries, abdominal pain, bloating, nausea, constipation, hematemesis, age of menarche, amenorrhea, oligomenorrhea, infertility, intolerance of cold temperature, hair loss, dry skin, and fractures.
   b. **Assessment of individuals with obesity associated with BED** should include questions about potential medical complications of obesity (including hypertension, hyperlipidemia, diabetes mellitus, coronary artery disease, degenerative joint disease, and sleep apnea).

2. **Physical examination should include measurement of height and weight, vital signs, and evaluation of potential complications of weight changes, or inappropriate compensatory behaviors.** An individual with bulimia nervosa will commonly have a normal physical examination.
   a. **Patients with eating disorders should be weighed and measured on initial evaluation;** for anorexia nervosa, weights should be monitored routinely throughout treatment. The members of the team managing the patient should agree who will follow weights, how often they will be checked, and how they will be communicated with the team. Clinicians should be sensitive to the discomfort individuals with eating disorders may experience when being weighed, but should avoid estimating weights since individuals with anorexia nervosa commonly wear clothing in such a way so as to disguise their weight.
   b. **Blood pressure, pulse, and temperature should be evaluated periodically** since hypotension, bradycardia, and hypothermia are common among individuals with anorexia nervosa and bulimia nervosa.
   c. **Assessment of individuals with anorexia nervosa should include examination for** dry skin, yellow skin (due to carotenemia), lanugo, hair loss, acrocyanosis, mitral valve prolapse, arrhythmia, decreased bowel sounds, and peripheral neuropathy.
   d. **Assessment of individuals with bulimia nervosa or binge-eating/purging anorexia should include examination for** parotid gland enlargement, submandibular adenopathy, dental caries, hand abrasions (Russell's sign), decreased or increased bowel sounds, and rectal prolapse.
3. **Laboratory analysis should routinely include initial and periodic assessment of serum electrolytes for any individual with purging behavior** since hypokalemia and hypomagnesemia are commonly seen in this population. Laboratory examination **for individuals with anorexia nervosa** should also **include a serum glucose** (since hypoglycemia is common in this population) **and a complete blood count** with differential, since leukopenia, neutropenia, anemia, and thrombocytopenia may be seen in association with anorexia nervosa.
   a. Assessment of individuals with electrolyte disturbances and symptomatic arrhythmias, or for those in whom psychopharmacologic intervention is planned, should include an electrocardiogram to evaluate whether the QT interval is prolonged or if any other abnormalities are present.
   b. Although amenorrhea associated with anorexia nervosa is most often due to decreased gonadotropin releasing hormone pulsatility (leading to hypogonadotropic hypogonadism and low estradiol levels), other causes (e.g., pregnancy) should be excluded.
   c. Since significant osteopenia occurs in half of women with anorexia nervosa, which poses a risk for fractures and kyphosis, women with anorexia nervosa should have a dual-energy X-ray absorptiometry (DEXA) evaluation of lumbar spine bone density to assess severity of bone loss.

B. Nutritional Assessment

Nutritional assessment includes the evaluation of appropriateness of body weight and adequacy of caloric and nutrient intake. Assessment of appropriateness of weight for height can be made by comparing weight and height against the Metropolitan Life Insurance Height-Weight Table or by calculation according to one of two formulas.

1. **Body mass index (BMI) is calculated by the formula:**

$$\mathbf{BMI} = \frac{\mathbf{Weight(kg)}}{\mathbf{Height(m)^2}}$$

   BMI can be used for adult men or women of all heights or weights. A BMI of ≤ 17.5 reflects a weight range consistent with anorexia nervosa. A BMI of 20–25 is considered to be within normal range.
2. **An alternate estimation of an appropriate body weight for height** for adults is made by calculation of the ratio of actual body weight to desirable body weight (percent expected body weight, or % EBW) as follows:

   Women: [100 lb. for the first 5 feet + 5 lb./inch above 5 feet] ± 10%

   Men: [106 lb. for the first 5 feet + 6 lb./inch above 5 feet] ± 10%

   % EBW of less than 85% is a weight for height consistent with anorexia nervosa.

C. Psychiatric Evaluation

Psychiatric evaluation of the eating-disordered patient includes establishing the type and severity of the eating disorder and excluding other psychiatric etiologies of appetite or weight changes (e.g., major depression), evaluating co-morbid psychiatric illness, and evaluating psychiatric risk.

1. **History of the present illness should evaluate dietary patterns** (i.e., restrictive or binge-pattern eating) **and modalities, frequencies, and durations of any inappropriate compensatory behaviors to lose weight or prevent weight gain, as well as the psychosocial context of the illness.** Educational information about the medical risks posed by these behaviors should be communicated at this time. For example, many patients are unaware of the extremely serious risks associated with ephedra or ipecac use.
   a. Inquire about self-induced vomiting, and whether or not syrup of ipecac is or has been used to induce emesis.
   b. Inquire about laxative abuse, including frequency of episodes and number of laxatives typically used per episode.
   c. Inquire about use of enemas.
   d. Inquire about use of diuretics.

e. Inquire about inappropriate use of diet pills, stimulants, or other medications (e.g., methylphenidate or insulin). Also inquire about use of ephedra-containing supplements.
f. Inquire about excessive exercise; determine how many hours daily or weekly the individual exercises and whether the individual is likely to exercise when sick or injured.
g. Inquire about fasting, meal-skipping, or restrictive patterns of eating.
h. Inquire about binge-pattern eating. **Clinically, a binge is defined as consuming an unusually large amount of food in a discrete period of time while experiencing a lack of control over the eating.**
i. Inquire about psychosocial precipitants to symptoms.
j. Evaluate the need for patient and family education and for family intervention.

2. **Psychiatric history** should include questions about previous treatment, as well as history of other psychiatric illness. **Eating disorders are commonly seen in association with mood, anxiety, substance abuse, or personality disorders.**
   a. Major depression, dysthymia, and obsessive-compulsive disorder are associated with anorexia nervosa.
   b. Major depression, bipolar disorder, substance abuse, anxiety disorders, and personality disorders are commonly seen with bulimia nervosa.
   c. Major depression, panic disorder, substance abuse, and personality disorders are associated with BED.
3. **A mental status examination should exclude other possible causes** (such as mood or anxiety symptoms) **of anorexia or hyperphagia,** should evaluate for the presence of co-morbid psychiatric illness, and should assess suicidal ideation. Suicidal ideation and behavior are relatively common among individuals with eating disorders.

V. Treatment

Treatment for eating disorders ideally addresses medical, psychological, and nutritional needs, and utilizes a multidisciplinary team approach. Members of the team do not need to be at the same institution or location, but ideally they should communicate regularly and openly with one another about symptoms and therapeutic interventions.

A. Medical Treatment

Unless there is a psychiatric emergency, the initial goals of treatment often include medical and nutritional stabilization. Potential complications of low weight (and sometimes overweight) or inappropriate compensatory behaviors are addressed. Regardless of the severity of the disorder, an individual with an eating disorder should be followed routinely by a primary care clinician to monitor weights, vital signs, and, when appropriate, serum electrolytes. Individuals with moderate to severe symptoms will need to be evaluated on a regular basis so that medical interventions can be made when necessary.

1. **Weight restoration is a primary medical goal for the treatment of anorexia nervosa;** a goal weight should be determined at the outset of treatment that is within normal range and adequate to regain reproductive function and to reverse bone demineralization. Individuals with anorexia nervosa are as a rule reluctant to gain weight, so weight restoration generally requires active and collaborative intervention among primary care clinician, mental health specialist, and nutritionist. Patients often respond to behavioral, educational, and psychotherapeutic interventions.
   a. Enteral or total parenteral feeding are utilized only in severe cases of anorexia nervosa that fail to respond to the above interventions.
   b. Weight gain in severely malnourished individuals must be carefully monitored since complications of re-feeding include hypophosphatemia, cardiac arrhythmia, congestive heart failure, and delirium.
2. **Correction of hypokalemia and other electrolyte disturbances is necessary** in this population to prevent cardiac arrhythmias.
3. **Vitamin supplementation** is indicated for individuals with poor nutrition and should include calcium 1,000–1,500 mg/day (if dietary sources of calcium are inadequate) and a multivitamin to provide 800 IU vitamin D daily.
4. **A combination of estrogen and progestin** has *not* been shown to be effective in correcting osteopenia in women with anorexia nervosa.
5. Despite menstrual abnormalities and associated infertility seen with anorexia nervosa and bulimia nervosa, pregnancy can occur. Because a variety of obstetric complications are associated with these disorders, **patients should be counseled to avoid conception until the illness has been treated.**
6. Stool softeners or non-cathartic, bulk-forming laxatives may be helpful in treating the severe constipation associated with chronic laxative abuse and withdrawal.
7. **Dental care** is indicated for individuals who induce vomiting because of the increased risk of dental caries.
8. **Weight loss treatment is contraindicated for individuals with active bulimia nervosa.** However, it may benefit some individuals with obesity and BED. For those with a history of repeated weight cycling or early-onset BED, it may be optimal to control the binge-pattern eating before embarking upon weight loss treatment.

B. Nutritional Counseling

Nutritional counseling is a helpful and often necessary adjunct to medical and psychiatric interventions.

1. **Dietary patterns and weights can be monitored** in this setting and communicated with other members of the team.

2. **Caloric requirements and nutritional deficiencies should be clarified** for patients and clinicians; counseling and suggested meal plans and supplements can be offered to patients who need to gain or lose weight.
3. **Behavioral strategies for establishing healthful patterns of eating can be introduced or reinforced** in this setting (i.e., patients can be assisted with self-monitoring of dietary patterns and identifying and avoiding cues to restrict, binge, or purge).

C. Mental Health Treatment

Mental health treatment for eating disorders addresses affective states, emotional conflicts, interpersonal tensions, traumatic losses, and/or maladaptive coping styles that have resulted in disordered patterns of eating and/or excessive preoccupation with body, food, and weight and helps the individual to normalize eating and eliminate inappropriate compensatory behaviors. Psychotherapy is the treatment of choice for these disorders. Pharmacologic therapy is often useful as an adjunctive treatment. Because restricting, bingeing, and purging symptoms are often used to modulate unpleasant affective states, some patients (especially those with serious co-morbid illness) will not tolerate their rapid eradication before alternate defenses and coping strategies are in place, and may even revert to more dangerous behaviors, such as substance abuse or self-mutilation, if eating behaviors are acutely controlled. Depending on degree of associated medical compromise, some teams will elect to avoid abrupt or premature control of disordered eating if a patient (a) risks psychiatric decompensation as a result and (b) can be monitored safely for medical complications. If the risk of psychiatric or medical compromise is high, patients may require inpatient or partial hospital care.

1. **Cognitive-behavioral therapy** (CBT) is the best-studied and best-established treatment for bulimia nervosa and for BED. **CBT appears more effective than medication for both of these disorders.** Less is known about its efficacy for anorexia nervosa.
   a. The mean reduction of binge-eating associated with bulimia nervosa with CBT is 73–93%, and the mean remission is 51–71%.
   b. The mean reduction of purging symptoms associated with bulimia nervosa with CBT is 77–94%, and the mean remission is 36–56%.
2. **Interpersonal psychotherapy** (IPT) has been shown to be equally (but not as rapidly) effective as CBT for the treatment of bulimia and has been shown effective for the treatment of BED.
3. **Psychodynamic psychotherapy, dialectical behavioral therapy, motivational enhancement therapy, guided imagery, and guided self-change have all been shown to be efficacious in treating bulimia nervosa.** Given that clinical goals are often broader than those measured in clinical trials and given the limited generalizability of findings from clinical outcome trials investigating efficacy of CBT for bulimia nervosa, a flexible and sometimes eclectic approach may best suit clinical populations characterized by serious symptoms, history of treatment failures, or psychiatric co-morbidity.
4. **Family therapy** is an effective therapy for the treatment of early-onset, non-chronic anorexia nervosa and is a useful modality of adjunctive therapy for other eating disorders as well, particularly for adolescents and young adults.
5. **Group psychotherapy** is also a useful adjunctive therapy for anorexia and bulimia nervosa. Group CBT or IPT is effective in the treatment of BED as well.

D. Pharmacotherapy

The indications for pharmacotherapy for eating disorders depend largely upon diagnosis, severity, and co-morbid psychiatric illness. Medication management of eating disorders is optimally offered as an adjunctive treatment to, and not a replacement for, psychotherapy. Because both individuals with anorexia and bulimia nervosa may be at risk for hypotension, dehydration, hypokalemia, hypomagnesemia, and cardiac arrhythmias among other medical complications, medication therapy may pose additional risks among this population and should be weighed carefully against potential benefits. Because there is a lack of data on efficacy and safety of medication to treat eating disorders in children and adolescents, the recommendations below apply only to an adult population.

1. **There is no medication that has been shown to be generally useful for the primary symptoms of anorexia nervosa in randomized, controlled, double-blind clinical trials.**
   a. There is some evidence that fluoxetine (60 mg/day) may be helpful in stabilizing *weight-recovered* individuals with anorexia.
   b. Sertraline (50–100 mg/day) has been shown to reduce cognitive traits associated with anorexia nervosa in one open controlled study; however, no between group differences in impact on weight were detected.
   c. Case reports of risperdal and olanzapine and one open trial of olanzapine (10 mg/day) suggest that these medications may be helpful in promoting weight gain and possibly other clinical improvement in anorexic patients.
   d. Other medications that effect weight gain are not routinely used, although zinc gluconate (100 mg/day) has been shown to accelerate weight gain among anorexic in-patients. However, safety and efficacy of prolonged zinc supplementation has not been established for patients with anorexia nervosa. The potential for weight gain with any pharmacologic intervention should be openly discussed with anorexic patients. There is also potential that such weight gain would precipitate

compensatory purging, exercise, or restricting-pattern eating.

e. Co-morbid psychiatric illness or symptoms (e.g., depression or anxiety) should be treated with appropriate pharmacologic therapy, but may have limited efficacy in severely underweight patients. Given medical complications associated with anorexia nervosa (e.g., electrolyte disturbances, hypotension, orthostasis, prolonged QTc, and constipation), side-effect profiles of medications should be evaluated so as to avoid either exacerbation of these conditions or other serious medical risk.

2. **The symptoms associated with bulimia nervosa are moderately responsive to a variety of antidepressant medications in the short-term, although remission rates are relatively low. CBT has been shown to be more effective than medication for the treatment of bulimia nervosa, but the addition of medication to psychotherapy is often clinically useful.** The average reduction of bingeing frequency among bulimic individuals on one of the medications shown to be effective is approximately 56% as compared with 11% on placebo; the reduction of frequency of self-induced vomiting is probably similar. Of the agents demonstrated to be effective, no particular medication has been shown to have superior efficacy, so it is recommended that a medication be chosen based on its side-effect profile and history of patient response. Consecutive trials of agents may be necessary to treat an individual with a poor response to an initial trial.

a. **Fluoxetine is the best studied among the medications effective against bulimia nervosa and is the only FDA-approved medication for its treatment.** It is generally well tolerated in this population. The recommended dosage is 60 mg/day. Other serotonin-specific reuptake inhibitors have not been studied in controlled trials but are in routine clinical use.

b. **Desipramine and imipramine** (in standard antidepressant dosages of up to 300 mg/day, as tolerated) **are effective in reducing the frequency of bingeing and purging in bulimia nervosa.** Amitriptyline has not been found effective in the treatment of bulimia nervosa, and other tricyclic antidepressants have not been studied in controlled trials.

c. **Ondansetron (24 mg/day in six divided doses) has been found effective in subjects with severe bulimia** in one controlled study.

c. **Trazodone (up to 400 mg/day) has been found effective in the treatment of bulimia nervosa** in one study but it is not routinely used given its associated sedation.

d. **High-dose (200–300 mg/day) naltrexone** was also found effective in treatment-resistant bulimic individuals in one study, but it is not recommended for routine use because of the risk it poses for hepatotoxicity.

e. **Despite proven efficacy of isocarboxazid and phenelzine in reducing bingeing and purging symptoms associated with bulimia nervosa,** they may pose an increased risk for a hypertensive crisis in this population and should generally be avoided if possible. Spontaneous hypertensive crises have been reported, but the risk may also be increased by dietary indiscretion or dyscontrol and the use of ephedra-containing products.

f. **Bupropion,** despite efficacy in one controlled study for symptoms of bulimia nervosa, was associated with an elevated seizure risk in bulimic subjects and **is also contraindicated for treatment in individuals with an eating disorder.**

g. **Lithium and carbamazepine have also been studied,** but they have not been found effective for the treatment of bulimia nervosa; other mood stabilizers and benzodiazepines have not been studied for its treatment.

3. **Medication management of BED** has not been studied as extensively for bulimia nervosa.

a. **Fluvoxamine** (50–300 mg/day in divided doses) **has been found effective in the treatment of BED** in one controlled study.

b. **Sertraline** (50–200 mg/day) **has been found effective in the treatment of BED.**

E. Indications for Inpatient Management

Although eating disorders can often be adequately managed in an outpatient setting, inpatient care or partial hospitalization may be required for some patients.

1. **Indications for inpatient management include:** serious medical risk (e.g., significant hypokalemia or dehydration, ongoing ipecac abuse); very low weight (e.g., ≤ 75% expected body weight) or rapid weight loss; growth arrest; psychiatric risk (e.g., risk of self-harm or psychosis); escalating or severe symptoms (e.g., inability to eat, frequent purging throughout the entire day); or failure of outpatient management.
2. It is often helpful to review medical and psychiatric parameters at the onset of treatment, which may signal a need for intensified care with the patient. In such instances, a treatment contract to which all members of the multidisciplinary team caring for the patient must agree in advance is helpful in the event of patient deterioration, non-adherence, and/or splitting.

VI. Conclusions

Eating disorders are common among young adult women, although they can affect both men and women and can occur from childhood into old age. They are often associated with co-morbid psychiatric illness, as well as with sometimes life-threatening medical complications. Successful treatment requires collaborative team management with medical, nutrition, and psychiatric intervention (Table 21-1).

Table 21-1. Summary of Assessment and Management of Eating Disorders

	Assessment	*Management*
General	*Determine onset, course, and patterning of:* • Binge or restrictive pattern eating • Purging or compensatory behaviors • Weight loss, gain, or cycling • Excessive concern and/or distress associated with eating, body, or weight *Exclude* • Alternative medical and psychiatric causes of anorexia, hyperphagia, and weight dysregulation	*Team members should:* • Clarify roles in treatment to patient and to one another • Communicate about symptoms and therapeutic interventions • Identify parameters signaling psychiatric or medical danger or treatment failure and review with the patient
Medical	*Evaluate for complications of purging, excessive exercise, starvation, and/or underweight or overweight with:* • Directed history • Vital signs • Physical exam • Laboratory analyses include: For bulimia nervosa: routinely, serum electrolytes; when indicated, EKG. For anorexia nervosa: routinely, serum electrolytes, glucose, and CBC; when indicated, EKG and DEXA of the lumbar spine. Beta-hCG, FSH, and/or prolactin may be useful in evaluating amenorrhea associated with these disorders	*Routinely monitor:* • Weights and vital signs • Serum electrolytes for patients with purging behaviors *Treat and follow:* • Medical complications initially present or as weight, diet, purging symptoms, or inappropriate compensatory behaviors change *Refer:* • Individuals with self-induced vomiting for dental care
Nutritional	*Evaluate:* • Dietary patterns/caloric and nutrient intakes • Appropriateness of weight (by tables or calculation of % EBW or BMI)	*Introduce and support:* • Nutritional guidelines for weight restoration or control and general health • Behavioral strategies to assist in symptom control
Psychological	*Evaluate:* • Excessive concern with and distress about eating, body shape, or weight • Psychosocial context of symptoms • Co-morbid psychiatric illness and suicidality	*Initiate:* • Psychotherapy *Consider:* • Medication (as an adjunctive therapy when appropriate and for co-morbid psychiatric illness)

Suggested Readings

American Psychiatric Association. (1994). *Diagnostic and statistical manual of mental disorders* (4th ed., pp. 539–550, 729–731). Washington, DC: American Psychiatric Press.

American Psychiatric Association. (2000). Practice guideline for the treatment of patients with eating disorders (revision). *American Journal of Psychiatry, 157,* 1–39.

Becker, A.E. (2003). Update on the outpatient management of eating disorders in adults. *Current Women's Health Reports, 3,* 221–229.

Becker, A.E., Grinspoon, S.K., Klibanski, A., & Herzog, D.B. (1999). Eating disorders. *New England Journal of Medicine, 340,* 1092–1098.

Becker, A.E., Hamburg, P., & Herzog, D.B. (1998). The role of psychopharmacologic management in the treatment of eating disorders. In D.L. Dunner, & J.F. Rosenbaum (Eds.), *Psychiatric Clinics of North America: Annual Drug Therapy,* pp. 17–51. Philadelphia: W.B. Saunders.

Brownell, K.D., & Fairburn, C.G. (Eds.). (1995). *Eating disorders and obesity.* New York: Guilford Press.

Faris, P.L., Kim, S.W., Meller, W.H., et al. (2000). Effect of decreasing afferent vagal activity with ondansetron on symptoms of bulimia nervosa: A randomised, double-blind trial. *Lancet, 355,* 792–797.

Fichter, M.M., Quadfleig, N., & Gnutzmann, A. (1998). Binge eating disorder: Treatment outcome over a 6-year course. *Journal of Psychosomatic Research, 44,* 385–405.

Grilo, C. (2002, November 23). A controlled study of cognitive-behavioral therapy and fluoxetine for binge eating disorder (abstract). *Eating Disorders Research Society Annual Meeting Scientific Program and Abstracts.* Charleston, South Carolina.

Hudson, J.I., McElroy, S.L., Raymond, N.C., et al. (1998). Fluvoxamine in the treatment of binge-eating disorder: A multicenter placebo-controlled, double-blind trial. *American Journal of Psychiatry, 155,* 1756–1762.

Jimerson, D.C., Herzog, D.B., & Brotman, AW. (1993). Pharmacologic approaches in the treatment of eating disorders. *Harvard Review of Psychiatry, 1,* 82–93.

Kohn, M.R., Golden, N.H., & Shenker, I.R. (1998). Cardiac arrest and delirium: Presentations of the refeeding syndrome in severely malnourished adolescents with anorexia nervosa. *Journal of Adolescent Health, 22,* 239–243.

McElroy, S.L., Casuto, L.S., Nelson, E.B., et al. (2000). Placebo-controlled trial of sertaline in the treatment of binge-eating disorder. *American Journal of Psychiatry, 157,* 1004–1006.

Newman-Toker, J. (2000). Risperidone in anorexia nervosa [Letter to the editor]. *Journal of the American Academy of Child and Adolescent Psychiatry, 39,* 941–942.

Paige, D.M. (Ed.). (1983). *Manual of clinical nutrition.* Pleasantville, NJ: Nutrition Publications.

Powers, P.S., Santana, C.A., & Bannon, Y.S. (2002). Olanzapine in the treatment of anorexia nervosa: An open label trial. *International Journal of Eating Disorders, 32,* 146–154.

Santonastaso, P., Friederici, S., & Favaro, A. (2001). Sertraline in the treatment of restricting anorexia nervosa: An open-controlled trial. *Journal of Child and Adolescent Psychopharmacology, 11,* 143–150.

Shisslak, C.M., Crago, M., & Estes, L.S. (1995). The spectrum of eating disturbances. *International Journal of Eating Disorders, 18,* 209–219.

Sullivan, P.F. (1995). Mortality in anorexia nervosa. *American Journal of Psychiatry, 152,* 1073–1074.

Chapter 22

Sleep Disorders

PATRICK SMALLWOOD AND THEODORE A. STERN

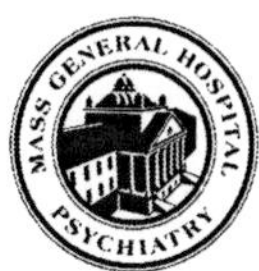

I. Introduction

Sleep, when restorative, becomes so routine as to warrant little more than a passing thought. If altered in even the slightest fashion, however, this once routine process shifts from a benign to a disordered state that can significantly impair any or all facets of daily life. In this chapter, normal sleep (including sleep stages, cycles, rhythm, and biological mechanisms) is examined. The three major classes of sleep disorders recognized by the *Diagnostic and Statistical Manual, Fourth Edition–Text Revision* (DSM-IV-TR) are then reviewed, with special emphasis placed on dyssomnias and parasomnias.

II. Normal Sleep

A. History

While the quest to understand sleep is as old as mankind itself, most of what is known about it has occurred in only the last 60 years. During that time, sleep has been re-defined as an active state, complete with stages, cycles, and rhythms that are as complex as the waking state. **Loomis (1935) observed that electroencephalographic (EEG) changes were prevalent throughout sleep. Aserinsky and Kleitman (1953) detected various types of eye movements during sleep,** most notably slow rolling eye movements occurring early in sleep and disappearing as sleep progressed, and rapid eye movements associated with irregular breathing and increased heart rate. They named **the sleep phase associated with the slow rolling rhythmic eye movements non-rapid eye movement (NREM) sleep,** and **the sleep phase associated with the fast erratic eye movements rapid eye movement (REM) sleep. In 1955, Dement and Kleitman discovered that REM sleep was associated with dreaming,** and, 2 years later, that REM and NREM sleep cycled over the course of the night.

B. Polysomnography

Polysomnography, the method used to objectively evaluate sleep, **involves the simultaneous recording of multiple physiological variables in a standardized fashion known as a polysomnogram (PSG). The parameters recorded by the PSG include,** but are not limited to, the following:

1. **Electroencephalogram (EEG):** a recording of the electrical activity of cortical neurons via scalp electrodes that are placed in standardized positions according to the International 10–20 System.
2. **Electrooculogram (EOG):** a recording of eye movements.
3. **Electrocardiogram (ECG):** a recording of heart rhythm.
4. **Electromyogram (EMG):** a recording of the activity of the left and right tibialis anterior muscles and the submental chin muscles.
5. **Respiratory efforts:** a recording of nasal and oral airflow by means of nasal thermistors, and thoracoabdominal movements by means of strain gauges.
6. **Pulse oximetry:** a recording of oxygen saturation in the blood.
7. **Snore monitor:** a recording of snoring by means of a microphone placed on the lateral aspect of the neck.

By employing polysomnography, wakefulness, sleep onset, NREM sleep, and REM sleep can be defined and studied. Table 22-1 summarizes the sleep stages, as well as the EEG, EMG, and EOG findings that define them.

C. Sleep Cycle and Architecture

NREM and REM do not occur randomly throughout the night, but **alternate in a rhythmic fashion known as the NREM-REM cycle.** In normal healthy individuals, this cycle begins with NREM 1 and progresses to NREM 2, 3, 4, 3, 2, and then REM. **This pattern generally repeats itself at 90–120-minute intervals** about three to four times a night. **NREM 3 and 4 are most prominent in the first half of the night** and diminish in the latter half of the night. **REM sleep,** however, is less prominent in the first half of the night and **increases as the night progresses. Sleep latency,** which is usually 10–20 minutes, is the time from lights out to the first NREM 2. **REM latency** is the time from sleep onset until the first REM, and is usually 90–100 minutes. **Sleep efficiency** is: [(total sleep time)/(total sleep record time)] × 100.

Sleep architecture is the pattern and distribution of sleep stages across an average night and is summarized in Table 22-1.

D. Circadian Rhythm

The circadian rhythm or "biological clock" is **an endogenous rhythm of bodily functions that is influenced by environmental cues, or *Zeitgebers*.** This cycle, unique to each person, **averages 25 hours,** but can be as long as 50 hours for some. Sleep disorders related to the circadian rhythm emerge when an individual's circadian rhythm clashes with environmental and societal expectations.

E. Sleep Across the Lifespan

The amount of time spent in the different stages of sleep varies with age. Infants, e.g., spend more than two-thirds of their day sleeping, whereas adults spend

Table 22-1. Human Sleep Stages and Distribution across the Night

	EEG Findings	*EMG Findings*	*EOG Findings*	*Distribution over the Night*
Wake	Alpha waves (8–14 Hz)	Muscle tone and activity present	Variable eye movements	<5%
NREM 1	Theta waves (4–7 Hz)	Muscle tone and activity present	Slow rolling eye movements	2–5%
NREM 2	Theta waves (4–7 Hz); sleep spindles (12–14 Hz ≥ 0.5 sec); K-complexes (triphasic)	Muscle tone and activity present, but slowing	Slow rolling eye movements	45–55%
NREM 3 and 4	Delta waves (0.5–2 Hz) present ≥ 50% of the time	Marked decrease in muscle tone and activity	Slow rolling eye movements	13–23%
REM	Relatively low-voltage mixed-frequency waves	Absence of muscle activity	Conjugate rapid eye movements	20–25%

less than a third of their day sleeping. **The elderly,** on the other hand, **experience a reduction in the intensity, depth, and continuity of sleep,** because of age-related degenerative changes in the sleep mechanisms of the central nervous system (CNS). Specific sleep changes in the elderly include:

1. Increased sleep latency
2. Reduced NREM 3 and 4
3. Decreased REM latency
4. Reduced total REM amount
5. Frequent awakenings
6. Decreased sleep efficiency

Table 22-2 summarizes sleep patterns across the lifespan.

F. Neuroanatomic Basis for Sleep

The actual neuroanatomic **basis for the sleep-wake cycle remains elusive.** Most of what is known has been inferred through the observations of early electrolytic lesion studies, which suggest that specific regions of the brain are critical for wakefulness and sleep. By drawing on these results and observing the effects of disease states, Hobson (1974) arrived at the most currently accepted neuroanatomic model for wakefulness and sleep. Hobson proposed that:

1. Wakefulness is maintained by the ascending reticular activating system (RAS).
2. Sleep occurs through decreased activity of the ascending RAS and activation of a hypnagogic sleep system.
3. REM arises through active processes in both the nucleus coeruleus and the gigantocellular tegmental field.

Current research supports this model, as disruption of any of these regions leads to alterations in the sleep-wake cycle, and invariably to sleep disorders.

III. Sleep Disorders

While several classification systems for sleep disorders exist, the DSM-IV-TR classification is perhaps the simplest and easiest to understand. The DSM-IV-TR divides sleep disorders into three major categories: primary sleep disorders, sleep disorders related to another mental disorder, and other sleep disorders. Of the three, primary sleep disorders are the most common and are therefore emphasized.

A. Primary Sleep Disorders

The DSM-IV-TR subdivides the primary sleep disorders into the **dyssomnias** and the **parasomnias.**

Table 22-2. Sleep Patterns Across the Lifespan

Age	*Time in Bed*	*Time Asleep*	*Stage 1*	*Stages 3 and 4*	*REM*
Birth	17–24 hours	16 hours	5%	–	50%
12 years	8.5 hours	8 hours	–	15–20%	20%
25–45 years	7.5 hours	7 hours	–	–	20%
Old age	8.5 hours	6.5 hours	15%	0%	20%

1. **Dyssomnias are primary sleep disorders that result in complaints of either sleeping too little (insomnia) or too much (hypersomnia). The DSM-IV-TR subcategorizes dyssomnias into six groups** based in part upon the pathophysiological mechanisms felt to underlie them. The groups include primary insomnia, primary hypersomnia, narcolepsy, breathing-related sleep disorder, circadian rhythm disorders, and dyssomnia not otherwise specified.

   a. **Primary insomnia. Insomnia is the subjective complaint of deficient, inadequate, or unrefreshing sleep. To qualify as a primary insomnia, there must be objective daytime sleepiness and/or subjective feelings of not being rested,** and an absence of psychiatric or medical conditions that better account for it. With **primary insomnia,** the classic form of insomnia, sufferers complain of decreased daytime functioning, and are frequently over-aroused and anxious at bedtime. **Sleep-state misperception,** also known as **subjective insomnia** and **non-restorative sleep,** is a primary insomnia **in which sufferers complain of inadequate and/or poor sleep, but objective findings on the polysomnogram are lacking.** Invariably, patients with sleep-state misperception under-estimate total sleep time and efficiency, and over-estimate sleep latency. **Idiopathic insomnia is chronic insomnia present from childhood** and is most likely the result of an underlying innate process.

      Primary insomnia is perhaps the hardest group of sleep disorders to treat. Once a careful assessment is completed, treatment involves selecting a specific modality based on etiology. Non-pharmacological techniques, such as good sleep hygiene, should be attempted first. If this is unsuccessful, brief intermittent use of sedative-hypnotics may be appropriate. Table 22-3 provides a list of basic sleep hygiene techniques.

   b. **Primary hypersomnias. The hallmark of all primary hypersomnias is the complaint of somnolence and excessive daytime sleep.** Other complaints include difficulty waking, sleep drunkenness, headache, intellectual dysfunction, and Raynaud's phenomenon. Like primary insomnias, primary hypersomnias are not the direct result of underlying medical or psychiatric conditions and are confirmed by objective PSG findings. **Recurrent hypersomnia,** also known as **Kleine-Levin syndrome,** is a rare, often self-limiting condition that **primarily affects adolescent males. Symptoms include hypersomnia, hyperphagia, and hypersexuality.** While the exact etiology is unknown, it often follows an acute viral infection. Treatment is controversial, but it includes the use of psychostimulants, SSRIs, and MAOIs.

   c. **Narcolepsy. Narcolepsy is defined by the following tetrad:**

      i. **Sleep paralysis** that occurs upon falling asleep or waking up.

      ii. **Sleep attacks** with sleep-onset REM periods (SOREMPs). These are usually brief (10–15 minutes), occur in inappropriate circumstances, and **are effectively treated with psychostimulants** (dextroamphetamine, methylphenidate, and pemoline).

      iii. **Cataplexy** (a condition of sudden and transient bilateral weakness or paralysis) triggered by strong emotion, often laughter, anger, or surprise. It frequently lasts only seconds and is **effectively treated with imipramine.**

      iv. **Hypnagogic hallucinations.**

      Narcolepsy is rare, with an incidence of 0.07%. The **onset** is usually in **the late teens and early twenties,** and the course is often chronic. **Genetic factors play a role,** as between 90% and 100% of Asian and Caucasian narcoleptics possess the human leukocyte antigen HLA-DR2 and DQwl phenotypes, compared with 20% to 40% of Asian and Caucasian non-narcoleptics; in addition, the probability of developing narcolepsy is 40 times greater if an immediate family member suffers from it. Although sufferers have increased daytime sleepiness with decreased night sleep, total sleep time does not increase over a 24-hour period.

   d. **Breathing-related sleep disorder. The hallmark of sleep-related breathing disorders is apnea.** Prior to a discussion of sleep apnea syndromes, several terms must be defined. **Apnea is the cessation of nasobuccal airflow for greater than 10 seconds Hypopnea is a 50% reduction of either nasobuccal airflow or thoracoabdominal movements during sleep,** resulting in either a wake pattern on the EEG or at least a 4% decrease in oxygen saturation on the pulse oximeter. The **apnea index** (AI) is the number of clinically significant apneas per hour of sleep;

Table 22-3. Basic Sleep Hygiene

- Limit in-bed time to the amount present before the sleep disturbance
- Lie down only when sleepy, and sleep only as much as necessary to feel refreshed
- Use the bed for sleep only
- Maintain comfortable sleeping conditions and avoid excessive warmth and cold
- Wake up at a regular time each day
- Avoid daytime naps
- Exercise regularly, but early in the day
- Limit sedatives
- Avoid alcohol, tobacco, and caffeine near bedtime
- Eat at regular times daily and avoid large meals near bedtime
- Eat a light snack, if hungry, near bedtime
- Practice evening relaxation routines, such as progressive muscle relaxation, meditation, or taking a very hot, 20-minute body temperature-raising bath near bedtime

likewise, the **hypopnea index** (HI) is the number of clinically significant hypopneas per hour of sleep. The **respiratory disturbance index** (RDI), perhaps the most sensitive of the indices, **is the sum of the AI and the HI.** An AI > 5, or RDI > 10 is considered pathologic and warrants treatment.

i. **Obstructive sleep apnea** (OSA), the quintessential sleep-related breathing disorder, **is the most common organic disorder of excessive daytime sleepiness,** accounting for 40–50% of all patients seen in sleep disorder centers. The estimated **prevalence is 1–2%** of the adult male population in the United States; **it increases to 8.5% of men between the ages of 40 and 65 years.** Women account for 12–35% of OSA patients, with the majority of them being postmenopausal. Nocturnal symptoms include snoring, choking, enuresis, reflux, and cardiac dysrhythmias; daytime symptoms include headaches, hypersomnolence, automatic behavior, and neuropsychiatric abnormalities. The most significant risk factors are male sex, age between 40–65 years, obesity, smoking, alcohol use, and poor physical health. **The principle defect is occlusion of the upper airway at the level of the pharynx during wake-sleep transitions and sleep proper. First-line therapy includes nasal continuous positive airway pressure** (nCPAP) **and bilevel positive airway pressure** (BiPAP). Mortality rates for OSA depend on the apnea index and treatment modalities. For patients who receive no treatment and have an apnea index > 20, the probability of a cumulative 8-year survival is reported at 0.63 ± 0.17. With the use of nCPAP, regardless of the initial apnea index, the probability of a cumulative 8-year survival rises to 1.0.

ii. Two other types of sleep apnea are recognized based on etiology and the presence or absence of respiratory effort during apneic events. **Central sleep apnea is a condition of repetitive apneas in which there is cessation of airflow without an attempt to initiate thoracoabdominal respiratory effort.** The etiology of the central sleep apnea, while debated, is felt to lie in abnormal CNS system processes. **Mixed sleep apnea,** as the name implies, is combined repetitive central and obstructive apneas. To qualify as a mixed apnea, an obstructive event must follow a central apnea.

e. **Circadian rhythm sleep disorders emerge when societal expectations conflict with an individual's preferred circadian rhythm.** As a result, the timing of sleep, not its quality and architecture, is adversely affected. The most frequently encountered circadian rhythm disorders are **jet lag syndrome, shift-work sleep disorder, delayed sleep phase disorder ("night owls"), advanced sleep phase disorder ("larks"), and non-24 hour day (or hypernyctohemeral) syndrome.** Treatment for these disorders includes gradually delaying sleep until one achieves the new schedule, or using light therapy, or melatonin. Virtually all circadian rhythm disorders are self-limited and resolve as the individual adjusts to the new sleep-wake schedule.

f. **Dyssomnias not otherwise specified.**

i. **Periodic limb movement disorder** (PLM) is a common dyssomnia affecting up to 40% of people over the age of 65 years, and 11% of people who complain of insomnia. **PLM manifests as brief (0.5–5 seconds) stereotypic contractions of the lower limbs,** frequently the dorsiflexors of the foot and flexors of the lower legs contract, **at intervals of 20–60 seconds.** Contractions appear more commonly during sleep stages 1 and 2, and although patients are unaware of them, the EEG demonstrates frequent awakenings. **Sleep is often unrefreshing, and hypersomnia is the most common complaint.** While the etiology of PLM is unknown, medications, electrolyte abnormalities, and anemia exacerbate it. Dopaminergic agents, such as L-dopa, pergolide, and bromocriptine, and benzodiazepines, particularly clonazepam, provide some relief, but definitive treatment is lacking.

ii. A closely related disorder to PLM is **restless leg syndrome** (RLS). RLS **is a movement disorder characterized by deep sensations of creeping or aching inside the legs and calves when lying or sitting that produce an overwhelming urge to move them.** The disorder is rarely painful, and movement or massage often provides temporary relief. Like PLM, RLS occurs in association with a number of medical problems, especially renal failure, diabetes, iron-deficiency anemia, and peripheral nerve injury. Unlike PLM, it affects sleep initiation more than sleep maintenance. Medications, especially serotonin reuptake inhibitors, can exacerbate the condition. Pharmacological agents such as L-dopa, bromocriptine, and clonazepam can provide symptomatic relief.

iii. **Post-traumatic hypersomnia** is hypersomnia that occurs within one year of a head trauma.

iv. **Idiopathic hypersomnia,** as the name implies, is hypersomnia of unknown origin. It is frequently confused with narcolepsy, but can be distinguished from it by the absence of cataplexy and by immediate-onset REM sleep. This condition is chronic and often treatment-resistant.

2. **Parasomnias are sleep disorders in which undesired activities are performed during sleep (however, when performed during waking hours, they are considered normal); they arise during specific sleep stages or at the transition between wakefulness and sleep.** Unlike dyssomnias, patients with parasomnias complain mainly about the event itself rather than the quality of sleep. These events are generally bizarre, but they are not taken seriously by

either the patient or the physician. **Children are affected more often than adults, and several different parasomnias may occur in the same individual. Typically, individuals are difficult to arouse during an episode, and once awakened, frequently have poor recall for the episode.** Common parasomnias include **sleepwalking, night terrors, and enuresis.**

a. **Wake-sleep transition disorders. Sleep starts and rhythmic movement disorder** are the most common disorders in this group of parasomnias. Sleep starts, or **hypnogogic jerks,** involve involuntary contractions of the legs and/or arms at the moment in which the individual enters sleep. This condition is benign, and requires no treatment, other than reassurance. **Rhythmic movement disorder (jactatio capitis nocturna) involves head-banging at sleep-onset,** and occurs almost exclusively in children. It is often self-limited and, if treatment is warranted, reduction of stress, benzodiazepines, tricyclic antidepressants (TCAs), and behavioral modification are the treatments of choice.

b. **Light sleep stage disorders.** This group of parasomnias **arises during NREM 1 and 2, and includes sleeptalking and bruxism.**
   i. **Sleep-talking (somniloquism),** as the name implies, **involves vocalizations** ranging from simple words and phrases to complete conversations. It is frequently spontaneous, but may be elicited by speaking to the sleeper. No treatment is warranted.
   ii. **Bruxism is repeated tooth-grinding during sleep,** and is often the result of underlying stress or dental conditions. Mouth guards are the treatment of choice.

c. **NREM sleep disorders.** This group of disorders **occurs mainly in NREM 3 and 4 (slow wave) sleep.** The most commonly encountered NREM sleep disorders **include sleepwalking, and night terrors.**
   i. Sleepwalking (somnambulism) occurs predominantly during the first third of the night and upon partial emergence from delta sleep. Individuals may walk for some distance and carry out semi-purposeful activities, such as running and eating. **While most patients are quite adept at avoiding obstacles, serious accidents, such as tripping or falling out of open windows, have been reported.** Sufferers are frequently unresponsive to efforts to wake them, and, once awakened, are amnestic to the event. Sleepwalking begins in childhood and often resolves spontaneously by adolescence. Common treatments include reassurance, provision of a safe sleep environment, and hypnosis.
   ii. **Night terrors (pavor nocturnus),** like sleepwalking, **occur during partial arousal from delta sleep,** but can begin in NREM stage 2. Patients generally scream, flail about, sit up in bed, and experience autonomic activity, including tachypnea, tachycardia, and mydriasis. These episodes, often 1–10 minutes in duration, take place early in the night, when NREM duration is at its longest. As with sleepwalking, **patients are often amnestic to the episode.** In children, it is often not associated with psychiatric illness, but in adults, it can be associated with post-traumatic stress disorder, generalized anxiety disorder, and borderline personality disorder. Treatment options include psychotherapy, stress reduction, and low-dose benzodiazepine (often clonazepam) to suppress delta sleep.

d. **REM sleep disorders.** This group of parasomnias **arises exclusively during REM sleep, and includes nightmare disorder and REM behavior disorder.**
   i. **The hallmark of nightmare disorder is terrifying dreams whose content is often remembered by the patient.** Unlike sleep terror, **nightmare disorder lacks autonomic arousal, frequently occurs late in the night as REM intervals increase, and demonstrates muscle atonia.** Nightmares are associated with increased emotional stress; therefore, the treatment of choice is to decrease the underlying stress.
   ii. **REM behavior disorder** is perhaps the most dramatic of all the sleep disorders. Essentially, **patients appear to be acting-out dream content through simple to quite complex movements** that result from the loss of muscle atonia during REM sleep. In contrast to sleepwalking, which occurs during the first third of the night during delta sleep, REM behavior disorder occurs during the second half of the night during REM sleep, with patients often recalling their dreams in vivid detail. Although 60% of cases are idiopathic, **up to one-third are due to brainstem pathology and alcoholism.** The disorder is more common in the elderly, and affects males nine times more frequently than females. Low-dose clonazepam can be helpful by decreasing REM sleep density and by suppressing the amount of REM sleep.

e. **Diffuse sleep disorders.** As the name implies, these disorders appear in any or all sleep stages.
   i. The most common is **nocturnal enuresis, a condition in which involuntary micturition occurs without conscious arousal.** It affects children more than adults, and, while a source of great embarrassment to sufferers, is often self-limited. Treatment involves first ruling out medical causes, such as primary enuresis, and, if none are present, using either behavioral methods, such as bladder training, or low-dose tricyclic antidepressants.
   ii. The final category is **sleep-related seizures,** which is a rare, but important, entity in this group of parasomnias. **Seizures occur mainly during light NREM sleep and usually the first 2 hours of sleep.** Because of their similarity to other sleep disorders, nocturnal seizures are often confused for enuresis, night terror, and sleepwalking. The treatment for sleep-related seizures is, as with most forms of seizures, anticonvulsants.

B. Secondary Sleep Disorders

The DSM-IV-TR separates secondary sleep disorders into those related to mental disorders, medical disorders, and to use of substances.

1. **Sleep disorders related to another mental disorder.** This group is further subdivided into insomnia types and hypersomnia types. **As a rule, however, sleep disorders resulting from psychiatric disorders most often present with insomnia rather than with hypersomnia as a chief complaint.** Because the mental disorder is the etiology for the sleep disorder, treatment consists of treating the primary psychiatric condition, with occasional symptomatic relief of the sleep complaint. The classic sleep findings associated with each major mental disorder are provided below.
   a. **Psychotic disorders.** The most prevalent findings are difficulty with sleep initiation and maintenance, which are most common in the acute phase of these illnesses. Total sleep time and sleep efficiency are often decreased, and REM is disrupted early in the episode. Medication side effects must be ruled out, as many of the medications used for treating psychotic disorders can also cause sleep disturbances.
   b. **Mood disorders.** Depression is perhaps the best studied of this group. Classic sleep findings attributed to depressions include early morning awakening, decreased delta sleep, decreased REM latency, a long first REM period, increased REM density, and nocturnal restlessness. However, with atypical depressions, there is often hypersomnia, as well as an increase in appetite. With bipolar illness, the percentage of REM sleep increases during the depressed phase and decreases during the manic phase.
   c. **Anxiety disorders are the most common psychiatric cause of insomnia.** Sleep disturbances associated with anxiety include increased pre-sleep worry with difficulty initiating sleep, decreased sleep efficiency, and poor sleep maintenance.
2. **Sleep disorders related to a general medical condition.** General medical conditions can induce sleep disturbances that mimic virtually any primary sleep disorder. **As a rule, the most frequent sleep complaint is insomnia,** rather than hypersomnia or parasomnia. To make the diagnosis, the history and physical examination must demonstrate a clear connection between the sleep disorder and the underlying medical problem. As with sleep disorders due to mental conditions, **the definitive treatment for this group of sleep disorders is to treat the underlying medical condition.** Although the list of medical conditions resulting in sleep disorders is rather lengthy, **the more common ones include seizures, cluster headaches, abnormal swallowing, cardiovascular disease, metabolic disorders, asthma, and gastroesophageal reflux.** A rare condition is **sleep-related hemolysis,** or **paroxysmal nocturnal hemoglobinuria,** which is an acquired hemolytic anemia exacerbated by sleep. Rather than a particular sleep disturbance, however, sufferers complain of rust-colored morning urine.
3. **Substance-induced sleep disorders. Substances, whether prescription medications or recreational drugs, can cause a wide range of sleep abnormalities that are often confused for primary sleep disorders.** To make the diagnosis, the DSM-IV-TR states that the history, physical, or laboratory examination must demonstrate that the substance is related to the sleep complaint and that the sleep disorder developed during or within a month of intoxication or withdrawal from the substance. Generally, if the substance is a CNS depressant, intoxication causes sedation and withdrawal causes insomnia. Likewise, if the substance is a CNS stimulant, intoxication results in insomnia and withdrawal results in sedation. Because the list of substances is immense, alcohol will be the only substance discussed.

   Alcohol is a widely used and abused CNS depressant. In small to moderate amounts, it is sedating, and, while it induces sleep, it also causes frequent awakenings. **In acute intoxication, alcohol decreases REM sleep and increases stages 3 and 4 sleep, while acute withdrawal produces insomnia, increases REM sleep, and decreases stages 3 and 4 sleep. Paradoxically, chronic use frequently results in insomnia,** and, if alcohol abuse or dependence is particularly long-standing, insomnia may persist for months or up to a year after detoxification. If the suspected agent of a sleep disorder is alcohol, sleeping preparations are contraindicated, as the combined use of alcohol and sedatives can be additive or synergistic, and result in severe CNS depression, respiratory suppression, and death.

Suggested Readings

American Psychiatric Association. (2000). *Diagnostic and statistical manual of mental disorders* (4th ed., Text Revision). Washington, DC: American Psychiatric Press.

Aserinsky, E., Kleitman, N. (1953). Regularly occuring periods of eye motility and concomitant phenomena during sleep. *Science, 118,* 273–274.

Bootzin, R.R., Lahmeyer, H., & Lillie, J.K. (Eds.). (1994). *Integrated approach to sleep management: The healthcare practitioner's guide to the diagnosis and treatment of sleep disorders.* Belle Mead, NJ: Cahners Healthcare Communications.

Carskadon, M.A., & Dement, W.C. (2000). Normal human sleep: An overview. In M.H. Kryger, T. Roth, & W.C. Dement (Eds.), *Principles and practice of sleep medicine* (3rd ed., pp. 15–25). Philadelphia: W.B. Saunders.

Moore, C.A., Williams, R.L., & Hirshkowitz, M. (2000). Normal sleep and sleep disorders. In B.J. Sadock, & V.A. Sadock (Eds.), *Kaplan and Sadock's comprehensive textbook of psychiatry* (7th ed., pp. 1677–1700). Baltimore, MD: Lippincott, Williams, and Wilkins.

Smallwood, P. (1998). Obstructive sleep apnea revisited. *Medical Psychiatry, 1,* 42–52.

Stern, T.A. (1990). Sleep disorders. In S.E. Hyman, & M.A. Jenike (Eds.), *Manual of clinical problems in psychiatry,* pp. 140–150. Boston: Little, Brown.

Chapter 23

Impulse Control Disorders

KATHY M. SANDERS

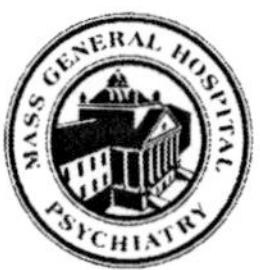

I. Introduction

This category of diagnoses in the *Diagnostic and Statistical Manual, Fourth Edition* (DSM-IV) is a "residual." **Diagnoses in this category include kleptomania, pyromania, pathological gambling, trichotillomania, intermittent explosive disorder, and impulse control disorder, not otherwise specified (NOS).**

Each of these conditions involves a drive, or a temptation, to perform some act that is harmful to the person or to others, or involves the failure to resist an impulse. Other associated features include an increase of tension (with dysphoria or arousal intensity) before committing an act that is followed by a release of tension, a sense of gratification, or a sense of pleasure and relief during and after the act. There may also be a sense of guilt, regret, or self-reproach following the behavior.

Whether these conditions are distinct diagnoses or variants of another Axis I disorder remains controversial. In some ways they are similar to obsessive-compulsive disorder (OCD), substance dependence, mood disorders, and mental disorders due to a general medical condition. Since similar treatments have been efficacious, a similar etiology has been postulated (OCD, eating disorders, mood disorders, paraphilias, and alcohol and substance abuse disorders).

A patient diagnosed with impulse control disorder has an increased risk of being diagnosed with a substance abuse disorder, OCD or another anxiety disorder, an eating disorder, or a mood disorder. Moreover, there is an increased incidence of substance abuse disorders and mood disorders in family members of patients with these impulse control disorders.

Theories place impulse control disorders on a spectrum of affective disorders, as a variant of OCD, or a blend of mood, impulse, and compulsive disorders. While historically these disorders were thought to result from psychodynamic conflicts, recently, since improvement of impulsive symptoms has accompanied use of the serotonergic antidepressants, more biological hypotheses are being explored.

II. Kleptomania

A. Definition

1. More than 150 years ago, kleptomania was recognized as an **out-of-character behavior of "nonsensical pilfering"** in which worthless items were stolen. A characteristic increase in tension was relieved only by the act of stealing. Individuals with this disorder were not known to have a lifestyle of stealing or pre-meditated thievery. Since its initial description, few systematic or rigorous studies have been conducted.
2. **Diagnostic criteria** according to the DSM-IV include:
   a. A repetitive failure to resist the urge to steal objects that are not needed for personal use or for monetary value.
   b. An increase in tension immediately before committing a theft.
   c. A sense of pleasure, gratification, or relief associated with performing a theft.
   d. The absence of anger or vengeance while stealing; thefts are not in response to a delusion or hallucination.
   e. Absence of diagnostic criteria for a conduct disorder, a manic episode, or an antisocial personality disorder.

B. Epidemiology

1. **Little is known about the epidemiology of kleptomania.** Few studies have been published on this subject.
2. That said, **the prevalence within the general population is estimated to be 6 out of 1,000.** Less than 5% of shoplifters meet criteria for kleptomania.
3. Women are more likely than are men to be diagnosed with kleptomania.
4. There is often a lag time of many years (up to several decades) between the onset of the behavior and an individual's presentation for treatment. Women with this disorder tend to seek treatment in their thirties, while men seek treatment in their fifties.

C. Evaluation/Examination

1. **This disorder tends to begin in late adolescence, followed by chronic, intermittent episodes of stealing** over many years.
2. **Patients generally come to professional attention via court referral or by disclosure during treatment for a related psychiatric disorder.**
3. Ego-dystonic reactions to the behavior and to the unpremeditated nature of the stealing episodes should be examined.
4. **Differential diagnosis** includes:
   a. Criminal acts of shoplifting or stealing
   b. Malingering to avoid prosecution for theft
   c. Antisocial personality disorder
   d. Conduct disorder
   e. Manic episode
   f. Schizophrenia
   g. Dementia

D. Treatment

1. Treatment successes are hard to pinpoint.
2. Treatment modalities include:
   a. Insight-oriented psychotherapy

b. Behavioral therapies that use covert and aversive sensitization

c. Somatic therapies, including electroconvulsive therapy (ECT) and pharmacotherapy, particularly with serotonergic antidepressants

III. Pyromania

A. Definition

1. **Pyromania is pathological fire-setting without evidence of secondary (e.g., monetary or political) gain, intense emotional expression, or fire-setting as a criminal act.**
2. **DSM-IV diagnostic criteria** include:
   a. The deliberate act of setting a fire in a purposeful manner on more than one occasion.
   b. An increase in tension and/or affective arousal associated with the act.
   c. Fascination, attraction, and curiosity about fires.
   d. Obvious pleasure, gratification, or relief while setting fires, or when witnessing or participating in the aftermath of fire-setting.
   e. The motivation for fire-setting is not due to monetary gain, as an expression of sociopolitical ideology, as a means of concealing criminal activity, as a means of expressing anger or vengeance, as a means of improving one's living circumstances, as a response to a delusion or hallucination, or as a result of impaired judgment (e.g., from dementia, mental retardation, or substance intoxication).
   f. Conduct disorder, a manic episode, or antisocial personality disorder must be ruled out.

B. Epidemiology

1. **True pyromania is rare.**
2. Pyromania is assumed to have a preponderance in males; often a fascination with fires dates back to childhood or early adolescence.

C. Differential Diagnosis

1. Intentional fire-setting for profit, for political interests, or for revenge preclude the diagnosis.
2. Delusions or hallucinations associated with schizophrenia or another psychotic disorder must be ruled out.
3. Fire-setting cannot be due to a manic episode with poor impulse control.
4. Dementia or another mental disorder caused by a medical condition may result in behavior due to an impaired ability to acknowledge consequences of an act.
5. Conduct disorder in children and an antisocial personality disorder in adults must be considered in the differential.

D. Treatment

There is no definitive treatment for fire-setting. Typically several modalities (behavioral therapy, pharmacotherapy, family therapy [especially where children are concerned]) are used simultaneously.

IV. Pathological Gambling

A. Definition

1. **Pathologic gambling involves a failure to resist the impulse to gamble in the face of a severe disruption in personal, family, or vocational functioning.** This disorder is most similar to addiction disorder; similarities to alcoholism are also noted.
2. **DSM-IV diagnostic criteria include:**
   a. **Persistent and recurrent maladaptive gambling as indicated by five (or more) of the following:**
      i. Preoccupation with gambling (e.g., re-living past gambling experiences, planning the next venture, or thinking about ways to get money to continue gambling).
      ii. The need to gamble with increasing amounts of money to achieve the desired excitement.
      iii. Repeated and unsuccessful efforts to control, cut back, or to stop gambling.
      iv. Restlessness or irritability during attempts to cut down or to stop gambling.
      v. Gambling as a means to escape from problems or to relieve dysphoric mood (e.g., feelings of helplessness, guilt, anxiety, or depression).
      vi. Increased gambling activity after losing money ("chasing" one's losses).
      vii. Lying to family members, to one's therapist, or to others, to conceal the extent of involvement with gambling.
      viii. The commission of illegal acts (such as forgery, fraud, theft, or embezzlement) to finance gambling.
      ix. Jeopardizing or losing a significant relationship, job, or educational or career opportunity because of gambling.
      x. Reliance on others to provide money to relieve a desperate financial situation caused by gambling.
   b. The gambling behavior is not better accounted for by a manic episode.

B. Epidemiology

1. **The incidence of pathological gambling may be as high as 3% in the general population.**
2. One-third of pathological gamblers are women who make up only 2–4% of Gamblers Anonymous membership.
3. Cultural and sociological factors play a role in the specific manifestation of behavior of the pathological gambler (e.g., cock fights, horse racing, the stock market, mah-jongg, pai go, or bingo).

C. Evaluation

1. **Consideration must also be given to social gambling and professional gambling.**
2. As with all impulse control disorders NOS, **the clinician must make sure the behavior is not due to a manic episode or to an antisocial personality disorder.**
3. Since pathological gamblers exhibit tolerance and withdrawal associated with episodes of gambling, evidence of **irritability, restlessness, poor concentra-**

tion, and dysphoria can be detected when a gambling episode is delayed or disrupted.

4. Increasingly, bets are made and risks taken as the need for excitement and arousal is chased.
5. Associated alcoholism, work-aholic behavior, mood disorders, and antisocial, narcissistic, and borderline personality disorders may be noted.

D. Treatment

1. **Treatment for compulsive gambling is difficult** and the course is characterized by frequent relapses, financial difficulties, and legal problems that work against a commitment to ongoing therapy.
2. No specific treatment modality has been shown to work predictably.
3. Treatment modalities include psychodynamic psychotherapy, behavioral therapy, cognitive therapy, pharmacotherapy, and electroconvulsive therapy (ECT).
4. The use of Gamblers Anonymous and the associated 12-step programs, Gam-Anon and Gam-a-teen, are important resources in breaking the addiction cycle.

V. Trichotillomania

A. Definition

1. **The term trichotillomania was introduced** to medical literature by the French dermatologist, **François Hallopeau in 1889** as a compulsive urge to pull out one's own hair.
2. The DSM-IV defines it as:
   a. **Recurrent pulling out of one's hair that results in significant hair loss.**
   b. **Increased tension that occurs immediately before pulling out the hair or when attempting to resist the behavior.**
   c. **The experience of pleasure, gratification, or relief occurs when pulling out the hair.**
   d. The disturbance is not better accounted for by another mental disorder and is not due to a general medical condition (e.g., a dermatological condition).
   e. The disturbance causes clinically significant distress or impairment in social, occupational, or other areas of functioning.

B. Epidemiology

1. **Initially considered rare,** there is evidence **that 1–3% of the population have this disorder.**
2. There is **a bimodal presentation.** Some individuals present before six years of age; in this group, boys and girls are evenly presented and they are managed with behavioral interventions. This type is time-limited and treatable. **The second cluster begins in adolescence and occurs predominately in girls. This disorder is chronic and poorly treated.**
3. The site of the hair pulling is commonly the scalp (in two-thirds of cases), but it can include eyelashes, eyebrows, facial hair, and pubic hair.
4. **Co-morbidity with other psychiatric diagnoses is common.** Mood disorders, psychotic disorders, eating disorders, anxiety disorders, and substance abuse disorders are prevalent.
5. Trichotillomania can be a symptom of other major mental illnesses (e.g., OCD, mental retardation, schizophrenia, depression, and borderline personality disorder). This has raised the controversy whether trichotillomania is a separate diagnostic entity.

C. Evaluation

1. It is important to **differentiate trichotillomania from OCD.** Look for impulsive urges as opposed to goal-associated ideation about the hair pulling.
2. **Factitious disorder** to get medical attention **should be ruled out.**
3. **Alopecia secondary to an organic cause is most difficult to rule out.**
4. Any Axis I mental disorder that has hair-pulling due to command hallucinations or delusional beliefs must be considered.

D. Treatment

1. As is the case with most of the impulse control disorders, **many different treatment modalities have been used with variable success.**
2. Psychodynamic psychoanalytic psychotherapy has been successful in anecdotal case reports.
3. **Behavioral treatment has been more successful.** Techniques include:
   a. **Focus on hair-pulling as a habit** and substituting other responses.
   b. **Positive reinforcement** for not pulling hair and negative reinforcement for hair-pulling, aversive conditioning, relaxation, and competing response training are some of the behavioral techniques.
   c. Hypnotherapy.
   d. **Psychopharmacology** with serotonergic antidepressants, neuroleptics, or lithium.
   e. **Personal appearance problems require** both psychotherapeutic and psychopharmacologic interventions for lasting efficacy of treatment.

VI. Intermittent Explosive Disorder

A. Definition

1. Impulsive and episodically violent behavior that cannot be better defined by a specific organic cause or due to a concomitant psychiatric diagnosis.
2. **The violence associated with this condition is characteristically out of proportion to the precipitating stressor.**
3. **DSM-IV diagnostic criteria include:**
   a. **Several discrete episodes of failure to resist aggressive impulses that result in serious assaultive acts or destruction of property.**

b. The degree of **aggressiveness** expressed during the episodes **is distinctly out of proportion to any precipitating psychosocial stressors.**

c. The aggressive episodes are not better accounted for by another mental disorder (e.g., antisocial personality disorder, borderline personality disorder, a psychotic disorder, a manic episode, conduct disorder, or attention deficit hyperactivity disorder) and are not due to the direct physiological effects of a substance (e.g., a drug of abuse, a medication) or a general medical condition (e.g., head trauma, Alzheimer's disease).

B. Epidemiology

1. Episodic violence of any type is common in our society. When applying strict diagnostic criteria, **this disorder is considered rare.**
2. **Men account for 80% of the cases.**
3. Intermittent explosive disorder and personality change due to a general medical condition, aggressive type, are the current diagnoses available to label a patient with episodic violent behavior.

C. Evaluation

1. **Most violent behavior can be accounted for by psychiatric and medical conditions.**
2. **The most common diagnosis associated with violence is personality change due to a general medical condition (e.g., seizures, head trauma, neurological abnormality, dementia, delirium),** aggressive or disinhibited type.
3. Personality disorders of the borderline or antisocial type must be ruled out.
4. Psychosis from schizophrenia or a manic episode may cause this episodic violence.
5. Aggressive outbursts while intoxicated or while withdrawing from a substance of abuse rule out the diagnosis of intermittent explosive disorder.

D. Treatment

1. **Psychopharmacology is commonly employed** in the chronic management of this disorder. **Anticonvulsants, lithium, beta-blockers, anxiolytics, neuroleptics, antidepressants (both serotonergic and polycyclic agents), and psychostimulants are used** with varying results.
2. **The acute management of aggressive and violent behavior may involve the use of physical restraint and the use of a combination of parenteral neuroleptics and benzodiazepines.**
3. Long-term outpatient management of intermittent explosive disorder requires attention to the therapeutic alliance between the clinician and the patient.

VII. Impulse Control Disorder NOS

A. Definition

1. This category of disorders does not meet diagnostic criteria for any of the previously discussed impulse control disorders or for another mental disorder having the features involving impulse control.
2. Included in this category are diagnoses such as **pathological spending, pathological shopping, repetitive self-mutilation, compulsive sexual behavior, and compulsive face-picking.**

B. Epidemiology

1. **Most of the literature on this category focuses on repetitive self-mutilation.**
2. It is **more common in women than in men.** However, it is considered endemic in male prisons.
3. **Two-thirds of self-mutilators have a history of sexual and physical abuse in childhood.**
4. The disorder starts in adolescence and is characterized by severe psychosocial morbidity.

C. Evaluation and Differential

1. The theories about the causes of self-mutilation range from psychodynamic to psychobiologic.
2. Self-mutilation gives a quick sense of relief and is often likened to an addiction.
3. **Differential diagnosis includes:**
   a. A component of borderline, narcissistic, and antisocial personality disorders
   b. Mental retardation, as caused by Lesch-Nyan and de-Lange syndromes
   c. Hallucinations or delusions from a psychotic disorder
   d. Sexual sadomasochism
   e. OCD

D. Treatment

1. Multi-modal treatment is currently recommended.
2. Prognosis is guarded and it worsens with co-morbidity, with eating disorders, and with substance abuse disorders. Intentional or accidental suicide is common.
3. **Psychopharmacology includes serotonergic enhancing drugs, and the narcotic antagonist, naltrexone.**
4. Other modalities include psychodynamic psychotherapy, behavioral therapy, and involvement in self-help and 12-step programs.

Suggested Readings

American Psychiatric Association. (1994). *Diagnostic and statistical manual of mental disorders* (4th ed., pp. 609–621). Washington, DC: American Psychiatric Press.

Beck, J.C. (1998). Legal and ethical duties of the clinician treating a patient who is liable to be impulsively violent. *Behavioral Science Law, 16*(3), 375–389.

Burt, V.E. (1999). Impulse-control disorders not elsewhere classified. In B.J. Sadock, & V.A. Sadock (Eds.), *Kaplan and Sadock's comprehensive textbook of psychiatry* (7th ed.). Baltimore, MD: Lippincott Williams and Wilkins.

Coccaro, E.F., Kavoussi, R.J., Berman, M.E., & Lish, J.D. (1998). Intermittent explosive disorder-revised: Development, reliability, and validity of research criteria. *Comprehensive Psychiatry, 39*(6), 368–376.

DeCaria, C.M., Hollander, E., Grossman, R., et al. (1996). Diagnosis, neurobiology, and treatment of pathological gambling. *Journal of Clinical Psychiatry, 57*(suppl. 8), 80–84.

McElroy, S.L., Hudson, J.I., Pope, H.G., Jr., et al. (1992). The DSM-III-R impulse control disorder not elsewhere classified: Clinical characteristics and relationship to other psychiatric disorders. *American Journal of Psychiatry, 149*(3), 318–327.

McElroy, S.L., Pope, H.G., Jr., Keck, P.E., Jr., et al. (1996). Are impulse-control disorders related to bipolar disorder? *Comprehensive Psychiatry, 37*(4), 229–240.

McElroy, S.L., Soutullo, C.A., Beckman, D.A., et al. (1998). DSM-IV intermittent explosive disorder: A report of 27 cases. *Journal of Clinical Psychiatry, 59*(4), 203–210.

Stein, D.J., Hollander, E., & Liebowitz, M.R. (1993). Neurobiology of impulsivity and the impulse control disorders. *Journal of Neuropsychiatry and Clinical Neuroscience, 5*(1), 9–17.

Wise, M.G., & Tierney, J.G. (2003). Impulse control disorders not elsewhere classified. In R.E. Hales, & S.G. Yudofsky (Eds.), *The American Psychiatric Publishing textbook of clinical psychiatry* (4th ed.). Arlington, VA: American Psychiatric Publishing.

Chapter 24

Adjustment Disorders, Grief, and Bereavement

ALICIA POWELL

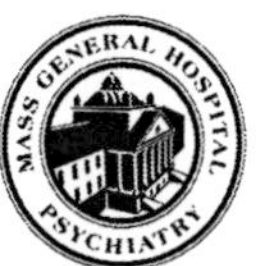

I. Introduction

Adjustment disorders are defined as stress-related phenomena in which the sufferer experiences significant dysfunction and symptoms that are relieved when the stressor is removed or a new state of adaptation is reached.

Epidemiologic studies report that **two to five percent of outpatients** are given the diagnosis of adjustment disorder, and 11–21% of general hospital patients seen in psychiatric consultation receive the diagnosis.

II. Clinical Features

In contrast to other disorders listed in the *Diagnostic and Statistical Manual, Fourth Edition* (DSM-IV), **no specific set of symptomatic criteria exist** that define an adjustment disorder.

Symptoms may be emotional or behavioral and **must occur within three months of the onset of an identifiable stressor.** The **symptoms must be either in excess of what would be expected from the stressor, or must cause significant impairment in social or occupational functioning.** Somatic concerns may be present.

Adults usually, but not always, present with depressed mood and/or anxiety. Pediatric patients typically present with behavioral symptoms, but they can also have emotional symptoms.

III. Evaluation and Differential Diagnosis

The stress-related problem may not meet criteria for another Axis I disorder, and cannot represent an exacerbation of a previously diagnosed Axis I or Axis II disorder. When presenting a case of adjustment disorder for the Board examiners, it is better to include the appropriate Axis I and/or Axis II disorders as rule out diagnoses than to exclude them altogether.

The stressor cannot be the loss of a significant person or object; if it is, bereavement (see below) would likely be diagnosed.

The DSM-IV categorizes adjustment disorders based on the predominant symptoms: depressed mood, anxiety, mixed anxiety and depressed mood, disturbance of conduct (seen frequently in pediatric populations), mixed disturbance of conduct and emotions, or not otherwise specified (NOS).

IV. Management of Adjustment Disorders

A. **Treatment of adjustment disorder lies in interventions that reduce the stressor (if possible), strengthen coping mechanisms, and maximize the patient's support system.**

B. **Psychotherapy,** especially supportive individual and/or family therapy, can help the patient express concerns in a safe environment and obtain needed support. For certain common stressors, such as an illness, support groups can provide a network of information and support.

C. Although not a primary treatment modality, **psychopharmacologic intervention may be indicated to reduce severe symptoms of anxiety or depression.** Treatment should not be withheld just because a patient does not meet strict criteria for a major Axis I disorder. Indeed, some patients diagnosed with adjustment disorder are in the early phase of an Axis I disorder.

V. Introduction to Grief and Bereavement

A. **Grief is a variable but normal response to a significant loss.** The terms **grief, mourning, and bereavement are often used interchangeably. The experience and expression of grief are affected by many factors: cultural norms, personality style, abruptness of loss, significance of the lost person or object to the grieving survivor, extent of preparation for the loss, and the type of death** (natural vs. unnatural).

B. **A complicated grief reaction is one which causes more severe or protracted suffering and loss of functioning** due to inability to grieve appropriately, or the presence of a second psychiatric disorder.

VI. Clinical Features

A. Surveys of bereavement reveal that **most grieving persons are able to cope and recover well from the process,** and few seek psychiatric attention. However, if the survivor does not proceed through a grieving process normally, that person is at risk for development of secondary somatic and emotional problems.

B. **Grief often appears as a temporary depressive syndrome with sadness, insomnia, diminished appetite, and interests.** The survivor may feel guilty about not having done more for the deceased. A passive wish to die may be present, especially as a desire to be with the deceased.

C. **The process of grief** may be organized into phases:
   1. **The initial phase, lasting hours to days, is marked by shock and disbelief.** Early denial is a protective and normal defense against the pain of acute loss.

2. **The next phase may occupy the next several months and usher in a gradual realization of the loss.** The bereaved person often expresses a variety of emotions, including sadness, anger, hopelessness, emptiness, and helplessness. During this period the survivor may experience many symptoms of major depression, including the feeling that life is no longer worth living. **Active suicidality with plan, intent, or gesture, should be taken as a sign of a complicated grief reaction and managed with appropriate attention to the patient's safety.**
3. **Usually between six months and one year after the loss, a final phase of grief ensues.** Symptoms of the second phase begin to resolve but may persist, especially if the bond to the deceased was extremely important to the survivor. **The bereaved person fully accepts the reality of the loss during the final phase, and begins to return to a functioning life.** It is normal for the survivor to re-experience symptoms from the first two phases when reminded suddenly of the loss. It is also normal for feelings of anger and anxiety to continue during the final phase. The important measure of the severity of these feelings is the survivor's level of functioning, which usually will be restored during the final phase. If not, the person may be experiencing a complicated grief reaction.

VII. Evaluation and Differential Diagnosis

A. **Evaluation should include an assessment of the severity of depression, the presence of psychotic symptoms, alcohol or drug abuse, and suicidal ideation.** Additionally, if the survivor witnessed the death, symptoms of post-traumatic stress disorder may appear.

1. **Pay particular attention to those who are bereaved as the result of suicide,** since data suggest that this group of survivors are themselves at increased risk for suicide.
2. **Inquire about the patient's network of social supports.**

B. **Symptoms of a second psychiatric condition,** if present, **should be investigated** appropriately. The diagnosis of major depression can be difficult in the setting of grief, but if neurovegetative symptoms and signs are severe, or if suicidal ideation is present, the examiner should consider the diagnosis of depression. **Remember that hearing the voice or seeing the face of the deceased may be an accepted symptom of grief in some cultures,** such as Latin cultures.

C. **Board examinees should not underestimate the power and importance of simple human compassion for the bereaved.** Examiners will expect you to be able to accept and tolerate the patient's feelings. **A listening presence is usually more helpful than directive phrases** like, "Be strong for your children," or false empathy such as, "I know what you're going through." Be sure, however, to **address the patient's grief directly during the interview, and offer a word of sympathy for the patient's loss.**

VIII. Management of Grief and Bereavement

A. Whether or not the grief reaction proceeds normally, **management consists of treatment of dysfunctional symptoms** (like insomnia), or any superimposed disorders, and facilitation of the mourning process. Any intervention should be tailored to the individual, as grief is a personal and variable process.

B. **Psychopharmacological treatment is not the primary treatment for grief, but it may promote sleep or relieve anxiety.** Unless a secondary depressive or psychotic disorder is present, antidepressants and antipsychotics have no role in the treatment of grief.

C. **Mild sedation with benzodiazepines may be indicated for severe anxiety or insomnia.** Avoid oversedating the patient, as this only impedes the grieving process. Since rapid relief is desired, avoid agents, such as antidepressants or buspirone, which can take weeks to work.

D. **If major depression, substance abuse, anxiety disorders, or psychosis is present in the grieving person, medical evaluation should be undertaken and the treatment for the disorder initiated.**

Suggested Readings

Clayton, P., Desmarais, L., & Winokur, G. (1968). A study of normal bereavement. *American Journal of Psychiatry, 125*(64), 168–178.

Strain, J.J., Newcorn, J., Fulop, G., & Sokolyanskaya, M. (1999). Adjustment disorder. In R.E. Hales, S.C. Yudofsky, & J.A. Talbott (Eds.), *The American Psychiatric Press textbook of psychiatry* (3rd ed., pp. 759–771). Washington, DC: American Psychiatric Press.

Weisman, A. (1998). The patient with acute grief. In T.A. Stern, J.B. Herman, & P.L. Slavin (Eds.), *The MGH guide to psychiatry in primary care,* pp. 177–180. New York: McGraw-Hill.

Chapter 25

Personality Disorders

PATRICK SMALLWOOD

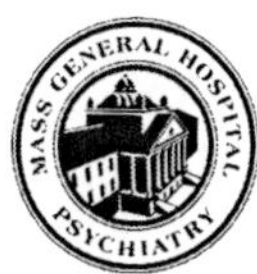

I. Introduction

Defining personality is as frustrating a task as is trying to untie the Gordian knot. To begin this seemingly impossible task, we offer the following **definition of personality: an enduring pattern of perceiving, relating, and thinking about the environment and oneself that is seen in a wide range of social and personal situations.** Personality is relatively stable and predictable, and, as such, characterizes the individual in ordinary situations. When normal, it is flexible and adaptable. **When disordered, it is implacable, maladaptive, deeply ingrained, and often distressing for both the patient and significant others.** Because individuals with this disorder are often manipulative, personality disorders often are not considered valid illnesses; those who make the diagnoses may place partial or full responsibility onto the patient. However, to ignore them as valid illnesses or to choose not to recognize them out of a misguided sense of protecting the patient from a perjorative label does a serious injustice and contributes to inadequate treatment.

A. Classification System

Because certain personality disorders share common features, the *Diagnostic and Statistical Manual of Mental Disorders, Fourth Edition-Text Revision* (DSM-IV-TR) has grouped them into three clusters. The **Cluster A personality disorders,** which include paranoid, schizoid, and schizotypal, appear to be odd and eccentric ("weird"). The **Cluster B personality disorders,** which include antisocial, borderline, histrionic, and narcissistic, share the common features of being dramatic, emotional, and erratic ("wild"). Finally, the **Cluster C personality disorders,** which include avoidant, dependent, and obsessive-compulsive, have a tendency to be anxious and fearful ("wimpy"). The remaining group, although not a cluster and share no common features, comprises personality disorders not otherwise specified. In general, patients frequently exhibit traits of more than one personality disorder, and, if criteria for more than one disorder are met, then each disorder should be diagnosed in a hierarchical manner in order to identify which disorder is primary. Of note, personality disorders are diagnosed on Axis II. For the sake of brevity, only the salient features of each personality disorder will be reviewed in this chapter, and the reader is referred to the DSM-IV-TR for specific diagnostic criteria.

B. Epidemiology

Personality disorders are common in the general population, **with an estimated prevalence of 10–18%.** Consequently, these disorders are encountered in a variety of clinical settings. In outpatient populations, for example, the prevalence is estimated at 30–50%, and on inpatient units, over 50% have a co-morbid personality disorder. **Of patients with Axis I diagnoses, 34%,** most notably anxiety disorders and alcohol abuse, **have co-morbid personality disorders.** For patients who demonstrate recurrent suicidal gestures and acts, the prevalence is 48–65%. Of importance, males and females are equally represented.

C. Etiology

Many theories abound as to the etiology of personality disorders. While each provides helpful constructs, none fully explains so complex a process. There is evidence to suggest that genetics play a role. For example, **Cluster A personality disorders are more common in relatives of schizophrenic patients, patients with Cluster B personality disorders have more family members with mood disorders,** and **patients with Cluster C personality disorders appear to have more relatives with anxiety disorders.**

Psychoanalytic theory, however, is by far the best-recognized theory for explaining the etiology of personality and personality disorders. **Freud** believed that personality traits were the product of fixation at a particular stage of psychosexual development. Wilhelm **Reich,** on the other hand, suggested that the personality arose from the particular pattern of defense mechanisms (unconscious mental processes that the ego uses to resolve conflict and thereby reduce anxiety and stress) that the individual consistently used. In non-disordered patients, these defenses are flexible and adaptable. For the disordered patient, they are inflexible and not easily given up, resulting in the impairments that often prompt them to seek treatment. By recognizing the pattern of defense mechanisms that a patient uses, the clinician should be able to determine the personality disorder, and thereby offer appropriate treatment. **Table 25-1 lists the more common defense mechanisms.**

D. Treatment

Because personality disorders are deeply ingrained and ego-syntonic, individuals with these disorders often resist treatment. The conventional treatment methods for these disorders are psychoanalysis and psychodynamic psychotherapy. The principal goals with these modalities are to help the patient identify and address the manner in which personality style is maladaptive, and thereby promote change by transforming what is an ego-syntonic state into an ego-dystonic state. Recently, pharmacotherapy has been explored. Here, the rationale is to identify those biological dimensions of personality that may respond to medication (such as aggression, impulsivity, anxiety, depression, and psychosis), and treat those symptoms with appropriate

Table 25-1. Common Defense Mechanisms

Defense Mechanism	*Description*
Projection	Unacceptable impulses and feelings are perceived and reacted to as though outside the self
Splitting	Objects are divided into "all good" and "all bad," with rapid shifting from one extreme to another
Regression	An attempt to return to an earlier stage of functioning to avoid tension and conflict at the present level of development
Fantasy	An autistic retreat involving the creation of imaginary lives to avoid conflict and obtain gratification
Dissociation	A temporary and drastic replacement of an unpleasant mood state (or current personal identity) with a more pleasant mood state (or alteration in one's sense of personal identity)
Intellectualization	Excessive use of intellectual processes to avoid expression of affect
Isolation	Separation of a cognitive process from its accompanying affect
Reaction formation	An unacceptable impulse is transformed to the opposite
Repression	A process by which an unwanted idea or feeling is held outside the conscious mind
Acting out	Direct observable action on an unconscious conflict in order to avoid being conscious of either the conflict or the affect that is associated with it
Passive aggression	Aggression toward others is expressed through passivity, masochism, and anger toward oneself

medications. Other popular modalities include cognitive-behavioral methods that attempt to modify specific behaviors (e.g., impulse control, frustration tolerance, and impaired cognitions) with strategies, such as relaxation, role-playing, and correction of distorted cognitions.

II. Cluster A Personality Disorders

A. Paranoid Personality Disorder

1. **Core features.** The core feature of paranoid personality disorder is **a pervasive, persistent, and inappropriate mistrust of people**. These individuals are reluctant to confide in others; they assume that most people will harm or exploit them in some manner. In new situations, they search for confirmation of these expectations, and view even the smallest slight as significant. They unjustifiably question the loyalty of friends and significant others, and consequently are often socially isolated and avoid intimacy. They pride themselves on being rational and objective, but they appear to others as unemotional, affectively restricted, and hypervigilant. **Put simply, these individuals bear grudges, collect injustices, and make mountains out of molehills.** Their preferred defense mechanisms include projection, denial, and rationalization. One note of caution: once challenged or stressed in any significant way, these individuals can show profound anger, hostility, and referential thinking, or experience brief psychotic states that warrant acute psychiatric treatment.
2. **Differential diagnosis.** The most common differential diagnoses for paranoid personality disorder include delusional disorder (paranoid type), schizophrenia (paranoid type), and schizoid and avoidant personality disorders. With delusional disorder and schizophrenia, reality testing is lost, as opposed to paranoid personality disorder, wherein reality testing remains intact. With schizoid and avoidant personality disorder, the amount and degree of paranoia are significantly less, which distinguishes it from paranoid personality disorder.
3. **Prevalence.** The prevalence of paranoid personality disorder **in the general population is between 0.5% and 2.5%,** increasing to 2–10% in outpatient settings, and 10–30% in inpatient settings. There appears to be **an increased incidence in families with schizophrenia and delusional disorder.** By far, the diagnosis is more common in males than females. There is a higher incidence of this disorder in minority groups, immigrants, and the deaf.
4. **Course.** The course of paranoid personality disorder is often **life-long,** with the best prognosis existing for those individuals with good ego strength and with a solid outside support system. A poorer prognosis includes individuals who not only have poor insight and little to no support system, but also those who have comorbid Axis I diagnoses (especially schizophrenia and substance abuse).
5. **Treatment.** Treatment is difficult at best, as these individuals frequently avoid it. If a patient does engage in treatment, **psychotherapy is the preferred modality, with the focus being supportive, consistent, and straightforward.** Due to trust issues and a need for distance, groups are ineffective for these patients. Recent studies support the use of low-dose antipsychotic agents and short-term benzodiazepines for psychotic paranoid ideation, and at times of stress when se-

vere anxiety, hostility, and psychotic decompensation emerge. Long-term pharmacotherapy rarely results in robust improvement, especially for non-psychotic and ego-syntonic paranoid ideation.

B. Schizoid Personality Disorder

1. **Core features. Individuals with schizoid personality disorder are eccentric loners who are emotionally detached and indifferent to the world around them.** They have little desire for relationships or emotional ties, even with family members. **In social situations, they withdraw, rarely make eye contact, and avoid spontaneous conversation.** Their lack of fashion seems to reflect this pervasive disinterest in the world, as they often don uncoordinated and outdated clothing. With respect to employment, they prefer non-competitive and isolative jobs with non-human themes, such as mathematics, philosophy, or astronomy. For hobbies, they enjoy solitary pursuits, such as computer games and puzzles. As perhaps a compensation for their lack of involvement in the world, these patients have extraordinary fantasy lives, which also includes their sexual experiences. Despite the apparent oddities, however, they possess clear thinking and intact reality testing. The best caricature of the schizoid personality would be the single, unfashionable, laboratory-oriented, absent-minded professor.
2. **Differential diagnosis.** The differential diagnosis for schizoid personality disorder includes schizophrenia, as well as paranoid, obsessive-compulsive, and avoidant personality disorders. Intact reality testing, normal abstracting ability, and the absence of formal thought disorder distinguish schizoid personality disorder from schizophrenia. Patients with paranoid personality disorder experience more social involvement than do schizoid patients. Unlike patients with schizoid personality disorder, patients with obsessive-compulsive and avoidant personality disorders, while often socially isolated, view loneliness as ego-dystonic and enjoy a richer interpersonal history.
3. **Prevalence. Schizoid personality disorder affects about 1–7.5% of the population, with males diagnosed twice as often as females.** As with paranoid personality disorder, incidence of psychotic disorders in the relatives of these patients is higher, although this association is less robust. There is also a slightly higher incidence of this disorder in people with solitary and night jobs.
4. **Course.** The onset of schizoid personality disorder is in early childhood, and generally persists throughout life. Most individuals function reasonably well and have few problems that require intervention. In a few cases, however, this disorder may progress to schizophrenia or other psychotic states.
5. **Treatment. Psychotherapy is the treatment of choice.** As these patients have the capacity for introspection, they may remain in therapy for quite a long time. Supportive therapy is the mainstay, yet some patients respond to insight-oriented psychotherapy. These patients generally do not desire group therapy, but after tolerating the interaction with others, groups may provide a means of improving social skills for some. Pharmacotherapy is often ineffective for the character pathology itself, and it should be reserved for co-morbid Axis I diagnoses.

C. Schizotypal Personality Disorder

1. **Core features. The essential features of the schizotypal personality are cognitive, perceptual, and behavioral eccentricities. Patients with this personality disorder frequently embrace beliefs, such as telepathy, clairvoyance, and magical thinking, to a degree that exceeds cultural and subcultural norms.** Socially, they are inept and uncomfortable, and therefore, prefer to be alone. The style of their clothing may be inappropriate and strange, further reflecting their eccentric nature. Their speech is often vague, digressive, or inappropriately abstract, and they may talk to themselves in public. The content of that speech may also reflect ideas of reference, bodily illusions, and paranoia, but there is usually an absence of formal thought disorders, and reality testing is intact. Under periods of stress, however, these patients may decompensate into brief psychotic states.
2. **Differential diagnosis.** The differential diagnosis for schizotypal personality disorder includes schizophrenia and several personality disorders. Paranoid and schizoid personality disorder share many of the core features of schizotypal personality disorder, but differ by degree and by absence of eccentricity. Borderline personality disorder shares unusual speech and an odd perceptual style, but it is associated with a stronger affect and connection to others. Patients with avoidant personality disorder, while uncomfortable and inept in social settings, are not eccentric, and they crave contact with others. Schizophrenia differs from schizotypal personality disorder in that the schizotype possesses good reality-testing and lacks psychosis.
3. **Prevalence. Schizotypal personality disorder affects about 3% of the population. There is no known gender ratio, but it is felt to be more prevalent in males.** Although there is no known genetic etiology, there appears to be a higher occurrence of this disorder in the biological relatives of schizophrenic patients.
4. **Course. The prognosis for this personality disorder is guarded.** Some patients are able to establish stable relationships, marry, and form families, despite their eccentricities. Others may experience periods of brief reactive psychosis or schizophrenic decompensation, leading some clinicians to believe that schizotypal personality is a precursor to schizophrenia. About 10% of these patients commit suicide.

5. **Treatment. The treatment for schizotypal personality disorder is mainly psychotherapy.** Because these patients avoid social contact, the first and most difficult task is to establish an alliance. Once accomplished, supportive therapy with social skills training becomes the mainstay for treatment, as these patients are often unable to tolerate exploratory, insight-oriented, or group psychotherapy. **Pharmacotherapy should target co-morbid Axis I disorders, with low-dose antipsychotics being used for brief psychotic decompensations.**

III. Cluster B Personality Disorders

A. Antisocial Personality Disorder

1. **Core features. The key features of antisocial personality disorder are repetitive unlawful acts and socially irresponsible behaviors that began prior to the age of 15 years.** These individuals are so **unconcerned with the feelings and rights of others that they are morally bankrupt and lack a sense of remorse.** Superficially, they are charming and engaging, yet beneath the facade lie individuals who live in a world filled with illegal activity, deceit, promiscuity, substance abuse, and assaultive behavior. Because patients with this disorder are indifferent to how their actions impact others, antisocial personality disorder is perhaps the most resistant to treatment.
2. **Differential diagnosis.** The differential diagnosis for antisocial personality disorder includes antisocial behavior, other Cluster B personality disorders, mania, psychosis, substance abuse disorders, mental retardation, and personality changes due to general medical conditions. With antisocial behavior, the actions are similar, but the history lacks a sense of degree and pervasiveness in the activities. Patients with borderline personality disorder may perform illegal acts, yet they tend to demonstrate more repetitive suicidal and parasuicidal behaviors, as well as intense affect and self-loathing. Narcissistic personality-disordered patients for the most part adhere to the law as a means to meet their selfish needs. Bipolar mania can be difficult to separate from antisocial personality disorder, as patients with antisocial personalities can also have co-morbid bipolar disorders. For the most part, however, patients with bipolar disorder often lack the degree of childhood conduct problems, and their antisocial behavior is usually limited to manic episodes. Once the mania is resolved, bipolar patients frequently display a sense of remorse. Patients with psychotic disorders may also perform criminal acts, but these acts are usually in response to delusions or hallucinations. Substance abuse disorders can be especially difficult to differentiate from antisocial personality disorder, as patients with antisocial personality disorder invariably engage in substance use. However, criminal behaviors associated with substance abuse disorders generally center around using and obtaining the drugs. Patients with mental retardation may perform criminal acts, but they may be unable to appreciate the illegal nature of the actions. Finally, patients with personality changes due to general medical conditions can display antisocial actions, but, for the most part, these individuals lack a criminal history prior to the precipitating condition.
3. **Prevalence.** The National Institute of Mental Health Epidemiological Catchment Area study indicates that **the prevalence of antisocial personality disorder is approximately 3% for men and 1% for women.** Although encountered more commonly in poor urban areas, up to 75% of the prison population carry the diagnosis. Patients with this disorder have an onset of conduct disorder before the age of 15 years, and frequently suffer co-morbid attention deficit hyperactivity disorders, polysubstance disorders, and somatization disorders. While the exact etiology is unknown, it occurs five times more commonly in first-degree relatives of males with the disorder.
4. **Course.** Early indicators of emerging antisocial personality disorder include multiple delinquent acts before the age of 10 years, and conduct disorder before the age of 15 years. The course is variable. Some improve during middle age as they come to the realization that society will no longer tolerate their behavior. Others end up in prison, experience the complications of drug dependency, or suffer violent deaths from injury, homicide, or suicide.
5. **Treatment.** As mentioned earlier, **this disorder is difficult, if not impossible, to treat.** Unfortunately, the most effective form of treatment appears to involve placement in confined settings or sustained incarceration, such as prison, where external constraints can substitute for their moral deficits. If psychotherapy is attempted, behavioral therapy with a strong emphasis on legal sanctions is the most effective method of treatment. Pharmacotherapy should target co-morbid Axis I disorders or dangerous behaviors toward self and others.

B. Borderline Personality Disorder

1. **Core features.** Borderline personality disorder is perhaps the best studied of all the personality disorders. **The salient features include affect instability with rapidly shifting mood swings, impulsivity, identity disturbance (described as chronic boredom or emptiness), recurrent manipulative suicidal and parasuicidal behaviors (e.g., self-mutilation), and idealization/devaluation ("splitting"). Central to this disorder is an impaired capacity to form stable interpersonal relationships.** Once there is real or perceived separation in those relationships, these patients

often react with intense fear and anger. If the fear of abandonment is realized, or if they experience significant stress, the borderline patient may also experience brief reactive psychotic states (also known as "micropsychotic episodes") or dissociative phenomena.

2. **Differential diagnosis.** The differential diagnosis for borderline personality disorder includes other personality disorders, an identity problem, bipolar spectrum disorders, and psychotic disorders. Borderline patients lack the peculiarity and referential thinking found in those with schizotypal personality disorder and the extreme suspiciousness seen in those with paranoid personality disorder. Histrionic, narcissistic, and dependent individuals have stable identities, are capable of forming solid interpersonal relationships, and rarely engage in self-mutilation or chronic suicidal behavior. Identity problems differ from borderline personality disorder in that the former are usually time-limited and linked to a developmental stage (late adolescence or early adulthood). Bipolar spectrum disorders can be difficult to distinguish from borderline personality disorder, as the two may co-exist. However, the mood swings displayed by the borderline patient cannot meet criteria for manic or hypomanic episodes. Finally, while the borderline may experience transient psychotic states, patients with major psychotic disorder generally experience a persistent impairment in reality testing.
3. **Prevalence. Borderline personality disorder occurs in 2–3% of the population, with a 2:1 female/male ratio. It is the most prevalent personality disorder in all clinical settings (12–15%), accounting for 51% of all inpatients and 27% of all outpatients with a personality disorder.** These patients are at increased risk for co-morbid mood disorders, as well as eating disorders, substance abuse, and post-traumatic stress disorder. Additionally, up to 10% will have completed suicide by the age of 30 years. There is an increased prevalence of mood disorders in families of borderline patients, as well as an increased prevalence of this disorder in mothers of affected children.
4. **Course.** Borderline personality disorder is usually diagnosed before the age of 40 years. While the course can be variable, it rarely changes over time. Some patients improve in middle age and revisit core symptoms only during periods of significant stress.
5. **Treatment.** Depending on the level of personality organization, patients with borderline personality disorder can engage in several modes of psychotherapy, including exploratory, insight-oriented, supportive, and cognitive-behavioral. One popular form of cognitive-behavioral treatment for the treatment of borderline personality disorder is dialectical behavioral therapy (DBT). This form of therapy focuses on opposing statements and views for almost every subject, with the primary point being that for every subject there is an opposing view. The dialectical clinician works to help the patient achieve synthesis rather than validation of opposite views. In addition to individual therapy, patients engage in highly structured skills training groups designed to enhance coping with identity diffusion, distress tolerance, interpersonal relationships, affect regulation, and crisis management. **The greatest barrier to therapy is the intense countertransference reactions that these patients instill in their treaters, and caution must be taken not to give in to those feelings.** Medications by themselves rarely make dramatic changes in this disorder, but they are useful adjuncts to psychotherapy. Target symptoms that respond to medication include impulsivity, emotional lability, intermittent psychosis, and mood symptoms. Vigorous use of pharmacological agents may be necessary for those periods when these patients pose a significant risk of harm to self or others.

C. Histrionic Personality Disorder

1. **Core features. The most notable features of histrionic personality disorder are pervasive overconcern with appearance and attention, exaggerated emotional response, poor frustration tolerance that ends in outbursts, and impressionistic speech that lacks detail. They view physical attractiveness as the core of their existence,** and, as such, are often provocative in dress, flamboyant in mannerisms, and inappropriately seductive in behavior. While they appear superficially charming, others tend to view them as vain and lacking in genuineness.
2. **Differential diagnosis.** The differential diagnosis for histrionic personality disorder includes other personality disorders, and somatization disorder. Borderline personality disorder differs from histrionic personality disorder in that the borderline displays more despair and suicidal/parasuicidal behaviors. Likewise, the narcissistic patient is more preoccupied with grandiosity and envy than is the histrionic individual. The dependent personality-ordered patient, while sharing the need for acceptance and reassurance, lacks the degree of emotionality seen in histrionic personality disorder. Somatization disorder can co-exist with histrionic personality disorder, but it is distinguished by the greater emphasis on physical complaints.
3. **Prevalence. Histrionic personality disorder occurs in 2–3% of the general population. While women receive the diagnosis more often, many clinicians feel that men are under-diagnosed.** This disorder is more common in first-degree relatives of people with this disorder.
4. **Course.** As is the case with most personality disorders, the course is variable. Some experience an attenuation or softening of the core symptoms with age.

Others may experience a complicated course, including co-morbid somatization, dissociative, sexual, and mood disorders. A few may experience brief reactive psychotic states under stressful situations.

5. **Treatment. Individual psychodynamic psychotherapy, with emphasis on emotional clarification, practical problem-solving, and adherence to structure and detail to counter their diffuse cognitive style, is the treatment of choice for this disorder.** Long-term pharmacotherapy is reserved for co-morbid Axis I disorders. Low-dose benzodiazepines are useful for transient emotional states, and low-dose antipsychotics are often necessary for episodes of dissociation and brief psychotic states.

D. Narcissistic Personality Disorder

1. **Core features. The hallmark of narcissistic personality disorder is an overwhelming and pathological self-absorption.** These individuals possess a grandiose sense of self-importance and feel that the people with whom they associate also need to be special and unique. **They are blindly ambitious, often breaking conventional rules and exploiting others to meet their self-serving ends. They lack empathy for others, and react with disappointment and rage when another's tragedy compromises their plans.** Beneath the facade of self-sufficiency and arrogance lies a fragile individual who is so hypersensitive to issues of self-esteem such that, if they are criticized in even the slightest manner, they react with intense emotion or brief psychotic decompensation.
2. **Differential diagnosis.** What makes the differential diagnosis for narcissistic personality disorder so difficult is that other Cluster B personality disorders often co-exist. Nonetheless, a few distinguishing features are helpful. **The borderline patient differs from the narcissist in that the former is more impulsive, has a less cohesive identity, and lives a more chaotic life.** The histrionic patient, unlike the narcissistic patient, is more emotional and deeply involved with others. While the narcissistic and antisocial patient both exploit people, the primary motivation for the narcissistic patient is mainly power rather than material gain.
3. **Prevalence.** The exact prevalence for this disorder is unknown. **The best estimates are that it occurs in less than 1% in the general population and between 2% and 15% in the clinical population. There are no data concerning familial patterns or gender ratio.**
4. **Course. The course of this illness is chronic.** These patients frequently suffer co-morbid mood disorders, particularly major depression and dysthymia. Under stress, they may also experience brief reactive psychosis. Aging is the ultimate blow to their self-esteem, as many of the things that they hinge their identity around (e.g., career, health, beauty, and youth) must naturally begin to fade. Consequently, the narcissistic patient is prone to severe mid-life crises.
5. **Course. The treatment of choice for narcissistic personality disorder is individual psychodynamic psychotherapy, including analysis and insight-oriented techniques.** These patients do not tolerate group settings. Pharmacotherapy should target co-morbid Axis I disorders, particularly depression. Lithium is helpful for mood swings, and antipsychotic agents are useful for transient psychotic states.

IV. Cluster C Personality Disorders

A. Avoidant Personality Disorder

1. **Core features. The core feature of avoidant personality disorder is an excessive discomfort or fear in intimate and social relationships that results in pathological avoidance as a means of self-protection.** For example, to guard against potentially unpleasant situations, these individuals frequently exaggerate the risks of ordinary unplanned tasks so as not to deviate from a safe daily routine. While genuinely desiring relationships, they are unwilling to enter them due to real or perceived signs of humiliation, rejection, or negative feedback. If, however, they manage to negotiate a relationship, it is only with assurance of uncritical acceptance. Because of this pervasive awkwardness and shyness, they suffer from incredibly low self-esteem.
2. **Differential diagnosis.** The differential diagnosis for avoidant personality disorder includes other personality disorders and social phobia. Patients with schizoid personality disorder, unlike patients with avoidant personality disorder, do not desire relationships with others. While dependent personality disorder shares many features with avoidant personality disorder, the former has greater fear of abandonment, and embraces, rather than avoids, relationships. Social phobia can be very difficult to distinguish from avoidant personality disorder, and many clinicians consider them one and the same. Other clinicians argue, however, that the distinction between the two is that patients with social phobia tend to have specific fears around social performances.
3. **Prevalence. Avoidant personality disorder is common, occurring in about 1–10% of the general population.** Temperament and disfiguring physical illnesses may be predisposing factors. It occurs equally among men and women.
4. **Course.** As long as the environment is perceived safe and protective, patients with avoidant personality disorder are able to function in relationships, marry, and have families. As with most personality disorders, they are prone to mood disorders, especially depression and dysthymia. Due to the special nature of this disorder, however, they are at especially high risk for anxiety disorders and social phobia.

5. **Treatment.** Treatment for this disorder can be difficult, due to these patients' fear of humiliation and rejection. Once assured of acceptance and safety, they respond to virtually all forms of therapy. Current practice focuses on group settings with a strong cognitive-behavioral emphasis. Anxiolytics are helpful in managing situational anxiety, and monoamine oxidase inhibitors (MAOIs) and selective serotonin reuptake inhibitors (SSRIs) are effective for treating co-morbid anxiety and depression.

B. Dependent Personality Disorder

1. **Core features. Individuals with dependent personality disorder have a strong desire for others to care for them and an extreme preoccupation with abandonment.** They fear being alone and will go to extreme lengths to preserve any relationship, no matter how physically or emotionally abusive it may be. They are submissive and passive toward others, and fear that any direct expression of anger will end in rejection. Subsequently, they often volunteer for unpleasant tasks, agree with others who may even be wrong, or look to others for assurance about simple daily decisions, to assure being liked or cared for.
2. **Differential diagnosis.** Dependent personality disorder can be difficult to distinguish from other psychiatric conditions, as many disorders have dependency as an underlying feature. The differential diagnosis for dependent personality disorder includes other personality disorders and agoraphobia. Patients with histrionic personality disorder have issues of dependency, but shorter and more numerous relationships. Borderline patients express more affect and anger around real or perceived abandonment, whereas dependent patients become more placating. When faced with rejection or termination of a relationship, avoidant patients withdraw from further contact, unlike dependent patients, who quickly seek out a new relationship to fill the void. Agoraphobia patients, while displaying dependency, tend to demonstrate a higher-level fear around leaving safe environments.
3. **Prevalence. Dependent personality disorder occurs in 2–4% of the general population, and accounts for about 2.5% of all personality disorders,** with females more commonly affected than men. Patients with a history of childhood separation anxiety or chronic illness may be predisposed. There is no known familiar pattern of inheritance.
4. **Course. Many patients with this disorder suffer co-morbid dysthymia, major depression, and alcohol abuse.** Because of their dependency and lack of assertiveness, they may also become victims of physical and emotional abuse. Careers are unlikely to advance, due to these patients' need for direction and an inability to make decisions without excessive reassurance.
5. **Treatment.** These patients respond well to various forms of individual psychotherapy. Group therapy with emphasis on cognitive techniques, assertive training, and social skills, can be highly useful. Pharmacotherapy should target co-morbid Axis I disorders, with benzodiazepines and SSRIs being the most effective medications.

C. Obsessive-Compulsive Personality Disorder

1. **Core features. The major features of obsessive-compulsive personality disorder are perfectionism and lack of compromise.** These individuals are so preoccupied with rules, efficiency, trivial details, and procedures that the purpose of the activity is often lost or the job is uncompleted. **They maintain an inflexible adherence to their own internally strict and unattainable standards, and subsequently dislike delegating tasks for fear that others will not meet those standards.** While mindful of the chain of command, they possess a strong need for control and resist the authority and autonomy of others. To their superiors, they appear diligent, as they will tolerate protracted work, even at the cost of pleasure and interpersonal relationships. To their equals or subordinates, they are harsh taskmasters with escalating criteria for job perfection, who are stingy with emotions and compliments.
2. **Differential diagnosis.** The principal differential diagnosis for obsessive-compulsive personality disorder is obsessive-compulsive disorder. While the two are often confused for each other, they differ significantly: patients with obsessive-compulsive disorder have true obsessions and compulsions that they find ego-dystonic, whereas patients with the personality disorder find their behaviors ego-syntonic and rewarded by others. Occasionally, the two disorders co-exist, requiring a diagnosis for each. Several features of narcissistic personality disorder overlap with obsessive-compulsive personality disorder, particularly the desire for perfection, the need to dominate others, and a drive for achievement. However, patients with narcissistic personality disorder engage in these behaviors as a means to achieve status and recognition, whereas patients with obsessive-compulsive personality disorder do so in order to fulfill their internal idealized standards.
3. **Prevalence.** This personality disorder is common in the general population, with males receiving the diagnosis more often than females. While the mode of transmission is unknown, it is more common among first-degree relatives of patients with this disorder. There is also an increased concordance in identical twins.
4. **Course.** The course for obsessive-compulsive personality disorder is **variable**. Some patients are able to negotiate intimate long-term relationships, but have

few friends, if any, outside those relationships. Others may mellow with age, becoming warm, caring, and generous to those around them. Often, however, depression, somatoform disorders, and alcohol dependence emerge as complications.

5. **Treatment. Unlike other personality disorders, individuals with this disorder often realize the impact of their behavior and seek treatment on their own.** They tend to improve with any number of treatment modalities, but particularly value a non-directive approach. Group therapy may be especially advantageous, as it permits others to point out bothersome behaviors and call for change. While there are few data to support pharmacotherapy, anecdotal evidence suggests that benzodiazepines may be useful in reducing the anxiety associated with their behaviors.

V. Personality Disorder Not Otherwise Specified

The diagnosis of personality disorder not otherwise specified is reserved for persistent personality dysfunction that results in significant impairment, but it does not reach full criteria for a single personality disorder, or meet criteria for one of the proposed personality disorders in Appendix B of the DSM-IV-TR. These proposed disorders include passive-aggressive and depressive personality disorders.

A. Passive-Aggressive Personality Disorder

The major feature of passive-aggressive personality disorder is passive resistance to authority figures and to any request for adequate performance. This resistance, viewed as covert aggression, reveals itself as obstructionism and procrastination. These patients fail to ask important questions concerning adequate performance expectations, and become sullen or argumentative if those expectations arise. When requested to carry out tasks, they become deliberately inefficient, may make excuses for delays, and frequently complain of being misunderstood or underappreciated. Often, others must pick up their slack.

B. Depressive Personality Disorder

The essential features of depressive personality disorder are pervasive pessimism, anhedonia, and mirthlessness. Patients with this disorder are invariably passive, serious, moralistic, self-denigrating, and suffer from low self-esteem. Since many patients with Axis I dysthymic disorder share similar presentations, some clinicians believe that this personality disorder and dysthymia are one and the same.

Suggested Readings

American Psychiatric Association. (2000). *Diagnostic and statistical manual of mental disorders* (4th ed., Text Revision). Washington, DC: American Psychiatric Press.

Bender, S., Dolan, T., Skodol, E., et al. (2001). Treatment utilization by patients with personality disorders. *American Journal of Psychiatry, 158*(2), 295–302.

Cloninger, R.C., & Svrakic, D.M. (2000). Personality disorders. In B.J. Sadock, & V.A. Sadock (Eds.), *Kaplan and Sadock's comprehensive textbook of psychiatry* (7th ed., pp. 1723–1764). Baltimore, MD: Lippincott, Williams, and Wilkins.

Phillips, K.A., & Gunderson, J.G. (1999). Personality disorders. In R.E. Hales, S.C. Yudofsky, & J.A. Talbott (Eds.), *The American Psychiatric Press textbook of psychiatry* (3rd ed., pp. 795–823). Washington, DC: American Psychiatric Press.

Stone, M.H. (1993). Long-term outcome in personality disorders. *British Journal of Psychiatry, 162,* 299–313.

Tyrer, P., Casey, P., & Ferguson, B. (1991). Personality disorder in perspective. *British Journal of Psychiatry, 159,* 463–471.

Chapter 26

Psychiatric Disorders Associated with the Female Reproductive Cycle

HELEN G. KIM, ADELE C. VIGUERA, AND BENITA DIEPERINK

I. Introduction

Women have higher rates of major depression compared to men in every age group. The National Co-morbidity Study reported lifetime prevalence rates of major depression of 21.3% in women and 12.7% in men. Studies have consistently found the highest rates of depression in women during the childbearing years. This observation has inspired a field of research examining psychiatric syndromes associated with reproductive events, such as menses, pregnancy and menopause. Contrary to popular lore, research has not revealed a consistent association between female reproductive hormones and psychiatric symptoms, but rather supports a more complicated interplay between biological, psychiatric, and psychosocial factors.

II. Premenstrual Syndrome and Premenstrual Dysphoric Disorder

A. Background

1. **Premenstrual syndrome (PMS)** is a variably defined constellation of emotional and physical symptoms that occurs during the luteal phase, i.e., between ovulation and menses. **Approximately 80% of women report at least one physical or emotional premenstrual symptom.**
2. **Only 2–8% of women have PMS symptoms severe enough to meet criteria for premenstrual dysphoric disorder (PMDD). This condition is defined by DSM-IV research criteria** and includes the following symptoms, timing, and parameters for severity:
   a. In most menstrual cycles during the past year, five or more of the following symptoms occur during the last week of the luteal phase with partial remission shortly after the onset of menses and complete remission postmenses. One of the symptoms must include (i), (ii), (iii), or (iv):
      i. Markedly depressed mood, hopelessness, or self-deprecating thoughts
      ii. Marked anxiety, feeling "keyed up," or "on edge"
      iii. Affective lability
      iv. Marked anger, irritability, or interpersonal conflicts
      v. Decreased interest in usual activities
      vi. Difficulty concentrating
      vii. Decreased energy
      viii. Changes in appetite, overeating, or specific food cravings
      ix. Sleep disturbance
      x. Feeling out of control/overwhelmed
      xi. Other physical symptoms (e.g., breast tenderness or swelling, joint or muscle pain, "bloating")
   b. Symptoms interfere with social or occupational functioning and are not merely an exacerbation of an Axis I diagnosis, such as major depression, panic disorder, or dysthymic disorder.
   c. Quality and timing of symptoms must be confirmed by prospective daily ratings during at least two consecutive symptomatic cycles.

B. Etiology

1. **Biological theories**
   a. **The neurotransmitter serotonin (5-HT) most likely plays a role in PMDD as it does in other mood and anxiety disorders.** Disruptions in 5-HT function have been associated with PMDD symptoms, such as mood lability, irritability, and increased carbohydrate cravings. In addition, medications that increase 5-HT have been shown to be effective in treating these PMDD symptoms. Steiner and Pearlstein (2000) have suggested that women with PMDD have a heightened sensitivity in the 5-HT system that renders them more vulnerable to normal hormone fluctuations around menses.
   b. Other theories have proposed a connection between PMDD and the gamma-aminobutyric acid (GABA), adrenergic, and opioid systems.
   c. **There is no consistent evidence that PMS/PMDD is associated with abnormal levels of sex steroid hormones (e.g., estrogen, progesterone, and testosterone). Studies suggest that certain subgroups of women may be susceptible to mood or anxiety symptoms during periods of normal reproductive hormone flux.** In one study, Schmidt (1998) treated women with PMS and controls with leuprolide, a gonadotropin-releasing hormone (GnRH) agonist that suppresses the hypothalamic-pituitary-gonadal (HPG) axis and ceases menstrual cyclicity. Women who had remission of their PMS symptoms were treated with estrogen or progesterone add-back therapy that subsequently induced recurrence of their PMS symptoms. In contrast, controls who were treated with the same regimen of leuprolide and estrogen or progesterone add-back had no PMS symptoms. In this study, women with PMS and controls had differential responses to changes in hormones rather than absolute hormone levels.
2. **The precise role of genetic and environmental factors (e.g., diet and stress) in predisposing women to PMS/PMDD is unknown.**

C. Assessment of the Patient with Premenstrual Complaints

1. **Rule out underlying medical conditions**. Review the medical history for syndromes that could mimic PMDD. For example, endometriosis may cause significant mood symptoms and pelvic discomfort prior to and during menses. In addition, certain conditions, such as migraines, epilepsy, and herpes, may have premenstrual worsening. Careful screening and a physical examination by an internist or gynecologist should be part of the evaluation of dysmenorrhea.
2. **Assess the reproductive endocrine status.** To determine the presence of luteal phase symptoms, one needs to determine whether the patient has regular ovulatory cycles. A patient with a history of spontaneous, regular menstrual cyclicity likely has normal menstrual function. To confirm regular ovulatory cycles, a woman can chart her basal body temperature to document a rise in temperature just after ovulation. Alternatively, a patient can measure urine LH using an over-the-counter kit to detect the LH surge prior to ovulation.
3. **Rule out underlying psychiatric conditions**. Review of the psychiatric history should include a patient's experience during periods of hormone fluctuations, such as during pregnancy and the post-partum period, which may reflect increased vulnerability to PMDD. In addition, different Axis I or II diagnoses can be exacerbated premenstrually rather than constitute PMDD. Excessive alcohol or drug use may also affect mood and anxiety states. Axis I diagnoses should be treated to see if symptoms resolve in the follicular phase but persist in the luteal phase.
4. **Recommend prospective daily rating scales.** After ruling out an underlying medical or psychiatric condition, patients should fill out prospective daily rating scales over two consecutive cycles. Less than 50% of women who present with a history of PMDD actually have a premenstrual pattern of symtoms on prospective scales (Rubinow, 1984). Careful prospective documentation of symptoms throughout the cycle is critical in making an accurate diagnosis and also helps to monitor the effect of treatment on symptoms.

D. Treatment

1. **Non-pharmacologic treatments**
   a. The role of dietary changes has not been well studied; however, **some women report some symptomatic improvement after making nutritional changes.** Anecdotally, women have benefited from decreasing salt consumption to decrease fluid retention, or avoiding caffeine to decrease breast tenderness. Consuming more complex carbohydrates during the late luteal phase may also improve PMS symptoms by increasing synthesis of brain serotonin.
   b. **Calcium (1,200 mg/day) and magnesium (360 mg/day) supplements have both been shown to be helpful in reducing PMDD symptoms.** Evidence is more controversial regarding other nutritional supplements that include vitamins B_6 and E.
   c. There have been no prospective studies of the effects of exercise on PMDD; however, **aerobic exercise often elevates mood** and certainly has many health benefits. For mood symptoms, women with PMS/PMDD could try regular aerobic exercise, especially through the luteal phase.
   d. **Circadian rhythm manipulations**, such as through sleep deprivation and light therapy, are other anecdotal PMS/PMDD treatments. A recent small study found that luteal phase treatment with light therapy for thirty minutes per day decreased PMS symptoms.
   e. Studies of **cognitive therapy** suggest decreased premenstrual psychiatric symptoms compared to wait-listed controls. Relaxation techniques and other forms of therapy may also help alleviate premenstrual symptoms.
2. **Hormonal treatments**
   a. **Oral contraceptive pills (OCPs) are commonly used to treat PMDD** with the hope that constant levels of estrogen and progestin throughout the menstrual cycle will eliminate premenstrual symptoms. However, there is lack of consistent evidence for their efficacy and they should not be considered a first-line treatment. Continuous adminstration of OCPs throughout the month (without a placebo week) may be helpful to some patients. OCPs may decrease the severity of the physical symptoms, but **may not affect, or may even worsen, premenstrual depression.**
   b. Although once a popular treatment for PMDD, **progesterone has failed to show consistent superiority over placebo in treating PMDD.**
   c. **Gonadotropin-releasing hormone agonists and synthetic androgens** to suppress ovulation may be useful in treating PMDD; however, **both have significant side effects and risks associated with prolonged anovulatory cycles.**
   d. Without further research, **no definitive statements can be made about the utility or safety of hormonal treatments for PMDD.**
3. **Psychotropic medications**
   a. **Multiple randomized controlled trials have demonstrated the efficacy of elective serotonin reuptake inhibitors (SSRIs) in treating PMDD. Given the weight of the evidence, SSRIs (fluoxetine [20 mg qd], sertraline [50 to 100 mg qd], paroxetine [20 mg qd], and citalopram [20 mg qd]) should be considered first-line treatments in treating PMDD.**

      SSRIs often decrease symptoms of PMDD within days of treatment rather than after weeks as is the case with major depression. This observation has lead to several studies using luteal phase dosing, also referred to as intermittent-dosing, of SSRIs for PMDD. The antidepressant is administered either one to two weeks prior to the anticipated menses. **Randomized, placebo-controlled, prospective studies of fluoxetine, sertraline and citalopram have shown that luteal phase dosing is effective and well-tolerated.**

b. Buspirone, a 5-HT_{1A} serotonin receptor partial agonist, at mean doses of 25 mg/day, was shown to be effective in a small, placebo-controlled, double-blind study, though larger controlled trials are needed to confirm this finding.

c. Studies of alprazolam for PMS/PMDD have shown mixed results in reducing psychiatric symptoms.

4. **Treatment of physical symptoms**

a. For bloating and weight gain, patients could try **decreasing salt intake and adding calcium and magnesium supplements**. For mastalgia, patients can try using support bras and **decreasing caffeine intake**.

b. For myalgias, arthralgias, or headache, **non-steroidal anti-inflammatory drugs (NSAIDs)** can be used as needed.

III. Psychiatric Illnesses During Pregnancy

A. Introduction

Despite early assumptions about the protective effects of pregnancy on women's psychological health, approximately **10% of women experience significant depressive symptoms during pregnancy.** Treatment of depressed pregnant patients involves a careful risk/benefit analysis of different pharmacologic and non-pharmacologic treatment options. Psychiatrists must help patients weigh the risk of prenatal exposure to psychotropic medications against the risk of unmedicated psychiatric illness. While there is increasing data to help inform these difficult decisions, there still remain many unanswered questions.

B. Categories of Risk Associated with Pharmacotherapy

1. **Risk of teratogenesis**. Teratogenesis is the dysgenesis of fetal organs leading to structural or functional anomalies. Fetal organ formation occurs primarily during the first trimester. The baseline risk of congenital malformations is estimated at 3–4%. Drugs are considered teratogenic if *in utero* drug exposure increases the frequency of congenital malformations above this baseline risk.

2. **Risk of perinatal toxicity**. Perinatal syndromes refer to symptoms present in the neonate that are frequently associated with drug exposure at or near delivery. Different syndromes have been described following *in utero* exposure to antidepressants, antipsychotics, and benzodiazepines. Potential contributing factors include drug withdrawal syndromes, prolonged drug effects secondary to immature hepatic microsomal activity, and increased free drug levels from decreased plasma protein levels and protein binding.

3. **Risk of behavioral teratogenesis**. Behavioral teratogenesis refers to the long-term effects of *in utero* drug exposure on neurobehavioral development. These long-term effects may have even more important consequences for patients than specific structural anomalies.

C. Risk of Untreated Maternal Psychiatric Illness

1. **Maternal psychiatric symptoms may jeopardize the well-being of both mother and fetus.** For instance, disabling depression and anxiety may lead to decreased self-care, poor appetite, and increased suicidality, which may all undermine compliance with prenatal care.

2. **Untreated depression and anxiety have been associated with poor compliance with prenatal care, poor neonatal outcomes (e.g., decreased birth weight and APGAR scores) and higher rates of obstetric complications (e.g., pre-term delivery).**

3. **Relapse of psychiatric illness** may increase the risk for recurrent affective illness or increased refractoriness to treatment.

D. Psychotropic Medications During Pregnancy

Patients commonly under-estimate the risks of untreated maternal psychiatric illness while over-emphasizing potential teratogenicity of their psychotropic medications. In one study, women exposed to non-teratogenic drugs estimated their teratogenic risk to be 25%, which is far above the baseline risk of 3–4% and more in the range of known teratogens, such as thalidomide. **Misperception about risk can lead both physicians and patients to terminate otherwise wanted pregnancies or avoid needed pharmacotherapy.** By informing patients about the nature and magnitude of drug exposure risk as well as the risks of untreated illness, psychiatrists can help patients reach their own decisions.

1. **Antidepressants**

a. **Tricyclic antidepressants (TCAs)**. Both prospective and retrospective studies have found no association between *in utero* TCA-exposure and increased risk of major congenital malformations. There have been case reports of perinatal toxicity including jitteriness, irritability, bowel obstruction, and urinary retention.

b. **Selective serotonin reuptake inhibitors (SSRIs). Among the SSRIs, reproductive safety data is most adundant for fluoxetine**. Prospective and retrospective studies as well as the manufacturer's database have reported approximately 3,000 fluoxetine-exposed pregnancies; no increased risk of major congenital malformations has been found. **Prospective studies of citalopram, sertraline, paroxetine, and fluvoxamine have to date not revealed an increased risk of major malformations; however, larger samples are required to corroborate these findings.**

c. One prospective study by Chambers (1996) found an increased risk of minor malformations and perinatal toxicity following *in utero* fluoxetine exposure; however, this study was complicated by a poorly matched control group and by non-blinded raters. Several other studies have also found an association between SSRI-exposure and premature delivery and perinatal toxicity, such as respiratory distress, hypoglycemia, jitteriness, and poor neonatal adaptation. In general, however, reports of **perinatal toxicity and pre-term delivery following *in utero* SSRI exposure have been limited to case reports and small studies. The incidence of these adverse events is probably low and discontinuing treatment in advance of labor and delivery, may place the mother at risk for relapse (especially as she enters the post-partum period, a time of well-established risk for relapse).**

d. **To date we have limited information about long-term neurobehavioral toxicity following *in utero* TCA and SSRI-exposure.** In an important prospective study, Nulman (1997) found no effect on language, behavior, and global IQ in pre-school children who had been exposed during the first trimester to TCAs or fluoxetine. In a recent follow-up study Nulman et al. (2002) found that even when exposed throughout pregnancy to TCAs or fluoxetine, pre-school children had no difference in temperament, language, and intellectual development compared to non-exposed children. In fact, rather than any medication effect, Nulman found that it was maternal depression itself that negatively impacted cognitive and language development in children. This finding underscores the importance of considering the risks of untreated maternal psychiatric illness as well as risks of *in utero* medication exposure on child development.

e. **Prospective data about reproductive safety for other antidepressants, including venlafaxine, nefazodone, mirtazapine, bupropion, MAO inhibitors (MAOIs), and stimulants, remain limited or unavailable.**

2. **Mood stabilizers**

a. **Lithium use during the first trimester has been associated with a 10–20 times greater risk for Ebstein's anomaly.** With the baseline risk for Ebstein's anomaly at 1/20,000, **the risk for Ebstein's anomaly following first trimester lithium exposure is between 1/2,000 (0.05%) and 1/1,000 (0.1%).** Thus, although the relative risk of Ebstein's anomaly is increased, the absolute risk following first trimester lithium exposure is small.

b. **Lithium has also been associated with perinatal toxicity including case reports of hypotonia, cyanosis, neonatal goiter, and diabetes insipidus, however the incidence of these adverse events is generally low and if they do occur, the symptoms are transient.**

c. **If prescribed during pregnancy, lithium should be given in divided doses to avoid high peak levels.** Patients should also have a **second trimester level II ultrasound to screen for congenital anomalies, especially cardiac dysmorphology.** In addition, clinicians should closely **follow maternal lithium levels around the time of delivery given the large volume changes seen during the post-partum period.**

d. **Prior to discontinuing lithium, one must consider the severity of the illness** (e.g., chronicity, presence of impaired judgment, or psychosis). **For women with severe illness, the risk of recurrence during pregnancy may overshadow the relatively small risk of Ebstein's anomaly.** For such women, maintenance lithium during pregnancy may be the most appropriate course. For women with less compelling histories, slowly tapering off lithium and reintroducing lithium later in the second or third trimesters may be the most prudent treatment.

e. A few studies have demonstrated that women with bipolar disorder are at high risk for relapse in pregnancy (> 50% risk), especially in the setting of discontinuing their mood stabilizer. It is well established that the post-partum period represents a time of very high risk for relapse (the risk ranges from 50–70%). Because of this high risk, post-partum prophylaxis, with a mood stabilizer at least a few weeks before delivery is recommended. Several studies have demonstrated the efficacy of lithium prophylaxis post-partum to reduce the risk of relapse.

f. The higher teratogenic risk associated with valproic acid and carbamazepine compared to lithium suggests that psychiatrists should **consider a lithium trial for women with bipolar illness who are planning to get pregnant.** Women who have not responded to lithium obviously have more limited choices, and have to consider the stability afforded by particular mood stabilizers, the teratogenic risks of these medications, and the risk of relapse.

g. **First trimester valproic acid and carbamazepine have well-established risks of neural tube defects of 5% and 1%, respectively.** Carbamazepine is also a competitive inhibitor of prothrombin precursors and may increase risk of neonatal hemorrhage. Psychiatrists should review potential teratogenic risks and the importance of contraception when taking these medications. In addition, **all pregnant patients, particularly those on valproic acid or carbamazepine, should take additional folate to mitigate the risk of neural tube defects.**

h. Other mood stabilizers, such as gabapentin, lamotrigine, topiramate, and verapamil have limited reproductive safety data.

3. **Antipsychotics**

a. **High-potency neuroleptics** have not consistently demonstrated increased teratogenicity following first trimester exposure. Low-potency phenothiazines should be avoided in pregnancy given their association with an increased risk of congenital malformations.

b. **We have limited information about the reproductive safety of atypical antipsychotics,** such as olanzapine, clozapine, risperidone, and quetiapine.

c. **Perinatal toxicity has been reported following neuroleptic exposure,** including motor restlessness, tremor, poor feeding, hypertonicity, and dystonia. Most case reports describe these symptoms as resolving within days or weeks.

d. We have limited **information regarding the long-term behavioral teratogenicity of *in utero* neuroleptic exposure.** Animal studies have found behavioral abnormalities in rats exposed to antipsychotics during pregnancy. However, these findings are of questionable relevance to humans and contradict two prospective studies of children exposed *in utero* to chlorpromazine which found no significant behavioral difference compared to nonexposed controls. Given the lack of well-designed prospective studies, no firm conclusions can be drawn regarding the long-term neurobehavioral effects of *in utero* antipsychotic exposure.

e. Patients and their psychiatrists have to consider whether discontinuing a particular antipsychotic poses unacceptable risks associated with psychosis during pregnancy, such as non-compliance with prenatal care, increased drug and alcohol use, and other high-risk behaviors.

4. **Benzodiazepines.** Early studies of first trimester benzodiazepine-use reported a ten-fold increase from baseline risk of oral cleft palate of 0.06%. However, significant controversy exists about the extent of risk associated with benzodiazepine use. Benzodiazepine use during pregnancy has also been associated with case reports of perinatal toxicity, including temperature dysregulation, apnea, depressed APGAR scores, hypotonia, and poor feeding. Long-term neurobehavioral data following *in utero* benzodiazepine exposure is unavailable.

E. Electroconvulsive therapy (ECT)

The safety of ECT during pregnancy has been widely reported in the literature. ECT has been used during pregnancy for more than 50 years. **For high-risk situations, such as psychotic depression or mania, which require expeditious treatment to protect both mother and fetus, ECT is the treatment of choice.** The safe and effective use of ECT during pregnancy requires coordination of care among the patient's psychiatrist, obstetrician, and anesthesiologist.

F. Psychotherapy

1. **Interpersonal therapy** (IPT) is a brief therapy that focuses on four different areas including role transitions, grief, and interpersonal disputes and deficits. A pilot study of 13 pregnant women found IPT decreased depressive symptoms and was associated with continued remission post-partum.
2. **Supportive, cognitive-behavioral and integrative psychotherapy** have been shown anecdotally to help with depression and anxiety during pregnancy.
3. **Light therapy** for three to five weeks decreased depression in a small pilot study of 16 pregnant women with major depression.

IV. Post-partum Psychiatric Illnesses

A. Introduction

Post-partum psychiatric syndromes are conceptualized along a continuum of symptom severity. Appropriate treatment of these illnesses not only alleviates maternal psychiatric symptoms, but also promotes healthy mother-infant attachment and infant development.

B. Overview

1. Post-partum **blues (PPB) are a self-limited constellation of symptoms which affects 50–85% of all women post-partum. These symptoms usually begin two to three days post-partum and consist of depressed mood, crying spells, mood lability, irritability, and anxiety.** These symptoms generally represent a normal part of the post-partum period. However, when symptoms persist beyond two weeks or significantly impair function, they may represent an evolving major depression.
2. **Post-partum depression (PPD) has been estimated to occur in 10–15% of all post-partum women depending on the diagnostic criteria used.** These prevalence rates are similar to those of non-puerperal cohorts. **Although only 60% of women have symptom onset within 6 weeks, the DSM-IV classifies PPD as major depression that occurs within 4 weeks post-partum.** The course of PPD is highly variable and ranges from 3 to 14 months. Clinical features include all the signs and symptoms of major depression. In addition, women with PPD often have prominent anxiety symptoms.
3. **Post-partum psychosis (PPP) is a rare condition that occurs in 1–2 of every 1,000 post-partum women. PPP generally begins acutely within the first 48–72 hours post-partum and represents a medical emergency.** Clinical features can include delirium, memory impairment, irritability, lability, and psychosis. PPP is a medical emergency that requires immediate hospitalization and treatment in order to protect both the mother and the infant.

C. Risk Factors

1. **Many theories of post-partum psychiatric symptoms have centered on the tremendous hormonal changes during the post-partum period. Although reproductive hormones have significant neuromodulatory effects, studies have consistently found no association between different hormones and post-partum psychiatric symptoms.**
2. The **multi-factorial** nature of post-partum psychiatric illnesses supports a more integrated theory in which

hormonal factors play an important causative role only in women with particular vulnerability to psychiatric illness. This predisposition to psychiatric illness may be biological (evidenced by personal or family history of psychiatric illness), psychological (evidenced by character pathology or limited coping skills), or environmental (evidenced by lower occupational/social functioning).

3. Studies have shown that the **following factors are associated with increased risk for post-partum psychiatric illness:**
   a. **Depression during pregnancy**
   b. **History of affective illness**
   d. **Family history of psychiatric illness**
   e. **Limited social support and interpersonal distress**, such as marital conflict and childcare stress
   f. **Negative life events** during and after pregnancy

D. Treatment

1. **Post-partum blues**. Women often benefit from education about the normalcy of certain mood symptoms during the post-partum period. They should also be informed of the signs and symptoms of an evolving major depression and the importance of prompt treatment. Most women with the post-partum blues also benefit from reassurance and supportive interventions, such as childcare assistance and referrals to support agencies.
2. **Post-partum depression**
   a. **Psychotherapy**. Pilot studies of **interpersonal therapy (IPT)** suggest that this time-limited therapy may help treat mild to moderate post-partum major depression. Another small study comparing **cognitive-behavioral therapy (CBT)** and fluoxetine proved that CBT is an effective treatment for post-partum depression.
   b. **Supportive interventions**. Grassroots national organizations, such as Depression after Delivery (DAD) and Visiting Moms can provide invaluable assistance to women with post-partum depression. Other options for surrogate family support include the services of a doula, a professional caregiver who is trained to help mothers adjust to the responsibilities of motherhood. Some doulas assist in the childbirth, while others provide critical support during the first post-partum weeks by helping with childcare or household tasks.
   c. **Pharmacotherapy**
      i. **Antidepressants**. Despite the high prevalence of post-partum psychiatric illness, there are only a limited number of medication treatment studies. To date, fluoxetine, sertraline, and venlafaxine have proven efficacious in the treatment of post-partum depression. Women at increased risk for post-partum depression should consider initiating prophylactic antidepressants either in late pregnancy or early postpartum. Alternatively, women may elect a wait-and-see approach; however, patients, their loved ones, and psychiatrists should be vigilant for early signs of relapse in order to institute prompt treatment.
      ii. **The most prudent antidepressant choice depends upon the patient's past history of medication response.** If a patient plans to nurse, clinicians must facilitate a careful risk/benefit analysis of taking psychotropic medication while nursing.
      iii. **Hormonal therapy**. Few studies have looked at the efficacy of estrogen and progesterone treatment for post-partum depression. Despite one small open study, progesterone has not proven to be an effective treatment for depressive symptoms. Three studies of estrogen alone or as an adjunct to antidepressants concluded that estrogen improved depressive symptoms; however, these studies had significant methodological issues that limit their generalizability.

E. Breastfeeding

All psychotropic medications are secreted in the breast milk. Physicians should **advise nursing women on psychotropic medications to monitor infants for behavioral changes.** In infants who are pre-term or develop signs of drug toxicity, one should consider avoiding nursing while taking medication and/or obtaining an infant drug level. In asymptomatic infants, obtaining drug levels is debatable since many variables determine drug concentration including breast milk concentration, infant absorption, hepatic metabolism, renal clearance and transmission across the blood-brain barrier. In addition, even if no infant drug level is detectable, there still may be trace amounts present that potentially have neurodevelopmental effects on the infant.

1. **Antidepressants**. There have been isolated case reports of elevated infant levels and toxicity with nursing mothers on doxepin and fluoxetine; however, the limited studies of TCAs and SSRIs do not reveal a consistent association between maternal dose and infant serum levels or toxicity. Unfortunately even less is known about the safety of nursing while taking other antidepressants (e.g., venlafaxine, bupropion, serzone, and mirtazapine). In helping patients assess the risks of antidepressants while nursing, clinicians should remind patients that information is limited to case reports and to very small studies.
2. **Mood stabilizers. Breastfeeding while taking lithium is considered a relative contraindication. Since infant serum lithium levels are about 50% of the mother's serum plasma level, the concern is that in the event of dehydration, the infant would be at increased risk for lithium toxicity. Other concerns that deserve further investigation are the risk for thyroid and renal dysfunction in the infant exposed to lithium via nursing.**

   Although not considered a contraindication in nursing mothers, the anticonvulsants, such as valproate and carbamazepine, have been associated with infant anemia and thrombocytopenia.

V. Menopause

A. Introduction

Although some women experience peri-menopausal psychiatric, cognitive, or somatic symptoms, no specific psychiatric disorder has been associated with menopause itself. The relationship between declining estrogen levels and mood symptoms remains controversial. Some studies have demonstrated that certain subgroups of women with histories of mood or anxiety disorders may be more vulnerable to relapse during this phase. As with PMS and post-partum psychiatric disorders, fluctuations in reproductive endocrine function rather than absolute hormone levels may drive this increased risk for affective symptoms.

B. Definitions

1. **Menopause is defined as the cessation of menses for 12 consecutive months.** Women naturally enter menopause with advancing age, usually between the ages of 41 and 59 years, with an average age of 51 years. Women can also experience menopause as a result of exogenous hormone treatment or following bilateral oophorectomy.
2. **Peri-menopause refers to the 5- to 10-year transition from regular menstrual functioning to menopause.** Hormonal changes during this period include declining estrogen levels, which are increasingly unopposed by progesterone due to anovulatory cycles.
3. Women enter the post-menopause, which can account for roughly one-third of a woman's entire lifespan. **While the female/male ratio of depression increases after the age of 45 years, the rate of depression in women throughout all ages declines in the post-menopausal period.**

C. Etiology

1. **Hormonal theories of menopause-associated depression remain controversial.** Support for "estrogen withdrawal" theories includes the increased rate of depression after bilateral oophorectomy compared to women undergoing natural menopause. Some emphasize the potential depressogenic effects of an abrupt decline in estrogen, while others counter that, following surgical menopause, many other complicated hormonal changes also occur, including falling testosterone and progesterone levels.
2. The "domino theory" of menopause-related affective disorders suggests that certain somatic symptoms, such as sleep disturbance from nocturnal hot flashes, may lead to mood disturbance. This has led some to wonder whether the positive effect on mood some women experience on hormone therapy (HT) results from a direct effect or from the psychological relief they experience as their menopausal somatic symptoms abate.
3. **Women with a history of major depression appear to be at greatest risk for peri-menopausal depression,** which furthers the debate over whether peri-menopause-associated depression represents a separate diagnosis or merely an exacerbation of recurrent major depression.
4. **Psychosocial theories often indict the stress of the life changes that mark the peri-menopausal transition.** Some of these psychosocial factors include losing one's reproductive potential, changing family roles, aging, and the onset of physical illnesses. While these factors may be associated with peri-menopausal depression, **a causal role for psychosocial factors in peri-menopausal depression has yet to be established.**

D. Evaluation

1. **Psychiatric assessment**
   a. **Screen for menopause-associated physical and psychological symptoms,** including whether they reflect minor nuisances or severely impair social and occupational function (see Table 26-1).
   b. **Consider creating mood charts** to determine the pattern and severity of symptoms. Both affective and somatic symptoms, such as hot flashes and vaginal dryness, should be monitored.
   c. **Obtain a thorough psychiatric history.**
   d. **Screen for alcohol and drug use** that may exacerbate psychiatric symptoms.
2. **Medical assessment**
   a. **Assess reproductive endocrine status.** Hormonal changes in menopause include a decrease in estrogen with subsequent elevations of luteinizing hormone (LH) and FSH. The endocrine profile of menopause is typically defined as an FSH level above 40 IU/l and an estradiol level below 25 pg/ml.

Table 26-1. Physical and Psychological Symptoms Associated with Menopause

Vasomotor symptoms
Hot flashes, night sweats, palpitations
Affective symptoms
Depressed mood, anxiety, mood swings
Cognitive symptoms
Poor memory or concentration
Somatic symptoms
Fatigue, headache, joint pain, paresthesias, vaginal dryness, dyspareunia

b. **Rule out underlying medical conditions, such as thyroid disease or cardiac arrhythmia, that can present with anxiety or depression.**

c. **Gynecologic history** should include whether a patient has had a chemically- or surgically-induced menopause versus a natural menopause. Patients who have had bilateral oophorectomy may experience more difficulties with mood and anxiety. Determine whether or not the woman still has her uterus, since estrogen replacement may increase the risk of uterine and breast cancer.

d. **Laboratory tests**, such as thyroid function, FSH, and estradiol levels, may be indicated.

E. Treatment Strategies

1. Pharmacologic strategies

a. **Hormone therapy (HT)**. HT may alleviate mild mood symptoms, along with certain physical symptoms, such as vaginal dryness and hot flashes. However, before prescribing HT clinicians should consider recent evidence from the Women's Health Initiative (WHI), a large multicenter prospective study of post-menopausal women. From 1993 to 1998, the WHI enrolled 161,809 post-menopausal women into a set of clinical trials including two HT arms. In July 2002, researchers stopped the WHI trial of estrogen-plus-progesterone because of the increased incidence of breast cancer, coronary heart disease, and thromboembolic events. Although the estrogen-only arm of the WHI continues, estrogen has been associated with an increased risk of uterine and breast cancer.

The cardioprotective effects of HT were also called into question by the Heart and Estrogen/Progestin Replacement Study (HERS), a large, randomized controlled trial comparing estrogen plus progestin in women with known coronary heart disease. The HERS results suggested an increased risk during the first year for coronary heart disease. **The WHI and HERS findings confirm that we still have much to learn about the short- and long-term risks and benefits of HT and treatment with HT should be based on the individual needs of the patient.**

b. **Antidepressants**. For menopause-associated major depression, standard antidepressant treatment should be initiated.

2. Psychotherapy strategies

Cognitive-behavioral, supportive, and psychodynamic therapy alone or in combination with pharmacotherapy may alleviate depression or anxiety symptoms.

3. **Psychoeducation**. Patients often benefit from reassurance that **menopause is not a disease** but a natural developmental transition. Psychiatrists should also educate patients about the hormonal changes and potential vasomotor, cognitive, and psychological symptoms that sometimes accompany menopause. Patient education should also include clear distinctions between these normal symptoms and more disabling conditions, such as major depression and Axis I anxiety disorders.

Suggested Readings

Burt, V.K., Suri, R., Altshuler, L., et al. (2001). The use of psychotropic medications during breast-feeding. *American Journal of Psychiatry, 158*, 1001–1009.

Chambers, C.D., Johnson, K.A., Dick, L.N., et al. (1996). Birth outcomes in pregnant women taking fluoxetine. *New England Journal of Medicine, 335*, 1010–1015.

Grady-Weliky, T.A. (2003). Premenstrual dysphoric disorder. *New England Journal of Medicine, 348*(5), 433–438.

Kessler, R.C., McGonagle, K.A., Schwartz, M., et al. (1993). Sex and depression in the National Co-morbidity Survey I: Lifetime prevalence, chronicity, and recurrence. *Journal of Affective Disorders, 29*, 85–96.

Miller, L.J. (1994). Use of electroconvulsive therapy during pregnancy. *Hospital Community Psychiatry, 45*(5), 444–450.

Nonacs, R., & Cohen, L.S. (2002). Depression during pregnancy: Diagnosis and treatment options. *Journal of Clinical Psychiatry, 63*(suppl 17), 24–30.

Nulman, I., Rovet, J., Stewart, D.E., et al. (2002). Child development following exposure to tricyclic antidepressants or fluoxetine throughout fetal life: A prospective, controlled study. *American Journal of Psychiatry, 159*(11), 1889–1995.

Nulman, I., Rovet, J., Stewart, D.E., et al. (1997). Neurodevelopment of children exposed in utero to antidepressant drugs. *New England Journal of Medicine, 336*, 258–263.

Patton, S.W., Misri, S., Corral, M.R., et al. (2002). Antipsychotic medication during pregnancy and lactation in women with schizophrenia: Evaluating the risk. *Canadian Journal of Psychiatry, 47*(10), 959–965.

Schmidt, P.J., Nieman, L.K., Danaceau, M.A., et al. (1998). Differential behavior effects of gonadal steroids in women with and in those without premenstrual syndrome. *New England Journal of Medicine, 338*(4), 209–216.

Schmidt, P.J., & Rubinow, D.R. (1991). Menopause-related affective disorders: A justification for further study. *American Journal of Psychiatry, 148*, 844–852.

Spinelli, M.G. (1997). Interpersonal psychotherapy for depressed antepartum women: A pilot study. *American Journal of Psychiatry, 154*, 1028–1030.

Steiner, M., & Pearlstein, T. (2000). Premenstrual dysphoria and the serotonin system: Pathophysiology and treatment. *Journal of Clinical Psychiatry, 61*(suppl 12), 17–21.

Viguera, A.C., & Cohen, L.S. (1998). Approach to the patient entering menopause. In T.A. Stern, J.B. Herman, & P.L. Slavin (Eds.), *The MGH guide to psychiatry in primary care*. New York: McGraw-Hill.

Viguera, A.C., Nonacs, R., Cohen, L.S., et al. (2000). Risk of recurrence of bipolar disorder in pregnant and nonpregnant women after discontinuing lithium maintainance. *American Journal of Psychiatry, 157*(2), 179–184.

Writing Group for the Women's Health Initiative Investigators. (2002). Risks and benefits of estrogen plus progestin in healthy postmenopausal women: Principal results from the Women's Health Initiative randomized controlled trial. *Journal of the American Medical Association, 288*(3), 321–333.

Chapter 27

HIV Infection and AIDS

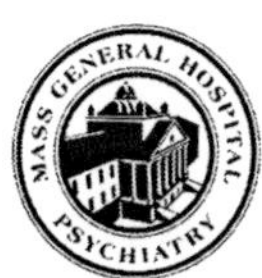

JOHN QUERQUES AND JONATHAN L. WORTH

I. Overview

A. **Human immunodeficiency virus type 1 (HIV-1) is a lentivirus, a type of retrovirus that causes slow, but progressive, immunologic and neurologic disease.** By depleting CD4 T-helper lymphocytes, infection with HIV-1 causes severe immunosuppression that can ultimately lead to fatal opportunistic infections (OIs), neoplasms, and dementing illness, and to a diagnosis of acquired immunodeficiency syndrome (AIDS).

1. Although the majority of AIDS cases in the United States are caused by infection with HIV-1, HIV-2 is responsible for some AIDS cases in West Africa. Therefore, this chapter focuses on HIV-1; for convenience we use the simpler abbreviation, HIV.
2. Different strains of HIV are grouped into three categories: M (main), O (outlier) and N (non-M, non-O). The M group is further classified into **subtypes** (different subtypes share less than 75% of their genetic material) and **variants** (called **circulating recombinant forms** [CRFs] because they form when different subtypes' genetic material blend). Currently, 11 subtypes and 13 CRFs have been identified.

B. **HIV infects certain neural cells within hours of infection,** and, through a variety of direct and indirect means, causes damage throughout the brain, though **subcortical structures and deep white matter are principal targets.**

C. **Provision of care for patients with HIV/AIDS may be complicated** by:

1. The emotional burden of seeing severe, critical illness, often in young patients
2. Countertransference reactions to, and prejudice against, patients from socially marginalized demographic groups
3. Fear of HIV transmission

D. **Owing largely to the availability of highly active antiretroviral therapy (HAART), HIV infection in the United States has become a chronic, treatable illness.** During the first 15 years of the pandemic, a diagnosis of HIV infection meant certain death; patients faced the grim reality of a ravaging, unrelenting illness, against which they and their doctors were defenseless. With the advent of protease inhibitors in 1996, patients began living with HIV infection, and even with AIDS, and thus with the stresses and burdens associated with other chronic medical problems.

E. **This chapter addresses key elements of the diagnosis and treatment of psychiatric disorders in HIV-infected and AIDS patients and the neurologic complications of HIV disease.** Because of the rapid pace of research in this area, we caution the reader that some information presented here may be outdated by the time of publication.

II. Epidemiology

A. The first case of AIDS was reported in 1981, but HIV infection was probably present—but unrecognized—as early as the 1960s.

B. According to the United Nations, HIV has infected more than 60 million people worldwide, two-thirds of whom are currently living with the virus. In 2002, 5 million people became newly infected with HIV, and more than 3 million died of the infection. The region most severely affected by the pandemic is sub-Saharan Africa, where an estimated 29.4 million people are currently infected.

C. In North America, nearly one million people are currently living with HIV infection/AIDS. Whereas the numbers of new *AIDS* cases (AIDS incidence) in the United States declined in the late 1990s (due to the availability of protease inhibitors in 1996), new *HIV* cases (HIV incidence) have consistently totaled 40,000 per year during the past decade. Compared with the early years of the pandemic, recent years have seen decreasing (but still significant) incidence among men who have sex with men (MSM) and injection drug users (IDUs), but increasing numbers among women, adolescents, and members of racial and ethnic minority groups.

1. 70% of new HIV infections occur in men.
   a. Homosexual exposure: 60%
   b. Exposure through injection drug use: 25%
   c. Heterosexual exposure: 15%
2. 30% of new HIV infections occur in women.
   a. Sexual exposure: 75%
   b. Exposure through injection drug use: 25%

D. One-third of HIV-infected people are unaware of their serostatus; only half have access to medical care.

E. **AIDS is still most prevalent among MSM, followed by IDUs and people who acquire the disease through heterosexual contact, despite decreases in the former two groups and increases in the latter since 1996.**

F. People at high risk for HIV infection include older adolescents and young adults, MSM, IDUs and their sexual partners, sexually active heterosexuals living in geographic areas where HIV is prevalent, people with chronic severe mental illness, racial and ethnic minorities, and children born to women in the above groups. Because these same demographic groups are also at high risk for psychiatric disorders, patients with HIV/AIDS frequently manifest psychopathology that is unrelated and antecedent to their retroviral illness.

1. The HIV Cost and Services Utilization Study found that nearly half of a nationally representative sample of 2,864 HIV-positive adults screened positive for major depression, dysthymic disorder, generalized anxiety disorder, or panic attack during the preceding year; 12% screened positive for substance dependence.
2. People with substance use, bipolar, and severe personality disorders are at increased risk for HIV infection because of impulsivity, impaired judgment, and the likelihood of bartering sex for drugs of abuse.
3. People at high risk for HIV infection may be more prone to psychiatric illness because these individuals typically have poor social supports and are disenfranchised, isolated, and socially marginalized.

G. The Centers for Disease Control and Prevention (CDC) first published criteria for AIDS diagnosis in 1987. The revision that followed in 1993 expanded the definition and led to an upturn in the number of AIDS cases. This revised classification system is based on the CD4 count and the presence of complications of HIV infection. **A CD4 count < 200 (or < 14% of total lymphocytes) or the presence of one of the illnesses listed in Table 27-1 defines AIDS.**

Table 27-1. AIDS-Defining Conditions

Recurrent pneumonia
Recurrent *Salmonella* septicemia
Mycobacterial infection
Pneumocystis carinii pneumonia
Coccidioidomycosis
Candidiasis
Cryptococcosis
Histoplasmosis
Toxoplasmosis of brain
Isosporiasis
Cryptosporidiosis
Cytomegalovirus infection
Herpes simplex virus infection
Progressive multifocal leukoencephalopathy
Kaposi's sarcoma
Lymphoma
Invasive cervical cancer
HIV-associated dementia
Wasting syndrome

III. General Approach to the Psychiatric Care of the Patient with HIV/AIDS

A. The differential diagnosis of psychiatric disturbance in a patient with HIVinfection/AIDS is wide. **Affective, behavioral, and cognitive symptoms may be due to primary psychiatric illness, primary effects of HIV in the central nervous system (CNS), secondary effects of systemic HIV disease on the CNS, and side effects of HAART and other medications used to treat HIV-related illnesses.** Because two or more of these conditions can co-exist and because features of these conditions overlap extensively, diagnosis is often challenging and the etiology of mental status changes may be described as multi-factorial (see Table 27-2).

B. When symptoms are due to HIV CNS infection, systemic HIV disease, or adverse medication effects, response to conventional psychotropic medications is worse, risk of side effects is greater, and tolerability is reduced, when compared with the use of these agents in patients with primary psychopathology.

C. Optimum HIV treatment, targeted at systemic and CNS manifestations, is essential. Such treatment enhances response to psychotropics and lowers the risk of side effects.

D. Important data to know include the severity of the CNS infection, the severity of the systemic HIV disease, the presence of active illness, the medication regimen, the presence of premorbid psychiatric illnesses, and the mode of retroviral infection.

1. **In general, the worse the systemic disease, the more compromised and more vulnerable the CNS is, and the greater the likelihood is that psychiatric symptoms are due to secondary causes** (e.g., medication side effects, OIs).
   a. Stage of systemic HIV disease can be determined by CD4 count, viral load, and history of HIV-related illnesses.
      i. When CD4 counts are < 500, patients are at risk of symptoms.
      ii. When CD4 counts are < 200, the rate of AIDS-defining illnesses increases markedly, and prophylaxis for OIs is instituted.

Table 27-2. Differential Diagnosis of Alteration in Mental Status in Patients with HIV Infection/AIDS

• Psychiatric disorders	**Bacteria**
• Psychoactive substance intoxication or withdrawal	*Mycobacterium avium-intracellulare*
• Primary HIV syndromes	*Mycobacterium tuberculosis*
Seroconversion illness	*Listeria monocytogenes*
HIV CNS infection	Gram-negative organisms
HIV dementia	*Treponema pallidum*
• CNS opportunistic infections	*Nocardia asteroides*
Fungi	• Neoplasms
Cryptococcus neoformans	Primary CNS non-Hodgkin's lymphoma
Coccidioides immitis	Metastatic Kaposi's sarcoma (rare)
Candida albicans	Burkitt's lymphoma
Histoplasma capsulatum	• Medication side effects (see Table 27-3)
Aspergillus fumigatus	• Endocrinopathies and nutrient deficiencies
Mucormycosis	Addison's disease (CMV, *Cryptococcus,* HIV-1, ketoconazole)
Protozoa/parasites	Hypothyroidism
Toxoplasma gondii	Hypogonadism
Amebas	Vitamin A, B_6, B_{12}, and E deficiencies
Viruses	• Anemia
JC virus	• Metabolic abnormalities
Cytomegalovirus (CMV)	• Hypotension
Adenovirus type 2	• Complex partial seizures
Herpes simplex virus	• Head trauma
Varicella zoster virus	• Non-HIV-related illnesses

2. **An answer to the question, How did you become infected?, asked in a non-judgmental tone, often reveals who the patient is as a person, how he/she feels about the way he/she was infected, and how he/she has coped with his/her seropositive status. Gathering this information not only helps to forge an alliance with the patient but also directs appropriate management.**

IV. Psychiatric Illness in the Patient with HIV/AIDS

A high index of suspicion should be maintained for "organic" causes of psychiatric symptoms in the patient with HIV infection/AIDS, especially at advanced stages of illness. In general, mental status changes that are gradual in onset are likely attributable to the primary effects of HIV on the CNS, whereas systemic complications of HIV disease more often cause acute neuropsychiatric disturbances.

This section discusses the diagnostic and therapeutic features of common psychiatric conditions that are distinctive to HIV infected/AIDS patients. For discussions of these disorders in the general population, the reader is referred to the appropriate chapters in this book.

A. Delirium

One of the most frequent psychiatric complications in hospitalized, HIV-infected patients, **delirium can occur at any stage of HIV infection, but it is more common in patients with advanced disease or with HIV-associated dementia.**

1. **Etiology.** In patients with asymptomatic HIV infection or with a CD4 count > 500, delirium is less likely to be due to HIV infection itself and more likely to be related to abuse of substances (e.g., alcohol, narcotics, steroids, testosterone). In symptomatic patients or in those with a CD4 count < 500 (especially < 100), HIV-related conditions and medication side effects are likely culprits, though the cause may be multi-factorial.
2. **Differential diagnosis.** Table 27-2 lists the conditions that may be responsible for delirium and other mental status changes in patients with HIV infection/AIDS. Table 27-3 lists the neuropsychiatric side effects of medications commonly used in HIV infection/AIDS treatment.

Table 27-3. Neuropsychiatric Side Effects of Medications Commonly Used in Patients with HIV Infection/AIDS

Nucleoside reverse transcriptase inhibitors	
Zidovudine (AZT)	Headache, restlessness, agitation, insomnia, mania, depression, irritability, delirium, somnolence, peripheral neuropathy
Didanosine (ddI)	Insomnia, mania, peripheral neuropathy
Zalcitabine (ddC)	Peripheral neuropathy
Stavudine (d4T)	Mania, peripheral neuropathy
Lamivudine (3TC)	Similar to AZT
Abacavir (ABC)	Headache
Non-nucleoside reverse transcriptase inhibitors	
Nevirapine	Headache
Delavirdine	Headache
Efavirenz	False-positive cannabinoid test, agitation, insomnia, euphoria, depression, somnolence, abnormal dreams, confusion, abnormal thinking, impaired concentration, amnesia, depersonalization, hallucinations
Tenofovir	Asthenia, anorexia
Protease inhibitors	
Indinavir	Headache, asthenia, blurred vision, dizziness, insomnia
Ritonavir	Circumoral and peripheral paresthesias, asthenia, altered taste
Saquinavir	Headache
Nelfinavir	Headache, asthenia
Amprenavir	Headache
Lopinavir/ritonavir combination	Asthenia, headache, insomnia
Other antivirals	
Acyclovir	Headache, agitation, insomnia, tearfulness, confusion, hyperesthesia, hyperacusis, depersonalization, hallucinations
Ganciclovir	Agitation, mania, psychosis, irritability, delirium
Antibacterials	
Cotrimoxazole	Headache, insomnia, depression, anorexia, apathy
Trimethoprim-sulfamethoxazole	Headache, insomnia, depression, anorexia, apathy, delirium, mutism, neuritis
Isoniazid	Agitation, depression, hallucinations, paranoia, impaired memory
Dapsone	Agitation, insomnia, mania, hallucinations
Antiparasitics	
Thiabendazole	Hallucinations, olfactory disturbance
Metronidazole	Agitation, depression, delirium, seizures (with IV administration)
Pentamidine	Hypoglycemia, hypotension, confusion, delirium, hallucinations
Antifungals	
Amphotericin B	Headache, agitation, anorexia, delirium, diplopia, lethargy, peripheral neuropathy
Ketoconazole	Headache, dizziness, photosensitivity
Flucytosine	Headache, delirium, cognitive impairment
Others	
Steroids	Euphoria, mania, depression, psychosis, confusion
Cytosine arabinoside	Delirium, cerebellar signs

3. **Evaluation.** Focused on identification of the underlying cause(s) of delirium, **the history and physical examination are the cornerstones of evaluation of the delirious patient.** Findings dictate the need for laboratory studies, which may include neuroimaging, electroencephalography (EEG), cerebrospinal fluid (CSF) analysis, and blood tests.
4. **Treatment. The hallmark of management is treatment of the underlying cause(s).** Neuroleptics (often given as the equivalent of haloperidol 0.5–5 mg daily) can be used empirically and for symptomatic control of agitation.
   a. High-potency agents are superior to medium- and low-potency neuroleptics, which can worsen delirium because of their anticholinergic effects.
   b. However, **the incidence of extrapyramidal side effects (EPS) from use of high-potency neuroleptics is increased in patients with advanced HIV disease.** Patients with AIDS and, in particular, those with HIV dementia are at increased risk for neuroleptic malignant syndrome. Alterations in the blood-brain barrier and subcortical injuries seen in HIV dementia may be responsible for the increased frequency of side effects in this population.
   c. With intramuscular administration, thrombocytopenia, coagulopathy, and reduced muscle mass need to be considered.
   d. Short-acting benzodiazepines may be combined with neuroleptics to control agitation, but they should not be used alone in the treatment of delirium.

B. Major Depression

Although major depression is one of the most frequent serious psychiatric complications of HIV infection, whether the occurrence of depression is due to HIV risk factors, the virus itself, or the chronicity of the illness is unknown. While individual studies comparing rates of depression in HIV-positive and -negative groups have not consistently found a higher rate in the former group, a recent meta-analysis did. While CD4 cell depletion per se is not associated with mood disorders, viral effects in prefrontal-subcortical circuits may contribute to the high rates of depression seen in HIV infection.

1. **Etiology.** Depression can occur at any stage of illness. **In patients with asymptomatic infection or with a CD4 count > 500, depression is likely to be primary.** A recurrence of a pre-morbid mood disorder or a first depressive episode may be precipitated by an HIV-related stressor, including unresolved bereavement. **In patients with symptomatic infection or with a CD4 count < 500, depression is more likely to be secondary** to HIV-related complications (see Table 27-2), medication side effects (see Table 27-3), HIV dementia, or substance use.
2. **Differential diagnosis**. The differential diagnosis includes grief, primary depression, new-onset or recurrent; delirium; HIV-associated dementia or minor cognitive-motor disorder (MCMD); delirium; an anergic-apathetic-fatigue state; and secondary causes associated with advanced HIV disease (adrenal dysfunction, euthyroid-sick syndrome, and hypogonadism with low testosterone).
   a. HIV infection can cause anergic-apathetic-fatigue states that are due to release of somnogenic lymphokines. They may not be characterized by significant depressive symptoms or by cognitive impairment.
3. **Evaluation.** Evaluation focuses on identification of psychosocial stressors, medication changes, substance use, and, in advanced cases, underlying conditions that may cause or worsen depression. Laboratory investigations are guided by history and physical findings.
4. **Treatment**
   a. **Pharmacotherapy with tricyclic antidepressants (TCAs) and serotonin reuptake inhibitors (SRIs) is the first line of therapy.** Regardless of agent, start with low doses and increase them slowly. Avoid sedating, anticholinergic, and anti-alpha-adrenergic agents (the latter especially in advanced HIV disease when hypotension is frequent).
   b. TCAs, especially nortriptyline, are particularly useful in patients with diarrhea, dehydration, wasting, and other causes of volume shifts because serum levels can be used to guide dosage.
   c. Bupropion or desipramine may be helpful for depression with marked fatigue and concentration difficulty, though the use of bupropion is complicated by the heightened seizure risk in HIV-infected patients.
   d. **Psychostimulants may be used as single or adjuvant agents for fatigue, apathy, and anorexia.** They may be used as first-line agents when depression is characterized by apathy more than by sadness and when patients have a history of intolerance to other agents.
      i. Because dextroamphetamine can cause severe tremor or persisting movement disorder in patients with advanced disease, some authorities prefer methylphenidate in this population. Pemoline may also be used.
   e. **Anticipate treatment intolerance or resistance and the need for polypharmacy in patients with unresolved grief, secondary mood disorders, and advanced HIV disease.**
   f. **Psychotherapy** is helpful, especially when psychosocial stressors are evident.
   g. **Electroconvulsive therapy** may also be beneficial.

C. Suicide

1. **Many people who are at risk for HIV infection are also at high risk for suicide,** probably because of psychiatric disturbance, substance use, and social disenfranchisement (see II.C.). Suicide may be the second leading cause of death among members of high-risk groups who ultimately become infected, second only to AIDS. For many, especially soon after

seroconversion, suicidal ideation or a suicide attempt may be an expression of fear and anger about reduced quality of life.

2. Broadly speaking, **reasons for these dramatic suicide rates can be categorized as due to pre-morbid psychiatric history, psychosocial stressors related to HIV infection, and neuropsychiatric complications of HIV infection.**
   a. **Risk may be most strongly related to concurrent depression.**
   b. Other risk factors include personality disorders, active substance use, bereavement, pain, coping with a homosexual orientation, HIV-related difficulties at home or at work, fear of and actual disease progression, loss of independence and autonomy, and feeling hopeless, worthless, and burdensome to others.
3. **Evaluation.** Determination of severity of suicidal thought, patient safety, and underlying diagnosis and identification of psychosocial stressors are key elements of the evaluation.
4. **Treatment.** Ensure safety, treat the underlying disorder(s), and provide psychotherapy and psychosocial interventions for stressors.

D. Difficulty Coping

Many people who are at risk for HIV infection have substance use disorders, poor self-esteem, and little education. In addition, they may be socially isolated, disenfranchised, illiterate, and impoverished. All are risk factors per se for poor coping. Even those with good preparation may have difficulty coping with HIV infection, in part because having a chronic and potentially critical illness is not an appropriate life-stage situation for many patients.

1. **The stressors faced by patients with HIV infection/AIDS are myriad:**
   a. **Diagnosis and treatment of HIV infection/AIDS:** testing seropositive; serial determination of CD4 count and viral load; initiation of HAART; initiation of prophylaxis for OIs; first hospitalization; transfer to hospice care
   b. **Experience of symptoms of HIV infection/AIDS:** wasting; diarrheal illness; treatment-resistant pain and insomnia; vision-impairing disease (e.g., cytomegalovirus retinitis); cognitive and motor dysfunction; side effects of medications (e.g., protease-inhibitor fat re-distribution syndrome)
   c. **Psychosocial consequences of HIV infection/AIDS:** disclosure of HIV serostatus; disclosure of sexual orientation (in some cases); loss of health insurance and employment; application for welfare and disability insurance; financial and social impoverishment
2. For patients on HAART, coping with the considerable side-effect burden and complicated dosing schedules of medications they will take life-long often prove the most pressing challenges.
3. **Differential diagnosis.** Ineffective coping with these stressors may present as major depression, substance use disorders, acute stress disorder, panic attacks, adjustment disorder, bereavement, or decompensated personality disorders. **If anxious symptoms are prominent, secondary causes** (e.g., hypoxia, hypoglycemia, anemia, medication side effects) **should be considered, especially in patients with symptomatic HIV infection or with a CD4 count < 500. "Anxiety" should also raise suspicion for fear, akathisia, and complex partial seizures.**
4. **Evaluation.** Identify the stressors. Use the "marathon model" to identify areas of weakness in the patient's ability to deal with those stressors, and diagnose the psychiatric disorder spawned by the faulty coping mechanism.
   a. **The "marathon model" assesses** the following four areas necessary for effective coping. Deficits in any one may compromise coping.
      i. **Training.** How did you cope with prior adversity? Assess how well these strategies will work with HIV infection.
      ii. **Personal team.** Does the patient recognize faces in the crowd along the marathon course? Who specifically comprises the patient's personal support system?
      iii. **Pit stops.** Can the patient take respite from HIV infection (e.g., with drug holidays or a week off without doctors' appointments)?
      iv. **Corporate support.** Does the patient have a primary care physician, HIV specialist, psychiatrist, hospital, health insurance, and employer?
5. **Treatment**
   a. **Non-pharmacologic treatment with supportive and psychoeducational psychotherapy and community- and government-based interventions should focus on establishment of missing components of the "marathon model" and maintenance and strengthening of those elements already present.**
   b. **Pharmacologic treatment** should provide symptomatic control.
      i. Short-term use of **high-potency benzodiazepines** in low doses is helpful for acute anxiety disorders. Long-term use can be problematic because of the potential for abuse and dependence in a population at risk for such disorders. High doses of benzodiazepines risk cognitive and motor side effects, especially in patients with HIV-associated dementia and intracranial lesions.
      ii. **Buspirone** is the treatment of choice in patients with a history of substance abuse or dependence and anxiety.
      iii. **TCAs** and **SRIs** can be used for chronic anxiety disorders.

E. Substance Use Disorders

1. As a powerful stressor, HIV infection/AIDS complicates both establishment and maintenance of abstinence. **Because substance abuse and dependence occur frequently in patients with HIV infection/AIDS, regardless of risk group, these disorders (including withdrawal states) should be considered in the differential diagnosis of any Axis I disorder.**
2. **Active abuse or dependence compromises treatment compliance and promotes high-risk behavior.**
3. **Methadone increases zidovudine (AZT) levels and decreases didanosine (ddI) and stavudine (d4T) levels.** Nevirapine, efavirenz, ritonavir, nelfinavir, amprenavir, and lopinavir can decrease methadone concentrations.

F. Psychosis

One study found that patients with HIV infection/AIDS and psychosis have a higher mortality rate and tend to have greater global neuropsychiatric impairment when compared to patients without psychosis.

1. **Etiology. In patients with asymptomatic HIV disease or a CD4 count > 500, psychotic symptoms are most likely due to a primary psychosis or to substance use (e.g., steroids, cocaine). In patients with symptomatic disease or a CD4 count < 500, secondary causes should be strongly considered.**
2. **Differential diagnosis.** Secondary causes are identical to those that cause delirium (see Table 27-2). Notable among these are: HIV CNS infection; cytomegalovirus and herpes simplex virus infections; advanced HIV-associated dementia; complex partial seizures; and medication side effects (see Table 27-3).
3. **Evaluation.** Laboratory tests (e.g., neuroimaging, EEG, CSF analysis, blood tests) are ordered as clinically indicated.
4. **Treatment. Management of psychosis proceeds along the same lines as that of delirium** (see IV.A.4.). Treatment of the underlying cause is the primary goal; symptoms are controlled with neuroleptics, usually with one-tenth to one-third of the dose required for acute "functional" psychoses.
   a. **Low doses of neuroleptics may be adequate to treat psychosis (and delirium) in HIV-infected patients because of HIV-related damage to subcortical structures, including the basal ganglia. Such injury may also explain the increased sensitivity to EPS in patients with HIV-related psychosis.**
   b. Clozapine should be avoided because of its hematopoietic toxicity.
   c. Risperidone is effective and well tolerated.
   d. Olanzapine's propensity to cause hyperglycemia, dyslipidemia, and considerable weight gain makes this agent an unfavorable choice in patients on HAART, which also causes significant metabolic disturbances (e.g., fat redistribution syndrome).
   e. The role of quetiapine, ziprasidone, and aripiprazole in patients with HIV infection/AIDS is yet to be clarified.
   f. Combination therapy with anticonvulsants and neuroleptics may be helpful.

G. Mania

1. **Etiology. In early stages of HIV disease, mania is usually due to pre-morbid bipolar disorder, substance use, or medication side effects** (see Table 27-3). **In more advanced disease,** these are still possibilities, but **new-onset mania should immediately raise suspicion for secondary causes,** including OIs, toxic/metabolic insults, and CNS space-occupying lesions (see Table 27-2). Mania can also be symptomatic of HIV dementia.
2. **Evaluation.** After determination of medication changes and assessment for substance use, **evaluation focuses on detection of underlying secondary causes.** Cranial magnetic resonance imaging (MRI) and CSF analysis should proceed if the patient has AIDS or a CD4 count < 100.
3. **Treatment. With more advanced disease, there is greater unresponsiveness to, and intolerance of, treatment.**
   a. **Lithium plus a neuroleptic is often ineffective and poorly tolerated in patients with advanced HIV disease.** Poor response may be predicted by any brain MRI abnormality, including atrophy.
      i. If lithium is used, be aware of volume shifts secondary to diarrhea and dehydration as these may raise serum lithium levels.
      ii. Lithium toxicity can occur in HIV-infected patients, even when levels are "therapeutic."
      iii. If a neuroleptic is used, guidelines for the use of these agents in patients with HIV infection/AIDS, as outlined above, should be followed (see IV.A.4.).
   b. Carbamazepine should be used cautiously, if at all, because of hematopoietic toxicity. It also decreases AZT levels.
   c. **Treatment with the Depakote® brand of valproate is highly effective and is better tolerated than standard combination therapy with lithium and neuroleptics in patients with advanced HIV disease who have abnormalities on neuroimaging studies.**
      i. Aim for symptom control or a low "therapeutic" level.
      ii. Valproate raises AZT levels.
      iii. The clinical significance of valproate's enhancement of viral replication *in vitro* is currently unclear.
   d. The role of gabapentin, lamotrigine, and topiramate in treating mania in patients with HIV infection/AIDS is yet to be clarified.
   e. Clonazepam is helpful, either alone or with valproate.

H. Insomnia

As the CD4 count falls, sleep quality often diminishes, night-time sleep fragments, sleep-onset delays, and early morning awakening becomes more frequent.

1. **Differential diagnosis.** Diagnoses include depression, anxiety, fear, pain, systemic HIV disease, HIV CNS infection, and medication side effects (see Table 27-3).
2. **Evaluation.** Assess the severity with visual or numeric analog scales, determine the cause(s), and diagnose co-morbid conditions that may worsen the sleep problem. In most cases, a clinical evaluation will suffice and polysomnography is not needed.
3. **Treatment**
   a. Teach patients the principles of sleep hygiene (see Chap. 22).
   b. Consider using low doses of sedating TCAs, trazodone, and nefazodone.
   c. Use of low doses of medium-potency neuroleptics for several days can help with the near-delusional fear at sleep initiation that grips some patients with HIV-associated dementia.
   d. Reserve use of benzodiazepines for short-term treatment of insomnia due to acute pain, exacerbations of chronic pain, adjustment disorders, acute stress disorder, and exacerbations of chronic sleep disorders. When benzodiazepines are used long-term for otherwise treatment-refractory cases, different agents should be used alternately (e.g., monthly) to avoid accommodation to any single agent. Avoid agents with long-acting, active metabolites (e.g., diazepam, chlordiazepoxide).

I. Pain

This symptom is frequent in advanced stages of HIV disease.

1. **Pain is most commonly due to a peripheral neuropathy,** which presents as a distal symmetric sensory polyneuropathy with numbness, tingling, and burning in the feet.
   a. It may be due to HIV infection itself or to nucleoside ART (AZT, didanosine, zalcitabine, stavudine). Didanosine is a more frequent culprit than are the others; it sometimes causes an irreversible neuropathy.
2. **Acute demyelinating neuropathy (Guillain-Barré syndrome)** is a self-limited, rapidly evolving symmetrical paralysis with variable sensory signs, beginning in the lower limbs, that sometimes complicates the flu-like illness that accompanies HIV seroconversion.
3. **A chronic progressive or relapsing inflammatory demyelinating polyneuropathy** may complicate the course of advanced HIV disease.
4. **Other causes of pain are herpes zoster, postherpetic neuralgia, myopathy, and headache.**
5. **Evaluation.** Determine the cause(s) and diagnose co-morbid conditions that amplify pain (e.g., depression, anxiety, and fear).
6. **Treatment.** Treat the cause(s) and the co-morbid conditions and address the bias that may be present among caregivers toward patients with a history of substance use. The approach is similar to that for any chronic pain syndrome.
   a. **Opiates.** Narcotics are recommended only for short-term use for acute pain and for exacerbations of chronic pain.
   b. **TCAs.** Low doses of nortriptyline or desipramine can be helpful.
   c. **Anticonvulsants.** Low doses of clonazepam can be beneficial, especially for hyperpathia. Carbamazepine should be used cautiously, if at all, because of hematopoietic toxicity. Valproate is generally less effective than is carbamazepine.
   d. **Lidocaine.** This agent is useful for herpes zoster and postherpetic neuralgia.
   e. As-needed dosing can be difficult for cognitively impaired patients and may result in dangerous overuse.
   f. For patients on methadone for opiate dependence, it is preferable to use another analgesic to control pain rather than increase the methadone dose.
   g. **Acupuncture.** This technique may be helpful when combined with pharmacotherapy.

V. Neurologic Manifestations of HIV/AIDS

The neurologic manifestations of HIV/AIDS are either primary (i.e., due to HIV itself or to the immunopathological changes precipitated by the retrovirus) **or secondary** (i.e., due to metabolic or toxic derangements, OIs, or neoplasms).

Primary manifestations include HIV-associated dementia, HIV meningitis, vacuolar myelopathy, and neuropathies, the most important of which for the psychiatrist is HIV-associated dementia.

Secondary manifestations include toxoplasmosis, cryptococcal meningitis, cytomegalovirus encephalitis, primary CNS lymphoma, and progressive multifocal leukoencephalopathy.

A. HIV-Associated Dementia

Known by many other names (e.g., AIDS dementia complex, HIV encephalopathy, HIV-1-associated dementia complex), **HIV-associated dementia presents as a subcortical dementing process caused by HIV CNS infection. Its incidence parallels the progression of systemic disease and depends on the effectiveness of HAART within the CNS, which may serve as a reservoir of active viral replication despite peripheral viral suppression. Therefore, it is most likely to occur in patients with other AIDS-defining illnesses or a CD4 count < 200.**

1. **Course.** Generally, HIV dementia is slow in onset and of mild to moderate severity, especially when HAART is CNS-effective. The longitudinal course varies; some patients experience progressive deterioration, whereas others follow a stable course. Sometimes a long period of relative stability ends in a precipitous decline, but **not all patients with subtle cognitive deficits or MCMD progress to the full-blown syndrome.** As

with other dementing illnesses, any degree of cognitive impairment renders a patient vulnerable to subsequent neurological insults (e.g., infection, metabolic derangement, sleep deprivation), which, in turn, lead to transient worsening of the cognitive deficits.

2. **Symptoms. HIV-associated dementia is characterized by affective, behavioral, cognitive, and motor symptoms and signs.**
   a. **Affective** features include apathy, depressed mood, fatigue, insomnia (see IV.H.3.c), and, in severe cases, depression, mania, or psychosis.
   b. **Behavioral** features include a change in social behavior, social withdrawal, anergia, and, in severe cases, agitation (associated with delirium).
   c. **Cognitive** features include deficits in attention, concentration, short-term memory, word-finding, visuospatial abilities, and completion of multiple-step activities. Patients may complain that previously automatic activities require effortful concentration. **Aphasia, agnosia, and apraxia occur very late in the course of HIV-associated dementia,** even though the fourth edition of the *Diagnostic and Statistical Manual of Mental Disorders* requires one of these deficits or executive dysfunction for the diagnosis of dementia due to HIV disease.
   d. **Motor** features include clumsiness, slowing of movements, and changes in gait and handwriting.
3. **Neurologic examination.** Typical findings include frontal release signs, hyperreflexia, disturbed smooth-pursuit eye movement, and incoordination and weakness (both worse in the lower limbs).
4. **Neuropsychological testing.**
   a. **Psychomotor slowing is the hallmark of HIV-associated dementia,** followed by impaired divided attention and concentration. Therefore, **Part B of the Halstead-Reitan Trail-Making Test is an ideal screening tool for HIV-associated dementia** because it is sensitive to impairments in psychomotor speed and divided attention and is easy to administer.
   b. At the bedside, the HIV Dementia Scale affords a quick survey of registration, recall, attention, psychomotor speed, and construction.
   c. In contrast, the Folstein Mini-Mental State Examination, because it mainly tests non-frontal *cortical* areas, is not particularly sensitive for HIV-associated dementia, which affects *sub-cortical* structures.
5. **Evaluation.** Because HIV dementia is a diagnosis of exclusion, **evaluation focuses on exclusion of other causes of altered mental status** in a patient with HIV infection/AIDS (see Table 27-2). Laboratory investigations include neuroimaging, CSF analysis, blood tests, and an EEG.
   a. Cranial **computed tomography** (CT) typically shows cerebral atrophy, ventricular enlargement, and white matter lucencies.
   b. Cranial **MRI** reveals cerebral atrophy, ventricular enlargement, and T_2-weighted hyperintense white matter lesions. There is a poor relationship between degree of abnormality on MRI and the severity of dementia.
   c. The white matter abnormalities on both CT and MRI occur as multiple punctate lesions or in large confluent areas.
   d. 75% of AIDS patients have evidence of brain pathology at autopsy, including:
      i. Reactive gliosis
      ii. Multi-nucleated giant cells
      iii. White matter pallor
      iv. Atrophy in subcortical structures and in frontal, parietal, and temporal cortices
      v. Sulcal and ventricular prominence
   e. However, decreased brain weight has not been shown to correspond with the severity of dementia. Moreover, neuropathological changes can also be seen in brains of HIV-infected patients who do not have dementia.
   f. CT and MRI are able to exclude focal lesions, but they are insensitive to the subtle changes detected by functional neuroimaging studies.
   g. In early dementia, **functional neuroimaging** studies demonstrate subcortical hypermetabolism, especially in the basal ganglia and thalamus. Later stages are characterized by cortical hypometabolism.
   h. **CSF analysis** shows only non-specific findings and should be ordered only if symptoms are progressive, or severe, or if the CD4 count is < 200.
   i. **Blood tests** should be ordered to exclude anemia, electrolyte derangements, endocrinopathies, OIs, syphilis, and vitamin B_{12} deficiency.
   j. An **EEG** may show mild, non-specific slowing; it is generally helpful only if a seizure disorder is suspected by virtue of manic symptoms, atypical panic attacks, or formed visual hallucinations.
6. **Treatment.** Treatment is four-pronged:
   a. **Optimize HAART for primary HIV CNS infection.**
      i. **Nucleoside antiretrovirals.** AZT may be the most effective of these agents because it achieves the highest concentration in the CSF. The treatment of choice for HIV-associated dementia, AZT improves cognitive function in the short-term and may retard cognitive decline. A full effect may not occur before 2–3 months; moreover, clinical improvement in the long-term may be limited by the development of viral resistance to AZT. Stavudine, lamivudine, and abacavir also readily traverse the blood-brain barrier.
      ii. **Non-nucleoside antiretrovirals.** Nevirapine and efavirenz achieve inhibitory concentrations in the CNS.
      iii. **Protease inhibitors.** Because the incidence of HIV-associated dementia parallels the severity of systemic HIV disease, the potent ability of these new agents to decrease viral load may prevent or decrease the

symptoms of dementia. Indinavir reaches inhibitory levels in the CNS; however, ritonavir, saquinavir, and nelfinavir weakly penetrate the blood-brain barrier.

b. **Control symptoms with psychotropic medications** (see appropriate sections above for management of specific psychiatric syndromes).

c. **Provide supportive psychotherapy** to help patients cope with cognitive and functional losses.

d. **Modify patients' activities to capitalize on preserved cognitive strengths.** Maintenance of routine, completion of one task at a time, and reduction of external stimuli are important elements of behavior modification. Neuropsychological test performance can help determine specific modifications.

B. HIV Meningitis

Usually self-limited, but potentially chronic, this aseptic meningitis is a rare complication of the flu-like illness that occurs during seroconversion in one-third of HIV-infected people.

C. HIV Vacuolar Myelopathy

A complication of later stages of HIV infection/AIDS, this condition presents with bilateral leg weakness, ataxia, loss of vibration and position sense in the lower extremities, as well as bowel and bladder incontinence.

D. HIV Neuropathies (see IV.I.)

E. Toxoplasmosis

The most common HIV-related opportunistic neurologic illness, infection with the protozoan, *Toxoplasma gondii*, causes encephalitis and abscesses in immunodeficient hosts, whereas many immunocompetent people are infected but remain asymptomatic.

1. **Symptoms and signs.** These include a rapidly progressive change in mental status, headache, and focal neurologic signs.
2. **Neuroimaging.** CT shows multiple ring-enhancing brain abscesses. T_2-weighted MRI scans demonstrate multiple foci of increased signal that have a predilection for the basal ganglia and are difficult to distinguish from lymphomatous lesions.
3. **Treatment. Pyrimethamine** and **sulfadiazine** lead to clinical and radiologic improvement, but suppressive therapy with pyrimethamine must continue for life because the infection cannot be eradicated.

F. Primary CNS Lymphoma

This neoplastic disease is the second leading cause of neurologic illness in HIV infected/AIDS patients. It presents as a slowly progressive neurocognitive disorder that can be mistaken for dementia before multi-focal signs and elevated intracranial pressure supervene.

1. **Symptoms and signs.** These features depend on the site(s) of the lesion(s).
2. **Neuroimaging.** Lymphoma can be difficult to distinguish from toxoplasmosis.
3. **Treatment.** There is no effective specific therapy, but **radiation** is used to decrease intracranial pressure.

G. Cryptococcal Meningitis

This type of meningitis is caused by the yeast, *Cryptococcus neoformans*.

1. **Symptoms and signs.** Fever, meningismus, cranial nerve abnormalities, and papilledema develop.
2. **Neuroimaging.** CT and unenhanced MRI can be unremarkable, but MRI with gadolinium can show meningeal enhancement.
3. **Treatment. Amphotericin B** and **flucytosine** are effective, but relapse is common; suppressive treatment with amphotericin B or **fluconazole** is required.

H. Cytomegalovirus Encephalitis

A complication of late-stage HIV infection/AIDS, this condition may be difficult to distinguish from HIV-associated dementia.

1. **Symptoms and signs.** Features include a rapidly progressive delirium, seizures, and fever.
2. **Neuroimaging.** MRI may show periventricular and subependymal abnormal signals.
3. **Treatment. Ganciclovir.**

I. Progressive Multifocal Leukoencephalopathy (PML)

Due to **infection with the JC papovavirus,** which is common in the immunocompetent population, PML follows a rapid downhill course in HIV infected/AIDS patients.

1. **Symptoms and signs.** Multi-focal neurologic signs are dependent on lesion location; a progressive delirium is common.
2. **Neuroimaging.** CT shows sub-cortical non-enhancing lucencies. MRI shows patchy areas of high signal in sub-cortical white matter.
3. **Treatment.** No specific therapy exists, but temporary improvement may be achieved with **cytosine arabinoside.**

VI. Treatment Considerations

Clinicians must be aware of: the neuropsychiatric side effects of antiretroviral medications and agents used to treat secondary opportunistic infections; the drug interactions between antiretroviral agents and psychotropics; the differences in response to psychiatric medications manifested by patients with HIV infection/AIDS; and the psychotherapeutic challenges in this population.

A. The antiretroviral armamentarium includes nucleoside reverse transcriptase inhibitors, nonnucleoside reverse transcriptase inhibitors, and, as of 1996, protease inhibitors (PIs).

1. ART is effective in slowing disease progression when the CD4 count is < 500. Combination therapy (i.e., HAART) is more effective than monotherapy.
2. The myriad neuropsychiatric side effects of these medications and others used to treat patients with HIV infection/AIDS are reviewed in Table 27-3.

B. Many antiretroviral agents are metabolized by the cytochrome P450 system; many are also inducers or inhibitors of this enzymatic pathway and thus may alter the metabolism of co-administered psychotropic medications.

1. **The three non-nucleoside reverse transcriptase inhibitors are metabolized by, and interact with, the P450 system, primarily the 3A4 isoform. Nevirapine induces the 3A4 isoform, delavirdine inhibits 3A4, and efavirenz is a mixed 3A4 inducer-inhibitor.**
   a. **Agents whose co-administration with nevirapine requires careful monitoring:** midazolam, oral contraceptives, and triazolam
   b. **Agents whose co-administration with efavirenz is not recommended:** ergot alkaloids, midazolam, pimozide, and triazolam
   c. **Agents whose co-administration with delavirdine is not recommended:** alprazolam, amphetamines, ergot alkaloids, midazolam, pimozide, and triazolam
2. **PIs are metabolized by and inhibit the P450 3A4 isoenzyme; of these, ritonavir is the most potent inhibitor.** In addition, ritonavir inhibits the 2D6 and 2C9 isoforms and induces 3A4 and 1A2; nelfinavir inhibits the 2C19 and 2D6 isoforms; and saquinavir inhibits the 2C9 isoform.
   a. **Agents that should not be co-administered with PIs:** ergot derivatives, midazolam, pimozide, St. John's wort, triazolam
   b. **Agents that should not be co-administered with ritonavir but can be (in low doses) with other PIs:** alprazolam, clorazepate, clozapine, diazepam, estazolam, flurazepam, meperidine, propoxyphene, and zolpidem
   c. **Agents whose co-administration with PIs requires low doses and testing of levels:** carbamazepine, clonazepam, hydrocodone, neuroleptics, oxycodone, psychostimulants, selective SRIs, and TCAs
   d. **Additional agents whose co-administration with ritonavir requires low doses:** maprotiline, nefazodone, trazodone, and venlafaxine
   e. **Agents whose levels may decrease with PIs:** alprazolam (with ritonavir), codeine, ethinyl estradiol (with ritonavir and nelfinavir), hydromorphone, lorazepam, methadone, morphine, oxazepam, and temazepam
   f. **Agents that decrease PI levels:** carbamazepine, phenobarbital, phenytoin, rifabutin, and rifampin, venlafaxine
   g. **Agents that increase PI levels:** fluvoxamine, nefazodone, norfluoxetine
   h. When low doses are indicated, a practical approach is to start with half the usual dose.
3. Trizivir® is a newly released combination product of abacavir, lamivudine, and zidovudine.

C. Patients with HIV infection/AIDS have less lean body mass, metabolize drugs more slowly, and are sensitive to drug side effects. Because of blood-brain barrier compromise, the HIV-infected brain may "see" higher levels of drug than serum levels may predict.

1. Aim for low therapeutic levels.
2. Start with low doses and increase them slowly.
3. Avoid anticholinergic, anti-alpha-adrenergic, and sedating medications.
4. In patients with cognitive impairment, avoid as-needed dosing because patients may accidentally overdose on dangerous medications.

D. Issues that arise in psychotherapy with HIV-infected/AIDS patients include self-blame, low self-esteem, death, guilt, health care decisions, and feelings of being punished.

1. Psychotherapists must be aware of their feelings about HIV-infection risk factors (e.g., substance abuse, homosexual sex, sex for trade) and be prepared to ask straightforward, non-judgmental questions about lifestyles unfamiliar to them.

VII. Legal Considerations

A. The patient's written informed consent is necessary before HIV antibody testing.

1. Statutes vary, but, in some jurisdictions, this permission may be obtained from the patient's attorney or the closest relative if the patient is incapacitated.

B. In psychiatric settings, staff are obligated to protect others by monitoring and restricting privileges of HIV-seropositive patients who engage in, or attempt to engage in, high-risk activities while in the hospital.

C. In some jurisdictions, physicians may have a legal requirement to disclose a patient's HIV serostatus against the patient's wishes to protect others without direct identification of the patient. In some jurisdictions, the physician must tell the patient that this information was disclosed. Because statutes vary by geography, clinicians should consult their local medical societies in these cases.

VIII. Conclusions

A. Infection with HIV exerts powerful biological, psychological, and social effects on patients and, directly or indirectly, is responsible for a panoply of affective, behavioral, and cognitive symptoms.

B. The care of these patients, therefore, taps all of a psychiatrist's skills. Not only must the psychiatrist be aware of the differences in the diagnosis and treatment of psychiatric syndromes in HIV-infected patients and the neurologic manifestations of HIV-related illnesses and treatments, he or she must be sensitive to the often fragile and chaotic psychosocial milieu in which many of these patients live.

Useful Internet Resources

AEGIS (self-proclaimed largest HIV/AIDS Internet site in the world)
aegis.com

American Psychiatric Association AIDS Resource Center
psych.org/aids/index.html

Centers for Disease Control and Prevention
cdc.gov

HIV/AIDS Treatment Information Service
hivatis.org

Joint United Nations Programme on HIV/AIDS
unaids.org

Journal of the American Medical Association HIV/AIDS Information Center
ama-assn.org/special/hiv/hivhome.htm

Project Inform (HIV information for the lay public)
projectinform.org

Suggested Readings

Agenerase (amprenavir) Product Information (1999, April). www.agenerase.com.

American Psychiatric Association. (1994). *Diagnostic and statistical manual of mental disorders* (4th ed., pp. 123–163). Washington, DC: American Psychiatric Press.

American Psychiatric Association. (2000). Practice guideline for the treatment of patients with HIV/AIDS. *American Journal of Psychiatry, 157*, 1–62.

Bing, E.G., Burnam, M.A., Longshore, D., et al. (2001). Psychiatric disorders and drug use among human immunodeficiency virus-infected adults in the United States. *Archives of General Psychiatry, 58*, 721–728.

Breitbart, W., Rosenfeld, B., Kaim, M., & Funesti-Esch, J. (2001). A randomized, double-blind, placebo-controlled trial of psychostimulants for the treatment of fatigue in ambulatory patients with human immunodeficiency virus disease. *Archives of Internal Medicine, 161*, 411–420.

Centers for Disease Control and Prevention. (1992). 1993 revised classification system for HIV infection and expanded surveillance case definition for AIDS among adolescents and adults. *Morbidity and Mortality Weekly Report, 41*(No. RR-17), 1–4, 15.

Centers for Disease Control and Prevention. (2002). Guidelines for using antiretroviral agents among HIV-infected adults and adolescents: Recommendations of the Panel on Clinical Practices for Treatment of HIV. *Morbidity and Mortality Weekly Report, 51*(No. RR-7), entire issue.

Centers for Disease Control and Prevention. (2001). HIV prevention strategic plan through 2005. Available: www.cdc.gov/nchstp/od/hiv_plan/default.htm.

Centers for Disease Control and Prevention. (2002). Update: AIDS—United States, 2000. *Morbidity and Mortality Weekly Report, 51*, 592–595.

Ciesla, J.A., & Roberts, J.E. (2001). Meta-analysis of the relationship between HIV infection and risk for depressive disorders. *American Journal of Psychiatry, 158*, 725–730.

Cournos, F., & Forstein, M. (Eds.). (2000). What mental health practitioners need to know about HIV and AIDS. *New Directions for Mental Health Services, 87*, 1–136.

Drugs for HIV infection. (1997). *Medical Lettres, 39*, 111–116.

Flexner, C. (1998). HIV-protease inhibitors. *New England Journal of Medicine, 338*, 1281–1292.

Grant, I., & Atkinson, J.H. (1995). Psychiatric aspects of acquired immune deficiency syndrome. In H.I. Kaplan, & B.J. Sadock (Eds.), *Comprehensive textbook of psychiatry VI* (6th ed., pp. 1644–1669). Baltimore: Williams and Wilkins.

Greenberg, D.B., & Beckett, A. (1999). Neuropsychiatric aspects of cancer and AIDS in the intensive care unit. In R.S. Irwin, F.B. Cerra, & J.M. Rippe (Eds.), *Intensive care medicine* (4th ed., pp. 2433–2440). Philadelphia, PA: Lippincott-Raven.

Grinspoon, S.K., & Bilezikian, J.P. (1992). HIV disease and the endocrine system. *New England Journal of Medicine, 327*, 1360–1365.

Grunfeld, C., Pang, M., Doerrler, W., et al. (1993). Indices of thyroid function and weight loss in human immunodeficiency virus infection and the acquired immunodeficiency syndrome. *Metabolism, 42*, 1270–1276.

Halman, M.H., Worth, J.L., Sanders, K.M., et al. (1993). Anticonvulsant use in the treatment of manic syndromes in patients with HIV-1 infection. *Journal of Neuropsychiatry and Clinical Neuroscience, 5*, 430–434.

Hinkin, C.H., Van Gorp, W.G., & Satz, P. (1995). Neuropsychological and neuropsychiatric aspects of HIV infection in adults. In H.I. Kaplan, & B.J. Sadock (Eds.), *Comprehensive textbook of psychiatry VI* (6th ed., pp. 1669–1680). Baltimore, MD: Williams and Wilkins.

Hriso, E., Kuhn, T., Masdeu, J.C., et al. (1991). Extrapyramidal symptoms due to dopamine-blocking agents in patients with AIDS encephalopathy. *American Journal of Psychiatry, 148*, 1558–1561.

Joint United Nations Programme on HIV/AIDS and World Health Organization. (2002, December). AIDS epidemic update. Available: www.unaids.org.

McDonald, C.K., & Kuritzkes, D.R. (1997). Human immunodeficiency virus type 1 protease inhibitors. *Archives of Internal Medicine, 157*, 951–959.

Melton, S.T., Kirkwood, C.K., & Ghaemi, S.N. (1997). Pharmacotherapy of HIV dementia. *Annals of Pharmacotherapy, 31*, 457–473.

New drugs for HIV infection. (1996). *Medical Letter, 38*, 35–37.

Panel on Clinical Practices for Treatment of HIV Infection. (1998, December). *Guidelines for the use of antiretroviral agents in HIV-infected adults and adolescents*. Available: www.hivatis.org (HIV/AIDS Treatment Information Service).

Physicians' desk reference. (1999). (53rd ed., pp. 464–469, 484–487, 1204, 1343, 1762–1766, 2675–2680, 2685–2688). Montvale, NJ: Medical Economics.

Piscitelli, S.C., & Gallicano, K.D. (2001). Interactions among drugs for HIB and opportunistic infections. *New England Journal of Medicine, 344*, 984–996.

Power, C., Selnes, O.A., Grim, J.A., & McArthur, J.C. (1995). HIV dementia scale: A rapid screening test. *Journal of Acquired Immune Deficiency Syndromes and Human Retrovirology, 8*, 273–278.

Robinson, M.J., & Qaqish, R.B. (2002). Practical psychopharmacology in HIV-1 and acquired immunodeficiency syndrome. *Psychiatric Clinics of North America, 25*, 149–175.

Schaerf, F.W., Miller, R.R., Lipsey, J.R., et al. (1989). ECT for major depression in four patients infected with human immunodeficiency virus. *American Journal of Psychiatry, 146*, 782–784.

Sepkowitz, K.A. (2001). AIDS—The first 20 years. *New England Journal of Medicine, 344*, 1764–1772.

Sewell, D.D., Jeste, D.V., Atkinson, J.H., et al. (1994). HIV-associated psychosis: A study of 20 cases. *American Journal of Psychiatry, 151*, 237–242.

Singh, A.N., Golledge, H., & Catalan, J. (1997). Treatment of HIV-related psychotic disorders with risperidone: A series of 21 cases. *Journal of Psychosomatic Research, 42*, 489–493.

Stern, Y., McDermott, M.P., Albert, S., et al. (2001). Factors associated with incident human immunodeficiency virus-dementia. *Archives of Neurology, 58*, 473–479.

Three new drugs for HIV infection. (1998). *Medical Lettres, 40*, 114–116.

Worth, J.L. (1997). HIV/AIDS patients. In N.H. Cassem, T.A. Stern, J.F. Rosenbaum, & M.S. Jellinek (Eds.), *Massachusetts General Hospital handbook of general hospital psychiatry* (4th ed., pp. 545–569). St. Louis, MO: Mosby Year Book.

Worth, J.L., & Boswell, S.L. (1998). Approach to the patient with HIV infection. In T.A. Stern, J.B. Herman, & P.L. Slavin (Eds.), *The MGH guide to psychiatry in primary care*, pp. 385–400. New York: McGraw-Hill.

Worth, J.L., & Halman, M.H. (1996). HIV disease/AIDS. In J.R. Rundell, & M.G. Wise (Eds.), *The American Psychiatric Press textbook of consultation-liaison psychiatry*, pp. 833–877. Washington, DC: American Psychiatric Press.

Chapter 28

Catatonia, Neuroleptic Malignant Syndrome, and Serotonin Syndrome

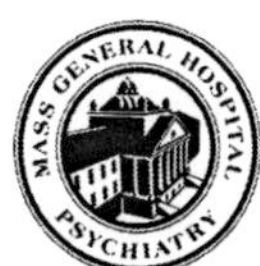

BRAD REDDICK AND THEODORE A. STERN

I. Introduction

The syndromes described in this chapter all allude to the complex interaction of motor, behavioral, and systemic manifestations derived from unclear mechanisms of neurochemical aberration. The clinical similarities among neuroleptic malignant syndrome (NMS), catatonia, and serotonin syndrome have led some to hypothesize a common pathophysiology. Many believe that NMS is but one point along a spectrum of clinical presentations, essentially being an extreme form of catatonia. As our psychopharmacologic armamentarium grows and as drugs potent in their modulation of monoamine action proliferate, the diagnosis and management of these complex disorders becomes even more important.

II. Catatonia

A. Definition

Few disorders are as enigmatic as catatonia. It has been described as a subtype of schizophrenia, but is reported to be more common in affective disorders. Its phenomenology includes a characteristic excitement as well as stupor.

The syndrome of catatonia (derived from the Greek word *katateinein*, to stretch tightly), is made up of an array of motor and behavioral signs and symptoms that often occur in relation to neurochemical insults. The syndrome was **characterized as early as 1874 when Karl Kahlbaum first described 21 patients** thought to have the disorder, which he proposed was a process of several stages corresponding to symptom severity. **Kraeplin included catatonia as a subgroup of** deteriorating psychotic disorders termed **"dementia praecox."** With the rise in neuroleptic use, catatonia as a subtype of schizophrenia has declined, and a greater proportion of affected patients suffer from affective disorders and general medical conditions.

B. Etiology

The potential etiologies of catatonia are many and are outlined in Table 28-1. The importance of prompt diagnosis is highlighted by the **potential complications** associated with catatonia (Table 28-2) and the existence of effective treatments, which may prevent such complications and interrupt progression of the illness.

C. Epidemiology

1. At least one study has looked at the incidence of catatonia upon hospital admission and found **its frequency among newly admitted psychiatric inpatients to be approximately 9%** (Rosebush et al., 1990).
2. The **exact prevalence of catatonia is unknown,** although the frequency of catatonic signs arising in affective disorders has remained unchanged since 1922.
3. This is in contrast to the observed decline in prevalence of catatonia associated with schizophrenia from 14% to 8%, which has been attributed to changing patterns in the diagnosis of schizophrenia or to a hypothesized decline of some viral infective disorder which may be involved in the pathogenesis of schizophrenia.
4. Several studies have attempted to outline the association between catatonia and affective disorders. Taylor and Abrams (1986) found that **25–50% of patients with catatonic signs and symptoms also met criteria for affective disorder.**
5. Roughly **20% of patients with bipolar illness** exhibit one or more catatonic characteristics. Approximately **5–10% of schizophrenic patients will have catatonic features.**

D. Diagnosis

1. The ***Diagnostic and Statistical Manual, Fourth Edition* (DSM-IV) outlines criteria for catatonia** in association with major depressive disorder (MDD), mania, mixed affective state, or schizophrenia; **at least two of the following must be present:**
   a. **Motor immobility**
   b. **Excessive motor activity**
   c. **Extreme negativism or mutism**
   d. **Peculiar voluntary movement**
   e. **Echolalia or echopraxia**
2. The syndrome is thought to be the result of a general medical condition when:
   a. The disturbance does not occur during the course of delirium.
   b. The disturbance is not better accounted for by another mental disorder.
   c. There is evidence from history, physical examination, or laboratory findings that the disturbance is the direct physiological consequence of a general medical condition.
3. In addition to the criteria outlined in the DSM-IV, it is important to consider subtypes of the syndrome to facilitate management and treatment. **Catatonic stupor** is characterized by psychomotor withdrawal, whereas **catatonic excitement** involves psychomotor hyperactivity. Another subtype, **malignant catatonia,**

Table 28-1. Potential Etiologies of the Catatonic Syndrome

Primary psychiatric
Acute psychoses
Conversion disorder
Dissociative disorders
Mood disorders
Obsessive-compulsive disorders
Personality disorders
Schizophrenia

Secondary neuromedical
Cerebrovascular
Arterial aneurysms
Arteriovenous malformations
Arterial and venous thrombosis
Bilateral parietal infarcts
Temporal lobe infarct
Subarachnoid hemorrhage
Subdural hematoma
Third ventricle hemorrhage
Hemorrhagic infarcts
Other central nervous system causes
Akinetic mutism
Pellagra
Alcoholic degeneration and Wernicke's encephalopathy
Cerebellar degeneration
Cerebral anoxia
Cerebromacular degeneration
Closed head trauma
Frontal lobe atrophy
Hydrocephalus
Lesions of thalamus and globus pallidus
Narcolepsy
Parkinsonism
Post-encephalitic states
Seizure disorders
Surgical interventions
Tuberous sclerosis

Neoplasm
Angiomas
Frontal lobe tumors
Gliomas
Langerhans' carcinoma
Paraneoplastic encephalopathy
Periventricular diffuse pinealoma

Poisoning
Coal gas
Organic fluorides
Tetraethyl lead poisoning

Infections
Acquired immunodeficiency syndrome
Bacterial meningoencephalitis
Bacterial sepsis
General paresis
Malaria
Mononucleosis
Subacute sclerosing panencephalitis
Tertiary syphilis
Tuberculosis
Typhoid fever
Viral encephalitides (especially herpes)
Viral hepatitis

Metabolic and other medical causes
Acute intermittent porphyria
Addison's disease
Cushing's disease
Diabetic ketoacidosis
Glomerulonephritis
Hepatic dysfunction
Hereditary coproporphyria
Homocystinuria
Hyperparathyroidism
Hyperthyroidism
Idiopathic hyperadrenergic state
Multiple sclerosis
Systemic lupus erythematosus
Thrombotic thrombocytopenic purpura
Uremia

Drug-related
Neuroleptics; typical and atypical (e.g., clozapine, risperidone)
Non-neuroleptics
Alcohol
Anticonvulsants (tricyclics, monoamine oxidase inhibitors, and others)
Anticonvulsants (e.g., carbamazepine)
Aspirin
Disulfiram
Metoclopramide
Dopamine depleters (e.g., tetrabenzine)
Dopamine withdrawal (e.g., levodopa)
Hallucinogens (e.g., mescaline, phencyclidine, and lysergic acid diethylamide)
Lithium carbonate
Morphine
Sedative-hypnotic withdrawal
Steroids
Stimulants (e.g., amphetamines, methylphenidate, and possibly cocaine)

Idiopathic

SOURCE: Adapted from Philbrick, K.L., & Rummans, T.A. (1994). Malignant catatonia. *Journal of Neuropsychiatry and Clinical Neuroscience, 6,* 1–13.

Table 28-2. Some Medical Complications Associated with Catatonia

Simple non-malignant catatonia
Aspiration
Burns
Cachexia
Dehydration and sequelae
Pneumonia
Pulmonary emboli
Thrombophlebitis
Urinary retention and sequelae
Urinary incontinence
Malignant catatonia
Acute renal failure
Adult respiratory distress syndrome
Aphasia and dysarthria
Cardiac arrest
Cheyne-Stokes respirations
Death
Disseminated intravascular coagulation
Electrocardiographic abnormalities
Gait abnormalities
Intestinal pseudo-obstruction
Laryngospasm
Myocardial infarction
Myocardial stunning
Necrotizing enterocolitis
Pneumomediastinum
Pseudomembranous colitis
Respiratory arrest
Respiratory stridor
Rhabdomyolysis and sequelae
Seizures
Sepsis
Severe dysphagia due to muscle spasm
Severe hepatocellular damage
Sudden, profound hypoglycemia
Unresponsiveness to pain
Upper gastrointestinal tract bleeding

suggested by Philbrick and Rummans (1994), is used when catatonia is complicated by autonomic instability or hyperthermia.

E. Differential Diagnosis

With the great number of medical and neurological illnesses that may potentially precipitate catatonia, differentiating among the possible etiologies can be a formidable task. Table 28-1 outlines **the many potential etiologies of catatonia** that must be considered when the syndrome arises.

F. Pathophysiology

The complex array of symptoms and the potential etiologies make discussion of the mechanism by which the syndrome of catatonia develops difficult. **Clinical features (e.g., rigidity) suggest involvement of the basal ganglia and its associated projections.** Given the clinical similarities among neurologic illness involving the frontal lobes, which produce akinetic mutism and idiopathic catatonia, **involvement of dopamine and inhibitory γ-aminobutyric acid (GABA) in the pre-frontal cortex has been implicated.** Alternatively, subtle **ictal events** involving the pre-frontal cortex and the basal ganglia have been postulated, since use of intravenous benzodiazepines (which have antiseizure effects) can treat catatonia.

G. Evaluation

1. **A thorough neuromedical work-up is essential** so that prompt treatment can be initiated and further medical and psychiatric complications can be prevented.
2. **An amobarbital interview may be helpful,** especially in stuporous catatonia; a temporary recovery from catatonic symptoms suggests psychiatric illness.
3. **A physical examination may reveal signs of medical complications. Findings associated with the catatonia syndrome associated with psychiatric illness** (idiopathic catatonia) include:
   a. Normal optokinetic responses
   b. Normal pupillary responses
   c. Normal ocular nystagmus on cold caloric tests
   d. Extreme negativism
   e. Mutism
   f. Waxy flexibility
   g. Autonomic instability (in the case of malignant catatonia and NMS)
   h. A rise in basal body temperature with hyperthermia as the extreme (in the case of malignant catatonia and NMS)
4. **History will often reveal clues to the existence of a pre-morbid psychotic disorder or underlying medication trial or medical condition,** such as those outlined in Table 28-1. When catatonic mutism precludes obtaining a thorough history, administration of intravenous lorazepam can bring on a temporary lucid interval that may facilitate data collection.

   Interviewing the catatonic patient can prove a challenge; it often relies on keen observation of behavior. Many have used rating scales such as **the modified Bush-Francis Catatonia Rating Scale,** which requires two of fourteen behavioral signs to make the diagnosis.
5. **Studies**
   a. **An electroencephalogram (EEG) is needed to detect a potential underlying seizure disorder.** Although a nor-

mal EEG may suggest idiopathic catatonia, many psychiatric patients display non-specific abnormalities on the EEG.

b. **Neuroimaging studies can rule out mass lesions, central nervous system (CNS) ischemic events, and underlying neuromedical illness** that confer vulnerability, although a normal imaging study does not rule out an underlying neuromedical etiology.

c. **Laboratory tests can illuminate clues to both catatonia and the risk factors for the development of NMS.** Like the physical examination, results of electrolytes, renal function, and the hematocrit may suggest dehydration and raise suspicion for NMS. **An elevated creatine phosphokinase (CPK) typically occurs in both malignant catatonia and NMS;** knowledge of its presence can guide therapy in terms of preventing subsequent renal failure from rhabdomyolysis.

H. Treatment

1. **Pharmacology**
   a. **Discontinuation of any potential offending pharmacologic agent** (e.g., dopamine blockers, such as neuroleptics, Compazine, or metoclopramide), which can cause or worsen catatonia, should be considered.
   b. **Review of the medication record should be accomplished** to determine if dopamine agonists have been withdrawn and consideration given to their resumption.
2. Since **electroconvulsive therapy** (ECT) continues to be a powerful and important treatment of catatonia, it **should be considered.** Frequently two to three treatments will suffice, although four to six treatments are usually given to prevent relapse.
3. **Medical/supportive care is essential;** it includes adequate hydration, nutrition, mobilization, and anticoagulation (to prevent thrombophlebitis and pulmonary embolism). Aspiration precautions are also important. Once catatonia is suspected, close observation and frequent vital sign checks are warranted. Throughout the course, a high index of suspicion should be sustained for the development of medical complications.
4. **If hyperthermia, autonomic instability, or malignant catatonia emerge, treatment in an intensive care unit may be indicated.**

III. Neuroleptic Malignant Syndrome (NMS)

A. Definition

NMS is a rare complication of neuroleptic therapy that confers high mortality if not treated in a prompt and skillful manner. It is a syndrome defined by its symptoms.

B. Epidemiology

1. **Lack of uniform diagnostic criteria, concurrent use of other medications, and methodological differences used in epidemiology studies have made estimating the frequency of NMS difficult;** its incidence is estimated from 0.07% to 2.2%.
2. Although there are clinical similarities between NMS and malignant hyperthermia (associated with general anesthesia), **patients with a history of either NMS or malignant hyperthermia do not appear to be at increased risk for developing the other.**
3. **Mortality rates for patients with NMS have decreased from 20% (prior to 1984) to 11.6%** currently, a decrease thought to be secondary to a greater awareness of the syndrome and its signs and symptoms.

C. Diagnosis

1. **Universally accepted criteria exist for NMS are lacking.** However, several attempts have been made to group signs and symptoms into major and minor categories.
2. **Currently the DSM-IV defines NMS as the development of severe muscle rigidity and elevated temperature in association with two or more of the following: diaphoresis, dysphagia, tremor, incontinence, changes in level of consciousness, mutism, tachycardia, elevated or labile blood pressure, leukocytosis, and laboratory evidence of muscle injury (elevated CPK).**
3. Making the diagnosis implies that the symptom complex cannot be better accounted for by a mood disorder with catatonic features, or a general medical or neurological illness.
4. Attempts to discover risk factors for the development of NMS have been ongoing. Keck and associates (1989) examined 18 patients with NMS in a case-controlled fashion. When compared with controls, they identified **several risk factors,** including:
   a. A greater degree of **pre-morbid psychomotor agitation**
   b. **Higher doses of neuroleptics** with greater rates of dose increase
   c. A higher number of **intramuscular injections**
   d. Concurrent use of **lithium**

D. Differential Diagnosis

1. As the clinical features of NMS resemble those of a host of medical and neurological illnesses, the diagnosis of NMS requires attention to the plethora of potential neuromedical etiologies.
2. Table 28-3 outlines common disorders to consider when the diagnosis of NMS is entertained.
3. Of particular note are those illnesses which present with hemodynamic changes, systemic manifestations, and clouding of the sensorium, which may be confused with NMS.
   a. Although clinically similar to NMS, **malignant hyperthermia** differs from NMS in that it is associated with anesthesia and has a characteristic histologic appearance

Table 28-3. Differential Diagnosis of Neuroleptic Malignant Syndrome

Central nervous system disorders
Head trauma
Meningitis
Parkinson's disease
Status epilepticus
Systemic disorders
Hyperthyroidism
Pheochromocytoma
Malignant hyperthermia
Heat stroke
Polymyositis
Sepsis
Psychiatric disorders
Lethal catatonia
Toxic conditions
Anticholinergic syndrome
Serotonin syndrome
Monamine oxidase inhibitor/tricyclic combination
Withdrawal from alcohol or sedative hypnotic drugs
Sudden discontinuation of levodopa

of skeletal muscle fibers (i.e., they contract on exposure to halothane or caffeine).

b. **Anticholinergic delirium** is manifest by clouding of the sensorium, and an elevated temperature (like NMS), but not by diaphoresis. The diagnosis of anticholinergic delirium can be further clarified by the administration of physostigmine, which will temporarily ameliorate anticholinergic symptoms.

c. **Serotonin syndrome** is another condition which has similar clinical signs to those of NMS. However, in serotonin syndrome, tremor is a more common peripheral motor finding, fever is present less often, and the laboratory abnormalities seen in NMS are usually absent.

E. Pathophysiology

1. Although poorly understood, **the mechanism thought to be responsible for NMS involves blockade of dopamine receptors central (in the basal ganglia and the hypothalamus) and peripherally (in post-ganglionic sympathetic neurons and smooth muscle).**
2. Neuroleptics have been implicated in directly altering basal temperature regulation in the hypothalamus, which may play an added role in the development of fever.
3. Additionally, observations that dantrolene may be beneficial in the treatment of NMS raise the hypothesis that neuroleptics may directly affect skeletal muscle and result in increased cell metabolism and hyperthermia.
4. Some have postulated that the underlying pathophysiology more likely reflects an imbalance in central dopamine and serotonergic and/or adrenergic tone. Case reports of NMS developing from tricyclic antidepressants, selective serotonin reuptake inhibitors (SSRIs), and atypical antipsychotic agents point to the potential involvement of non-dopamine monoamines as well.

F. Treatment

1. Given the high morbidity and mortality associated with NMS, **prompt treatment is essential.**
2. Initial management should include transfer to a general hospital where **intensive hemodynamic monitoring and supportive care** can be initiated.
3. Medical and supportive care is crucial once the diagnosis of NMS is made. Suggested supportive measures include provision of **adequate intravenous hydration, active cooling, and close hemodynamic monitoring.**
4. **Electrolyte balance and renal function should be monitored** closely, given the increased risk of renal failure associated with NMS. Dialysis may be necessary.
5. A detailed history and chart review may reveal the use of either neuroleptic or non-neuroleptic dopamine antagonists, or withdrawal of dopamine agonists. Any dopamine antagonist (Table 28-4) should be removed and the agonists resumed.

G. Treatment Hierarchy

1. Discontinue neuroleptics and other dopamine antagonists.
2. Provide supportive care.
3. **Institute pharmacologic interventions.** These have included **dantrolene,** which may be helpful in reducing muscle rigidity, but it carries a risk of hepatotoxicity. **Bromocriptine** is thought to be effective through its action as a central D_2 agonist, although it may potentially worsen any underlying psychosis. **Other treatments that may be beneficial include amantadine, levodopa, clonazepam, benztropine, non-depolarizing paralytic agents, and ECT.**
4. **Controversy surrounds the assumption that the development of NMS confers greater risk of developing the syndrome if rechallenged with a neuroleptic.** Most investigators agree that reinstitution of antipsychotic medicines should be delayed for at least 2 weeks after an episode of NMS has resolved, and should include a neuroleptic of lower potency.

Table 28-4. Dopamine Antagonists

Antipsychotics (neuroleptics)
Phenothiazines
Chlorpromazine (Thorazine)
Triflupromazine (Vesprin)
Mesoridazine (Serentil)
Thioridazine (Mellaril)
Acetophenazine (Tindal)
Fluphenazine (Prolixin, Permitil)
Perphenazine (Trilafon)
Trifluoperazine (Stelazine)
Butyrophenones
Droperidol (Inapsine)
Haloperidol (Haldol)
Thioxanthenes
Chlorprothixene (Taractan)
Thiothixene (Navane)
Dibenzoxepines
Loxapine (Loxitane, Daxoline)
Clozapine (Clozaril)
Indolone
Molindone (Moban)
Diphenylbutylpiperidine
Pimozide (Orap)
Other dopamine antagonists
Antiemetics
Metaclopramide (Reglan)
Promethazine (Phenergan)
Prochlorperazine (Compazine)
Trimethobenzamide (Tigan)
Antihistamines
Hydroxyzine (Atarax, Vistaril)

IV. Serotonin Syndrome

A. Definition

1. Serotonin plays a major role in multiple psychiatric illnesses. As the number of agents that directly effect central serotonergic tone has increased, so has our understanding of the clinical features related to serotonin excess (serotonin syndrome) and the need for heightened clinical awareness in the prevention, recognition, and prompt treatment of the syndrome.
2. Although **its incidence is unknown,** serotonin syndrome is **most commonly the result of the interaction between serotonergic agents and monoamine oxidase inhibitors** (MAOIs), and commonly results in changes in mental status, restlessness, myoclonus, hyperreflexia, diaphoresis, shivering, and tremor.
3. The presumed mechanism involves the brainstem and spinal cord activation of the 1A form of serotonin receptor.
4. **Discontinuation of the serotonergic agents and institution of supportive treatment are the primary treatments,** although the 5-HT receptor antagonists may also play a role.
5. Once treatment is initiated, the syndrome usually resolves within 24 hours; associated confusion can last for days.

B. Clinical Presentation

1. Serotonin syndrome most commonly occurs in individuals with a history of a psychiatric disorder for which a psychotropic medicine has been prescribed, most commonly some combination of an SSRI, L-tryptophan, an MAOI, an antiparkinson agent, and lithium.
2. **Initially, patients experience tremor, mild confusion, and incoordination, followed by systemic signs (e.g., hyperreflexia, diaphoresis, shivering, and marked agitation).**
3. **In severe form patients may develop fever, myoclonus, and diarrhea.**
4. These clinical features can range in duration from 6 hours up to 44 hours after the initiation of treatment.
5. Table 28-5 outlines the clinical features of serotonin syndrome.

C. Pathophysiology

1. The preponderance of evidence, which relies mostly on animal studies and a few studies in humans, implicates the role of 5-HT in the pathogenesis of serotonin syndrome.

Table 28-5. The Most Common Clinical Features of the Serotonin Syndrome in Order of Frequency

- Mental status changes
- Confusion
- Hypomania
- Restlessness
- Myoclonus
- Hyperreflexia
- Diaphoresis
- Shivering
- Tremor
- Diarrhea
- Incoordination

2. The identification of receptor subtypes and subsequent research on the benefits of 5-HT antagonism, has implicated 5-HT_{1A} receptor activation as responsible for serotonin syndrome.
3. Other studies (as in NMS) have implicated both dopamine and serotonergic activation in the syndrome's pathogenesis, arguing that agents with a ratio of greater serotonergic properties to corresponding dopaminergic properties are most likely to precipitate the syndrome.
4. This hypothesis is further supported by peripheral manifestations of serotonergic activation (comprising a majority of symptoms observed in the syndrome), along with observations that 5-HT_{1A} receptors predominate in the caudal brainstem and spinal cord.
5. As these observations are based on animal models of neurotransmission, caution must be used in extrapolating these results to humans.

D. Epidemiology

1. The **incidence of serotonin syndrome is unknown,** and there are no data to suggest that sex or age differences confer any variability in predisposition to developing the syndrome.
2. Given the overlap of symptoms with NMS, serotonin syndrome is often mistaken for NMS and thus may be under-reported. Additionally, **the possible existence of varying gradations in symptom severity may also confound full recognition of this syndrome.**

E. Evaluation

1. As with NMS, a detailed history will often reveal concomitant use of at least two psychotropic medications, which confers greater risk for developing the syndrome. As NMS shares many clinical features with serotonin syndrome, prior use of neuroleptics and a history of psychosis are of particular importance.
2. Typically the history is most helpful in establishing a temporal relationship with the initiation of psychotropic agents.
3. **Laboratory testing** is useful to assess a patient's underlying nutritional and hydration status, to screen for elevated CPK raising suspicion of NMS, and to investigate the presence of an underlying medical condition which may raise the risk of developing the syndrome and subsequent complications.
4. Of note, certain monoamine secreting tumors (e.g., carcinoid tumors and oat cell lung malignancies) have been associated with the serotonin syndrome. With these rare malignancies in mind, gastrointestinal and lung roentgenograms may be helpful in the initial investigation.
5. As is the case in catatonia and NMS, an **EEG and neuroimaging** are useful in uncovering an underlying seizure disorder or neurological condition, although normal studies do not rule out the presence of a neuromedical illness.

F. Drug Interactions

1. **As is the case with NMS, drug effects and interactions are the most common precipitant of the syndrome.**
2. Case reports highlight the greater risk of SSRIs, L-tryptophan, and MAOIs in precipitating the syndrome. Specifically, case reports have centered around symptoms arising when SSRIs are combined with either L-tryptophan or an MAOI. Table 28-6 lists **the most common drug interactions associated with serotonin syndrome.**
   a. In general, when serotonergic reuptake inhibition is combined with MAO inhibition, the potential for induction of serotonin syndrome is greatly increased. Such a presentation has also been described in combining medications with MAOI properties with either L-tryptophan or lithium.
   b. Additionally, the syndrome can be precipitated by overdoses of MAOIs.
   c. The potential hazards of using an MAOI and a medicine with any serotonergic properties or reuptake inhibition demand vigilance when prescribing an MAOI.
   d. Current treatment practice includes a 2-week washout interval following the discontinuation of an MAOI. In the case of fluoxetine, a minimum of 5-week washout period is required following the discontinuation of fluoxetine and before the initiation of an MAOI.

G. Treatment

1. Given the non-existence of prospective studies evaluating the treatment of serotonin syndrome, **treatment strategies are derived primarily from case reports and data stemming from animal studies.**
2. To date, the literature addressing treatment indicates that **removal of the offending agent will often result in the resolution of symptoms within 24 hours.** The first step in treatment is always to discontinue the suspected offending agent.
3. **Supportive measures are essential in both treating and preventing potential medical complications** and often include antipyretics to combat fever, cooling blankets for the development of hyperthermia, clonazepam for myoclonus, anticonvulsants if seizures

Table 28-6. The Most Common Drug Interactions Associated with the Serotonin Syndrome in Order of Frequency

- L-Tryptophan and an MAOI (with lithium)
- Fluoxetine and an MAOI
- Fluoxetine and L-tryptophan
- Clomipramine and clorgyline
- Bromocriptine and L-dopa/carbidopa

arise, and antihypertensive agents, such as nifedipine, for severely elevated blood pressure. Rarely does the syndrome progress to respiratory failure (which is usually due to aspiration) that requires artificial ventilation.

4. Animal models have suggested that **prophylaxis is possible with pre-treatment using 5-HT$_1$ receptor antagonists.** Agents that confer non-specific 5-HT receptor antagonism and have demonstrated benefit in the treatment or prevention of the symptoms associated with serotonin syndrome include **methysergide** and **cyproheptidine.**
5. Beta-blockers may also be useful in treatment due to their 5-HT blocking properties. Specifically, **propranolol** has demonstrated 5-HT$_{1A}$ receptor antagonism in animal models, and, in at least one case report, it was successful in blocking the progression of the syndrome after a patient ingested varying amounts of L-tryptophan, isocarboxide, and lithium.

Suggested Readings

American Psychiatric Association. (1994). *Diagnostic and statistical manual* (4th ed., DSM-IV). Washington, DC: American Psychiatric Press.

Blumer, D. (1997). Catatonia and the neuroleptics: Psychobiologic significance of remote and recent findings. *Comprehensive Psychiatry, 38,* 193–201.

Bush, G., Fink, M., Petrides, G., et al. (1996). Catatonia. Treatment with lorazepam and electroconvulsive therapy. *Acta Psychiatr Scand, 93,* 137–143.

Fricchione, G., Bush, G., Fozdar, M., et al. (1997). Recognition and treatment of the catatonic syndrome. *Journal of Intensive Care Medicine, 12,* 135–147.

Keck, P.E., Pope, H.G., Cohen, B.M., et al. (1989). Risk factors for neuroleptic malignant syndrome. *Archives of General Psychiatry, 46,* 914–918.

Philbrick, K.L., & Rummans, T.A. (1994). Malignant catatonia. *Journal of Neuropsychiatry and Clinical Neuroscience, 6*(1), 1–13.

Pope, H.G., Jr., Jonas, J.M., Hudson, J.I., et al. (1985). Toxic reactions to the combination of monoamine oxidase inhibitors and tryptophan. *American Journal of Psychiatry, 142,* 491–492.

Prager, L., Millham, F., & Stern, T.A. (1994). Neuroleptic malignant syndrome: A review for intensivists. *Journal of Intensive Care Medicine, 9,* 227–234.

Rosebush, P.I., Hildebrand, A.M., Furlong, B.G., et al. (1990). Catatonic syndrome in a general psychiatric inpatient population: Frequency, clinical presentation, and response to lorazepam. *Journal of Clinical Psychiatry, 51,* 357–362.

Stern, T.A., Schwartz, J.H., & Shuster, J.L. (1992). Catastrophic illness associated with the combination of clomipramine, phenelzine, and chlorpromazine. *Annals of Clinical Psychiatry, 4,* 81–85.

Stern, T.A., Herman, J.B., & Slavin, P.L. (Eds.). (1998). *The MGH guide to psychiatry in primary care.* New York: McGraw-Hill.

Sternbach, H. (1991). The serotonin syndrome. *American Journal of Psychiatry, 148,* 705–713.

Taylor, M.A., & Abrams, R. (1986). Cognitive dysfunction in mania. *Comprehensive Psychiatry, 27*(3), 186–191.

Chapter 29

Neuroimaging in Psychiatry

DARIN D. DOUGHERTY AND SCOTT L. RAUCH

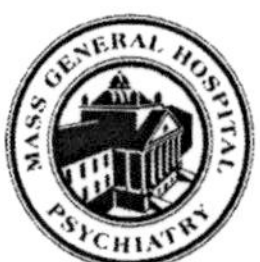

I. Introduction

In general, neuroimaging is used as an aid in the differential diagnosis of neuropsychiatric conditions; rarely does neuroimaging alone establish the diagnosis. When one is contemplating the use of neuroimaging, a variety of factors must be considered, including the indications, risks, costs, advantages, and limitations. This chapter reviews these factors and provides general guidelines for the use of neuroimaging in neuropsychiatric syndromes.

II. Modalities

A. Structural

1. **Computed tomography** (CT)
   a. Technology
      i. **CT uses X-rays that are differentially attenuated,** depending on the material through which they pass (higher attenuation in dense material, such as bone; lower attenuation in less dense material, such as air and fluid).
      ii. **CT uses serial X-rays acquired in an axial slab-wise (i.e., tomographic) manner.**
   b. **CT with contrast**
      i. Radiopaque iodine-based contrast material introduced intravenously **allows visualization of lesions that compromise the integrity of the blood-brain barrier** (e.g., cerebrovascular accident [CVA], tumor, inflammation).
      ii. **Contrast media** that enhance the visibility of pathology by CT **are either ionic or non-ionic.** Non-ionic contrast is many times more expensive than ionic contrast. However, **ionic contrast has a greater risk of side effects.**

         - **Idiosyncratic reactions occur in 5% of cases** and include hypotension, nausea, flushing, urticaria, and sometimes frank anaphylaxis. Risk factors include age of less than 1 year or greater than 60 years, and a history of asthma, allergies, cerebrovascular disease, or prior contrast reactions.
         - Chemotoxic reactions can occur in the brain and the kidney. **Chemotoxicity may present as impaired renal function or even renal failure,** with the main risk factor being pre-existing renal insufficiency. In the brain, **chemotoxic reactions manifest as seizures.** Such reactions occur in approximately 1 in every 10,000 cases, but develop in up to 10% of cases in which gross disruption of the blood-brain barrier is present.
   c. Newer CT Methods
      i. Spiral CT
      ii. CT angiography
   d. **Advantages and limitations**
      i. **CT offers excellent spatial resolution (< 1 mm).**
      ii. **CT is useful for the detection of acute bleeding** (less than 24–72 hours old), but is less helpful in subacute bleeding (more than 72 hours old) and in severely anemic patients (i.e., with a hemoglobin below 10 g/dL).
      iii. CT is not helpful in visualizing subtle white matter lesions.
      iv. CT uses ionizing radiation and so it is strongly contraindicated in pregnancy.
2. **Magnetic resonance imaging** (MRI)
   a. Technology
      i. **MRI exploits the magnetic properties of hydrogen atoms in water molecules to construct a representation of tissue.** Nuclei are excited; as they relax, they give off energy that is used to construct the images. Different components of the relaxation process exist and occur at different rates (called T_1 and T_2) in different tissues. Specific imaging parameters (T_1-weighted vs. T_2-weighted) are selected according to the clinical circumstances.

         - T_1-weighted images are used for optimal visualization of normal anatomy.
         - T_2-weighted images are used to detect areas of pathology.

      ii. **Diffusion-weighted imaging** (DWI) is a newer MRI technique that detects the tiny random movements of water molecules (diffusion) in tissue. This technique allows a map of the average apparent diffusion coefficient (ADC) to be calculated. Shortly after the onset of an ischemic stroke, the ADC of brain tissue is significantly reduced because of cytotoxic edema. Over several days, the rapid initial drop in ADC is followed by a return to "pseudonormal" values at approximately 1 week and then elevation above normal values subsequently. DWI is **remarkably sensitive in detecting and localizing acute ischemic brain lesions and allows differentiation of acute regions of ischemia from chronic infarcts.** DWI may soon become the modality of choice for clinical situations where acute ischemia is suspected.
   b. **MRI with contrast**
      i. **Gadolinium** is used as the contrast medium because of its paramagnetic properties. Like CT contrast, it is introduced intravascularly. The use of **MRI with con-**

trast material highlights vascular structures and aids in the detection of pathology in areas where blood vessel walls or the blood-brain barrier are compromised. Gadolinium causes fewer and less severe side effects than does CT contrast, with one reported death in over 5 million dosings.

c. **Advantages and limitations**

i. MRI provides **excellent spatial resolution and superior soft-tissue contrast** in comparison to CT (e.g., more useful for the visualization of white matter).

ii. MRI is **superior for surveying the posterior fossa and brainstem.**

iii. MRI does not use ionizing radiation, and so it is **preferable to CT in pregnancy** although it is still relatively contraindicated.

iv. MRI is **contraindicated in patients with metallic implants** for the following reasons:

- Metal can cause artifacts in MR images.
- Metal can shift position or absorb heat within the magnetic field, causing burn injuries.
- Mechanical devices, such as pacemakers, can malfunction within the magnetic field.

3. **CT versus MRI** (Table 29-1)

a. CT is more economical than MRI and is available at more centers.

b. CT is the modality of choice for patients with acute bleeds or acute trauma, **though DWI may soon become the modality of choice for assessing suspected acute brain ischemic events.**

Table 29-1. Summary Comparisons of CT and MRI

Consideration	*CT vs. MRI*
Economy	CT ≥ MRI
Availability	CT ≥ MRI
Speed	CT > MRI
Comfort	CT > MRI
Quality of visualization	
Bleeding	
Acute (< 48–72 h)	CT > MRI
Subacute (> 48–72 h)	MRI > CT
Ischemia	
Acute	DWI > MRI ≈ CT
Chronic	DWI ≈ MRI > CT
Bone	CT > MRI
Gray matter	MRI > CT
White matter	MRI > CT
Posterior fossa	MRI > CT
Spatial resolution	CT ≥ MRI

c. **MRI is superior to CT for the differentiation of white from gray matter and the identification of white matter lesions.**

d. **MRI is superior to CT for the detection of posterior fossa and brainstem pathology.**

e. CT is recommended if MRI is contraindicated (i.e., paramagnetic prostheses; inability to tolerate scanner time, noise, or confinement).

f. **MRI is recommended if radiation exposure is contraindicated** (i.e., young children or women of childbearing potential).

B. Functional

1. **Positron emission tomography** (PET)

a. Technology

i. **PET uses positron emission from administered radionuclides to measure cerebral blood flow** (e.g., oxygen-15) **or cerebral glucose metabolism** (e.g., fluorodeoxyglucose [FDG]), **both of which correspond to neuronal activity.**

ii. With PET one can use inhaled or intravenous radionuclides to look at the brain in the resting state or when activated by specific tasks.

iii. One can also use radioactive ligands to perform receptor characterization studies.

b. **Advantages and limitations**

i. PET is **the gold standard of functional neuroimaging modalities.**

ii. PET **offers excellent spatial resolution (4–8 mm).**

iii. PET **is very expensive and requires immediate access to the cyclotron,** which produces positron-emitting radionuclides.

2. **Single photon emission computed tomography** (SPECT)

a. **Technology**

i. **SPECT also uses radionuclides** (e.g., xenon-133, ^{99m}Tc-HMPAO) for functional imaging, but measures single photon emission rather than positron emission.

ii. As with PET, both inhaled and intravenous radionuclides are available, as are radioligands for measuring indexes of gross brain activity and performing receptor characterization.

b. **Advantages and disadvantages**

i. SPECT is **more affordable than PET** and does not require a cyclotron for production of radionuclides.

ii. SPECT **provides inferior spatial resolution (≥ 8 mm)** compared with PET.

iii. SPECT **resolution worsens as one attempts to image deeper brain structures.**

3. **PET versus SPECT** (Table 29-2)

a. **PET provides superior spatial resolution, especially for deeper brain structures.**

b. PET offers a broader array of radioligands for use in receptor studies and is the only modality that allows for the measurement of metabolism.

Table 29-2. Summary Comparisons of PET and SPECT

Consideration	*PET vs. SPECT*
Economy	
Institutional	SPECT » PET
Per scan	SPECT > PET
Availability	SPECT > PET
Spatial resolution	PET > SPECT
Temporal resolution	PET ≥ SPECT
Sensitivity	PET > SPECT
Signal/noise ratio	PET > SPECT
Variety of ligands	PET > SPECT

c. SPECT is less expensive than PET and is more widely available.

4. **Functional magnetic resonance imaging** (fMRI) **and magnetic resonance spectroscopy** (MRS)
   a. **These modalities remain research tools at this time,** although clinical applications are likely to evolve in the near future.

III. Indications

A. Structural

1. **Computed tomography**
   a. There have been numerous studies of the results of CT imaging in psychiatric populations. Across these studies, 12% of patients demonstrated focal abnormalities. **The likelihood of detecting an abnormal finding increased with age, with an abnormal neurologic examination, with an altered mental status, and with a history of head trauma or alcohol abuse.** Weinberger (1984) proposed **criteria for CT imaging in psychiatric settings:**
      i. **Confusion or dementia**
      ii. **New-onset psychosis**
      iii. **Movement disorder**
      iv. **Anorexia nervosa**
      v. **Prolonged catatonia**
      vi. **New-onset major affective disorder or personality change after age 50 years of age**
2. **Magnetic resonance imaging**
   a. When MRI became available in the 1980s, the neuroimaging literature reflected a shift toward the use of MRI in psychiatric populations.
   b. Many studies found an increased incidence of white matter lesions in psychiatric populations. However, **studies also revealed that 30% of normals over age 60 years have white matter abnormalities of no apparent clinical significance.**
   c. The largest study was done at McLean Hospital over a 5-year period and included all patients who received an MRI during that time (Table 29-3).

Table 29-3. Brain MRI Results in 6200 Psychiatric Inpatients: Unexpected and Potentially Treatable Findings

MRI Findings	*Number of Cases*	*%*
Multiple sclerosis	26	0.4
Hemorrhage	26	0.4
Temporal lobe cyst	22	0.4
Tumor	15	0.2
Vascular malformations	6	0.1
Hydrocephalus	4	0.1
Total	99	1.6

NOTE: Results from 6200 consecutive MR scans performed at McLean Hospital over a 5-year period. Patients receiving MR scans represent approximately 40% of the total number of patients seen during that period.

SOURCE: Adapted from Rauch, S.L., & Renshaw, P.F. (1995). Clinical neuroimaging in psychiatry. *Harvard Review of Psychiatry, 2,* 297–312.

   d. Finding a structural abnormality on neuroimaging is of questionable value if it does not alter the treatment or outcome.
3. **Pre-ECT therapy neuroimaging**
   a. Patients who require electroconvulsive therapy (ECT) often have a more treatment-refractory affective illness and may warrant a more thorough organic work-up.
   b. Pre-ECT neuroimaging may be helpful in identifying lesions that may lead to an adverse outcome with ECT (aneurysms, tumors, arteriovenous malformations, hydrocephalus, and basal ganglia infarction).
4. **General guidelines for structural neuroimaging**
   a. **Criteria**
      i. **Patients with acute changes in mental status** (including changes in affect, behavior, or personality) **plus one of three additional criteria:**
         - Age greater than 50 years
         - Abnormal neurologic exam (especially focal abnormalities)
         - **History of significant head trauma** (i.e., with extended loss of consciousness, neurologic sequelae, or temporarily related to mental status change in question)
      ii. New-onset psychosis
      iii. New-onset delirium or dementia of unknown cause
      iv. Prior to an initial course of ECT
   b. Considerations
      i. **Adherence to the criteria listed above should yield positive findings in 10–45% of cases. However, only 1–5% will produce findings that lead to specific medical intervention.**
      ii. If structural neuroimaging is indicated, one should use MRI unless the problem is an acute trauma, or if an acute bleed is suspected.

5. **Specific pathology**
   a. **Hydrocephalus**
      i. **In obstructive hydrocephalus, structural neuroimaging studies will reveal enlarged third and lateral ventricles,** small sulci, and possible lucencies at the tips of the ventricles that suggest obstruction of the aqueduct of Sylvius. Asymmetric ventricular enlargement suggests obstruction of the foramen of Monro or a portion of the ventricle.
      ii. **In non-obstructive hydrocephalus, structural neuroimaging will reveal enlargement of all four ventricles,** though the fourth ventricle will be less enlarged than the other ventricles.
   b. **Cerebral infarct**
      i. **Recent infarcts may not be demonstrable with early CT,** though there may be an irregular, low density in the region of the infarct. DWI shows promise in the diagnosis of acute cerebral infarction.
      ii. **Older infarcts are generally seen as sharp, semiregular areas of low density,** often abutting the cortical surface or the surface of a ventricle.
   c. **Cerebral hemorrhage**
      i. **Structural neuroimaging reveals a confluence of a dense area of blood with a surrounding rim of diminished density,** often with mass effect and blood in the subarachnoid space and ventricles.
      ii. Note that the scan may be normal in individuals with subarachnoid hemorrhage and lumbar puncture may be required for diagnosis.
   d. **Head trauma**
      i. **Structural neuroimaging of epidural hematomas is characterized by a lenticular-shaped, biconvex area of low density.**
      ii. **Structural neuroimaging of subdural hematomas is characterized by a crescent-shaped area of low density acutely and high density if chronic (aged blood).**
   e. **Calcification**
      i. If noted in the skull, possible etiologies include osteoma, Paget's disease, metastases, or meningioma.
      ii. **Calcification is normally found in the pineal gland, choroid plexus, habenula, and falx.**
      iii. **Calcification in other brain regions may indicate aneurysm, tumor** (especially meningioma, oligodendroglioma, or craniopharyngioma in the suprasellar region), **or infection** (especially fungal or parasitic).
   f. **Lytic lesions (holes) in the skull**
      i. **Single lytic lesions may indicate meningioma, hemangioma, or metastasis.**
      ii. **Multiple lytic lesions may be indicative of Paget's disease, myeloma, or metastases.**
   g. **White matter abnormalities**
      i. **May be indicative of multiple sclerosis, vasculitis, cerebritis, or leukoencephalitis.**

B. Functional

Most applications of functional neuroimaging in psychiatry occur in the field of research. However, a clinical role for functional neuroimaging in dementia and seizures is evolving and showing promise.

1. **Dementia**
   a. Characteristic neuroimaging profiles of various forms of dementia are emerging. **Some studies have indicated that functional neuroimaging can offer better than 90% sensitivity and specificity in distinguishing Alzheimer's disease from other kinds of dementia.**
   b. However, most forms of dementia are irreversible, and specific diagnoses may not affect the treatment. Furthermore, an adequate clinical examination often is the only thing necessary to reach a diagnosis of dementia.
2. **Seizures**
   a. Some seizures, especially complex partial seizures, are not always detected by the electroencephalogram (EEG). The EEG measures cortical surface electrical activity but it is less efficacious if the seizure focus is deep.
   b. **PET and SPECT images demonstrate ictal hyperactivity and interictal hypoactivity. This allows the detection of seizure foci during the predominant inter-ictal period.**
   c. To evaluate a possible seizure disorder, functional neuroimaging is performed in conjunction with EEG. **PET also is useful for more precise localization of seizure foci in a patient with a known seizure disorder** if neurosurgical intervention is indicated.
3. **Other**
   a. In addition, there is growing potential for the use of functional neuroimaging in the evaluation of movement disorders, stroke, and brain tumors.

IV. Psychiatric Neuroimaging Research

A. What Can We Measure?

1. **Structure**
   a. Volumetric parameters (morphometric MRI)
2. **Function**
   a. Indices of gross neuronal activity
      i. **Cerebral blood flow** (CBF)
         - SPECT: HMPAO
         - PET: oxygen-15 (water, CO_2, or butanol)
         - Functional MRI techniques can be divided into two classes:

         "Non-contrast" techniques that make use of endogenous physiological factors to detect changes in cerebral activation. This technique may use T_1-weighted pulse sequences to detect changes in blood flow or T_2-weighted pulse sequences to detect changes in the local concentration of paramagnetic deoxyhemoglobin (often referred to as "blood oxygen-level dependent" imaging, or BOLD).

"Contrast" techniques that utilize intravenous administration of a paramagnetic agent.

ii. **Glucose metabolism**

- PET: FDG

b. **Neurochemistry**

i. Receptor binding capacity: PET and SPECT

ii. Transmitter metabolism: PET

iii. Quantification of chemical concentrations: Magnetic Resonance Spectroscopy (MRS)

- Endogenous (e.g., *N*-acetylaspartate)
- Exogenous (e.g., fluoxetine, lithium)

B. Neuroimaging Research Paradigms

1. **Volumetric studies**

2. **Functional anatomy: PET, SPECT, fMRI**

a. Neutral state

b. Pre/post-treatment

c. Symptom provocation or symptom capture

d. Cognitive-behavioral activation

3. **Receptor characterization: PET, SPECT**

a. Pathophysiology

b. Candidate medications

4. **Moiety concentration quantification: MRS**

a. Endogenous

b. Exogenous

C. Neuroimaging and the Neurobiology of Psychiatric Diseases

1. **Dementias**

a. **Alzheimer's disease**

i. **Accelerated atrophy,** most prominent in temporal structures.

ii. **Hypoactivity in temporoparietal areas** bilaterally.

iii. Functional abnormalities may actually precede symptoms in asymptomatic individuals at genetic risk.

b. **Multi-infarct dementia**

i. **Multiple areas involved,** often both cortical and subcortical lesions with **patchy hypoactivity**

c. **Pick's disease**

i. **Frontotemporal wasting accompanied by frontotemporal hypoactivity**

ii. Often asymmetric or unilateral

d. **Parkinson's disease**

i. **Subtle nigrostriatal degeneration**

ii. **Hypoactivity exhibited in temporoparietal regions bilaterally**

iii. Most similar to Alzheimer's disease

e. **Huntington's disease**

i. **Striatal degeneration** with hypoactivity in striatum

f. **Progressive supranuclear palsy**

i. **Hypoactivity in frontal cortex**

2. **Major depression**

a. **Decreased dorsolateral pre-frontal cortical activity and increased ventral pre-frontal cortical activity** regardless of depressive subtype.

b. Magnitude of dorsolateral pre-frontal hypoactivity correlated to symptom severity.

c. **This hypoactivity resolves with resolution of symptoms.**

d. Increased amygdala activity as a trait phenomenon.

e. Anterior cingulate metabolism as a predictor of treatment response.

3. **Schizophrenia**

a. **Global volumetric abnormalities,** as well as decreased volume of left temporal lobe

b. **Decreased anterior to posterior activity ratio** (accentuated with frontal activation task, such as Wisconsin Card Sort)

c. **Increased basal ganglia to cortex activity ratio** (attenuated with neuroleptic treatment)

d. **Decreased frontal activity** correlated with negative symptoms

e. Hallucinations associated with activation in striatum, thalamus, limbic and paralimbic structures, as well as correspondent sensory cortex and language areas

f. Inconsistent findings regarding D_2 receptor density

4. **Anxiety disorders**

a. Inconsistent findings for panic disorder, generalized anxiety disorder, and simple phobia

b. Anxiety states non-specifically mediated by limbic and anterior paralimbic systems

c. **Obsessive-compulsive disorder** (OCD) studies yield convergent results

i. **Structural abnormalities involving caudate nucleus and white matter**

ii. Increased activity in components of a circuit implicated in the pathophysiology of OCD, including orbitofrontal cortex, caudate nucleus, thalamus, and anterior cingulate cortex

iii. Increased frontal and caudate activity normalize with successful treatment regardless of treatment modality (pharmacotherapy or behavioral therapy)

iv. Elevated anterior cingulate and orbitofrontal activities may predict poor treatment response

5. **Tourette's syndrome**

a. **Volumetric abnormalities in the striatum,** including replicated finding of rightward shift in lenticulate asymmetry.

b. Functional studies remain somewhat inconsistent, but converge to show hypoactivity within the basal ganglia.

c. Receptor studies implicate increased binding capacity of dopamine transporter sites.

6. **Attention deficit disorder** (ADD) **and attention deficit hyperactivity disorder** (ADHD)

a. **Volumetric abnormalities in the caudate,** with reduced and/or reversed laterality.

b. Functional studies have indicated a failure to normally recruit the anterior cingulate cortex during selective attention tasks.

c. Although stimulant medication has been shown to ameliorate symptoms, no specific or focal change in brain activity profile has been associated with stimulant treatment in ADD.

Suggested Readings

Albers, G.W. (1998). Diffusion-weighted MRI for evaluation of acute stroke. *Neurology, 51*(suppl. 3), S47–S49.

Bonte, F.J., Weiner, M.F., Bigio, E.H., et al. (2001). SPECT imaging in dementias. *Journal of Nuclear Medicine, 42,* 1131–1132.

Dougherty, D., & Rauch, S.L. (1997). Neuroimaging and neurobiological models of depression. *Harvard Review of Psychiatry, 5,* 138–159.

Dougherty, D.D., & Rauch, S.L. (2001). *Psychiatric neuroimaging research: Contemporary strategies.* Washington, DC: American Psychiatric Publishing.

Dougherty, D.D., Rauch, S.L., & Rosenbaum, J.F. (2003). *Essentials of neuroimaging for the practitioner.* Washington, DC: American Psychiatric Publishing.

Giedd, J.N., Blumenthal, J., Molloy, E., & Castellanos, F.X. (2001). Brain imaging of attention deficit/hyperactivity disorder. *Annals of New York Academy of Science, 931,* 33–49.

Hollister, L.E., & Shah, N.N. (1996). Structural brain scanning in psychiatric patients: A further look. *Journal of Clinical Psychiatry, 57,* 241–244.

Horowitz, A.L. (1992). *MRI physics for radiologists: A visual approach.* New York: Springer-Verlag.

Kasai, K., Shenton, M.E., Salisbury, D.F., et al. (2003). Progressive decrease of left superior temporal gyrus gray matter volume in patients with first-episode schizophrenia. *American Journal of Psychiatry, 160,* 156–164.

Kaufman, D.M. (2001). *Clinical neurology for psychiatrists* (5th ed.). Philadelphia, PA: W.B. Saunders.

Lyoo, I.K., & Renshaw, P.F. (2002). Magnetic resonance spectroscopy: Current and future applications in psychiatric research. *Biological Psychiatry, 51,* 195–207.

Malison, R.T., McDougle, C.J., Van Dyck, C.H., et al. (1995). [^{123}I]B-CIT SPECT imaging of striatal dopamine transporter binding in Tourette's disorder. *American Journal of Psychiatry, 152,* 1359–1361.

Osborn, A.G. (1994). *Diagnostic neuroradiology.* St. Louis, MO: Mosby Year Book.

Rauch, S.L., Jenike, M.A., Alpert, N.M., et al. (1994). Regional cerebral blood flow measured during symptom provocation in OCD using oxygen 15-labeled carbon dioxide and PET. *Archives of General Psychiatry, 51,* 62–70.

Rauch, S.L., & Renshaw, P.F. (1995). Clinical neuroimaging in psychiatry. *Harvard Review of Psychiatry, 12,* 297–312.

Reiman, E.M., Caselli, R.J., Yun, L.S., et al. (1996). Preclinical evidence of a genetic risk factor for Alzheimer's disease in apolipoprotein E type 4 homozygotes using PET. *New England Journal of Medicine, 324,* 752–758.

Renshaw, P.F., & Rauch, S.L. (1999). Neuroimaging in clinical psychiatry. In A.M. Nicholi, Jr. (Ed.), *The Harvard guide to psychiatry* (3rd ed.). Cambridge, MA: Belknap Press.

Silbersweig, D.A., Stern, E., Frith, C., et al. (1995). A functional neuroanatomy of hallucinations in schizophrenia. *Nature, 378,* 176–179.

Silverman, D.H., Small, G.W., Chang, C.Y., et al. (2001). Positron emission tomography in evaluation of dementia: Regional brain metabolism and long-term outcome. *Journal of the American Medical Association, 286,* 2120–2127.

Toga, A.W., & Mazziotta, J.C. (Eds.). (1996). *Brain mapping: The methods.* Boston, MA: Academic Press.

Weinberger, D.R. (1984). Brain disease and psychiatric illness: When should a psychiatrist order a CAT scan? *American Journal of Psychiatry, 141,* 1521–1527.

Chapter 30

Diagnostic Rating Scales and Psychiatric Instruments

David Mischoulon and Maurizio Fava

I. Introduction

A. Overview

When screening for psychiatric disorders, psychiatrists typically rely on information obtained from the clinical interview, from review of medical records, and from other sources. However, administration of various standardized diagnostic instruments can be helpful, and at times necessary. For example, the overwhelming majority of clinical research studies rely heavily on the use of diagnostic instruments. **In the clinical setting, a standardized questionnaire often serves as an adjunct to the clinical interview**, particularly in cases where the diagnosis is in doubt, or when the efficacy of a treatment is unclear. Psychiatric rating scales attempt to translate clinical observations into objective and (sometimes) quantifiable information. This chapter reviews some commonly used instruments and provides guidelines for the implementation of these instruments.

B. Uses for Diagnostic Psychiatric Instruments

1. To help ensure the accuracy of a diagnosis
2. To quantify the severity of symptoms
3. To quantify the effectiveness, or lack thereof, of a given treatment modality

C. Reliability and Validity

1. **Reliability refers to a scale's ability to convey consistent, reproducible information.** Diagnostic instruments are usually tested for their reliability by having more than one rater administer them, and then comparing the results (i.e., inter-rater reliability). If the instrument is designed to measure phenomena that are consistent over time, test-retest reliability is the measure used.
2. **Validity refers to the scale's ability to measure what it intends to measure.** For a diagnostic instrument to be valid, it must be reliable, although a reliable instrument may not necessarily be valid.

D. Types of Diagnostic Instruments: Self-Rated vs. Clinician-Rated

1. **Clinician-rated instruments.** These are diagnostic instruments that are administered by the clinician. These instruments are advantageous in that they are generally valid and reliable. Most diagnostic instruments are of this kind.
2. **Self-rated instruments.** These are instruments that the patient must complete. Self-rating scales have the advantage that they require less clinician time, which makes them especially useful for screening purposes. However, the reliability of self-rated scales is often difficult to assess, and some patients may be too impaired to complete them. The concordance rate between self-rating and observer scales is not well established.

E. Diagnostic Interviews

Structured clinical interviews were developed because of a perceived unreliability of psychiatric diagnoses. This problem was especially serious with regard to international studies, as psychiatrists from different countries or cultural backgrounds often had a different conceptualization of mental disorders. Several scales were developed, including:

1. The Present State Examination (PSE)
2. The Structured Clinical Interview for Axis I Diagnostic and Statistical Manual of Mental Disorders, Fourth Edition (SCID)
3. The Schedule for Affective Disorders and Schizophrenia (SADS)
4. The Diagnostic Interview Schedule (DIS)
5. The Composite International Diagnostic Interview (CIDI)
6. The Schedules for Clinical Assessment in Neuropsychiatry (SCAN)
7. The Mini-International Neuropsychiatric Interview (MINI)

The SCID will be reviewed here, as it is the most commonly used diagnostic instrument in psychiatry. The MINI will be reviewed as well.

II. General Psychiatric Diagnostic Instruments

A. The Structured Clinical Interview for DSM-IV (SCID)

1. **Overview of the SCID** (Note: the DSM-III-R version of SCID is still in use in research settings). **The SCID is essentially a semi-structured interview that applies DSM-IV criteria to a patient.** It is organized into modules that cover most of the major Axis I disorders (mood disorders, psychotic disorders, anxiety disorders, substance use disorders, somatoform disorders, post-traumatic stress disorder, adjustment disorders, and eating disorders).
2. **Administration of the SCID.** The SCID is administered by a clinician, sometimes as an exclusive diagnostic tool, often after the patient has already screened positive for a given disorder (e.g., depression) through a shorter, self-administered questionnaire (such as the Beck Depression Inventory). The SCID begins with a

general introductory section on demographics, general medical and psychiatric history, and use of medications. Questions here tend to be more open-ended. It then proceeds by modules to the different Axis I disorders. Questions here are asked exactly as written, and each is based on the individual criteria from DSM-IV. Answers are generally rated on a scale of 1–3 (1 = doubtful, 2 = probable, 3 = definite), and, based on the number of positive answers, a diagnosis is determined. A SCID-based interview may take up to 2 hours to complete, depending on how complicated a patient's history is, and on the patient's ability to provide a good history.

3. **Value of the SCID.** Because the SCID is a time-consuming instrument, **it is used almost exclusively in the research setting.** It is probably the most reliable means of diagnosing psychiatric disorders. In some instances, clinicians may use only a portion of the SCID, such as the mood disorder module.

B. The Mini-International Neuropsychiatric Interview (MINI)

1. **Overview and Administration of the MINI.** The MINI is a short, structured diagnostic interview for diagnosis of DSM-IV and ICD-10 disorders. It is similar to the SCID, and is administered by the clinician. **The MINI differs from the SCID in that it is more compact, and questions are answered on a "yes/no" basis rather than on a numerical scale**. The MINI can easily be administered in 15–30 minutes. Other differences from the SCID include the addition of a module on antisocial personality disorder and a section with detailed questions on suicidality. The MINI covers melancholic depression, but not atypical depression. There are a number of MINI-derived instruments, such as the MINI-Plus and the MINI-Kid.
2. **Value of the MINI.** The short and focussed, but accurate nature of the MINI, as well as its ease of administration, makes it especially useful in clinical trials, and in epidemiologic studies where a brief assessment may be required. Increasing numbers of researchers are implementing the MINI in randomized clinical trials. It may eventually find a niche in general clinical settings as well.

III. Depression Scales

A. Hamilton Rating Scale for Depression (HAM-D)

1. **Overview of the HAM-D. The HAM-D aims to quantify the degree of depression in patients who already have a diagnosis of major depression.** Questions focus on symptoms experienced only over the past week. It is administered by the clinician, and it generally does not require more than 20 minutes to complete. The HAM-D is a useful tool for measuring the progress of a patient during the course of treatment, in either the research or the clinical setting.
2. **Description of the HAM-D.** Several different versions of the HAM-D exist; they differ only in the number of questions included. The longest version includes 31 items; the shortest includes only six items. The longer versions include questions about atypical depression symptoms, psychotic symptoms, psychosomatic symptoms, and symptoms associated with obsessive-compulsive disorder (OCD). The standard form which is generally used in research studies is the 17-item Hamilton D (HAM-D-17).
3. **Scoring of the HAM-D.** There is a structured version of this instrument in which questions are asked exactly as written, and are rated on a scale of 0–4 or 0–2, depending on the answers given by the patient. Other versions allow more open-ended questioning. Scores on the HAM-D-17 typically fall into the following ranges:
   a. Not depressed: 0–7
   b. Mildly depressed: 7–15
   c. Moderately depressed: 15–25
   d. Severely depressed: over 25
4. **The HAM-D as a research tool.** Research studies rely on the Hamilton-D to quantify responses to a given treatment over time. Research studies will often cite a change in Hamilton-D score as a criterion for response. For example, a decrease of 50% or more in the Hamilton-D score is considered to be a positive response to treatment, whereas a score of 7 or less is considered typical of remission. The HAM-D is the most widely studied instrument for depression, and its reliability and validity are high.

B. Clinical Global Improvement (CGI) Scale

1. **Overview.** The CGI scale is a two-item instrument used as an adjunct in the treatment of psychiatric disorders. It is administered by the clinician after a history has been obtained, and after the HAM-D or other instruments have been completed and reviewed by the clinician. It measures, based on history and scores on other instruments:
   a. CGI-S (severity): the current condition of the patient on a scale of 1–7 (1 being normal, and 7 being among the most severely ill patients).
   b. CGI-I (improvement): the degree of improvement (as perceived by the clinician) since the start of treatment on a scale of 1–7, 1 being very much improved, and 7 being very much worse. Improvement in CGI ratings is also used in research to determine the degree of improvement over time with a given treatment.

C. Inventory of Depressive Symptomatology (IDS)

1. **Overview and Administration of the IDS. The IDS measures depressive signs and symptoms.** There is a clinician-administered version (IDS-C) and a patient administered self-report version (IDS-SR). There are 28-item and 30-item versions of these instruments.

The IDS has been shown to correlate well with the Hamilton-D scale, as well as the Beck Depression Inventory (BDI), but has the advantage of providing more thorough coverage of symptoms of atypical depression. **The IDS is thought to be a good instrument for measuring changes in symptom severity during antidepressant clinical trials.** It is thought to be useful for assessing most types of depression, including dysthymia.

D. Beck Depression Inventory (BDI)

1. **Overview of the BDI. This 21-item questionnaire for assessment of degree of depression is probably the most widely used self-rating scale;** it is self-administered by the patient, and can be completed in a few minutes. It is often used as a screening tool for determining the likelihood of a patient meeting criteria for major depression. A clinician may also use it to determine the degree of improvement over time. Questions are different from those found on the Hamilton-D, in that they focus more on cognitive symptoms of depression.
2. **Scoring of the BDI.** Patients generally must choose between four answers on each item (numbered 0–3 for degree of severity of depression). Scores correlate with severity of depression as follows:
   a. Normal: 0–7
   b. Mild depression: 7–15
   c. Moderate depression: 15–25
   d. Severe depression: over 25

The BDI has been shown to correlate well with the Hamilton-D and CGI, and, because of its sensitivity to change over time, it is often used in drug trials.

E. The Harvard Department of Psychiatry National Depression Screening Day Scale (HANDS) Scale

1. **Overview of the HANDS.** The HANDS questionnaire is a brief self-rating scale that a patient can self-administer in the office setting. It can be completed by the patient in a few minutes, and is then scored by the clinician. It is typically used as part of National Depression Screening Day, and by primary care physicians as an indicator for further evaluation of the patient, when depression is suspected.
2. **Scoring of the HANDS.** The screening form **includes 10 questions about symptoms of depression;** for each item, the patient must answer whether he or she feels this way "none or little of the time" (0 POINTS), "some of the time"(1 POINT), "most of the time" (2 POINTS), or "all of the time" (3 POINTS). Scores correlate with likelihood of depression as follows:
   a. Unlikely depression: below 8
   b. Likely depression: 9–16
   c. Very likely depression: 17–30

The HANDS questionnaire has been shown to be valid and reliable, but has not yet achieved widespread use in psychiatric research settings. It may prove very useful in the primary care setting, given its ease of administration. It is now routinely used in National Depression Screening Day.

IV. Schizophrenia Scales

A. Overview

The complexity of schizophrenia requires that clinicians use several different instruments to assess and study this illness. Scales have been designed to assess positive and negative symptoms, social and vocational adjustment, and medication side effects. **Virtually all schizophrenia scales must be administered by a clinician, as many patients would not be able to complete a self-rated form.**

B. Description of Scales

1. **Brief Psychiatric Rating Scale (BPRS).** The BPRS includes sixteen to twenty-four items, each rated on a scale of 1–7. Items primarily cover symptoms of psychosis, but also address depression, and anxiety symptoms. Ratings are expressed as a sum total of all items. The scale is brief and may be administered in 15–30 minutes. One limitation of the BPRS is that some definitions of items tend to be vague and are subject to interpretation. However, the scale has shown high inter-rater reliability.
2. **Positive and Negative Symptoms Scale (PANSS).** As its name implies, the PANSS, similar to the BPRS, focuses more on the positive and negative symptoms. This scale is frequently used in trials of antipsychotic drugs, largely because of its inclusion of negative symptoms. However, it requires more time to complete than does the BPRS. It has excellent inter-rater reliability and has been validated against other instruments.
3. **Scale for the Assessment of Positive Symptoms (SAPS).** The strength of the SAPS is its focus on formal thought disorder, which is less emphasized on the previously mentioned scales.
4. **Scale for the Assessment of Negative Symptoms (SANS).** The SANS was the first scale developed to assess negative symptoms, and it provides the standard against which other scales are compared. It focuses on five groups of symptoms, including alogia, affective flattening, avolition-apathy, anhedonia-asociality, and inattention. Ratings are based on clinical observations of the rater as well as of other staff and family members.

V. Anxiety Scales

A. Anxiety Disorder Interview Scale, Revised (ADIS-R)

The ADIS-R is a semi-structured interview used for arriving at DSM-III-R diagnoses of anxiety disorders. It provides information on panic, generalized anxiety, and phobic avoidance, and it also measures degree of disability. The scale includes the Hamilton-A and Hamilton-D scales for anxiety and depression, respectively. Its inter-rater reliability is high for most of the anxiety disorders, except generalized anxiety disorder (GAD).

B. Hamilton Rating Scale for Anxiety (HAM-A)
This is the most widely used scale for measurement of anxiety. It is used for patients with diagnosed anxiety disorders. It is similar to the HAM-D, in that it emphasizes somatic symptoms and experiences. It has reasonable validity and reliability.

C. Fear Questionnaire
This is a self-rated instrument used for assessing phobias, including agoraphobia, blood injury phobia, social phobia, and total phobia.

D. Yale-Brown Obsessive-Compulsive Scale (Y-BOCS)
The Y-BOCS is the most widely used scale for assessment of severity of obsessive-compulsive disorder (OCD) symptoms. It includes 10 items, and a symptom checklist. Inter-rater reliability is excellent. This scale has been used extensively in medication trials for measuring changes in severity of OCD symptoms.

VI. Mania Scales

A. Manic State Rating Scale (MSRS)
The MSRS is a 26-item scale; it is rated on a 0–5 scale, and is based on the frequency and intensity of symptoms, particularly elation-grandiosity and paranoid-destructiveness. The MSRS was designed primarily for use on inpatient units, and has been found to be reliable and valid.

B. Young Mania Rating Scale (Y-MRS)
This scale has 11 items, and is scored following a clinical interview. Four items (irritability, speech, thought content, and aggressive behavior) are given extra weight and scored on a 0–8 scale, whereas the other items are scored 0–4. The scale has a high inter-rater reliability; scores on the Y-MRS correlate well with length of hospital stay.

VII. Cognitive Impairment Scales

A. Overview
Cognitive scales are useful as an initial screen for organic psychopathology; results of these scales can help the clinician decide whether or not to request formal neuropsychological testing or imaging studies. These scales, however, may be influenced by the patient's intelligence, level of education, and literacy; consequently, clinicians need to be careful not to make erroneous conclusions based on scores of these scales.

B. Description of Scales

1. **Mini-Mental State Examination (MMSE). The MMSE is the most widely used instrument for measuring cognitive impairment.** It is a highly structured instrument, which may be administered by non-clinicians. It includes questions about orientation, memory, attention, naming, as well as ability to follow commands, write a sentence, and copy intersecting polygons. The MMSE may be administered in less than 10 minutes; it has established reliability and validity.
2. **Blessed Dementia Scale (BDS).** This instrument includes 50 items that assess orientation, recent and remote memory, and the ability to carry out activities of daily living. It is used primarily to diagnose Alzheimer's dementia.

VIII. Personality Disorder Scales

A. Overview
The accurate diagnosis of personality disorders is difficult under most circumstances. Most diagnostic scales have demonstrated poor reliability, largely due to the subjective quality of the criteria, patient unreliability, and the tendency for many patients to meet criteria for more than one disorder at a time. Diagnostic reliability of these scales needs to be improved.

B. Description of Scales

1. **Structured Clinical Interview for DSM-III-R Personality Disorders (SCID-II).** The SCID-II instrument is used for the diagnosis of personality disorders. As with the SCID-I, the SCID-II is organized around different personality disorders; questions are based on the criteria for each personality disorder, and are answered "yes" or "no." This instrument is time-consuming to administer; it is used almost exclusively for research purposes.
2. **Personality Disorder Examination (PDE).** The PDE is a lengthy and semi-structured interview consisting of 359 items; it is rated on a 3-point scale (absent, doubtful, or clinically significant). It requires 1–2 hours to complete and provides fairly rich information, which places less burden on the assessor's judgment.

IX. Substance Abuse Scales

A. CAGE Questionnaire
This brief instrument is widely used as a screening tool. The name of the scale is an acronym for:

1. Have you ever felt a need to cut down on drinking?
2. Have people annoyed you by criticizing your drinking?
3. Have you ever felt guilty about drinking?
4. Have you ever had an eye-opener?

Answering "yes" to two or more of these questions strongly suggests an alcohol-related problem, particularly in a male population.

B. Michigan Alcoholism Screening Test (MAST)
The MAST consists of 25 true-false questions that may be self-rated or administered by the clinician. Briefer versions have been developed, with comparable validity

to the original. The Drug Abuse Screening Test (DAST) is similar to the MAST, and may discriminate between alcohol and drug abusers.

C. Addiction Severity Index (ASI)

The ASI assesses severity of problems with drug and alcohol abuse, with medical illness, with the legal system, with the family system, as well as with one's system of support (social and employment). It appears to be a valid instrument that is useful in research as well as in treatment planning. It may be administered in less than an hour.

X. Social Functioning Scales

A. Overview

These scales are often used to assess the outcome of an illness or its overall effect on the patient.

B. Description of Scales

1. **Global Assessment of Functioning Scale (GAF).** The GAF is used on Axis V of the DSM-IV; it is based on collected information on psychological, social, and occupational function. It rates the patient on a scale of 1–100, with a higher score indicating higher function. Usually there are two ratings made: one for current function, and one for highest function in the past year.
2. **Social Adjustment Scale (SAS).** The SAS assesses social functioning during the past month. Subjects answer questions about work role, household role, parental role, extended family role, sexual roles, social and leisure activities, and overall well-being. This scale covers the widest domain of social function, but it may be less useful for severely dysfunctional patients, who may be unable to work and/or who have very limited social contacts.

XI. Drug Side Effect Scales

A. Abnormal Involuntary Movement Scale (AIMS)

The AIMS is **widely used to measure late-onset movement disorders**, such as tardive dyskinesia. Movements of the head, trunk, and extremities are observed, and rated on a scale of 1–5. It is routinely used in patients receiving antipsychotic medication; typically it is administered every 3–6 months.

B. The Udvalg for Kliniske Undersogelser (UKU) Scale

The UKU scale inquires about different psychotropic-induced side effects. It is composed of three sections. The first is a 48-item questionnaire that includes psychological, neurologic, and autonomic symptoms, among others, resulting from medications. Responses are rated on a scale from 0–3. The second section assesses the degree of interference that side effects cause in activities of daily living. The third section examines the consequences that the side effects have on continued treatment. It requires 30–60 minutes to administer, and is typically used in clinical trials for assessment of novel psychotropic medications.

XII. Conclusion

Diagnostic and psychiatric instruments can be useful diagnostic tools, both in psychiatric research as well as in the clinical setting. These tools may be used independently or in conjunction with a thorough clinical interview. They may serve to measure results in a research study, and to help the clinician ascertain the degree of illness and the response to treatment over time.

Suggested Readings

Andreasen, N.C. (1982). Negative symptoms in schizophrenia: Definition and reliability. *Archives of General Psychiatry, 39*, 784–788.

Baer, L., Jacobs, D.J., Meszler-Reizes, J., et al. (2000). Development of a brief screening instrument: The HANDS. *Psychotherapy and Psychosomatics, 69*, 35–41.

Beck, A.T., Ward, C.H., Mendelson, M., et al. (1961). An inventory for measuring depression. *Archives of General Psychiatry, 4*, 561.

Beigel, A., Murphy, D., & Bunney, W. (1971). The manic state rating scale: Scale construction, reliability, and validity. *Archives of General Psychiatry, 25*, 256.

Blessed, G., Black, S.E., Butler, T., & Kay, D.W. (1991). The diagnosis of dementia in the elderly. A comparison of CAMCOG (the cognitive section of CAMDEX), the AGECAT program, DSM-III, the Mini-Mental State Examination and some short rating scales. *British Journal of Psychiatry, 159*, 193–198.

Blessed, G., Tomlinson, B.E., & Roth, M. (1968). The association between quantitative measures of dementia and of senile change in the cerebral grey matter of elderly subjects. *British Journal of Psychiatry, 114*, 797–811.

Di Nardo, P., Moras, K., Barlow, D.H., et al. (1993). Reliability of DSM-III-R anxiety disorder categories. Using the Anxiety Disorders Interview Schedule-Revised (ADIS-R). *Archives of General Psychiatry, 50*, 251–256.

Endicott, J., Spitzer, R.L., Fleiss, J.L., & Cohen, J. (1976). The global assessment scale. A procedure for measuring overall severity of psychiatric disturbance. *Archives of General Psychiatry, 33*, 766–771.

Fenton, W.S., & McGlashan, T.H. (1992). Testing systems for assessment of negative symptoms in schizophrenia. *Archives of General Psychiatry, 49*, 179–184.

Folstein, M.F., Folstein, S.E., & McHugh, P.R. (1975). "Mini-mental state." A practical method for grading the cognitive state of patients for the clinician. *Journal of Psychiatric Research, 12*, 189–198.

Frank, E., Prien, R.F., Jarrett, R.B., et al. (1991). Conceptualization and rationale for consensus definitions of terms in major depressive disorder. Remission, recovery, relapse, and recurrence. *Archives of General Psychiatry, 48*, 851–855.

Goodman, W.K., Price, L.H., Rasmussen, S.A., et al. (1989). The Yale-Brown Obsessive Compulsive Scale. I. Development, use, and reliability. *Archives of General Psychiatry, 46*, 1006–1011.

Goodman, W.K., Price, L.H., Rasmussen, S.A., et al. (1989). The Yale-Brown Obsessive Compulsive Scale. II. Validity. *Archives of General Psychiatry, 46*, 1012–1016.

Gur, R.E., Mozley, P.D., Resnick, S.M., et al. (1991). Relations among clinical scales in schizophrenia. *American Journal of Psychiatry, 148*, 472–478.

Hamilton, M. (1959). The assessment of anxiety states by rating. *British Journal of Medical Psychology, 32*, 50.

Hamilton, M. (1960). A rating scale for depression. *Journal of Neurology and Neurosurgery in Psychiatry, 23*, 56–62.

Kay, S.R., Fiszbein, A., & Opler, L.A. (1987). The Positive and Negative Syndrome Scale (PANSS) for schizophrenia. *Schizophrenia Bulletin, 13*, 261–276.

Lewis, S.J., & Harder, D.W. (1991). A comparison of four measures to diagnose DSM-III-R borderline personality disorder in outpatients. *Journal of Nervous Mental Disorders, 179*, 329–337.

Lingjaerde, O., Ahlfors, U.G., Bech, P., et al. (1987). The UKU side effect rating scale. A new comprehensive rating scale for psychotropic drugs and a cross-sectional study of side effects in neuroleptic-treated patients. *Acta Psychiatr Scand, 334*(suppl), 1–100.

Loranger, A.W., Sartorius, N., Andreoli, A., et al. (1994). The International Personality Disorder Examination. The World Health Organization/Alcohol, Drug Abuse, and Mental Health Administration international pilot study of personality disorders. *Archives of General Psychiatry, 51*, 215–224.

Marder, S.R. (1995). Psychiatric rating scales. In H.I. Kaplan, & B.J. Sadock (Eds.), *Comprehensive textbook of psychiatry* (6th ed., pp. 619–635). Baltimore, MD: Williams and Wilkins.

Marks, I.M., & Matthews, A.M. (1979). Brief standard self-rating for phobic patients. *Behavior Research Therapy, 17*, 263–267.

Oldham, J.M., Skodol, A.E., Kellman, H.D., et al. (1992). Diagnosis of DSM-III-R personality disorders by two structured interviews: Patterns of comorbidity. *American Journal of Psychiatry, 149*(2), 213–220.

Overall, J.E., & Gorham, D.R. (1962). The Brief Psychiatric Rating Scale. *Psychology Report, 10*, 799.

Rush, A.J., Giles, D.E., Schlesser, M.A., et al. (1986, May). The Inventory for Depressive Symptomatology (IDS): Preliminary findings. *Psychiatry Research, 18*(1), 65–87.

Rush, A.J., Gullion, C.M., Basco, M.R., et al. (1996). The Inventory of Depressive Symptomatology (IDS): Psychometric properties. *Psychology in Medicine, 26*(3), 477–486.

Shear, M.K., & Maser, J.D. (1994). Standardized assessment for panic disorder research. A conference report. *Archives of General Psychiatry, 51*, 346–354.

Sheehan, D.V., Lecrubier, Y., Sheehan, K.H., et al. (1998). The Mini-International Neuropsychiatric Interview (M.I.N.I.): The development and validation of a structured diagnostic psychiatric interview for DSM-IV and ICD-10. *Journal of Clinical Psychiatry, 59*(suppl 20), 22–33; quiz 34–57.

Spitzer, R.L., Williams, J.B., Gibbon, M., & First, M.B. (1992). The Structured Clinical Interview for DSM-III-R (SCID). I: History, rationale, and description. *Archives of General Psychiatry, 49*, 624–629.

Williams, J.B. (1988). A structured interview guide for the Hamilton Depression Rating Scale. *Archives of General Psychiatry, 45*, 742–747.

Williams, J.B. (1990). Structured interview guides for the Hamilton Rating Scales. *Psychopharmacology Service, 9*, 48–63.

Williams, J.B. Gibbon, M., First, M.B., et al. (1992). The Structured Clinical Interview for DSM-III-R (SCID). II. Multisite test-retest reliability. *Archives of General Psychiatry, 49*, 630–636.

Young, R.C., Biggs, J.T., Ziegler, V.E., & Meyer, D.A. (1978). A rating scale for mania: Reliability, validity and sensitivity. *British Journal of Psychiatry, 133*, 429–435.

Zimmerman, M. (1994). Diagnosing personality disorders. A review of issues and research methods. *Archives of General Psychiatry, 51*(3), 225–245.

Chapter 31

Psychological Assessment

MARK A. BLAIS, STEVEN R. SMITH, AND SHEILA M. O'KEEFE

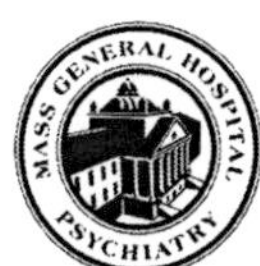

I. Introduction

The purpose of this chapter is to facilitate a better understanding of psychological assessment and testing. This will be accomplished by reviewing the methods used to construct valid psychological instruments, the major categories of psychological tests (including detailed examples of each category), and the application of these instruments in clinical assessment. In addition, issues related to the ordering of psychological testing and tips for understanding the final assessment report will be provided.

II. A Brief History of Modern Psychological Assessment

A. **In the late 1800s, the first generation of psychologists, such as Sir Francis Galton** (1822–1911), **focused their efforts on the measurement of sensorimotor functions** (e.g., reaction times) and tried to associate these measurements with life achievement (e.g., educational level, occupation, and social status).

B. **James McKeen Cattell,** an American psychologist, coined the term "Mental Test" in 1890.

C. At about the time that sensorimotor measurement was fading out, **Alfred Binet** (1857–1911) and **Theodore Simon** were commissioned by the French School Board to develop a test to identify students who might benefit from special education programs. **Binet's 1905 and 1908 scales form the basis of our current intelligence tests.** In fact, the development of Binet's 1905 scale marked the modern era of psychological testing.

D. The development of instruments to measure personality and psychopathology started around the time of the First World War. To aid in the war effort, **Woodworth developed a self-report test of psychopathology designed to screen army recruits** (called the Personal Data Sheet). Although this effort was unsuccessful, it provided the methodology for the later development of the Minnesota Multiphasic Personality Inventory (MMPI), a self-report test still in use today.

E. **Jung's Word Association Test** (1918) represents the prototype of the projective tests of psychopathology.

F. This was followed by both **Rorschach's Inkblot Test,** which was published in 1921, **and Murray's Thematic Apperception Test** (TAT), published in 1938. The second half of this century has seen intensive efforts focused on the further development of these initial breakthroughs.

III. Psychometrics and the Science of Test Development

A. Test Development Strategies

Three basic test development strategies have guided test construction: rational, empirical, and construct validation methods.

1. **Rational test construction relies on a theory of personality or psychopathology** (like the cognitive theory of depression) to guide item selection and scale construction. **Scales are developed that reflect a particular theory.**
2. **Empirically guided test construction uses a large number of items** (called an item pool) **and statistical tests to determine which items differentiate between well-defined groups of subjects** (this is called the empirical keying of items). The items that successfully differentiate one group from another are grouped together to form a scale regardless of their thematic content.
3. **The construct validation method combines aspects of both the rational and empirical test construction methodologies.** Within this framework, a large pool of items are written to reflect a theoretical construct (e.g., impulsivity), and then these items are tested to determine if they actually differentiate subjects who are either high or low on the construct (impulsive vs. nonimpulsive subjects). Items that successfully differentiate between the groups are retained for the scale. In addition, if theoretically important items do not differentiate between the two groups, this finding may lead to a revision in the theory. **The construct validation methodology is considered the most sophisticated strategy for test development.**

B. Reliability and Validity

To be useful, a psychological test must possess both adequate reliability and validity.

1. **Reliability represents the repeatability, stability, or consistency of a subject's test score. Reliability is usually represented as some form of a correlation coefficient ranging from 0 to 1.0.** Research instruments can have reliabilities as low as 0.70, while clinical instruments should have reliabilities in the high 0.80s to low 0.90s. This variation is because research instruments are interpreted as group measures, whereas clinical instruments are interpreted for a sin-

gle individual. A number of **reliability statistics** are available for evaluating a test:

a. **Internal consistency:** the degree to which the items in a test perform in the same manner.
b. **Test-retest reliability:** the consistency of a test score over time either a few days or a few weeks to a year later.
c. **Inter-rater reliability** for observer-judged rating scales; this is measured by Kappa, and reflects the degree of agreement between raters usually corrected for chance agreement.

Unreliability (the amount of error present in a test score) can be introduced by variability in the subject (subject changes over time), the examiner, or the test itself (given under different instruction).

2. **Validity** is a more difficult concept to understand and to demonstrate, than reliability. **The validity of a test reflects the degree to which the test actually measures the construct it was designed to measure.** Again, validity measures are usually represented as correlation coefficients ranging from 0 to 1.0. Multiple types of validity data are needed before a test can be considered valid.

Types of validity data include:

a. **Content validity,** which assesses the degree that an instrument covers the full range of the target construct (e.g., a test of depression that did not include items covering disruptions in sleep and appetite would have limited content validity).
b. **Predictive and concurrent validity,** which demonstrates how well a test either predicts future demonstration of the construct (predictive) or how well it correlates with other current measures of the construct (concurrent validity).
c. **Convergent and divergent validity,** which refers to the ability of a scale to demonstrate significant positive correlations with similar scales, while also having low or negative correlations with scales measuring unrelated traits. Taken together the convergent and divergent correlations indicate the specificity with which the scale measures the intended construct.

In a comprehensive review of the literature, Meyer et al. (2001) found that **psychological tests possess validity comparable to that of most widely used medical tests**. They also found that, in many circumstances, psychological tests provide **incremental validity** for detecting psychiatric disturbance over and above the diagnostic interview alone. However, it is important to realize that no psychological test is universally valid. Tests are considered valid or not valid for a particular purpose (e.g., detecting psychosis).

C. Definition of a Psychological Test

Ideally, a psychological test is a measurement tool made up of a series of standard stimuli (i.e., questions or visual stimuli). These test stimuli are administered following a standard format under a standard set of instructions. The patient's responses are recorded and scored according to a standardized methodology (insuring that a given response always scored the same way). The patient's test results are interpreted against a normative sample allowing for an accurate evaluation of the patient's performance.

IV. Major Categories of Psychological Tests

A. Intelligence Tests

1. **IQ testing.** Intelligence is a difficult construct to define and to measure. Wechsler wrote that "intelligence, as a hypothetical construct, is the aggregate or global capacity of the individual to act purposefully, to think rationally, and to deal effectively with the environment" (Matarazzo, 1979). This definition helps us see both what the modern tests of intelligence quotients (IQ) try to measure (adaptive functioning) and why intelligence or IQ tests can be important as aids in clinical assessment, particularly in treatment planning. If IQ reflects aspects of effective functioning, then IQ tests measure aspects of adaptive capacity. Although not the only tests available, the **Wechsler series** of IQ tests cover the majority of the human age range. The series starts with the **Wechsler Preschool and Primary Scale of Intelligence** (ages 4–6 years), progresses to the **Wechsler Intelligence Scale for Children-III** (5–16 years), and ends with the **Wechsler Adult Intelligence Scale-III** (16–89 years) (Wechsler, 1991, 1997). The recently developed **Wechsler Abbreviated Scale of Intelligence** (WASI; Wechsler, 1999) is a briefer scale of intelligence that provides an estimate of IQ based on two or four WAIS-III subtests thought to be central to the concept of intelligence.

   All the Wechsler scales provide **three major IQ tests scores: the Full Scale IQ, the Verbal IQ, and the Performance IQ.** All three IQ scores have a mean of 100 and a standard deviation (SD) of 15. This statistical feature means that a 15-point difference between a subject's Verbal IQ and Performance IQ can be considered both statistically significant and clinically meaningful. Table 31-1 presents an overview of IQ categories.

2. **Scoring of the IQ.** It is important to realize that IQ scores represent a patient's ordinal position, their percentile ranking as it were, on the test relative to the normative sample. These scores do not represent a patient's innate intelligence and there is no good evidence that they measure a genetically determined intelligence. They do reflect some degree of the patient's current adaptive functioning. Furthermore, because IQ scores are not totally reliable (all test scores contain some degree of unreliability) they should be reported with confidence intervals indicating the range of scores in which the subject's true IQ would fall.

   The Wechsler IQ tests are composed of 10 or 11 subtests which were developed to tap two intellectual

Table 31-1. IQ Categories with Their Corresponding IQ Scores and Percentile Distribution

Full-Scale IQ Score Percentile	*IQ Categories*	*Normal Distribution*
≥ 130	Very superior	2.2
120–129	Superior	6.7
110–119	High average	16.1
90–109	Average	50.0
80–89	Low average	16.1
70–79	Borderline	6.7
≤ 69	Mentally retarded	2.2

domains: **verbal intelligence** (vocabulary, similarities, arithmetic, digit span, information, and comprehension) and **non-verbal visual spatial intelligence** (picture completion, digit symbol, block design, matrix reasoning, and picture arrangement). Empirical studies have suggested that the Wechsler subscales can be re-organized to reflect three cognitive domains: verbal ability, visual-spatial ability, and attention and concentration (attention and concentration is tapped by the arithmetic, digit span, and by digit symbol subtests). Each of the Wechsler subtests is constructed to have a mean score of 10 and standard deviation of 3. Given this statistical feature we know that if two subtests differ by 3 or more scaled score points then the difference is significant. All IQ scores and subtest scaled scores are also adjusted for age.

B. Tests of Personality, Psychopathology, and Psychological Functioning

1. **Objective tests of personality and psychopathology.** Objective psychological tests, **also called self-report tests, are designed to clarify and quantify a patient's personality functioning and psychopathology.** Objective tests use a patient's response to a series of true/false or multiple choice questions to broadly assess psychological functioning. **These tests are called "objective" because their scoring involves little speculation.** Objective tests provide excellent insight into how the patient sees him- or herself and how he wants others to see and react to him.

   a. **The Minnesota Multiphasic Personality Inventory-2 (MMPI-2).** The MMPI-2 (Butcher et al., 1989) is a 567-item true/false, self-report test of psychological functioning. It was designed to provide an objective measure of abnormal behavior, to separate subjects into two groups (normals and abnormals), and then to further subcategorize the abnormal group into specific classes (Greene, 1991). The MMPI-2 contains **ten clinical scales** that assess major categories of psychopathology, and **three validity scales** designed to assess test-taking attitudes. MMPI-2 validity scales are **(L) Lie, (F) Infrequency, and (K) correction.** The MMPI-2 Clinical Scales include **(1) Hs, Hypochondriasis; (2) D, Depression; (3) Hy, Conversion Hysteria; (4) Pd, Psychopathic Deviate; (5) Mf, Masculinity/Femininity; (6) Pa, Paranoia; (7) Pt, Psychasthenia; (8) Sc, Schizophrenia; (9) Ma, Hypomania; and (0) Si, Social Introversion.** Over 300 "new" or experiential scales have also been developed for the MMPI-2. MMPI raw scores are transformed into T-score and a T-score of 65 or more indicates clinical psychopathology. The MMPI-2 is interpreted by determining the highest two or three scales, called a code type. For example, a 2-4-7 code type indicates the presence of depression (scale 2), anxiety (scale 7) and impulsivity (scale 4) and the likelihood of a personality disorder (Greene, 1991). (Computer scoring and interpretive reports for the MMPI-2 are available through NCS Assessments, P.O. Box 1416, Minneapolis, MN 55440, [1-800-627-7271].)

   b. **The Millon Clinical Multiaxial Inventory-III (MCMI-III).** The MCMI-III **is a 175-item true/false, self-report questionnaire designed to identify both symptom disorders (Axis I conditions) and personality disorders** (PDs) (Millon, 1994). The MCMI-III is composed of three Modifier Indices (validity scales), ten Basic Personality Scales, three Severe Personality Scales, six Clinical Syndrome Scales, and three Severe Clinical Syndrome Scales. **One of the unique features of the MCMI-III is that it attempts to assess both Axis I and Axis II psychopathology simultaneously.** The Axis II scales resemble, but are not identical to, the DSM-IV Axis II disorders. Computer scoring and interpretive reports are also available from NCS (see above). Given its relatively short length (175 items vs. 567 for the MMPI-2), the MCMI-III can have advantages in the assessment of patients who are agitated, whose stamina is significantly impaired, or who are just suboptimally motivated.

   c. **The Personality Assessment Inventory** (PAI) (Morey, 1991). The PAI is one of the newest objective psychological tests available. The PAI was developed using a construct validation framework with equal emphasis placed upon theory-guided item selection and the empirical functioning of the scales. The PAI **uses 344 items and a 4-point response format** (false, slightly true, mainly true, and very true) to make 22 non-overlapping scales. These 22 scales (4 validity scales, 11 clinical scales, 5 treatment scales, and 2 interpersonal scales) cover a range of clinically important Axis I and Axis II psychopathology and other variables relevant to interpersonal functioning and treatment planning (e.g., the PAI has scales designed to measure suicidal ideation, resistance to treatment, and aggression). The PAI possesses outstanding psychometric features and is an ideal test for broadly assessing multiple domains of relevant psychological functioning. (The PAI is marketed by Psychological Assessment Resources [PAR] P.O. Box 998, Odessa, FL 33556 [1-880-331-TEST].)

d. **Validity scales.** Certain response styles or sets can have a negative impact on the accuracy of a patient's self-report. **Validity scales are incorporated into all major objective tests to assess the degree to which a patient's response style may have distorted the findings of the self-report test. The three most typical response styles are careless or random responding (which may indicate that someone is not reading or understanding the test), attempting to "look good" by denying pathology, and attempting to "look bad" by over-reporting pathology (a cry for help or malingering).**

e. **Objective tests and the DSM-IV.** The computer-generated reports available from objective tests frequently provide suggested DSM diagnoses. At best these diagnoses are informed suggestions and at worse marketing gimmicks. **Psychological tests do not make clinical diagnoses, clinicians do.**

2. **Projective psychological tests.** Projective tests of psychological functioning differ from objective tests in that they **are less structured and require more effort on the part of the patient to make sense of, and to respond to, the test stimuli.** Even the instructions for the projective tests tend to be less specific than those of objective tests. As a result, **the patient is provided with a great degree of freedom to demonstrate his or her own unique personality characteristics and psychological organizing processes.** Although the objective test provides a view of the patient's "conscious" self-presentation, **the projective tests provide insights into the patient's typical style of perceiving, organizing and responding to ambiguous external and internal stimuli.** When combined together, data from objective and projective tests can provide a fairly complete picture or description of a patient's range of functioning.

a. **The Rorschach Inkblot Test.** The inkblot test, developed by Hermann Rorschach, is **a test of whole personality functioning** (Rorschach, 1942/1921). The Rorschach test **consists of ten cards** with inkblots on them (five are black and white, two are black, red and white, and three are various pastels) which are presented to the patient. The test is administered in two phases. First, the patient is presented with the ten inkblots one at a time and asked "what might this be." The responses are recorded verbatim and the examiner tries to get two responses to each of the first two cards. In the second phase, the examiner reviews the patient's responses and inquires **where on the card the response was seen** (known as "location" in Rorschach language) and **what made it look that way** (known as the "determinants") to the patient. For example, if a patient responded to card V with "A flying bat" (inquiry: "Can you show me where you see that?") "Here I used the whole card" ("What made it look like a bat?") "The color, the black made it look like a bat to me," this response would be coded: **Wo FMa.FC'o A P 1.0.**

In the past, Rorschach "scoring" has been criticized for being too subjective. However, over the last 20 years **John Exner, Jr.** (Exner, 1986, 1993) **and his colleagues have developed a Rorschach system (called the Comprehensive System) which has demonstrated acceptable levels of reliability.** Currently inter-rater Kappa scores of 0.80 or better are required for all Rorschach variables reported in published research studies. For comparison, Kappas in this range are equal to or better than the Kappas reported for structured interview DSM diagnoses. **Rorschach data are particularly useful for quantifying a patient's reality contact and the quality of their thinking.**

b. **Thematic Apperception Test (TAT).** The TAT **is useful in revealing a patient's dominant motivations, emotions, and core personality conflicts** (Murray, 1938). The TAT **consists of a series of 20 cards depicting people in various interpersonal interactions.** The cards were **intentionally drawn to be ambiguous.** The TAT is administered by presenting eight to ten of these cards, one at a time, with the instructions to **"Make up a story around this picture. Like all good stories it should have a beginning, middle, and an ending. Tell me how the people feel and what they are thinking."** While there is no one accepted standard scoring method for the TAT (making it more of a clinical technique than psychological test proper), when sufficient cards are present, reliable information can be obtained. A few standardized scoring methods have been developed for the TAT. However, these are limited to specific aspects of psychological functioning, such as level of defense operations and degree of psychological maturity. Psychologists typically assess TAT stories for:

i. Emotional themes
ii. Level of emotional and cognitive integration
iii. Interpersonal relational style
iv. View of the world (is it seen as a helpful or hurtful place). This type of data can be particularly useful in predicting a patient's response to psychotherapy and to the psychotherapist.

c. **Projective drawings.** Psychologists often employ projective drawings (free-hand drawings of human figures, or of a house, tree, and person) as a supplemental assessment procedure. They represent clinical techniques more than tests, as there are no formal scoring methods. In fact, the interpretation of these drawings often relies heavily upon psychoanalytic theory. Despite their poor psychometric properties, projective drawings can sometimes be very revealing. For example, psychotic subjects may produce human figure drawings that are transparent with internal organs. Still it is important to remember that projective drawings are less reliable and less valid than are other tests reviewed in this chapter.

3. **Behavior rating scales.** Behavior rating scales are the most commonly used form of measurement with children and adolescents. They are also useful for those populations that are unable to complete a self-report of personality, such as adults with severe psychotic disorders, dementia, or mental retardation. **Behavior rating scales have the benefits of being inexpensive, cost effective, and easy to administer.** Forms for teachers and parents allow psychologists to obtain ratings of patient behaviors that may differ across settings. Common examples of behavior rating scales are the **Child Behavior Checklist** (Achenbach, 1991), and the **Behavior Assessment System for Children** (Reynolds & Kamphaus, 1992).

V. Assessment of Children

Although advances in the psychological assessment of children have generally lagged behind those in adult assessment, more and more measures and procedures are being developed for use with younger patients. The assessment of children is often challenging due to several special issues, including difficulties with affective and cognitive labeling, developmental fluctuations, cognitive development, familial context, and reliance on others for accurate reporting. The **Rorschach Inkblot Test** can be used with children as young as five years, and TAT-style story-telling tests, such as the **Roberts Apperception Test** and the **Children's Apperception Test,** are very common. Projective drawing techniques, such as **House-Tree-Person** and **Kinetic Family,** are also used with young and non-verbal children. Several child and/or adolescent self-report measures are also available including the **MMPI-Adolescent** (Butcher et al., 1992), the **Youth Self-Report** (Achenbach & Edelbrock, 1991), and the **Personality Inventory for Youth** (Lachar & Gruber, 1995). However, as is stated earlier, the most common form of measurement with children is behavior rating scales.

VI. The Assessment Consultation Process and the Report

A. Obtaining the Assessment Consultation

The referral of a patient for an assessment consultation should be like the referral to any professional colleague. Psychological testing cannot be done "blind." The psychologist will want to hear relevant information about the case and will explore with you what question(s) you want answered (this is called the **referral question**) by the consultation. **Based upon this case discussion, the psychologist will select an appropriate battery of tests designed to obtain the desired information.** Most comprehensive psychological test batteries will include self-report (and/or parent report if the patient is a child) and projective measures of personality, as well as a measure of overall cognitive ability. Differing perspectives allow for a more comprehensive and valid picture of the patient's functioning.

It is helpful if you prepare your patient for the testing by reviewing with him or her why the consultation is desired and that it will likely take a few, perhaps three, hours to complete. You should expect the psychologist to evaluate your patient in a timely manner and to provide you with verbal feedback (a "wet read") within a few days after the testing. The written report should be available within two weeks.

B. Using the Test Results

You should review the relevant findings from the consultation with your patient. This helps confirm for the patient the value of the testing and the time they invested in it. If either you or your patient have any questions about the findings you should contact the psychologist for clarification. Ultimately, if necessary, the psychologist should be willing to meet with you or with the patient to explain the test results. It is generally not a good idea for the patient to read the professional report.

C. Understanding the Assessment Report

The report is the written statement of the psychologist's findings. It should be understandable and it should plainly state and answer the referral question(s). **The report should contain the following information:**

1. **Relevant background information**
2. **A list of the procedures used in the consultation**
3. **A statement about the validity of the test results and the confidence the psychologist has in the findings**
4. **A detailed description of the patient, based upon test data**
5. **Recommendations drawn from the test findings**

The test findings should be presented in a logical manner providing a rich integrated description of the patient (not a description of the individual test results). It should contain some raw data (e.g., IQ scores). This will allow any follow-up testing to be meaningfully compared to the present findings. It should close with a list of recommendations. To a considerable degree the quality of a report (and a consultation) can be judged from the recommendations provided. A good assessment report should contain a number of useful recommendations. You should never read just the summary of a test report; this results in the loss of important information, as the whole report is already a summary of a very complex consultation process.

Suggested Readings

Butcher, J., Dahlstrom, W., Graham, J., et al. (1989). *MMPI-2: Manual for administration and scoring*. Minneapolis: University of Minnesota Press.

Costa, P., & Widiger, T. (2002). *Personality disorders and the five factor model of personality* (2nd ed.). Washington, DC: American Psychological Association.

Exner, J. (1986). *The Rorschach: A comprehensive system* (Vol. 1 basic foundations, 2nd ed.). New York: Wiley & Sons.

Exner, J., (1993). *The Rorschach: A comprehensive system* (Vol. 1, 3rd ed.). New York: Wiley.

Greene, R. (1991). *The MMPI-2/MMPI: An interpretive manual.* Boston, MA: Allyn and Bacon.

Groth-Marnat, G. (1997). *Handbook of psychological assessment* (3rd ed.). New York: Wiley.

Hathaway, S.R., & McKinley, J.C. (1943). *The Minnesota Multiphasic Personality Inventory* (rev. ed.). Minneapolis: University of Minnesota Press.

Kamphaus, R.W., & Frick, P.J. (1996). *Clinical assessment of child and adolescent personality and behavior.* Needham Heights, MA: Allyn & Bacon.

Maruish, M. (1999). *The use of psychological testing for treatment planning and outcome assessment.* New Jersey: Lawrence Erlbaum Associates.

Matarazzo, J. (1979). *Wechsler's measurement and appraisal of adult intelligence.* New York: Oxford University Press.

Meyer, G.J., Finn, S.E., Eyde, L.D., et al. (2001). Psychological testing and psychological assessment: A review of evidence and issues. *American Psychologist, 56*(2), 128–165.

Millon, T. (1994). *Millon Clinical Multiaxial Inventory-III Manual.* Minneapolis, MN: National Computer Systems.

Morey, L. (1991). *The Personality Assessment Inventory: Professional manual.* Odessa, FL: Psychological Assessment Resources.

Murray, H. (1938). *Explorations in personality.* New York: Oxford University Press.

Wechsler, D. (1991). *Manual for the Wechsler Intelligence Scale for Children-III.* New York: Psychological Corporation.

Wechsler, D. (1997). *Manual for the Wechsler Adult Intelligence Scale* (3rd ed.). New York: Psychological Corporation.

Wechsler, D. (1999). *Wechsler Abbreviated Scale of Intelligence [WASI].* New York: Psychological Corporation.

Chapter 32

Neuropsychological Assessment

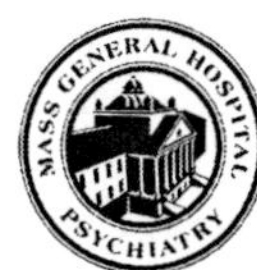

MARK A. BLAIS, JANET C. SHERMAN, AND DENNIS K. NORMAN

I. Introduction

Neuropsychology is a science dedicated to the study of brain-behavior relationships. In its clinical practice, neuropsychology is concerned with the behavioral expression of brain dysfunction. The aspect of behavior that is the focus of a neuropsychological assessment is cognition, with **the neuropsychologist's primary goal to establish which aspects of cognitive functioning are impaired for a patient, and which aspects are preserved.** The neuropsychologist relies on numerous reliable and well-standardized techniques in measuring a spectrum of cognitive behaviors. **The pattern of cognitive strengths and weaknesses identified in a neuropsychological evaluation can provide important information regarding the nature of the neurological impairment and its etiology and can also provide important prognostic and practical information** that can be utilized to inform possible therapeutic programs aimed at recovery of function.

II. History of Neuropsychological Tests

Neuropsychology and the field of neuropsychological assessment represent relatively recent developmental lines within applied psychology. The term "neuropsychology" was first introduced into psychological parlance by Karl Lashley (1936). Early approaches to the understanding of brain damage treated it as a unitary phenomenon of "organicity." Based on this approach, the assumption was made that some sort of common functional deficit would underlie all forms of cerebral dysfunction, with the concomitant assumption that patients with brain damage could be assessed and diagnosed based on a single test (e.g., Bender-Gestalt Test). As the scientific understanding of brain-behavior relationships improved, the global concept of "organicity" was increasingly seen as limited, with the recognition that **organic impairment could be present in a variety of cognitive functions.** This more advanced understanding of brain functioning and damage led psychologists to seek assessment instruments that could evaluate specific cognitive functions and possible sources of cognitive deficits. With this increased understanding as well as a greater need for neuropsychological assessment during World War II due to soldiers suffering head wounds, **Halstead (1947) developed one of the first neuropsychological test batteries. Reitan (1986) later refined this series of tests into the battery known today as the Halstead-Reitan (H-R) Neuropsychological Test Battery.**

III. Current Approaches to Neuropsychological Assessment

The modern neuropsychologist is trained to assess brain-behavior relationships utilizing a range of standardized neuropsychological instruments. Most neuropsychologists today utilize a **composite test battery, characterized by a range of tests that are designed to measure specific cognitive functions. The choice of particular tests utilized varies with the individual patient and the nature of the disorder.** In contrast to this approach, fixed batteries are also currently utilized.

A. The H-R battery is the oldest standardized neuropsychological assessment battery. **The H-R battery is an elaborate and time-intensive set of neuropsychological tests.** It was developed from over 27 tests used by Halstead in the 1940s to measure cerebral functioning and biological intelligence. The Halstead battery was refined by Reitan, and today **the standard H-R battery consists of eight core tests, with supplemental tests being added as indicated.** Analysis of an H-R battery is almost exclusively quantitative. The H-R profile is **interpreted at four levels:**
   1. Impairment Index (a composite score reflecting the subject's overall performance)
   2. Lateralizing
   3. Localizing signs
   4. Pattern analysis for inferences of etiology (see Reitan, 1986).

B. **The Luria-Nebraska Battery (L-NB)** was developed in an attempt to standardize the innovative work of Luria and his Russian colleagues. Although Luria's work represents a thorough and well-conceptualized approach to neuropsychological assessment, the degree to which the L-NB had been successful in standardizing this approach is not clear. **The L-NB is not widely used in the United States** and a number of prominent U.S. neuropsychologists have criticized the L-NB, suggesting that it is diagnostically unreliable.

C. **A newer and more flexible approach** to neuropsychological assessment is **The Boston Process Approach.** In this approach a **small core test battery** (usually containing one of the Wechsler IQ tests) **is administered and hypotheses regarding cognitive deficits are developed based on the patient's per-**

formance. Other instruments then are administered to test out and refine these hypotheses about the patient's cognitive deficits. The Boston approach focuses on both **quantitative** and **qualitative** aspects of a patient's performance, with the qualitative focus on the manner or style of the patient's performance, not just its accuracy. According to this approach, **review of how a patient failed an item or test can be more revealing than whether the item was passed or failed.** In this way the Boston approach reflects an integration of features from behavioral neurology and psychometric assessment.

IV. Goals of a Neuropsychological Assessment

The main goal of a neuropsychological evaluation is to relate a patient's test performance to both the functional status of their central nervous system (CNS) and their real world functional capacity. These questions arise for **any patient who has suffered neurological disease or damage, and for whom there is a question of possible behavioral dysfunction.** Individuals referred for a neuropsychological evaluation cover the entire age span, and include individuals with both **acquired impairments** and **developmental impairments. Acquired impairments are those deficits brought about by brain disease or damage, typically occurring after the CNS has already developed.** Included in this class of impairments are cerebral vascular accidents, head injury, dementing illnesses, toxic and viral conditions. Note that acquired impairments are more common in the adult than in the pediatric population. Moreover, the characteristics of acquired impairments in children are different than in adults with generalized CNS insults far more common in childhood and localized cerebral pathologies more common in adulthood. In addition, recovery profiles differ in the two populations due to both the greater plasticity of the brain in childhood as well as the greater vulnerability of the developing versus the mature brain. **Developmental impairments arise when the brain fails to develop normally, the cause of which is often unknown.** These disorders, which are far more common within the pediatric population than are acquired impairments include learning disabilities, attention deficit hyperactivity disorder, pervasive developmental disorder, and mental retardation. Questions concerning the functional impact of developmental disorders arise for adults as well as children, as the consequences of these impairments can become more apparent with increased school or work demands in adulthood.

The specific goals of a neuropsychological assessment include the following:

A. Diagnosis

The assessment seeks to determine if the patient's test performance provides evidence to suggest the presence of cortical damage or dysfunction; to localize cortical damage based on behavioral deficits (although given sophisticated neuroimaging techniques, this goal is less critical than in the past); to distinguish different neurological conditions based on the behavioral data; and to discriminate between psychiatric vs. neurological symptoms.

B. Prognosis

Cognitive deficits have been found to be highly predictive of a patient's outcome (Keefe, 1995). The precision of the data also allows for patients' neuropsychological status to be followed during the course of a disease over time (e.g., cognitive decline in the case of a dementia; recovery of function following surgical or psychopharmacologic intervention).

C. Patient Care and Planning

The precise descriptive information regarding a patient's cognitive status that is provided by a neuropsychological assessment can help in the appropriate management of many neurological disorders. Management questions where a neuropsychological assessment can be helpful include those pertaining to a patient's capacity for self-care, ability to benefit from a therapeutic program, ability to return to work, ability to make financial or legal decisions, and ability to make judgements required when driving. The information provided by a neuropsychological assessment can also be used to determine how a rehabilitation program should be structured. Finally, neuropsychological test results can be used to help improve self-awareness and to set realistic goals by informing a patient and their family members of a patient's cognitive strengths and limitations.

V. Methods Used in a Neuropsychological Assessment

The neuropsychologist relies on multiple sources of information, including the patient's history (i.e., medical, education, personal), qualitative observations of the patient's behavior, and quantitative methods (specifically tests designed to assess an individual's behavior in an objective and formalized manner). Tests used in a neuropsychological assessment have the following important characteristics: They are norm-referenced, and allow the examinee's performance to be compared with individuals who share important demographic characteristics with the patient (e.g., age, education, gender); they rely on standard scores (with raw test scores transformed to have a given mean and standard deviation), and standardized methods, such that tests are administered and scored in the same manner across all individuals in different settings. It is important to note that **the usefulness of neuropsychological test data can be limited by the quality of the norms employed.** Unfortunately, the quality of norms varies greatly from test to test. In a composite test battery, tests are chosen to sample a wide range of behaviors to obtain a comprehensive assessment of an individual's cognitive status. In assessing a patient with an acquired impairment, the neuropsychologist must also estimate the patient's pre-morbid level of cognitive functioning. Given that direct data (i.e., test scores obtained prior to onset of disease) are rarely available, the neuropsychologist relies on indirect methods in this determination. These methods include obtaining historical and observational data, including information regarding a patient's educational and occupational history, and using the "present ability approach," based on the fact that brain damage does not uniformly impact all aspects of cognitive functioning. Certain aspects of cognitive functioning, in particular vocabulary knowledge, and reading abilities tend to be resistant to effects of neurologic disease, thus providing a relatively reliable estimate of premorbid level of functioning.

A neuropsychological assessment includes assessment of intellectual functioning (IQ testing). Intelligence quotient (IQ) is a derived score used in many test batteries designed to measure a hypothesized general ability. While there is considerable controversy regarding what intelligence tests measure, there is a solid scientific basis for IQ testing, which has been shown to be the best available long-range predictor of outcome and adjustment. Within neuropsychology, it is important to recognize the important role that IQ testing plays as well as to recognize its limitations. Intelligence testing is essential in assessing individuals with developmental impairments, as it addresses the question of whether the child's deficit are more global or specific in nature. In acquired impairments, intelligence testing plays a valuable role in helping to determine the individual's overall level of cognitive functioning. However, it is important to recognize that IQ scores do not bear a direct relationship to size of brain lesion and they are often impervious to certain neuropsychological deficits. The most commonly used IQ measures (Wechsler Scales of Intelligence) include Verbal and Performance IQ scores, which provide a "rough" measure of left and right hemisphere functions.

In addition to the assessment of intelligence, a complete neuropsychological evaluation includes assessment of different aspects of cognitive functioning, including (1) attention and concentration, (2) language (expressive and receptive), (3) memory (immediate and delayed), (4) visual-spatial constructional, and (5) executive functioning and abstract thinking. Neuropsychological evaluations covers similar areas to those assessed in the mental status examination used in neurology and psychiatry, differing mainly in that it provides a more comprehensive, less subjective, and better quantified assessment of the major cognitive functions.

Below, we review some of the specific neuropsychological tests that might be used to compose a battery or to assess specific cognitive functions. (For a description of these tests see Lezak [1995] and Spreen and Strauss [1998].)

A. Attention and Concentration

Attention and concentration are **central to most complex cognitive processes,** and are among the most commonly impaired functions associated with brain damage. Some patients who complain of memory disorders are found to have impaired attention and concentration rather than memory dysfunction. Aspects of attention typically assessed in a neuropsychological assessment include measures of attentional capacity (e.g., digit span), sustained attention (e.g., continuous performance measures), divided attention (e.g., Paced Auditory Serial Addition Test), visual scanning (e.g., letter cancellation tasks; Trail Making Test, Part A), and alternating attention (e.g., Trails B).

B. Receptive and Expressive Language

Because of the importance of documenting deficits in communication skills secondary to brain insults, the evaluation of language functioning is an important part of a neuropsychological assessment. Language measures included in a neuropsychological evaluation assess **single word comprehension, confrontation naming, reading decoding, reading comprehension, verbal fluency, and writing. Frequently used measures of language functioning are the WAIS-III Verbal IQ Subtests, the Boston Naming Test, Controlled Oral Word Association Test (F-A-S; Category Fluency), reading (North American Adult Reading Tests [NAART], Gates or Nelson-Denny Reading Comprehension tests), and written expression (a writing sample).**

C. Memory Functioning

The assessment of memory is an essential component in a neuropsychological battery as impaired memory is both a major reason for referral and a strong predictor of treatment outcome. Memory impairment is also the hallmark and one of the earliest neuropsychological impairments in cortical dementia (i.e., dementia of the Alzheimer's type). Normative data utilized in a neuropsychological assessment can be extremely helpful in distinguishing age-related memory changes from those that characterize a dementia, and can also help distinguish memory complaints that accompany depression (pseudodementia) from those of dementia. **An evaluation of memory includes both assessment of visual and auditory memory, immediate and delayed recall (usually with a 30-minute delay), assessment of the pattern and rate of new learning, and explores whether memory impairments are due to difficulties with encoding, recall or retrieval deficits. A determination of the aspect of memory that is impaired provides important diagnostic information** (e.g., with frontal amnesia associated with impairments in encoding and impaired retention and retrieval of information associated with temporolimbic amnesia). Tests of memory commonly used in a neuropsychological assessment are reviewed below.

1. **The Wechsler Memory Scale-III (WMS-III)** (Wechsler, 1997) is one of the principal memory inventories. The WMS-III is composed of 11 subtests tapping auditory and visual memory at both immediate and 30-minute delayed recall. It also provides indications of auditory and visual learning efficiency (new learning ability). Like the Wechsler IQ scales, this memory test is well standardized. The age-adjusted mean performance for the major memory scores is set at 100 with a standard deviation of 15. The memory subscales all have a mean of 10 and a standard deviation of 3. These statistical properties allow for a fairly detailed evaluation of memory functioning. In fact, in the most recent revision of the Wechsler IQ and Memory Scales, these tests are co-normed, allowing for a meaningful comparison between IQ and memory performance.
2. The **Three Shapes and Three Words Memory Test** is **a less demanding test of language-based (written) and visual memory.** This brief test also provides measures of learning rate, and immediate and delayed recall phases; however, it is not well normed (Weintraub & Mesulam, 1985).

D. Visual-Spatial Constructional Ability

Many aspects of visual perception and construction can be impaired in acquired and developmental disorders. Assessment of these functions provides information as to the integrity of the right parieto-temporo-occipital network processing. These tests assess a patient's ability to make basic perceptual distinctions, including visual scanning and visual recognition (i.e., object or face recognition) and visual organization (ability to make sense of incomplete, ambiguous or fragmented visual stimuli). Ability to integrate visual and motor skills, typically assessed in visual construction tasks provides information concerning an individual's visual organization strategies as well as more basic perceptual and motor skills. **Tests that tap visual-spatial functioning include the Rey-Osterreith Complex Figure Test, Benton Visual Form Discrimination Test, Benton Judgement of Line Orientation Test, Hooper Visual Organization Test, and the Performance IQ Subtests of the WAIS-III.**

E. Executive Functions and Abstract Thinking

Executive functioning **refers to a number of higher-order cognitive processes, such as judgment, planning, logical reasoning, and the modification of behavior (or thinking) based upon external feedback.** These functions, associated with functioning of frontal-subcortical network processing are critical in enabling a person to engage in independent and purposive behaviors. Individuals with impaired executive functioning, even in the face of preserved cognitive functioning, may be incapable of self-care, working, or maintaining normal social relationships. Tests used to assess executive functioning must be novel, complex tasks that require the individual to integrate information. Tests commonly used to assess executive functioning are reviewed below.

1. One of the most frequently used tests of executive functioning is the **Wisconsin Card Sorting Test** (WCST), an abstract problem-solving task that requires the patient to sort 128 response cards that vary in three dimensions (color, form, number). The patient is not told the sorting criteria, nor is s/he told that the sorting criteria shift during the test. Instead, the patient must determine the predetermined correct responses based on the examiner's limited corrective feedback ("right" or "wrong" to each sort). One of the primary scores from the WCST is the number of perseverative errors committed, providing a measure of the patient's cognitive flexibility.
2. Other tests of executive functioning include **The Booklet Category Test,** the **Stroop Color Word Test,** and the **Similarities and Comprehension Subtests of the WAIS-III** (which provide information about abstract reasoning). Also, the patient's ability to utilize organizational strategies on complex learning tasks, such as **The California Verbal Learning Test-II** and the **Rey Complex Figure,** provide important information regarding executive functions.

F. Motor and Sensory Functioning

Measures of tactile sensitivity and motor strength and speed have long been important in the clinical or bedside neurological examination. Neuropsychologists also measure these functions, employing more sensitive instruments that allow a patient's performance to be compared to standardized norms. **Typically, neuropsychologists are interested in both the absolute magnitude of the patient's performance (how well did they perform compared to the test's norms) and any noted differences between the two body sides (the left-right discrepancies).**

1. **Tests of motor functioning** include the **Finger Tapping Test** (the average number of taps per 10 seconds with each hand), **Hand Dynamometer** (a test of grip strength), and **Grooved Pegboard Test** (a test of fine motor dexterity and speed).
2. **Sensory ability tests** include **Finger Localization Tests** (naming and localizing fingers on the subject's and examiner's hand) and **Two-Point Discrimination** and **Simultaneous Extinction test** (measures two-point discrimination threshold and the extinction or suppression of sensory information by simultaneous bilateral activation).

G. Emotional Function

Many psychiatric conditions, particularly anxiety and depression, can produce transient neuropsychological deficits. Therefore, depending on the referral question, a neuropsychological assessment may also include a self-report test of psychopathology, such as the MMPI-2 (see chapter 31), Beck Depression Inventory, and/or Beck Anxiety Scales. Including such tests in the battery allows the neuropsychologist to evaluate the possible contribution of psychopathology to the cognitive profile.

VI. Brief Neuropsychological Assessment Tools

A number of brief neuropsychological assessment tools are used in clinical practice today. Brief assessment tools are not a substitute for a comprehensive neuropsychological assessment, but they can be useful as screening instruments or when patients can not tolerate a complete test battery. Two such brief tests are the **Dementia Rating Scale (DRS)-II and the Neurobehavioral Cognitive Status Examination** (known as the **COGNISTAT**). **These tests provide a reasonable and brief assessment of the major areas of cognitive functioning (attention, memory, language, reasoning, and construction). Both tests employ a screening methodology** to evaluate these cognitive domains, with the patient first being presented with a moderately difficult item, and, if that item is passed, the rest of the items in that domain are skipped (with the examiner moving on to the next domain). However, if the screening item is failed, then a series of items are given to the patient to evaluate more fully the specific cognitive ability.

A. The **DRS-II is a useful tool for assessing elderly** (65 years and up) **patients who are suspected of having dementia of the Alzheimer's type (DAT).** The total score and the scores from the Memory and Initiation/Perseveration subscales have been shown to be useful in identifying patients with DAT. The DRS was designed to a low performance "floor." This means that the test contains many items tapping low levels of functioning, which allows the test to track patients further as their functioning declines. This quality makes the DRS a useful tool for monitoring DAT patients throughout their illness.

B. The **COGNISTAT** is conceptually similar to the DRS; however, it **was designed to be used with younger adults** (20–66 years old). This test **provides a rapid and standardized measure of the major areas of cognition.** It is a helpful tool for screening psychiatric patients for cognitive deficits and for assessing patients who are unable or unwilling to complete a comprehensive assessment battery.

VII. Common Neuropsychological Assessment Referral Questions

A. Depression vs. Dementia

The differentiation of depression from dementia in the elderly **is the most common neuropsychological referral question** (see chapter 31 for a discussion of "referral question"). Depression in the elderly is often accompanied by apparent cognitive deficits, making the diagnostic picture somewhat confused with that of early dementia. By evaluating the profile of deficits obtained across a battery of tests a neuropsychologist can help establish the differences between these two illnesses. For example, a depressed patient tends to have problems with attention, concentration, and memory (new learning and retrieval), whereas a patient with early dementia has problems with delayed recall memory (encoding) as well as word-finding or naming problems early on, attention and concentration are relatively preserved in patients with DAT. Each type of patient can display problems with frontal lobe/executive function. However, the memory performance in the depressed patient will often improve with cues or strategy suggestions while this typically does not help the patient with dementia. Although this general pattern will not always be true, it is this type of contrasting performance that allows neuropsychological assessment to aid in differential diagnosis.

B. Independent Living

Whether a patient is capable of living independently is a complex and often emotionally charged question. Neuropsychological test data provides one line of information needed to make a reasonable medical decision. In particular, **neuropsychological test data regarding memory functioning (both new learning rate and delayed recall) and executive functioning (judgment and planning) have been shown to predict failure and success in independent living.** However, any neuropsychological test data should be thoughtfully combined with information from an occupational therapy (OT) evaluation, assessment of the patient's psychiatric status, and family input (when available) before rendering any judgment about a patient's capacity for independent living.

C. Attention Deficit Disorder (ADD)

Neuropsychological assessment has a role in the diagnosis and treatment of adults and children with ADD. However, as with assessment of independent living status, it provides just a piece of the data necessary for diagnosing ADD. **The evaluation of ADD should include a detailed review of academic performance, including report cards and school records. When possible, parents should also be interviewed for their recollections of the patient's childhood behavior. The neuropsychological evaluation should focus upon measuring intelligence, academic achievement (expecting to see normal or better IQ with reduced academic achievement), and multiple measures of attention and concentration (with tests of passive, active [shifting] and sustained attention).** Although the neuropsychological testing profile might aid in the diagnosis of ADD in adulthood, the diagnosis can usually be made solely on historical data and symptom checklists. The neuropsychological test data or profile is often more useful in helping the patient, the family, and the treater understand the impact of ADD on the structure and organization of the patient's current cognitive abilities, as well as ruling out common co-morbid disorders, such as learning disabilities. Also, an understanding of the patient's cognitive strengths and weaknesses can be used to guide recommendations regarding possible interventions and accommodations.

D. Neuropsychological Assessment and Treatment Planning

Neuropsychological assessments can often aid in the treatment planning of patients with moderate to severe psychiatric illness. While this aspect of neuropsychological testing is somewhat under-utilized at present, in the years to come this may prove to be the most beneficial use of these tests. Neuropsychological assessment facilitates treatment planning by providing objective data and the test profile regarding the patient's cognitive skills (deficits and strengths). **The availability of such data can help clinicians and family members have more realistic expectations about the patient's functional capacity** (Keefe, 1995). This can be particularly helpful for patients suffering from severe disorders (e.g., schizophrenia). The current literature indicates that neuropsychological deficits are more predictive of long-term outcome in schizophrenic patients than are either positive or negative symptoms.

VIII. The Neuropsychological Assessment Report

In contrast to the written report following a personality assessment (reviewed in chapter 31), the written neuropsychological testing report tends to be less integrated. **The test findings are provided and reviewed for each major area of cognitive functioning (intelligence, attention, memory, language, reasoning, and construction). These reports typically contain a substantial amount of data (both raw and standardized scores)** which is crucial for meaningful retesting comparisons. However, the neuropsychological assessment report should provide a brief summary reviewing and integrating the major findings and also contains useful/meaningful recommendations. As with all professional consultations, the examining psychologist should be willing to meet with you and/or your patient to review the findings and their implications.

Suggested Readings

Keefe, R. (1995). The contribution of neuropsychology to psychiatry. *American Journal of Psychiatry, 152,* 6–14.

Kolb, B., & Whishaw, I.Q. (1996). *Fundamentals of human neuropsychology* (4th ed.). New York: W. H. Freeman and Company.

Lezak, M. (1995). *Neuropsychological assessment* (3rd ed.). New York: Oxford University Press.

Matarazzo, J. (1979). *Wechsler's measurement and appraisal of adult intelligence.* New York: Oxford University Press.

McCarthy, R.A., & Warrington, E.K. (1990). *Cognitive neuropsychology: A clinical introduction.* San Diego, CA: Academic Press.

Milberg, W., Hebben, N., & Kaplan, E. (1986). The Boston process neuropsychological approach to neuropsychological assessment. In I. Grant, & K. Adams (Eds.), *Neuropsychological assessment of neuropsychiatric disorders.* New York: Oxford University Press.

Reitan, R. (1986). Theoretical and methodological bases of the Halstead-Reitan neuropsychological test battery. In I. Grant, & K. Adams (Eds.), *Neuropsychological assessment of neuropsychiatric disorders.* New York: Oxford University Press.

Rentz, D.R. (2002, May). *Neuropsychological assessment of dementia.* Presented at Dementia: A Comprehensive Update. Cambridge.

Shallice, T. (1990). *From neuropsychology to mental structure.* New York: Cambridge University Press.

Snyder, P.J., & Nussbaum, P.D. (Eds.). (1998). *Clinical neuropsychology: A pocket handbook for assessment.* Washington, DC: American Psychological Association.

Spreen, O., & Strauss, E. (1998). *A compendium of neuropsychological tests.* (2nd ed.). New York: Oxford University Press.

Storand, T.M., & Vanden Bos, G. (1994). *Neuropsychological assessment of dementia and depression in older adults: A clinician's guide.* Washington, DC: American Psychological Association.

Wechsler, D. (1997). *Manual for the Wechsler Adult Intelligence Scale* (3rd ed.). New York: Psychological Corporation.

Wechsler, D. (1997). *Wechsler memory scale* (3rd ed.). New York: Psychological Corporation.

Weintraub, S., & Mesulam, M.-M. (1985). Mental state assessments of young and elderly adults in behavioral neurology. In M.-M. Mesulam (Ed.), *Principles of behavioral neurology.* Philadelphia: F. A. Davis.

Yozawitz, A. (1986). Applied neuropsychology in a psychiatric center. In I. Grant, & K. Adams (Eds.), *Neuropsychological assessment of neuropsychiatric disorders.* New York: Oxford University Press.

Chapter 33

Laboratory Tests and Diagnostic Procedures

MENEKSE ALPAY AND LAWRENCE PARK

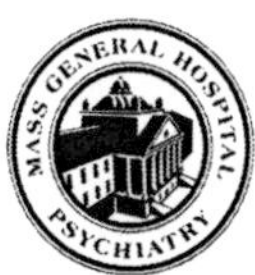

I. Introduction

A. Diagnoses in psychiatry are made by identification of symptom patterns that constitute psychiatric illnesses, as outlined in the *Diagnostic and Statistical Manual, Fourth Edition* (DSM-IV). They are not based on objective, biologically based tests and procedures. These procedures are used to exclude organic etiologies for psychiatric presentations, to help with the clinical diagnosis, and to monitor illness progression.

B. In the past, numerous attempts have been made to correlate psychiatric illnesses with certain biological tests, such as the dexamethasone suppression test (DST) in patients with depression. However, despite extensive research on the DST and other biological tests, a sensitive and reliable test for major depression has yet to be developed; in fact, a "gold standard" biological test or procedure does not exist for any psychiatric diagnoses.

C. Advances in technology have yielded powerful new methods of examination (e.g., neuroimaging, biochemical and genetic marker analysis). Advances in these techniques may fundamentally change our understanding of psychological states, and change how psychiatry is practiced.

This chapter covers the wide range of tests and procedures currently used for psychiatric assessment.

II. Diagnostic Tests

A. Overview

The initial and most important steps in any psychiatric assessment are a compilation of a comprehensive history, a physical examination, and a mental status examination. A carefully conducted initial assessment serves to characterize the nature of psychiatric symptomatology, to suggest an underlying organic etiology, and to direct further tests and studies. A carefully elicited history may reveal evidence of medical conditions, substance-related effects, history of medical or psychiatric illness, family history of medical or psychiatric illness, or psychosocial stressors that could precipitate or aggravate psychiatric symptoms. Physical examination may reveal further signs and symptoms indicative of an underlying medical condition.

B. In general, the initial onset of psychiatric symptoms after the age of 40 years suggests an organic etiology. A history of chronic medical illness, medication use, or alcohol or drug use raises the possibility of recurrence of an illness that presents with neuropsychiatric symptoms. A family history of certain genetic psychiatric illnesses (e.g., bipolar disorder or schizophrenia), or certain heritable medical conditions (e.g., Huntington's disease), is suggestive that these conditions are related to the presentation. The presence of endocrine and metabolic disorders (e.g., thyroid dysfunction, pheochromocytoma) also needs to be taken into consideration when making a psychiatric diagnosis.

C. Physical examination provides information that may facilitate making either a primary psychiatric diagnosis or an underlying medical diagnosis. Particularly important elements of the physical exam include vital signs and examination of the neurological and cardiac systems.

1. Elevated temperature (as well as a decreased temperature in infants and the elderly) indicates possible infectious etiology. If significant temperature abnormalities are present, localizing signs should be assessed to ascertain the location of the infection. Significantly elevated temperature, given the appropriate clinical circumstances, could also suggest neuroleptic malignant syndrome.
2. Body habitus (including weight and height) may indicate eating disorders.
3. Blood pressure and pulse are important as they serve as markers for cardiovascular function, and for adequate cerebral perfusion.
4. Assessment of level of consciousness can facilitate the diagnosis of a subdural hematoma.
5. Examination of the skin may reveal stigmata of syphilis, liver dysfunction, chronic alcohol use, or intravenous drug administration. New lesions may indicate recent trauma. Previous lesions may be examined to ascertain the severity of past attempts at self-injury.
6. Pupillary examination aids in the diagnosis of substance (particularly opiates) intoxication or withdrawal.
7. Chvostek's sign is an indication of hypocalcemia.
8. A Kayser-Fleisher ring around the pupil is a sign of Wilson's disease.
9. Papilledema, as seen on funduscopic examination, is associated with increased intracranial pressure.
10. In regard to examination of the neck, a positive Kernig or Brudzinski sign may suggest meningitis.
11. Palpation of the thyroid should be conducted to assess for any change in size or consistency, which might suggest thyroid dysfunction.

12. Respiratory and cardiac examinations assess the overall oxygenation of the body (including the brain). Any instability in either system could suggest possible cerebral hypoxia. In addition, respiratory and cardiac examination are important in distinguishing anxiety and panic from primary anxiety syndromes, and medical conditions, such as mitral valve prolapse or pheochromocytoma.
13. Examination of the abdomen may yield clues about possible renal, hepatic, gastrointestinal, or urinary tract involvement.
14. Neurological deficits are often associated with psychiatric presentations. Certain physical deficits may represent underlying focal lesions (e.g., vascular events, tumors) that could also explain psychiatric symptoms. In addition, certain other neurologic illnesses (e.g., seizure disorders, Parkinson's disease, Huntington's disease, multiple sclerosis) may have associated neuropsychiatric manifestations.

D. **The mental status examination is central to the initial evaluation insofar as it characterizes the nature of the patient's mental state. In addition, certain findings may be suggestive of organic dysfunction.**
1. Decline in level of consciousness or agitation may indicate a state of delirium with an underlying organic etiology.
2. Decline in memory or cognition may represent dementia.
3. Impairments of speech, cognition, or behavior may implicate specific areas of brain dysfunction.
4. Discrete psychiatric symptoms (such as visual hallucinations, delusions, and illusions) are also suggestive of an organic etiology.

III. Types of Studies

A. Laboratory Tests

The most common studies used by psychiatrists are laboratory tests, including analyses of serum chemistries and drug levels (see Tables 33-1 and 33-2). In addition, **endocrine studies** may be particularly important for those with a psychiatric presentation (see Table 33-3). **Serological studies,** including those for syphilis, human immunodeficiency virus (HIV), hepatitis, and rheumatic diseases, may help to detect infectious/immune-mediated etiologies of psychiatric presentations (see Table 33-4). **Hematological studies** include a complete blood count (CBC), erythrocyte sedimentation rate (ESR), bleeding studies, d-dimer, and Coombs test (see Table 33-5). **Analysis of other bodily fluids** (urine, cerebrospinal fluid [CSF]) **and stool** may be indicated as well (see Table 33-6).

B. Other Techniques

1. **Radiologic techniques**
2. Tests of cardiac function include an **electrocardiogram (EKG), echocardiography, and Holter monitoring.**
3. Tests of respiratory function include an **arterial blood gas (ABG), pulse oximetry, and pulmonary function tests.**
4. **Vascular studies,** such as carotid and/or transcranial Doppler ultrasonography, may be used to assess the integrity of the vascular system.
5. Other studies, such as **electroencephalography (EEG), electrophysiology, and polysomnography,** assess the function of the central (CNS) and peripheral nervous systems.

IV. Routine Screening and Test Choice

A. **In general, the decision to order a test should revolve around the likelihood that a test will be abnormal, as well as the clinical importance of an abnormal (or normal) result.** No clear consensus about routine screening for psychiatric presentations in medically healthy patients has been established.

In clinical practice routine screening tests include: CBC, serum chemistries, ESR, vitamin B_{12}, folate, thyroid stimulating hormone level (TSH), and rapid plasma reagen (RPR). The list of studies with relevance to psychiatric presentations is large. Table 33-7 presents studies that one might consider for the initial work-up of psychiatric symptoms.

B. **Beyond the initial routine screening, any further studies should be based on the specific clinical situation.** In those with a history of high-risk behaviors and a positive RPR, HIV infection should be assessed. A history of significant weight loss may indicate occult malignancy or infection and may require further work-up. In a malnourished patient, nutritional assessment, including the level of vitamins and minerals, should be assessed. Patients may demonstrate a decreased ESR in anorexia nervosa, while an increased aldolase may be present in bulimia; a positive phenolphthalein assay in stool or urine may indicate laxative abuse. Women of childbearing age should be assessed for pregnancy.

C. **Psychosis**

Initial presentation of psychotic symptoms warrants a full organic work-up. Multiple causes of psychosis must be excluded, including CNS lesions, CNS infections, seizure disorders, toxic effects of drugs, alcohol withdrawal, and metabolic or endocrine abnormalities. **Work-up should include comprehensive laboratory testing, lumbar puncture and CSF analysis, syphilis serology, neuroimaging, and an EEG.**

Table 33-1. Serum Chemistries

Test	*Indication*	*Comments*
Alanine aminotransferase (ALT)	Medical work-up	↑ Hepatitis, cirrhosis, liver metastasis ↓ Pyridoxine (B_6) deficiency
Albumin	Medical work-up	↑ Dehydration ↓ Malnutrition, hepatic failure, burns, multiple myeloma, carcinomas
Aldolase	Ψ: Eating disorders	↑ Ipecac abuse, schizophrenia
Alkaline phosphatase	Medical work-up Ψ: Psychotropic medication use	↑ Paget's disease, hyperparathyroidism, hepatic disease/metastases, heart failure, phenothiazine use ↓ Pernicious anemia (B_{12} deficiency)
Ammonia	Medical work-up	↑ Hepatic encephalopathy/failure, Reye syndrome, GI hemorrhage, severe congestive heart failure (CHF)
Amylase	Ψ: Eating disorders	↑ Bulimia nervosa
Aspartate aminotransferase (SGOT/AST)	Medical work-up	↑ CHF, hepatic disease, pancreatitis, eclampsia, cerebral damage, alcohol
Bicarbonate	Ψ: Panic, eating disorders	↑ Bulimia, laxative abuse, psychogenic vomiting ↓ Hyperventilation, panic, anabolic steroid use
Bilirubin, total	Medical work-up	↑ Hepatic, biliary, pancreatic disease
Bilirubin, direct	Medical work-up	↑ Hepatic, biliary, pancreatic disease
Blood urea nitrogen	Medical work-up Ψ: Psychotropic medication use	↑ Renal disease, dehydration, lethargy, delirium
Calcium	Medical work-up Ψ: Mood disorders, psychosis, eating disorders	↑ Hyperparathyroidism, bone metastasis ↑ Mood disorders, psychosis, eating disorders ↓ Hypoparathyroidism, renal failure ↓ Depression, irritability, delirium, chronic laxative use
Carbon dioxide	Ψ: Panic, eating disorders	↓ Hyperventilation, panic, anabolic steroid abuse/use
Ceruloplasmin	Medical work-up	↓ Wilson's disease
Chloride	Ψ: Eating disorders, panic	↓ Bulimia, psychogenic vomiting ↑ (Mild) hyperventilation, panic
Creatinine phosphokinase (CK, CPK)	Medical work-up Ψ: NMS, physical restraint, substance abuse	↑ Neuroleptic malignant syndrome (NMS), IM injection, rhabdomyolysis, restraints, dystonic reactions ↑ Antipsychotic use
Creatinine	Medical work-up	↑ Renal disease
Ferritin	Medical work-up	↓ Iron deficiency (most sensitive test)
Folate	Ψ: Alcohol, medications	↓ Psychosis, paranoia, fatigue, agitation, dementia, delirium ↓ Alcoholism, phenytoin, oral contraceptive estrogen
γ-Glutamyltranspeptidase (GGT)	Medical work-up Ψ: Alcohol	↑ Alcohol, cirrhosis, liver disease
Glucose	Medical work-up Ψ: Panic, anxiety, delirium, depression	↑ Delirium ↓ Delirium, agitation, panic, anxiety, depression
Iron-binding capacity	Medical work-up	↑ Fe deficiency anemia
Iron, total	Medical work-up	↓ Fe deficiency anemia

(continued)

Table 33-1. *(Continued)*

Test	*Indication*	*Comments*
Lactate dehydrogenase (LDH)	Medical work-up	↑ Myocardial infarction, pulmonary infarction, hepatic disease, renal infarction, seizures, cerebral damage, pernicious anemia; associated with RBC destruction
Magnesium	Medical work-up Ψ: Alcohol	↓ Alcohol; associated with agitation, delirium, seizures, ↑ Panhypopituitarism
Phosphorus	Medical work-up	↑ Renal failure, diabetic acidosis, hypoparathyroidism, hypervitaminosis D ↓ Cirrhosis, hyperparathyroidism, hypokalemia, panic, hyperventilation
Potassium	Medical work-up Ψ: Eating disorder	↑ Hyperkalemia acidosis, anxiety in cardiac arrhythmia ↓ Cirrhosis, metabolic alkalosis, laxative abuse, diuretic abuse, bulimia, psychogenic vomiting, anabolic steroid use
Protein, total	Medical work-up Ψ: Psychotropic medication use	↑ Multiple myeloma, myxedema, SLE ↓ Cirrhosis, malnutrition, overhydration May affect protein-bound medication levels
Sodium	Medical work-up Ψ: Use of lithium	↓ Hypoadrenalism, myxedema, CHF, diarrhea, polydipsia, carbamazepine (CBZ) use, SIADH, anabolic steroid use ↓ More sensitive to lithium use
Uric acid	Medical work-up	↑ Gout, hematological disorders, renal disorders, endocrine disorders, hypertension, Lesch-Nyhan
Vitamin A	Medical work-up	↑ Hypervitaminosis A, depression, delirium
Vitamin B_{12}	Medical work-up Ψ: Dementia, mood disorder	↓ Megaloblastic anemia, dementia, psychosis, paranoia, fatigue, agitation, dementia, delirium

SOURCE: Rosse, R.B., Deutsch, L.H., & Deutsch, S.I. (1995). Medical assessment and laboratory testing in psychiatry. In H.I. Kaplan, & B.J. Sadock (Eds.), *Comprehensive textbook of psychiatry*. Baltimore, MD: Williams and Wilkins.

↑, increase in lab value; ↓, decrease in lab value; Ψ, psychiatric indication.

SIADH, syndrome of inappropriate antidiuretic hormone.

D. Depression

Depression is a common psychiatric symptom. Even though it is often a primary psychiatric symptom, depression may also be associated with a number of medical conditions (e.g., thyroid dysfunction, folate deficiency, Addison's disease, rheumatoid arthritis, systemic lupus erythematosus [SLE], Parkinson's disease, dementia, and the use of certain medications and drugs).

E. Anxiety

Anxiety can be associated with a wide range of organic etiologies as well. Underlying medical conditions that may account for anxiety symptoms include seizure disorders, post-concussive syndrome, thyroid dysfunction, parathyroid dysfunction, hyperadrenalism, hypoglycemia, pheochromocytoma, drug effects, alcohol or barbiturate withdrawal, cardiac disease (e.g., myocardial infarction [MI], mitral valve prolapse), respiratory compromise (e.g., chronic obstructive pulmonary disease), menopause, and porphyria. **To exclude these organic causes, work-up may include pertinent laboratory testing, serum glucose or glucose tolerance testing, endocrine testing, a cardiac work-up, respiratory function tests, a chest X-ray, urine vanillymandelic acid [VMA], urine porphyrins, and an EEG.**

V. Special Populations

A. The Pediatric Population

In pediatric patients, psychiatric symptoms are relatively uncommon. When psychiatric problems occur in children, they are often secondary to organic etiologies. For instance, changes in mental status may occur from infec-

Table 33-2. Serum Toxicology

Class	*Substance*	*Presentation*
Drugs	Alcohol	Intoxication: delirium, psychosis, mood disturbance, anxiety, sexual dysfunction, sleep disturbance Withdrawal: delirium, psychosis, mood disturbance, anxiety, sleep disturbance Persistent use: dementia, amnesia
	Amphetamines	Intoxication: delirium, psychosis, mood disturbance, anxiety, sexual dysfunction, sleep disturbance Withdrawal: mood disturbance, sleep disturbance
	Caffeine	Intoxication: anxiety, panic, sleep disturbance Withdrawal: NA
	Cannabis	Intoxication: delirium, psychosis, anxiety Withdrawal: NA
	Cocaine	Intoxication: delirium, psychosis, mood disturbance, anxiety, sexual dysfunction, sleep disturbance Withdrawal: mood disturbance, anxiety, sleep disturbance
	Hallucinogens	Intoxication: delirium, psychosis, mood disturbance, anxiety
	Inhalants	Intoxication: delirium, psychosis, mood disturbance, anxiety Persistent use: dementia
	Nicotine	Withdrawal: anxiety
	Opioids	Intoxication: delirium, psychosis, mood disturbance, sexual dysfunction, sleep disturbance Withdrawal: sleep disturbance
	Phencyclidine	Intoxication: delirium, psychosis, mood disturbance, anxiety
	Sedative-hypnotics/ anxiolytics	Intoxication: delirium, psychosis, mood disturbance, sexual dysfunction, sleep disturbance Withdrawal: delirium, psychosis, mood disturbance, anxiety, sleep disturbance Persistent use: dementia, amnesia
Metals	Lead	Apathy, irritability, anorexia, confusion
	Mercury	Psychosis, fatigue, apathy, decreased memory, emotional lability, "mad hatter-like"
	Manganese	Parkinson-like syndrome, "manganese madness"
	Aluminum	Dementia
	Arsenic	Fatigue, blackouts, hair loss
	Copper	Wilson's disease
Bromides		Psychosis, hallucinations, dementia (especially if serum chloride is elevated)

SOURCE: Rosse, R.B., Deutsch, L.H., & Deutsch, S.I. (1995). Medical assessment and laboratory testing in psychiatry. In H.I. Kaplan, & B.J. Sadock (Eds.), *Comprehensive textbook of psychiatry.* Baltimore, MD: Williams and Wilkins.

tion, injury, and exposure to toxins (e.g., heavy metals). CNS infection may be excluded by lumbar puncture and CSF analysis (including culture, fungal, and viral studies). If there is a question of head injury, computed tomography (CT) or magnetic resonance imaging (MRI) may be crucial studies. Toxic exposures may be assessed through laboratory examination.

B. The Geriatric Population

In geriatric patients, there is an increased likelihood of having a concomitant medical condition. As a result, it is important to recognize that one (or more) organic causes may underlie psychiatric symptoms in the elderly. As is the case with younger patients, there is no consensus as to which studies to obtain. Kolman (1984) reported five tests of **relatively high usefulness in the elderly: a midstream urine (urinalysis, culture, and sensitivities), a chest X-ray, a serum vitamin B_{12}, an EKG, and a blood urea nitrogen (BUN).** Medical conditions that may contribute to psychiatric symptoms in the elderly include urinary tract infection, anemia, thyroid disease, and dementia.

Anemia affects more than 30% of all elderly patients, and can lead to weakness, fatigue, depression, lack of

Table 33-3. Endocrine Studies

Study	*Indication*	*Comments*
Thyroid TSH (thyroid-stimulating hormone)	Screening for thyroid dysfunction	↑ Hypothyroid ↓ Hyperthyroid
Other thyroid function tests	Thyroid dysfunction	↑ Hyperthyroid ↓ Hypothyroid
Parathyroid	Medical work-up Anxiety	↑ Variety of organic mental disorders ↓ Causes hypocalcemia, anxiety
Growth hormone	Schizophrenia, anorexia, depression	↑ Increased response to dopamine (DA) agonist in schizophrenia, anorexia Blunted response to insulin-induced hypoglycemia in depression
Prolactin	Antipsychotic medication use, cocaine, seizures	↑ Antipsychotic use, cocaine withdrawal, generalized seizure Lack of increase suggests pseudoseizure
β-HCG (β-human chorionic gonadotropin)	Pregnancy	↑ Pregnancy
GnRH (gonadotropin-releasing hormone	Psychiatric symptoms	↓ Schizophrenia, anorexia, depression, anxiety
LH (luteinizing hormone)	Panhypopituitarism; depression	↓ Panhypopituitarism, depression
FSH (follicle-stimulating hormone)	Panhypopituitarism, post-menopause, anorexia	↓ Panhypopituitarism ↑ Post-menopausal, anorexia (mild increase)
Estrogen	Menopause, PMS mood disturbance and anxiety	↓ Menopause, depression, PMS Variable changes with anxiety
Testosterone	Steroid/progesterone use, impotence, decreased sexual desire	↑ Anabolic steroid use ↓ Organic causes of impotence, decreased sexual desire, medroxyprogesterone treatment (sexual offenders)
Melatonin	Mood disorders	↓ Seasonal affective disorder
ACTH (adrenocorticotropin hormone)	Medical work-up	↑ Steroid use, seizures, psychosis, Cushing's, stress response
Cortisol	Medical work-up Mood disorders	↑ Cushing's disease, anxiety, depression
CCK (cholecystokinin)	Eating disorders	Blunted post-prandial response in bulimia (may normalize after antidepressant treatment)
Erythrocyte uroporphyrinogen-1-synthetase	Medical work-up; Psychosis	↑ Acute porphyria, psychosis

SOURCE: Rosse, R.B., Deutsch, L.H., & Deutsch, S.I. (1995). Medical assessment and laboratory testing in psychiatry. In H.I. Kaplan, & B.J. Sadock (Eds.), *Comprehesive textbook of psychiatry.* Baltimore, MD: Williams and Wilkins.

PMS, premenstrual syndrome.

motivation, agitation, or confusion. Although a CBC will document levels of hemoglobin and hematocrit, other studies also aid in the diagnosis of the anemia.

Thyroid disease is also common (especially in the elderly, and may be atypical in its presentation). Checking a serum thyroid-stimulating hormone (TSH) now constitutes thyroid screening. If the TSH is abnormal, additional thyroid function tests (TFTs) can be performed.

The National Institutes of Health Consensus Development Conference recommended a careful history

Table 33-4. Serology

Test	*Agent/Indication*	*Psychiatric Indication*	*Comment*
RPR, VDRL, FTA-ABS	Syphilis	Dementia, variable	Tertiary syphilis neurological involvement
ELISA, Western blot	HIV	Dementia, psychosis, personality disorder, mood disturbance, variable symptoms	CNS involvement
Hepatitis screen	Hep A antigen (Ag)	Anorexia, depression	Less severe, better prognosis than Hep B
	Hep B surface Ag	Depression	Active Hep B infection
	Hep B core Ag		Active Hep B infection
	Hep B surface antibody (Ab)		Previous infection/vaccination, immunity
Monospot	Epstein-Barr virus (EBV)	Mood disturbance, anxiety	Infectious mononucleosis (may present with depression, fatigue, personality change)
CMV	CMV	Mood disturbance, anxiety, confusion	
Lyme titer	*Borrelia burgdorferi*	Mental status changes	Erythema chronica migrans, meningitis, arthritis, cardiac problems
ANA	Antinuclear antibody	Delirium, psychosis, mood disturbance	Systemic lupus erythematosus (SLE), drug-induced lupus
LA	Lupus anticoagulant	Phenothiazine use	Elevated with phenothiazine use, especially chlorpromazine
LE cell preparation	Lupus erythematosus	Depression, psychosis, delirium, dementia	Associated with systemic LE

SOURCE: Rosse, R.B., Deutsch, L.H., & Deutsch, S.I. (1995). Medical assessment and laboratory testing in psychiatry. In H.I. Kaplan, & B.J. Sadock (Eds.), *Comprehensive textbook of psychiatry.* Baltimore, MD: Williams and Wilkins.

CMV, cytomegalovirus.

Table 33-5. Hematology

Test		*Indication*	*Comment*
CBC	Hemoglobin, hematocrit	Anemia	Associated depression, psychosis
	White blood cell count	Medical work-up, infection, psychotropic use	Leukocytosis associated with lithium, NMS Leukopenia, agranulocytosis associated with phenothiazine, carbamazepine, clozapine use
	Platelets	Medical work-up, psychotropic use	↑ Certain psychotropic medications (CBZ, clozapine, phenothiazine)
	Mean corpuscular volume	Alcohol history	↑ Alcohol, vitamin B_{12} or folate deficiency
	Reticulocyte count	Medical work-up, carbamazepine use	↑ Megaloblastic, iron deficiency anemia, anemia of chronic disease Monitor when using carbamazepine
ESR	Erythrocyte sedimentation rate	Medical work-up	↑ Non-specific infection, inflammation, autoimmune, malignant process
PT	Prothrombin time	Medical work-up	↑ Cirrhosis
Coombs test		Medical work-up	Hemolytic anemia associated with psychotropic medication use (chlorpromazine, phenytoin, levodopa, methyldopa)

SOURCE: Rosse, R.B., Deutsch, L.H., & Deutsch, S.I. (1995). Medical assessment and laboratory testing in psychiatry. In H.I. Kaplan, & B.J. Sadock (Eds.), *Comprehesive textbook of psychiatry.* Baltimore, MD: Williams and Wilkins.

Table 33-6. Urine, Stool, CSF Studies

Test	*Indication*	*Comment*
Urine	Urinalysis	Urinary tract infection, renal disease, diabetes, alcohol use, acute starvation, urinary tract bleeding, tumor
	Culture and sensitivities	Urinary tract infection
	Chemistries (osmolarity, Na, K, Cl, HCO_3, creatinine)	Renal disease, prelithium work-up
	Porphyrins, coproporphyrin, uroporphyrin	Porphyria
	Catecholamines, vanillylmandelic acid (VMA), myoglobin	Pheochromocytoma
	Copper	Wilson's disease
CSF	Opening pressure	↑ Infection, CNS mass, abscess, hematoma
	Appearance	Cloudy: infection Xanthochromic: CNS hemorrhage
	Glucose	↑ CNS infection
	Protein	↑ CNS infection
	Cells	+WBC: CNS infection +RBC: traumatic tap, CNS hemorrhage
	Culture and sensitivities	CNS infection
Stool	Culture and sensitivities	GI infection
	Ova and parasites	GI parasitic infestation
	Leukocytes	GI infection
	Clostridium difficile toxin	*Clostridium difficile* infection
	Heme	GI bleed
	Phenophthalein	Laxative use/abuse

SOURCE: Rosse, R.B., Deutsch, L.H., & Deutsch, S.I. (1995). Medical assessment and laboratory testing in psychiatry. In H.I. Kaplan, & B.J. Sadock (Eds.), *Comprehensive textbook of psychiatry.* Baltimore, MD: Williams and Wilkins.

and physical examination as the "best diagnostic test" for dementia since different dementing illnesses have different presentations. In addition, they recommended a **CBC, serum chemistries, TFTs, and possibly a screening test for syphilis, a vitamin B_{12} level, and folate levels. If clinically indicated, further testing could include neuroimaging (CT, MRI), an EEG, and an LP.** Others have suggested that a chest X-ray, carotid studies, HIV testing, immunologic screens, and screening for toxins/medications may also be useful. **Positron emission tomography (PET) may be useful for the recognition of atypical, early-onset dementias.**

C. Patients with Substance Abuse

Substance use (associated with intoxication, overdose, and withdrawal) is a major cause of mental status changes. Commonly, serum and urine are tested for substances (see Table 33-8). Alcohol is also routinely checked through breath analysis (breathalyzer). Other methods (e.g., analysis of hair or saliva) have also been developed but are not routinely used in clinical practice. Chronic alcohol use may damage the liver and elevate liver transaminases. In addition, liver damage is reflected by decreased serum proteins and by an elevated partial thromboplastin time (PTT). A macrocytic anemia may develop as a result of a decreased folate level. In advanced alcohol dependence, a global decrease in mass of the cortex and cerebellum often results and may be noted on brain-imaging studies. Clinical correlation may include Wernicke's encephalopathy or Korsakoff's amnestic syndrome. Regarding alcohol withdrawal, serum levels of alcohol do not correspond to the severity or timing of withdrawal symptoms.

VI. Neuroimaging

Neuroimaging is used to narrow the differential diagnosis and to determine the prognosis of patients with neuropsychiatric disorders. It is a non-invasive and powerful tool, that can assess brain structure and function. Contemporary neuroimaging modalities include structural and functional neuroimaging.

A. Structural Neuroimaging

1. **Computed axial tomography (CT or CAT scan) with or without contrast.** CT scanning uses X-ray beams to determine the attenuation when passing through differ-

Table 33-7. Studies to Consider for Psychiatric Presentations

First-line tests to consider	Serum/breath alcohol
CBC	Serum toxicology
Serum chemistry panel	Heavy metal screen
Thyroid function tests	Serum medication levels
Syphilis serology (RPR, VDRL)	ESR
	ANA
HIV	LP/CSF analysis
Vitamin B_{12} and folate	Serum/urine copper
UA	Serum ceruloplasmin
Urine toxicology	Monospot (EBV)
Urine uroporphyrins/ porphobilinogen	Blood cultures
	Skin test—tuberculosis, brucellosis
Erythrocyte uroporphyrinogen-1-synthetase	Pregnancy test
Serum ceruloplasmin	Urine uroporphyrins
CXR	Urine/serum osmolality
EKG	Polysomnography
Second-line tests to consider, if indicated	Nocturnal penile tumescence
CT—head	Evoked potentials
MRI—brain	Stool tests for occult blood
SPECT/PET scan-brain	ABG
Skull X-rays	
EEG	

SOURCE: Morihisa, J.M., Rosse, R.B., & Cross, C.D. (1994). Laboratory and other diagnostic tests in psychiatry. In *APA textbook of psychiatry*. Washington, DC: American Psychiatric Association.

ent densities of organ systems. The beams from different angles penetrate different organs. Detectors are arranged in a ring-like fashion (with the patient in the center) to generate images. During the process, the patient is advanced through the gantry of the scan after each slice is completed. On the films, areas of high attenuation (e.g., bone) appear white, those of low attenuation (e.g., gas) appear black, and those of intermediate attenuation (e.g., soft tissue) appear in shades of gray.

When contrast material is used, it travels intravascularly and leaks out in areas where the blood-brain barrier (BBB) is compromised. Contrast enhancement occurs in the CNS with tumors, bleeding, infection, inflammation, metastasis, and abscesses.

2. **Magnetic resonance imaging (MRI) with or without contrast.** MRI uses the magnetic properties of water molecules in the body. In the magnetic field of the MRI scanner, hydrogen atoms in water molecules become aligned as dipoles with or against the magnetic field. When radio-frequency is applied, some of the dipoles absorb the energy and align against the magnetic field (high-energy dipoles). When the radiofrequency is turned off, they return to a lower energy state where they are aligned with the magnetic field. This emission of energy (dipoles from high-energy alignment against the magnetic field to low-energy alignment with the magnetic field) is detected by a coil, and an MRI scanner measures the signal. Images are constructed by applying magnetic field gradients during the radio-frequency irradiation.

   MRI images are obtained using different acquisition parameters referred to as T_1 weight and T_2 weight. T_1-weighted images represent neuroanatomy clearly, whereas T_2-weighted images highlight areas of pathology. On T_2-weighed images, regions with extravasated blood appear dark, due to the paramagnetic effects of iron; areas with tumor, plaques, and edema appear light due to increased water content. As in CT, contrast material can be used to highlight areas of a compromised BBB.

   MRI is contraindicated in patients with paramagnetic prostheses or an inability to tolerate scanner time or confinement.
3. **When is structural neuroimaging indicated?** Decisions about when to obtain structural imaging need to be made on a case-by-case basis after a thorough evaluation of the patient. The following conditions and situations represent these in whom neuroimaging may detect a brain lesion associated with a treatable general medical condition:
   a. New-onset psychosis
   b. New-onset delirium
   c. New-onset dementia
   d. Onset of any psychiatric problem in patients > 50 years old
   e. Abnormal neurologic examination
   f. History of head trauma
   g. Initial work-up for electroconvulsive therapy
4. **Which one is indicated: CT or MRI?**
   a. A CT scan is preferred in:
      i. Acute hemorrhage and acute trauma
      ii. Identification of calcification
      iii. If MRI is contraindicated
   b. MRI is preferred when:
      i. Higher soft-tissue resolution is required
      ii. Posterior fossa pathology is suspected
      iii. Radiation exposure is contraindicated (e.g., children, young women)

B. Functional Neuroimaging

Functional neuroimaging modalities (positron emission tomography [PET] and single photon emission computed tomography [SPECT]) demonstrate neuronal activity, cellular metabolism, and neuroreceptor profiles with the

Table 33-8. Detection of Drugs in Urine

Class of Agent	*Agent*	*Serum*	*Urine*	*Hair*
Barbiturate		Variable	3 days to 3 weeks	—
Alcohol		1–2 days	1 day	—
Stimulant	Amphetamine	Variable	1–2 days	~90 days
	Cocaine (benzolecgonine)	Brief	2–3 days	~90 days
Opiate	Propoxyphene	8–34 hours (half-life)	1–2 days	~90 days
	Codeine, morphine, heroin	Variable	1–2 days	~90 days
	Methadone	15–29 hours (half-life)	2–3 days	~90 days
Anxiolytic	Benzodiazepine	Variable	2–3 days	—
Cannabinoids	Delta-9-THC	—	~30 days	~90 days
Phencyclidine		—	8 days	~90 days

SOURCE: Gastfriend, D.R., & O'Connell, J.J. (1998). Approach to the cocaine or opiate-abusing patient. In T.A. Stern, J.B. Herman, & P.L. Slavin (Eds.), *The MGH guide to psychiatry in primary care*. New York: McGraw-Hill.

use of radioactive substances (tracers), which are given intravenously or by inhalation. The tracer arrives in the CNS and is distributed according to regional blood flow, glucose metabolism, and receptor metabolism. It emits a signal that is detected by the scanner, and blood flow or glucose or receptor metabolism are recorded by tomographic imaging.

1. **PET scanning.** A PET scan requires an on-site cyclotron to prepare the positron emitter tracers, which have a short half-life. Its resolution is greater and more uniform when compared to SPECT, but it is much more expensive. It uses fluorodeoxyglucose (FDG) to assess glucose metabolism, oxygen^{15} to assess brain blood flow, and specific radioligands to assess receptors for specific neurotransmitters.
2. **SPECT scanning.** A SPECT scan uses single photon-emitting nucleotides rather than positron-emitting nucleotides. Major tracers used are xenon^{133}, ^{99m}Tc-MPAO to determine blood flow and, as in PET scanning, specific radioligands to assess receptors for specific neurotransmitters.
3. **Functional MRI (fMRI)** and **magnetic resonance spectroscopy (MRS)** are new imaging modalities that offer a great promise as tools for research and clinical applications in the future. **Functional imaging is helpful with each of the following:**
   a. **Seizures.** PET scanning is done in conjunction with EEG to determine the location of a seizure focus, especially in patients with complex partial seizures. During an ictus the seizure focus is hyperactive; interictally the focus will be hypometabolic. This EEG-PET combination is useful in localizing foci in the pre-operative assessment of neurosurgical intervention in patients with refractory seizure disorders.
   b. **Dementia.** Several profiles for dementias exist. Functional imaging studies of patients with Alzheimer's disease demonstrate decreased activity in bilateral parietal and temporoparietal cortices ("ear muff" sign). Parkinson's disease-related dementia mimics Alzheimer's disease. In vascular dementia, there are multiple areas of asymmetric cortical and subcortical hypoactivity. In Pick's disease, frontotemporal cortex hypoactivity is seen. In Huntington's disease caudate hypoactivity is present.
   c. **Major depression.** In patients with major depression, there is a decrease in anterolateral pre-frontal cortex activity, more on the left than on the right. The magnitude of decrease of this defect correlates with symptom severity. Functional neuroimaging is used in the differential diagnosis of major depression and other mood disorders, as well as dementia.
   d. **Schizophrenia.** In patients with schizophrenia, there is a decrease in the ratio of anterior to posterior metabolism. Decreased frontal activity correlates with negative symptoms. Hallucinations are associated with activation of Broca's area, the striatum, and the anterior cingulate cortex.
   e. **Obsessive-compulsive disorder.** There is increased activity in the orbitofrontal cortex-caudate nucleus-thalamus-anterior cingulate cortex circuitry. Increased frontal and caudate activity normalizes with successful treatment.
   f. **Post-traumatic stress disorder.** Hippocampal volume is decreased in patients with PTSD compared to healthy controls. Additionally, there is inadequate activation of the anterior cingulate and medial frontal cortex. There is an exaggerated activation of the amygdala in response to threat and exaggerated deactivation in Broca's area.

VII. Electrophysiology

A. Electroencephalogram (EEG)

1. **Waveforms.** The EEG records low-voltage electrical activity of the brain. In organic brain disease, there are changes in this electrical activity, and the EEG is helpful in the diagnosis and differential diagnosis of these disorders. The frequency of the electrical activity is measured in hertz (Hz), a measure of cycles per second. These frequencies are named with Greek letters.
   a. Delta: 0–4 Hz
   b. Theta: 4–8 Hz
   c. Alpha: 8–12 Hz
   d. Beta: > 12 Hz

   Amplitude refers to voltage of the EEG with a normal range of 10–100 μV (on a scalp EEG). Usually low-voltage fast activity indicates severe CNS pathology other than sleep and high-voltage slow activity is seen in delirium.
2. **Most frequently seen EEG patterns**
   a. **Normal:** posterior alpha rhythm, often low-voltage beta anteriorly, often low-voltage theta in frontotemporal or temporal region.
   b. **Sleep**
      i. **Stage 1:** drowsiness, disappearance of alpha rhythm, onset of frontal, central, and temporal beta
      ii. **Stage 2:** vertex sharp waves (high-voltage single or complex theta or delta waves), predominant runs of sinusoidal 12–14 Hz activity called **sleep-spindles**
      iii. **Stage 3–4:** delta (1–3 Hz) activity.
      iv. **Rapid eye movement (REM):** low-voltage fast with ocular movement artifacts
   c. **Seizure**
      i. **Generalized seizures:** bilateral, symmetric, synchronous, paroxysmal spike, and sharp waves followed by slow waves
      ii. **Absence: 3-Hz spike-wave complexes** accompanying blinking
      iii. **Complex partial seizures:** spikes, polyspikes, and waves over temporal region
      iv. **Pseudoseizures:** normal EEG
   d. **Delirium:** generalized theta and delta activity (generalized slowing); hepatic, and uremic encephalopathies both show **triphasic** waves.
   e. **Dementia:** Alzheimer's disease and vascular dementia show alpha slowing of the background (from 10–12 Hz to 8 Hz); with advanced disease the EEG becomes disorganized. Subacute sclerosing panencephalitis (SSPE) and Creutzfeldt-Jakob disease both show **periodic complexes accompanying myoclonic jerks.**
   f. **Locked-in syndrome:** normal EEG
   g. **Persistent vegetative state:** slow and disorganized EEG
   h. **Death:** electrocerebral silence
   i. **Medications:** benzodiazepines and barbiturates cause beta activity; neuroleptics and antidepressants may cause non-specific changes, recent research has shown that mood stabilizers (antiepileptic origin) may also slow EEG patterns.
   j. **Focal lesion:** focal slowing, usually delta, is referred to as polymorphic delta activity.
   k. **Increased intracranial pressure:** frontal, intermittent, rhythmic delta activity (FIRDA)

   The EEG should always be interpreted in concert with the clinical presentation. Final determination rests on the overall clinical picture. Activation with hyperventilation, photic stimulation, sleep, and sleep deprivation are helpful in activating seizure foci.

B. Evoked Potentials (EPs)

Any neural activity, internal or external, can cause small changes in the EEG. In EP recordings, stimuli are repeated many times and EEG changes are averaged and recorded to see deviations from the norm. In this way, the integrity of sensory and cognitive pathways can be assessed. For example, in multiple sclerosis (MS), when the myelin sheath is damaged, conduction will be slowed, and EPs will be delayed.

The main categories of EPs are:

1. **Brainstem EPs (auditory stimuli)**
2. **Somatosensory EPs (brief electrical stimuli)**
3. **Visual EPs (checkerboard stimuli: alternating black and white squares)**
4. **Auditory EPs (click)**
   a. During the assessment of auditory EPs, a click is applied, and the early component recorded is P 50. In healthy subjects, when a conditioned paired click is applied, the P 50 to the second click is reduced. In patients with schizophrenia, it is not. This is interpreted as a dysfunction of sensory gating in patients with schizophrenia.
   b. Another important EP for psychiatrists is the EP P 300. The P 300 is related to information-processing. It is seen in tasks requiring a behavioral response to a target stimulus. Several patient populations (e.g., demented individuals, patients with schizophrenia) show low amplitude and increased latency in P 300.

C. Polysomnography (PSG)

Many psychiatric disorders, especially depression, change the sleep pattern; these changes can be observed during an overnight sleep study at a sleep center and involve an EEG, an electro-oculogram, electromyography, and pulse oxymetry monitoring. This type of study is helpful to detect illnesses (such as sleep apnea) which, if left untreated, can cause many psychiatric symptoms.

D. Transcranial Magnetic Stimulation (TMS)

A very promising research tool for the treatment of mood disorders is TMS; it has been used for over 15 years in detection of MS plaques. A small electromagnet is placed on the scalp and the cortex is stimulated by a magnetic pulse. When the motor cortex is stimulated, lesions in the sub-clinical motor pathway can be identified. Additionally, researchers have used this tool to investigate language, vision, and memory systems. Currently, it is being researched in the treatment of mood disorders.

E. Procedures/Challenges

Diagnostic procedures are not regularly used in the clinical setting. Two types of procedures do exist: endocrine stimulation procedures, and sedative/hypnotic interviews.

1. **Endocrine stimulation procedures.**
   a. **Dexamethasone suppression test (DST).** The assumption behind the DST is that dysfunction of the hypothalamic-pituitary-adrenal axis underlies major depression, particularly melancholic depression. The test involves administration of an exogenous corticosteroid, dexamethasone 1 mg at bedtime. Then cortisol levels are drawn at various times throughout the next day (usually at 08:00, 16:00, and 23:00 hours). The normal effect is suppression of cortisol and other adrenocorticosteroid release. An abnormal effect is absence of suppression of cortisol release. Non-suppression is defined as a cortisol > 5 μg/dL. Non-suppression is thought to result because of dysfunction of the feedback loop, in which dexamethasone blocks the release of corticotropin-releasing factor from the hypothalamus.

   Although extensively tested, the sensitivity of the DST in detecting major depression is about 40–70% (with better correlation with severe psychotic affective disorders). Its specificity ranges from 70% to 90%. False positives may occur in a variety of medical conditions, including significant weight loss, alcohol use, and use of other drugs (e.g., barbiturates, anticonvulsants). Overall, the DST demonstrates only limited success in identifying major depression.

   b. **Thyrotropin-releasing hormone (TRH) stimulation test.** TRH normally stimulates the release of TSH from the pituitary. **It has been reported that a blunted response of TSH release is associated with major depression.** Sensitivity is low, with a blunted TSH response occurring in only 25% of depressed patients. In addition, **the blunted response is also seen with alcoholism, bulimia, borderline personality disorder, panic disorder, and hyperthyroidism.**

   c. **Panic provocation tests.** In panic provocation tests, it is theorized that relative states of **hypercarbia result in anxiety or panic.** Numerous agents have been shown to induce panic attacks in people with a history of panic attack. These agents include CO_2, intravenously (IV) administered lactate, IV caffeine, isoproterenol, β-carboline, and flumazenil administration. IV lactate infusion has been demonstrated to be 72% sensitive in detecting persons with panic disorder. Panic provocation tests are not typically used for clinical diagnostic purposes.
2. **Sedative/hypnotic interviews.** The sedative/hypnotic interview (e.g., the Amytal interview) continues to have a role in clinical diagnosis. This technique has been used to aid in differentiation between primary physical versus primary mental dysfunction. **The theory behind this technique is that administration of amobarbital (Amytal) or any sedative/hypnotic agent decreases the conscious guardedness and facilitates free communication.** While this procedure typically employs IV amobarbital infusion, any sedative/hypnotic agent is effective if sufficient sedation is achieved.

VIII. Monitoring Psychotropic Medications

A. Antidepressants

There are no established guidelines for monitoring levels of antidepressants. In the treatment of the medically ill, physicians should consider side effects of the antidepressants as well as the effects of the illness on the metabolism of psychotropics. In patients with liver disease, the antidepressant dosage needs to be carefully adjusted, and liver function tests (LFTs) need to be monitored for the possibility that increased LFTs may result from psychotropic use. Use of tricyclic antidepressants (TCAs) in the cardiac patient needs to be monitored closely (levels of TCAs and electrocardiogram [EKG] should be checked at baseline and during ongoing care) due to the effects of TCAs on cardiac conduction (PR, QRS, and QT_c prolongation), which may lead to lethal arrhythmias. **It is recommended that blood levels of TCAs be monitored in patients with:**

1. **Non-compliance**
2. **Poor response while taking a therapeutic dose for a reasonable time**
3. **Older age and medical illness**
4. **Serious depression (e.g., suicidal ideation)**

B. Mood Stabilizers

1. **Lithium.** Lithium is commonly used in patients with mood disorders, and it affects many organ systems including the kidneys, the thyroid, the heart, and the CNS. It is recommended that serum electrolytes, BUN, creatinine, thyroid function tests, and an EKG be checked routinely. Additionally, in patients with kidney problems, a 24-hour urine test for creatinine and protein clearance is recommended. Steady states of lithium are reached in 3 days ($t_{1/2}$ = 12 hours), or can be as long as 8 days in patients with kidney problems due to prolonged $t_{1/2}$.
2. **Carbamazepine.** Carbamazepine affects mainly hepatic, hemopoietic, and cardiac conduction systems. A fatal side effect is agranulocytosis. Therefore, it is important to check a CBC before the initiation of treatment, every 2 weeks for the first 2 months, and once every 3 months thereafter. Platelet count, reticulocyte count, serum electrolytes, an EKG, and liver function tests (aspartate aminotransferase [AST], alanine aminotransferase [ALT], lactate dehydrogenase [LDH], and

Table 33-9. Mood Stabilizers

Agent	*Half-life (hours)*	*Dose Range (mg/day)*	*Protein Binding*	*Blood Levels*
Lithium	24	300–2,400	Low	0.5–1.2 mEq/L (weekly × 1 month, monthly × 3 months, then every 3 months)
Valproic acid	16	200–2,000	Very high	50–100 µg/mL (weekly × 2 weeks, then every 3 months)
Lamotrigine	12	100–700	Medium	—
Gabapentin	6	900–1,800	None	—
Oxcarbazepine	8–11	600–2,400	High	10–35 mcg/ml
Topiramate	21	100–800	Medium	—
Carbamazepine	8–30 (variable due to autoinduction)	200–1,200	High	6–12 µg/mL (weekly × 2 weeks, then every 3 months)

alkaline phosphatase) need to be checked, before and 1 year after the initiation of treatment. In patients of childbearing age, a pregnancy test needs to be done before initiation due to the teratogenic side effects of carbamazepine.

Discontinuation is recommended when the white blood cell count is < 3,000/mm^3, hemoglobin is < 11 mg/dL, the platelet count is < 100,000/mm^3, or the reticulocyte is < 0.3%.

3. **Valproic acid.** Valproic acid mainly affects the liver, but it can also affect the hematopoietic system and the pancreas.

For details about mood stabilizers, see Table 33-9.

C. Antipsychotics

Clozapine is the only antipsychotic that requires close laboratory monitoring due to the possibility of agranulocytosis in 1% of patients taking this medication. Baseline and weekly CBCs are mandatory when prescribing this medication. If the white blood cell count (WBC) drops significantly (< 3,000), even though it may be in the normal range, or in case of mild leukopenia (WBC = 3,000–3,500), the patient needs to be monitored closely, and CBCs should be checked twice weekly. In the case of leukopenia (WBC = 2,000–3,000) or granulocytopenia (granulocytes = 1,000–1,500), the medication needs to be stopped, CBCs need to be checked daily, and the patient needs to be hospitalized. Clozapine therapy may be continued after normalization of the blood count. **If agranulocytosis develops (WBC < 2,000, or granulocytes < 1,000), clozapine is discontinued for life.** Under this condition, the patient needs to be hospitalized and placed under a hematologist's care. Use of other bone-marrow suppressants needs to be avoided; a biopsy may be necessary.

Additionally, an EEG may be helpful if the dosage of the clozapine needs to be raised beyond 600 mg because of an increased incidence of seizures. Clozapine can be reintroduced carefully in patients who experience clozapine-induced seizures.

In patients with cardiac disease, who are taking antipsychotics (e.g., thioridazine), the EKG needs to be checked due to the risk of serious cardiac conduction disturbances.

Table 33-10. Genetic Markers

Genetic Finding	*Disorder*	*Comments*
Chromosome 4, short arm	Huntington's disease	Autosomal dominant, 100% penetrance
Chromosome 21	Alzheimer's dementia	Near gene for amyloid precursor protein
X chromosome	Fragile X	Association with infantile autism, pervasive developmental delay
X chromosome	Fragile X carriers	Possible association with schizophrenic spectrum, chronic mood disorders
A1 allele of D_2 receptor	Alcoholism, Tourette's, ADHD, autism, PTSD	Mutation of allele may act as modifying gene

Table 33-11. Biological Markers

Biological Marker		*Comments*
Homovanillic acid (HVA) (plasma)	DA metabolite	Decrease with antipsychotic treatment predicts good treatment response
3-Methoxy-4-hydroxyphenylglycol (MHPG) (24-h urine)	NE activity	Lower levels in bipolar than unipolar depressed
		Low levels may predict imipramine response
		High levels associated with learned helplessness
		Low CSF levels may be associated with increased risk of suicidal behavior
5-Hydroxyindoleacetic acid (5-HIAA) (CSF)	5-HT metabolite	Low levels associated with suicidal behavior, aggression, impulsivity, disturbed childhood behavior, violent suicide attempts, depression, seizures, alcohol use
		High levels associated with anxiety, obsession, inhibited behavior
Tryptophan (serum)	Amino acid	Low levels reported in depression
		Low tryptophan diet precipitated some depression
Serine (serum)	Amino acid	High levels associated with some psychotics (serine hydroxymethyltransferase activity low)

IX. Genetic Testing and Biological Markers

Recently, research has focused on attempts to identify genetic markers that might underlie psychiatric illnesses. Although no firm relationships have been identified, some possible associations have been identified (see Table 33-10). A related area of research is attempting to identify biological markers of psychiatric illnesses. No firm relationships have been identified, but the list of potential markers is growing (see Table 33-11).

Suggested Readings

Anfinson, T.J., & Kathol, R.G. (1992). Screening laboratory evaluation in psychiatric patients: A review. *General Hospital Psychiatry, 14,* 248–257.

Boutros, N., & Braff, D. (1999). Clinical electrophysiology. In D.S. Charney, E.J. Nestler, & B.S. Bunney (Eds.), *Neurobiology of mental illness,* pp. 121–131. New York: Oxford.

Dolan, J.G., & Mushlin, A.I. (1985). Routine laboratory testing for medical disorders in psychiatric inpatients. *Archives of Internal Medicine, 145,* 2085–2088.

Falk, W. (1998). Approach to the patient with memory problems or dementia. In T.A. Stern, J.B. Herman, & P.L. Slavin (Eds.), *The MGH guide to psychiatry in primary care,* pp. 207–220. New York: McGraw-Hill.

Fenton, G.W. (1984). The electroencephalogram in psychiatry: Clinical and research applications. *Psychiatry of Deviance, 2,* 53–57.

Gastfriend, D.R., & O'Connell, J.J. (1998). Approach to the cocaine or opiate-abusing patient. In T.A. Stern, J.B. Herman, & P.L. Slavin (Eds.), *The MGH guide to psychiatry in primary care,* pp. 455–460. New York: McGraw-Hill.

Kolman, P.B.R. (1984). The value of laboratory investigations of elderly psychiatric patients. *Journal of Clinical Psychiatry, 45,* 112–116.

Morihisa, J.M., Rosse, R.B., & Cross, C.D. (1994). Laboratory and other diagnostic tests in psychiatry. In *APA textbook of psychiatry,* pp. 277–310. Washington, DC: American Psychiatric Association.

Rosse, R.B., Deutsch, L.H., & Deutsch, S.I. (1995). Medical assessment and laboratory testing in psychiatry. In H.I. Kaplan, & B.J. Sadock (Eds.), *Comprehensive textbook of psychiatry VI,* pp. 601–618. Baltimore, MD: Williams and Wilkins.

SECTION III

Neurologic Disorders

Chapter 34

Functional Neuroanatomy

Stephan Heckers

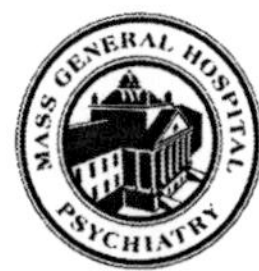

I. Overview

There are about 10^{11} neurons in the central nervous system (CNS), and each neuron establishes about 10^3–10^4 connections to other neurons. How are these neurons arranged to process information? This question may serve as a guide to understand, in a systematic fashion, the basic principles of human neuroanatomy.

II. Information Processing in the Brain

The processing of sensory information involves three steps: the collection of sensory information through perceptual modules, the creation of a representation, and the production of a response.

Sensory organs provide information about physical attributes of incoming information. **Details of physical attributes** (e.g., temperature, sound frequency, or color) **are conveyed through multiple segregated channels within each perceptual module.** The anatomical systems involved in reception are the sensory organs, the thalamus, and primary sensory cortex. **Integration of the highly segregated sensory information occurs at several levels.** The first integration occurs in **unimodal association areas** where physical attributes of one sensory domain are linked together.

A second level of integration is reached in multi-modal association areas, which link physical attributes of different sensory qualities together, and **a third level of integration is provided by the interpretation and evaluation of experience.** It is at this third level of integration that the brain creates a representation of experience that has the spatio-temporal resolution and full complexity of the outside world. The representation of experience is evaluated and interpreted, which involves conscious and non-conscious processes. Evaluation and interpretation involve comparison of new information with previously stored information. This allows the brain to classify information (e.g., as new or old, or as threatening or not threatening).

Based on the result of the evaluation and interpretation, the brain can then create a response through a variety of channels (e.g., language, affect, and motor behavior).

III. Anatomical Systems

A. Anatomical Areas

Four major anatomical systems are involved in the processing of information: the thalamus, the cortex, the medial temporal lobe, and the basal ganglia (Figure 34-1). The function of these four systems is modulated by several groups of neurons that are characterized by their use of a specific neurotransmitter. Most of psychopharmacology is aimed at strengthening or inhibiting these modulatory systems.

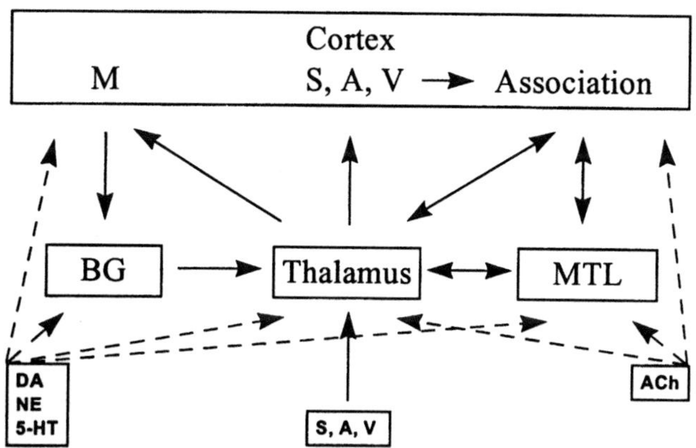

Figure 34-1. Basic circuitry of information processing.

1. **The thalamus is the gateway to cortical processing of all incoming sensory information:** somatosensory (S), auditory (A), and visual (V).
2. **Primary sensory cortex** (i.e., S1, A1, V1) **receives sensory information from the appropriate sensory modules** (sensory organ + thalamus). **The association cortex integrates information from primary cortices, from sub-cortical structures, and from brain areas affiliated with memory, to create the representation of experience.**
3. **The medial temporal lobe serves** two major functions in the brain: **to integrate multi-modal sensory information** for storage into and retrieval from memory, **and to attach limbic valence to sensory information** (e.g., pleasant or unpleasant, fight or flight).
4. **The basal ganglia are primarily involved in the integration of input from cortical motor areas.** They modulate the activity of thalamocortical projections, thereby creating a cortico-striato-thalamic loop.

B. Neurotransmitter Systems

Four groups of densely packed neurons provide diffuse projections to all areas of the brain to modulate their functions:

1. **Cholinergic neurons in the basal forebrain (BF) and brainstem**
2. **Dopaminergic neurons in the substantia nigra (SN) and ventral tegmental area (VTA)**

3. **Noradrenergic neurons in the locus coeruleus (LC)**
4. **Serotonergic neurons in the raphe nuclei (R)**

We will now review in some detail the four major anatomical systems (the cortex, the thalamus, the basal ganglia, and the medial temporal lobe) and their modulation by the neurotransmitter-specific projection systems.

IV. Cortex

The association cortex is a six-layered cortex, the so-called isocortex. **Layers 2 and 4** of the human isocortex **are defined by a high density of small interneurons** (i.e., neurons that do not send long-ranging projections to other cortical or sub-cortical areas). **In contrast, layers 3 and 5 are defined by a high density of pyramidal cells, which collect input through their dendrites and project to other cortical or sub-cortical areas. Interneurons are GABAergic cells** (GABA is γ-aminobutyric acid) **and exert an inhibitory influence on their targets** (via $GABA_A$ receptors), whereas **pyramidal cells are glutamatergic and have an excitatory influence.** Normal cortical function depends on an intricate balance of GABAergic inhibition and glutamatergic excitation. Seizures, e.g., are caused by a decrease of GABAergic tone and an increased firing of pyramidal cells. Sedation, on the other hand, can be caused by an increased GABAergic tone.

Cortical neurons are targets for many ascending fibers arising from the underlying white matter. Some of these inputs originate from other cortical areas or from the thalamus. Others arise from neurotransmitter-specific projection systems, such as the dopaminergic neurons of the ventral tegmental area (VTA) and the serotonergic neurons of the raphe nuclei. These two systems, the dopamine (DA) and the 5-hydroxytryptamine (serotonin, 5-HT) systems, modulate the function of cortical areas by specific effects on cortical neurons. **The effect of DA on cortical neurons is conveyed by three DA receptors, the D_1, D_4, and D_5 receptors. The D_1 and D_5 receptors are expressed primarily on pyramidal cells, whereas the D_4 receptor is primarily expressed on GABAergic interneurons.** The other important neurotransmitter-specific projection system in the cortex is the serotonergic system. One serotonergic receptor, **the $5\text{-}HT_{2A}$ receptor, is of particular relevance for the pathophysiology of psychosis.** Hallucinogens (e.g., lysergic acid diethylamide [LSD]) act as agonists at the $5\text{-}HT_{2A}$ receptor, and several antipsychotic compounds, especially the atypical neuroleptics, block the activity of this receptor. Modulation of cortical function, via the D_1, D_4, D_5, and $5\text{-}HT_{2A}$ receptors, leads to fine tuning of information-processing, e.g., by increasing the signal-to-noise ratio during corticocortical and thalamocortical neurotransmission. This modulation is one of the important mechanisms for the action of neuroleptic drugs.

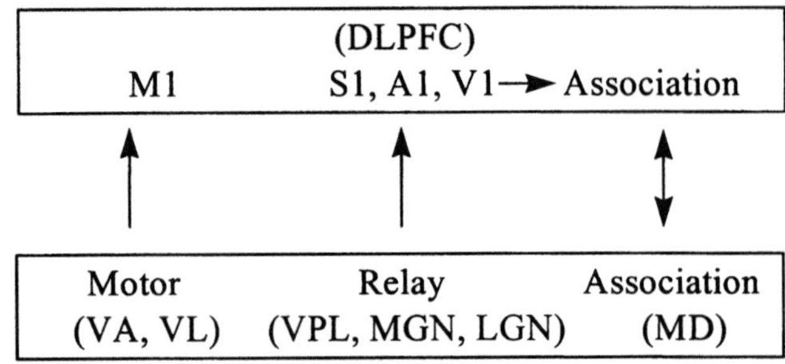

Figure 34-2. Thalamo-cortical connections.

V. Thalamus

The thalamus serves several important functions in information-processing in the human brain.

The relay nuclei (ventral posterior lateral [VPL], medial geniculate nucleus [MGN], and lateral geniculate nucleus [LGN]) convey sensory information from the sensory organs to the appropriate areas of the primary sensory cortex (S1, A1, and V1) (Figure 34-2).

The association nuclei, especially the mediodorsal nucleus, establish reciprocal connections with the association cortex.

The motor nuclei (i.e., ventral nuclei) relay input from the basal ganglia to the motor and premotor cortex.

VI. Basal Ganglia

The basal ganglia include the ventral striatum, the dorsal striatum (caudate and putamen), and the globus pallidus (Figure 34-3).

The dorsal striatum (caudate, putamen) receives input from motor cortex and projects to the globus pallidus. The globus pallidus relays the neostriatal input to the thalamus. The thalamus, in turn, projects back to the cortical areas that gave rise to the corticostriatal projec-

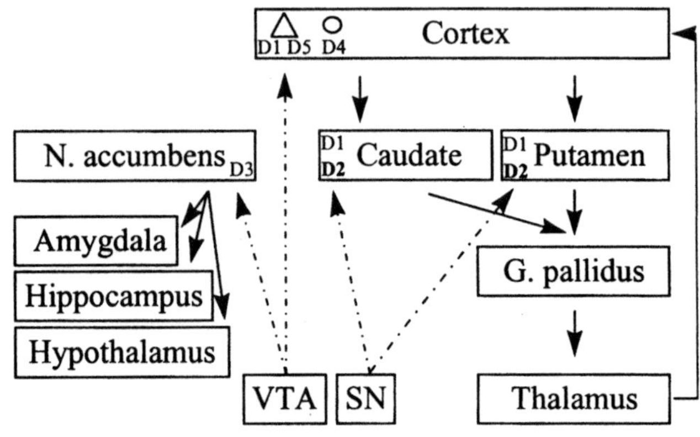

Figure 34-3. Basal ganglia circuitry.

tions, thereby closing the cortico-striato-pallido-thalamo-cortical loop. This loop is involved in the generation and control of motor behavior.

In contrast, **the ventral striatum (the nucleus accumbens) is connected with the amygdala, hippocampus, and hypothalamus and is therefore considered part of the limbic system.** Reward and expectancy behavior and their derailment during drug addiction involve the recruitment of the nucleus accumbens.

All basal ganglia structures are modulated by neurotransmitter-specific projection systems, in particular by dopaminergic neurons. Dopaminergic neurons of the SN project to the neostriatum (nigrostriatal fibers), and dopaminergic neurons of the VTA project to the nucleus accumbens (mesolimbic fibers) and cortex (mesocortical fibers). The two major DA receptors in the dorsal striatum are the D_1 and D_2 receptors. The nucleus accumbens expresses primarily the D_3 receptor.

VII. Medial Temporal Lobe

The medial temporal lobe contains the amygdala, the hippocampal region, and superficial cortical areas that cover the hippocampal region and form the parahippocampal gyrus (PHG) (Figure 34-4).

The hippocampal region can be subdivided into three sub-regions: the dentate gyrus, the cornu ammonis sectors, and the subiculum. The neurons of the human hippocampal region are arranged in one cellular layer, the pyramidal cell layer. Most pyramidal cell layer neurons are glutamatergic whereas the small contingent of non-pyramidal cells is GABAergic. The serial circuitry of the glutamatergic neurons provides the structural basis for long-term potentiation, a physiological phenomenon crucial for formation of memory. The glutamatergic receptor crucial for the creation of long-term potentiation is the NMDA (*N*-methyl-D-aspartate) receptor.

The PHG receives many projections from multi-modal cortical association areas and relays them to the hippocampal region. Intrinsic connections within the hippocampal region allow further processing before the information is referred back to the association cortex. Some authors have argued that the reciprocal connections between the hippocampal formation and one association area, the pre-frontal cortex (either directly or via the PHG), are particularly prominent.

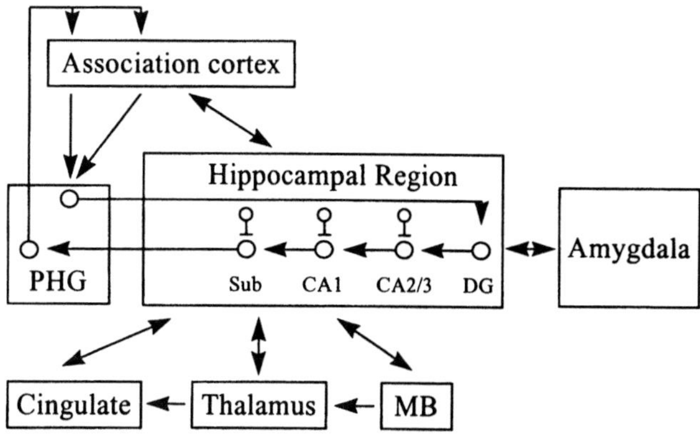

Figure 34-4. Medial temporal lobe circuitry.

The hippocampus is closely connected with the limbic system (e.g., via the Papez circuit). It has been proposed that the hippocampal formation is recruited via these connections to regulate emotion or to modulate information processing by attaching limbic valence to sensory stimuli.

Interactions between the frontal lobes and the medial temporal lobe are particularly important for declarative memory (i.e., the acquisition and retrieval of information about facts and events). An intricate balance of hippocampus and frontal lobes ensures that the constructive process of memory encoding and retrieval creates accurate representations of experience. Interactions between the hippocampus and the frontal cortex are crucial for the formation of memory, for conscious awareness, and for self-awareness.

Suggested Readings

Fogel, B.S., Schiffer, R.B. (1996). *Neuropsychiatry.* Baltimore, MD: Williams and Wilkins.

Kandel, E.R., Schwartz, J., & Jessel, T. (1996). *Principles of neural science* (4th ed.). New York: Elsevier.

Mesulam, M.-M. (2000). *Principles of behavioral and cognitive neurology.* New York: Oxford University Press.

Chapter 35

The Neurologic Examination

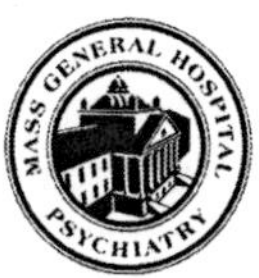

ANTHONY P. WEISS AND MARTIN A. SAMUELS

I. Introduction

A. The Importance of the Neurologic Examination in Psychiatric Practice

The neurologic examination, as taught in its unabridged form, can intimidate both medical students and seasoned clinicians alike. Filled with eponymic signs and a multitude of complex maneuvers, the standard neurologic examination is often a source of confusion. Perhaps for this reason, the neurologic exam is all too often omitted by the busy clinician. It has, unfortunately, become commonplace to see the entire examination summarized as "grossly intact."

Including a thorough neurologic examination as part of a patient evaluation is especially relevant to the practice of psychiatry for several reasons:

1. **Psychiatric symptoms (affective, behavioral, or cognitive) may result directly from underlying neurologic disease** (e.g., a stroke causing mood lability). Associated sensory-motor findings on examination may uncover the underlying illness.
2. **Psychiatric symptoms may be highly co-morbid in certain neurologic diseases** (e.g., the high rate of depression in Parkinson's disease and of psychosis in Huntington's disease). In some cases, the psychiatric symptoms may predate other features of the illness, and a thorough examination by the psychiatrist may lead to early recognition and treatment.
3. **The neurologic exam is crucial for distinguishing "real" neurologic deficits from simulated deficits associated with conversion disorders or malingering.** The psychiatrist will often be called upon to clarify this diagnostic dilemma.
4. **Many psychotropic medications affect the motor systems of the brain, and lead to neurologic side effects** (e.g., dystonias, and other movement disorders). Recognition of these adverse effects is critical in the overall management of the psychiatric patient.

This chapter presents a straightforward approach to the neurologic examination and provides the busy psychiatrist with the clinical tools necessary to handle the situations described above. This chapter assumes at least a rudimentary knowledge of neuroanatomy (see chapter 34). While a few pertinent clinical situations will be described, the reader is referred to other chapters for discussion of specific neurologic illnesses.

B. Overview of the Complete Neurologic Examination

The neurologic examination does not need to be comprehensive in every patient. Belief to the contrary has contributed to the notion that this examination is too time-consuming and cumbersome for the busy physician. The complete neurologic exam, like any new skill, needs to be taught and practiced in its entirety. While it may be intimidating to the trainee, it is the only way to learn all of the skills that may be called upon in clinical practice. Like a football team that learns an entire playbook only to use a small portion of it in any one game, the physician needs to be facile with all of the exam tools available to be able to use specific techniques when indicated. Examination of the snout reflex may be unnecessary (and perhaps off-putting) to the 20-year-old with a numb hand, but may be an important part of a dementia evaluation.

II. Mental Status

A. Overview of the Mental Status Examination

As with the general neurologic examination, the mental status examination can appear formidable when considered in its entirety. Indeed, formal neuropsychological testing can take several hours or even days to complete. This should not dissuade the clinician from assessing a few basic components of the patient's mental state.

Given the incredible complexity of human cognitive function, it should not come as a surprise that the full mental status exam has several components (Table 35-1). In this section we highlight a "bare bones" approach to the mental status; the reader is referred to chapter 2 for further detail.

B. The "Psychiatric" Mental Status

The mental status examination has historically been separated into "psychiatric" and "neurologic" components. While this division is clearly arbitrary, the distinction is used here for convenience. The main components of the psychiatric mental status evaluation include (Table 35-1):

1. **Observational assessment. This includes general observations of the patient's appearance, attitude toward the examiner, and overall demeanor. It also includes a description of the patient's speech and motor behavior.** These observations usually provide important clues into the patient's internal state. For example, a disheveled, unshaven man with minimal eye contact, sparse, hypophonic speech, and a general slowness of movement, might be expected to have a depressive disorder.
2. **Mood and affect.** These terms are analogous to the symptom and sign of emotional disturbance. **Mood represents how the patient feels, while affect is how the patient displays that mood to the world.** Incon-

Table 35-1. The Complete Mental Status Examination

- I. "Psychiatric"
  - A. Observational assessment
    - 1. Dress
    - 2. Demeanor
    - 3. Attitude toward examiner
    - 4. Speech (rate, volume, and prosody)
    - 5. Motor behavior
  - B. Mood/affect
  - C. Thought process
  - D. Thought content
    - 1. Obsessions
    - 2. Delusions
  - E. Perceptual disturbances
    - 1. Hallucinations
    - 2. Illusions
- II. "Neurologic"
  - A. Level of consciousness
  - B. Memory (verbal and non-verbal)
    - 1. Registration
    - 2. Recall
    - 3. Remote
  - C. Language
    - 1. Expression (spontaneous)
    - 2. Comprehension
    - 3. Repetition
    - 4. Naming
    - 5. Reading/writing
  - D. Visual-spatial/constructional
  - E. Calculation
  - F. Abstraction
  - G. Praxis
  - H. Right-left orientation
  - I. Face and object recognition

gruence of mood and affect, while not specific, is an important finding since it may be related to an underlying "organic" deficit.

3. **Thought process.** The expression of thought should be a goal-directed process, in which thoughts are connected and presented in a logical manner. **Abnormality of thought process lies on a continuum from subtle parenthetical comments to a complete lack of connection between ideas.** Such an abnormality will often leave the examiner confused or even wondering what question was originally asked.
4. **Thought content.** Our inner world of beliefs, convictions, and moment-to-moment ideas is hidden from even the savviest psychiatrist. **Thought content can therefore be assessed only by direct inquiry (What are you thinking about?), an analysis of speech, or inference from behavior.** While the line between normal and abnormal thought is sometimes blurry, most clinically relevant abnormalities (e.g., delusions) are clear.

C. The "Neurologic" Mental Status

This section of the mental status focuses on specific cognitive functions, and, as noted above, can involve hours or days of detailed testing (Table 35-1). **For routine purposes, the following four components comprise an adequate exam.** Unlike other features of the neurologic exam, **it is important that these components be done in order, since basic functions must be intact in order to perform more complex tasks.**

1. **Level of consciousness.** Consciousness lies on a continuum from full alertness to coma. While the two extremes are generally obvious, the middle ground of attentional deficit can be subtle. Since inattention is a hallmark of delirium (acute confusional state), a common and emergent medical condition, **attention should be tested in all patients.** Sustained attention is also a critical component for all other cognitive functioning. Some common tests of attention include:
   a. **Serial 7s.** Ask the patient to subtract 7 from 100, and then continue to serially subtract 7 from the remainder. This test is limited by its reliance on calculation, which may be more a function of education than attention.
   b. **Digit span.** Have the patient repeat a randomly presented list of digits. A normal capacity is between five and seven. Alternatively, have the patient spell a five-letter word (e.g., WORLD) backward.
2. **Language.** Language is the means by which we present our thoughts to each other. Like other cognitive functions, language can be extraordinarily complex, with entire texts of aphasiology dedicated to its study. **In general, three simple questions allow the examiner to draw valid conclusions about language in the individual patient:**
   a. **Is the language *fluent* or *non-fluent*?** Independent of the actual words, does the speech sound like a language? Loss of the normal inflection and spacing of normal speech leads to non-fluent language production.
   b. **Is *comprehension* normal or abnormal?** Does the patient seem to understand what you are saying? A request to complete a one- to three-step command (though complex commands may test more than just receptive language function) best assesses this. Asking simple yes/no questions (e.g., Were you born in Mexico? or Are we in the kitchen?) is another common method.
   c. **Is *repetition* normal or abnormal?** Have the patient repeat a phrase such as "no ifs ands or buts." This particular

phrase is quite sensitive, given the difficulty of repeating conjunctions.

3. **Memory.** Memory function is generally divided into three components:
   a. **Immediate recall.** This is the ability to hold information long enough to use it (remembering a phone number given by the operator long enough to dial it). Immediate recall is heavily dependent on attention and is tested by both digit span and phrase repetition (see above). Asking the patient to repeat three named items (e.g., piano, monkey, and blue) is another commonly used method.
   b. **Short-term memory.** Short-term memory involves the ability to store information for later use. Asking the patient to reproduce the three previously named items after a span of 2–5 minutes is a common test.
   c. **Long-term memory.** Long-term memory involves the recall of past events. This is nearly impossible to test accurately at the bedside, since the examiner is rarely privy to details of remote events from the patient's life. Asking about well-known national events or people (e.g., How did JFK die?) is dependent on the age and educational background of the patient. Accurate assessment often requires a standardized battery of questions available in full neuropsychological testing.
4. **Visual-Spatial Skills**
   a. **Writing.** Have the patient write his name, address, and a sentence about the weather. Look for grammatical errors, as well as errors in spacing and overall presentation.
   b. **Clock.** Have the patient fill in a circle with numbers in the form of a clock. Then ask him to set the hands at 10 minutes to 2. Abnormalities can occur in planning (poor spacing of numbers) or in positioning of the hands, which may belie a frontal lobe lesion. Complete absence of detail on one side of the clock (usually left) may represent a hemineglect syndrome associated with a (right) parietal lobe lesion.

III. Cranial Nerves

A. Olfactory Nerve (CrN I)

Testing of the first cranial nerve is almost uniformly neglected, with the entire cranial nerve examination often described as "II-XII WNL." This notation not only indicates little regard for the first cranial nerve, but also communicates little about the individual features of the exam. It should therefore be abandoned.

The first cranial nerve runs along the orbital surface of the frontal lobe, an area that is otherwise clinically silent. Lesions in this area (e.g., frontal lobe meningioma) may produce unilateral anosmia, occasionally as a unitary symptom. Routine testing of smell is therefore quite important.

Carrying a small vial of coffee is a simple and convenient method for testing smell. Each nostril should be tested separately.

B. Optic Nerve (CrN II)

The optic nerve and its posterior radiations run the entire length of the brain and produce different patterns of symptoms and signs depending on where they are compromised. **A thorough visual examination can therefore be quite informative, and involves five components:**

1. **Funduscopic examination.** The optic nerve is the only nerve that can be visualized directly. The physician should take advantage of this fact in assessing its integrity. A good funduscopic exam will also reveal much about the systemic vascular system and is a critical guide to the presence of increased intracranial pressure.
2. **Visual acuity.** Testing of visual acuity (i.e., the actual strength of vision) is frequently ignored in the adult patient. This is unfortunate since poor vision can profoundly impair a patient's functioning and is often reversible with corrective lenses or surgery. Acuity should be assessed in each eye separately while wearing current corrective lenses.
3. **Pupillary measurement.** Pupillary size represents the delicate balance between sympathetic and parasympathetic input to the ciliary muscles of the eye. The presence of abnormally large or small pupils reflects an imbalance, and may be an important sign of disease. Similarly, an inequality in pupillary size (anisocoria) can be an important hallmark of severe intracranial pathology. Each pupil should be measured in millimeters, with measurements clearly documented for further reference.
4. **Pupillary reaction.** The direct and consensual pupillary reaction to light, and the near reaction (accommodation), should be tested routinely. This will assess any damage in either the afferent or efferent pathways that comprise the pupillary response. A penlight and close observation are all that is necessary.
5. **Confrontational visual fields.** As noted above, the visual system runs from the retina to the occipital cortex, involving a substantial area of the central nervous system (CNS). Lesions anywhere along this pathway will lead to visual field cuts. Importantly, the patient is almost never aware of this abnormality of vision; careful testing is therefore required to elucidate it. Sit directly in front of the patient, and have him look in your eyes. Test each eye separately by bringing an object (pin or wiggling finger) into each visual quadrant. For the patient who is unable to cooperate in this fashion, simply having him count fingers displayed in each quadrant is another option.

C. Eye Movement (CrNs III, IV, and VI)

These three cranial nerves are considered together given their relation to innervation of the extraocular musculature involved in eye movement. **There are two main categories of eye movement:**

1. **Saccades.** These are rapid eye movements that allow for brisk transition between items in the visual field. Saccades are tested by having the patient look to the ceiling, floor, left, and right sequentially. Asking the patient to look quickly at your finger and then the opposite thumb is another method.
2. **Pursuits.** These are slow voluntary eye movements that allow for smooth tracking of a moving target. They are tested by having the patient follow your finger through a full range of motion (up, down, left, and right).

In assessment of eye movements, the examiner should take note of the resting position of the eye (is there a gaze preference?), the fullness of movement (are there any limitations in eye movement?), and the presence of any nystagmus (involuntary oscillation of the eyes). Any abnormality should be noted descriptively.

D. Trigeminal Nerve (CrN V)

The trigeminal nerve provides sensory innervation to the face (including the afferent limb of the corneal reflex) and motor innervation to the muscles of mastication. It is evaluated as follows:

1. **Facial sensation.** As with sensory testing in general (see V, below), testing sensory integrity of the face can be a frustrating exercise if the examiner insists on precision. Unless the patient has a specific sensory complaint (e.g., numb chin or facial pain), thorough testing of all sensory modalities is probably unnecessary. Testing light touch (by stroking the face with your fingers) or temperature sensitivity (using a cold metal tuning fork) is usually adequate. Asking the patient to "quantify" the degree of difference (If this side is a dollar, how much is this side?) is generally not a fruitful exercise. Simply asking, "Does this feel normal on both sides?" saves time and will generally detect any abnormalities worth further investigation.
2. **Corneal reflex.** The corneal reflex involves the direct and consensual blink response to corneal irritation. While it can be helpful in localization of brainstem dysfunction (usually in the comatose patient), it is unfortunately both non-specific and insensitive. It is therefore not done routinely. The reader is referred to other sources for more detailed information.
3. **Muscles of mastication.** The motor branches of the trigeminal nerve innervate the muscles that open and close the jaw. Denervation abnormalities lead to noticeable jaw malalignment. Palpation of the major muscles (masseter) and brief observation of jaw motion are sufficient in the patient without localized complaints.

E. Facial Nerve (CrN VII)

The facial nerve provides motor innervation to the muscles of facial expression. To assess its function, observe the overall appearance of the face, realizing that subtle facial asymmetries are common. Next, ask the patient to wrinkle her forehead, shut her eyes tightly, and smile (or show her teeth). Weakness in these muscle groups should be apparent.

The distinction between *central* and *peripheral* facial nerve palsies can be a source of great confusion (and frequent debates during morning rounds!). Central facial nerve palsy refers to a disruption of the upper motor neuron (corticobulbar) fibers that innervate the facial nuclei, while peripheral facial nerve palsy is a disruption of the facial nerve itself. Since there is bilateral corticobulbar innervation only to the portion of the facial nerve that subserves the forehead, a unilateral upper motor neuron (UMN) lesion will spare the forehead. A lesion of the facial nerve itself (Bell's palsy) will cause complete hemi-facial weakness. This differentiation is critical since a peripheral lesion is often benign, while the central lesion may represent important intracranial pathology.

F. The Acoustic/Vestibular Nerve (CrN VIII)

Lesions of this nerve are an important cause of dizziness. Examination of the dizzy patient, including an assessment of the eighth cranial nerve, is beyond the scope of this chapter.

G. Glossopharyngeal and Vagus Nerves (CrNs IX and X)

These two nerves innervate the palate, pharynx, and larynx and are critical for speech and swallowing. Lesions of CrNs IX and X are usually clinically obvious, since they produce dysarthric or hoarse speech and drooling (due to an inability to swallow secretions). The usual method of testing these nerves, the gag reflex, is highly variable and often unhelpful. Inspection of the oral cavity is probably sufficient in the asymptomatic patient.

H. Spinal Accessory Nerve (CrN XI)

This nerve provides motor innervation to two muscles: the trapezius and the sternocleidomastoid. A strong shoulder shrug and head turn provide evidence of intact innervation of each muscle, respectively.

I. Hypoglossal Nerve (CrN XII)

The hypoglossal nerve provides motor innervation to the tongue. Denervation is usually not subtle and will often cause an audible lisp. Have the patient protrude his tongue, and look for deviation to one side. Dyskinesias related to the use of neuroleptic medication (e.g., tardive dyskinesia) may be apparent. Small spontaneous movements of the protruded tongue can be a normal finding.

IV. The Motor Examination

A. Motor Tone

Motor tone refers to the resistance of a limb to passive movement through its normal range of motion. To examine for tone, have the patient fully relax her arms and/or legs to allow you to determine the degree of stiffness during passive motion. An increased level of tone, noted by rigidity or spasticity, is an important finding that may belie an UMN or extrapyramidal lesion (parkinsonism). Rigidity as a feature of Parkinson's disease is further discussed elsewhere in this book.

B. Muscle Bulk

Muscle atrophy is an important sign of lower motor neuron disease. Assessment of muscle bulk can be extraordinarily difficult, even for the seasoned clinician, due to natural variations in body habitus and the role of weightlifting or exercise (i.e., "bulking up"). Muscles that are unaffected by weightlifting or exercise (e.g., the facial muscles or the intrinsic muscles of the hand) may therefore provide the best estimate of overall muscle bulk.

C. Motor Power (Strength)

It is impractical (and unnecessary) to test each of the several hundred muscles in the human body. Should the patient have a focal motor complaint, knowledge of major muscle groups in the proximal and distal limbs becomes important. Muscle strength is graded from 0 (no motion) to 5 (normal strength).

Observation of gait is an excellent screening test for the patient without focal weakness. If the patient is able to rise briskly and independently from a seated position and walk independently, gross motor deficits can be confidently ruled out. The ability to walk on heels and toes further assures distal lower extremity strength. Gait must be tested in all patients, particularly in the elderly, for whom falls are a life-threatening event.

D. Abnormal Movements

Abnormal involuntary movements should be noted and described. They are discussed in detail in the chapter on movement disorders (see chapter 42).

V. The Sensory Examination

A. Primary Sensory Modalities

Sensation allows tactile exploration of our environment. Even the most thorough examiner could not test every square inch of the body for intact sensation, nor would this be necessary. Knowledge of the full sensory exam is important for the patient with a focal sensory complaint, and the reader is referred to other texts for detailed information on this peripheral nerve exam. The main sensory modalities include:

1. **Pain:** tested by pinprick (using disposable sterile pins).
2. **Temperature:** tested by touching the skin with a cold metal object (tuning fork).
3. **Light touch:** tested by simply brushing the patient's skin with your hand or a moving wisp of cotton.
4. **Vibration sense:** tested by applying a "buzzing" tuning fork to the distal lower extremities.
5. **Proprioception:** best tested by the Romberg maneuver (can be assessed during gait observation). Ask the patient to stand with his feet as close together as possible, while still maintaining stability. Ask him to close his eyes while assuring him that you will not let him fall. The patient with poor proprioception will begin to sway and lose balance after closing his eyes.

B. Cortical Sensory Modalities

The primary sensory modalities discussed above provide input to the brain about the external environment. The sensory cortex integrates these "building blocks" to form complex sensory experiences. Since higher level sensory processing requires reliable primary input, testing these cortical sensory modalities is unnecessary in the patient with primary sensory deficits. **Two types of advanced sensory processing are recognized:**

1. **Stereognosis:** the ability to reach into your pocket and distinguish a quarter from a dime is an example of stereognosis. Simply, it is the ability to recognize objects using touch. It is tested by simply placing common objects in the patient's hand and asking her to name them with her eyes closed.
2. **Graphesthesia:** the ability to recognize numbers or letters "written" on the skin, most often using the palm. As with stereognosis, primary sensory modalities must be intact for this test to have meaning.

VI. Coordination Testing

A. Gait Testing

Coordination reflects the ability to orchestrate and control movement, and is crucial in the translation of movement into productive activity. Although the cerebellum probably plays the lead role in motor coordination, several other structures (basal ganglia, red nucleus) are also clearly involved.

Walking is an extraordinarily complex motor skill that requires significant coordination of trunk and limbs. Its actual complexity makes it an ideal screening test for coordination ability. The human has a particularly narrow base when standing upright; with any degree of incoordination (ataxia), the patient will need to widen the base to remain upright. Balance becomes even more difficult when other sensory information is removed, forming the basis for the Romberg maneuver.

The sensitivity of screening is increased by having the patient walk heel to toe (as on a tightrope). The ability to do this smoothly and quickly rules out any major impairment in coordination.

B. Diadochokinesia

This term reflects the paired nature of agonist and antagonist muscle activity in coordinated limb movement. Abnormalities of this function are given the lengthy label dysdiadochokinesia, and are detected by several simple maneuvers:

1. **Finger to nose.** Have the patient alternate between touching your finger and touching her nose. Look for

inaccuracy of movement (dysmetria) and presence of tremor (intention tremor).

2. **Heel to shin.** Have the patient run the heel of one foot down the shin of the opposite leg (from knee to ankle) as accurately as possible.
3. **Rapid alternating movements.** Include rapid pronation/supination of the forearm (e.g., screwing in a lightbulb), finger tapping, or toe tapping. Having the patient tap out a rhythm is an excellent way to assess coordination ability. With cerebellar damage, the rhythm will be poorly timed, with emphases in the wrong places.

VII. Reflex Testing

A. Proprioceptive Reflexes

These reflexes, also known as deep tendon reflexes (DTRs), are based on the simple reflex arcs that are activated by stretching (or tapping). **Since they are influenced by the descending corticospinal tracts, DTRs can provide important information on the integrity of this pathway at several levels.** The reader is likely familiar with the methods used to elicit the five major DTRs: biceps, triceps, brachioradialis, quadriceps (knee), and Achilles (ankle). The grading of each reflex is on a 4-point scale, with 2 (2+) designated as normal.

B. Nociceptive Reflexes

These reflexes are based on reflex arcs located in the skin (rather than muscle tendons) and are therefore elicited by scratching or stroking. These include the abdominal reflexes, cremasteric reflex, and anal wink, none of which is extensively used clinically.

The major nociceptive reflex of clinical value is the plantar reflex. Stroking the sole of the foot should elicit plantar flexion of the toes. Babinski's sign, marked by an extensor response (i.e., dorsiflexion) of the toes, often with fanning of the toes and flexion of the ankle, is seen in pyramidal tract disease. It has become one of the most famous eponymic signs in all of medicine.

C. Primitive Reflexes (Release Reflexes)

These reflexes are present at birth but disappear in early infancy. Their reappearance later in life is abnormal and is often reflective of frontal lobe disease. Amongst others, they include:

1. **Grasp reflex.** Stroking the patient's palm will lead to an automatic clutching of your finger between his thumb and index finger.
2. **Snout reflex.** Gentle tapping over the patient's upper lip will cause a puckering of the lips. This may also elicit a **suck response,** or a turning of the head toward the stroking stimulus (**root reflex**).

VIII. Conclusion

The brain is an organ that is unmatched in its eloquence. Unlike the anginal grip of cardiac disease or the choking dyspnea of respiratory dysfunction, illness of the brain can send many different messages. Deciphering these messages, using the neurologic examination, can be complex, and at times bewildering. This should not discourage the practicing psychiatrist from using the examination described in this chapter as a routine part of every patient evaluation.

Suggested Readings

DeGowin, R.L. (1994). *DeGowin and DeGowin's diagnostic examination* (6th ed.). New York: McGraw-Hill.

Glick, T.H. (1993). *Neurologic skills.* Boston, MA: Blackwell Scientific.

Haerer, A.F. (1992). *DeJong's the neurologic exam* (5th ed.). Philadelphia: Lippincott-Williams and Wilkins.

Lishman, W.A. (1998). *Organic psychiatry* (3rd ed.). Oxford: Blackwell Science.

Samuels, M.A. (1996). *Videotextbook of neurology for the practicing physician: Vol. 2. The neurologic exam.* Boston, MA: Butterworth-Heinemann (Elsevier).

Samuels, M.A. (1999). *The manual of neurologic therapeutics* (6th ed.). Philadelphia, PA: Lippincott-Williams and Wilkins.

Samuels, M.A., & Feske, S. (1996). *Office practice of neurology* (2nd ed.). Philadelphia, PA: Churchhill-Livingstone (Elsevier).

Chapter 36

Neuropsychiatric Dysfunction

STEPHAN HECKERS

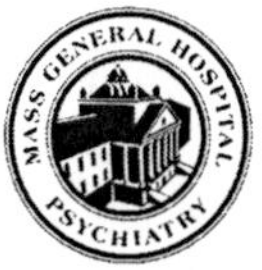

I. Introduction

Psychiatrists are often challenged to bridge the disciplines of medicine, neurology, and psychiatry when faced with a patient who has behavioral abnormalities. **The neuropsychiatric evaluation combines medical, neurologic, and psychiatric skills, and includes documentation of the history, examination of the patient, and often the ordering of additional tests.**

II. General Evaluation

A. Specific Features of the Neuropsychiatric Evaluation

1. **History**
   a. **An acute onset of behavioral change should always lead to a thorough search for traumatic events, including physical** (e.g., traumatic brain injury), **chemical** (e.g., hypoxia during stroke), **or psychological** (e.g., stress during a disaster) **insults. Often overlooked are neuropsychiatric sequelae of a medical condition that present some time after the initial symptoms have disappeared** (e.g., depression and anxiety after stroke).
   b. **The age of onset** of several neuropsychiatric disorders (e.g., autism, schizophrenia, mania, or dementia) is relatively well defined. When considering a diagnosis that is rare (e.g., late-onset schizophrenia or early-onset dementia), other more prevalent conditions should be ruled out.
   c. **The course and temporal pattern** (e.g., stable, progressively deteriorating, episodic, or ictal) of the expression of symptoms can provide clues for the diagnosis of specific disorders, such as seizures or dementia.
2. **Baseline mental functioning** of the patient. It is crucial to assess the degree of deficits, such as memory loss, language difficulties, or impaired judgment, and determine how this differs from the pre-morbid level of functioning.
3. **Findings of the physical and mental status exam. It is helpful to organize the pattern of behavioral abnormalities along the lines of cortical and subcortical structures.** If the patient demonstrates deficits in one behavioral domain, related functions should be examined (see Table 36-1).

B. Medical History

The history of present illness should document any recent surgical procedures or medical problems. For example, delirium is often seen post-operatively, after myocardial infarction, or with infections (especially when fever is present). Depression is frequently seen after stroke or can accompany a malignancy. **Particularly challenging are paraneoplastic syndromes,** such as limbic encephalitis, when neuropsychiatric deficits predate the onset of other signs of the underlying malignancy. **Any previous neurologic event or recurrent psychiatric illness,** such as psychotic disorder, anxiety disorder, mood disorder, or drug abuse, **should be documented. Any current drug use** (including prescription, over-the-counter, and illicit drugs) **should be documented.**

C. Examination

1. **Physical examination.** Abnormal **vital signs,** especially fever and tachycardia, should prompt a thorough search for systemic or central nervous system (CNS) abnormalities that could explain the neuropsychiatric dysfunction. If **signs of meningeal irritation** (neck stiffness, Kernig or Brudzinski signs) are present, a computed tomography (CT) scan of the head and lumbar puncture should be performed.
2. **Neurological examination.** The **examination of the cranial nerves** should include **a funduscopic exam** and the testing of extraocular movements, sensory **and motor function of the face, and the gag reflex.** Tests of smell are important in patients with a history of traumatic brain injury, if an orbitofrontal process (e.g., stroke or tumor) is suspected, or in patients reporting olfactory or gustatory hallucinations. **Abnormal muscle tone** and abnormal movements of face and limbs may be seen in patients with extrapyramidal movement disorders or in patients treated with psychotropic medication. Examination of reflexes typically includes deep tendon reflexes, Babinski reflex, and primitive reflexes (e.g., snout, grasp, glabellar, and palmomental as frontal release signs). **Coordination** can be tested easily with the finger-nose-finger test or heel-shin-heel test.
3. **Laboratory tests** to rule out many medical conditions that can lead to neuropsychiatric dysfunction should include **electrolytes, calcium, glucose, and tests of kidney, liver, and thyroid function, a complete blood count, levels of vitamins B_{12} and folate, lues serology (such as the rapid plasma reagin [RPR]), and a test for antibodies against the human immunodeficiency virus (HIV). Screening for drugs** (illicit, therapeutic, and over-the-counter) in serum, and for cocaine and marijuana (i.e., tetrahydrocannabinol [THC]) in urine, requires permission of the patient except in an emergency.

III. Evaluation of Behavioral Domains

A. Level of Consciousness

The alert patient responds promptly and appropriately to sensory stimulation. **Fluctuation of the level of**

Table 36-1. Mapping of Behavioral Abnormalities

	Region				
Behavior	*Frontal*	*Parietal*	*Temporal*	*Striatum*	*Thalamus*
Language	• Motor aphasia [L] • Confabulation	• Dyslexia [L] • Dysgraphia [L]	• Sensory aphasia [L]	• Dysarthria • [L] caudate nucleus: fluent aphasia	• Confabulation • Anterolateral thalamus: logorrheic aphasia
Affect	• Apathy • Inappropriate, disinhibited • Motor aprosodia [R]	• Sensory aprosodia [R]			
Memory	• Impaired working memory		• Impaired encoding/recall of information		• Impaired encoding/recall of information
Others	• Impaired attention • Poor planning, insight • Reduplicative paramnesia	• Impaired attention [R] • Dyscalculia [L]	• Prosopagnosia [L+R]		• Impaired attention
Motor	• Paresis • Abulia • Echopraxia • Perseveration • Frontal release signs	• Dyspraxia [R]		• Extrapyramidal movement disorder	

[L] and [R] indicate left (dominant) and right (non-dominant) hemisphere, respectively; in some right hemisphere dominant, left-handed subjects, the hemispheric asymmetry is reversed.

GLOSSARY

Abulia	Lack of will or motivation
Agnosia	Lack of sensory ability to recognize objects
Aphasia	Impairment of language function due to brain damage
Aprosodia	Lack of pitch, rhythm, and modulation in speech
Dysarthria	Disturbance of articulation
Dyscalculia	Difficulty in computing
Dysgraphia	Difficulty in writing
Dyslexia	Difficulty in reading
Dyspraxia	Difficulty in executing purposeful movements
Echopraxia	Involuntary imitation of movements made by another person
Prosopagnosia	Difficulty in recognizing faces
Reduplicative paramnesia	Delusion that a person is replaced by an imposter (Capgras syndrome)

consciousness between alertness, drowsiness, and stupor is a hallmark of acute confusional states (delirium). Hyperalertness can be seen in drug-induced states or severe anxiety.

B. Appearance and Psychomotor Activity

The patient's posture, hygiene, and clothing may provide valuable information about the patient's affect, thinking, and reality testing. **The patient's attitude** toward the physician and how he engages in the interview may provide information about his personality structure.

Abnormal motor behavior can be due to cortical, basal ganglia, cerebellar, or lower motor neuron disease. **Repetitive movements** may represent tremor, dyskinesia, or tics. **Psychomotor retardation** is often seen in depression but can also be due to hypokinetic movement disorders (e.g., Parkinson's disease), degenerative diseases (e.g., Alzheimer's disease), stroke, or catatonia. **Waxy flexibility** (i.e., the patient remains in a position modeled by the examiner) is sometimes seen in a catatonic state. **Increased psychomotor activity,** to the degree of agitation, is seen in anxious or psychotic patients, as a side effect of psychotropic medication (akathisia) mainly due to neuroleptics and selective serotonin reuptake inhibitors, or in the hyperactive form of delirium.

C. Speech

The flow, volume, and rate of speech should be noted.

Pressured speech often accompanies a manic state, whereas **a decreased rate of speech** may be due to depressed mood, and unexpected pauses may represent the psychotic symptom of thought blocking.

If speech is not coherent or goal-directed, more formal language testing (see below) and detailed examination of the thought process are warranted.

Prosody, the affective modulation of speech, is often impaired in patients with right hemisphere lesions, with parietal lesions affecting more the perception (sensory aprosodia) and frontal lesions more the production (motor aprosodia) of affectively modulated speech. However, aprosodia is also seen in depression or hypokinetic movement disorders.

Abnormalities of the larynx, tongue, or mouth can lead to **dysarthria,** a pure motor dysfunction which should be differentiated from aphasia.

D. Affect

The outward display of emotion, affect, should be differentiated from the internally felt emotion, mood. Affect is normally appropriate to the situation and congruent with mood and thinking.

Inappropriate and incongruent affect is seen in patients with schizophrenia or mania, or after frontal lobe damage. Pseudobulbar palsy can result in markedly inappropriate and incongruent affect, so-called pathological laughter or pathological crying. The range of affect and appropriate modulation can be restricted to a consistently dysthymic or anhedonic level, as in depression, or to a consistently elevated level, as seen in mania or frontal lobe damage.

E. Thought

Thinking is assessed appropriately by listening to the patient talking freely. The thought process should be coherent, logically organized, and goal-directed.

Loosely organized and **incoherent speech (flight of ideas and loose associations)** and an excessive use of words in response to a question, ending in the appropriate answer **(circumstantiality)** or not answering at all **(tangentiality)** are typically seen in mania. Also consider **aphasia** in a patient with incoherent speech (see below).

Poverty of thought with lack of associations is seen in depression, some forms of schizophrenia, after frontal lobe damage, and in basal ganglia disorders, such as Parkinson's disease. **The thought content is the material of the patient's conversation.** Excessively recurring themes might indicate a preoccupation or a delusion. It is important to question the patient about the character of his thoughts and rule out clearly psychotic symptoms, such as thought insertion or withdrawal, and ideas of reference (e.g., the television is sending messages specifically to the patient).

F. Perception

The correct reception and interpretation of sensory input can be altered due to abnormalities of the peripheral sensory organs, their projections to unimodal cortical areas, or higher-order cortical areas and sub-cortical structures. Sensory deficits can occur at any of these three levels.

Illusions typically occur with abnormalities of the sensory organs, in drug-induced states, or in acute confusional states.

Hallucinations are often seen in psychotic disorders, but can also be found in patients with seizure, stroke, or tumor, and secondary to drug intoxication or withdrawal.

G. Cognition

1. **Orientation. The patient should be oriented to person, place, and time. Orientation to person is almost always preserved,** even in acute confusional states.

   Non-aphasic patients disoriented to person should be evaluated for a dissociative disorder or malingering.

   Orientation to place (by asking for the name of the city, building, floor, and type of room) or time (by asking for year, month, day, and time of day) are often impaired in dementia, delirium, or an amnestic disorder. Orientation changes rapidly in acute confusional states and answers should be recorded to compare the degree of impairment.
2. **Attention. The attentional matrix provides the background for all other cognitive faculties and includes vigilance, perseverance, concentration, and resistance to interference. The reticular activating system, the thalamus, and the association cortical**

areas, primarily those of the frontal lobes, all contribute to the attentional matrix. Serial recitation tasks (such as the **serial 7s**) or the **digit span** test (repeating a string of numbers forward or backward, 6 ± 1 correct numbers in one string is normal) **are very helpful, easy-to-use tests to assess attention.**

Patients with frontal lobe damage, delirium, or metabolic encephalopathy often score very poorly on such tests. However, anxious and depressed patients might also do poorly. Poor attention is seen in patients with dementia, or in children, adolescents, and adults with attention deficit disorder.

One form of impaired attention, **unilateral neglect, is seen after lesions of the parietal cortex, the cingulate cortex, the frontal eye field, the thalamus, or the striatum.** Simple bedside tests (e.g., asking the patient to either bisect lines of varying lengths drawn on a piece of paper or cancel all letters of one type on a piece of paper covered with many different letters) are often better than testing for sensory extinction on one side after bilateral sensory stimulation.

3. **Language.** The disruption of language function interferes significantly with everyday functioning of the patient. **The assessment should include testing of repetition, comprehension, naming, reading, and writing.**
   a. Repetition can be tested with sentences such as **"No ifs, ands, or buts."** Repetition is impaired in all four major aphasic disorders involving perisylvian structures (**Broca's area** in motor aphasia, **Wernicke's area** in sensory aphasia, both areas in global aphasia, and the **arcuate fasciculus** connecting the two areas in conduction aphasia) (Table 36-2). Paraphasic errors while repeating should be recorded. Correct repetition does not mean comprehension of the language.
   b. **Comprehension can be tested by asking the patient to perform one-, two-, or three-step tasks.** Alternatively, especially when the patient is apraxic, simple yes/no questions or commands to point to body parts may be used. If a temporoparietal lesion involves Wernicke's area or its vicinity (as in lesions resulting in the sensory transcortical aphasia), comprehension will be impaired.
   c. **Naming is usually assessed by confrontation naming of objects or body parts.** Alternatively, words from a given category (e.g., animals) can be requested; normal subjects should be able to name about 12 in 1 minute. Word-finding difficulties (**dysnomia**) are also seen in metabolic encephalopathy, as a side effect of psychotropic medication, and in exhaustion, anxiety, and depression. It is then important to rule out other language deficits.
   d. **Reading should be tested** by asking the patient to read individual words, sentences, or paragraphs. **Alexia** is the inability to comprehend written material. Alexia is associated with agraphia if the lesion is located in the left inferior parietal lobule.
   e. **Writing tests** should include dictation of sentences rather than just phrases (e.g., "I'm fine"). Purely mechanical agraphia due to motor dysfunction should be excluded. Aphasia is typically associated with agraphia, but agraphia not always with aphasia.
4. **Memory. Short-term memory** may be tested by asking the patient to encode a list of three or four words and then testing the immediate and delayed recall after 5 minutes. Remote memory can be tested by asking for past events or famous people.

   Impaired memory is seen in psychiatric disorders and as a result of a neurologic insult. In psychogenic amnesia personal events cannot be recalled, but nonpersonal information of the same time period is often spared. Psychotic disorders and depression often lead to impaired encoding of memory.

   It is always important to distinguish between amnesia, an isolated memory deficit, and more global neuropsychiatric dysfunction, such as dementia or delirium, that affect more cognitive domains than just memory. Hippocampal damage due to hypoxia and hypoglycemia or damage to thalamus, mamillary bodies, and periventricular structures due to thiamine deficiency (i.e., Wernicke-Korsakoff syndrome) are well-known causes of amnestic syndromes.

Table 36-2. Differential Diagnosis of the Main Types of Aphasia

Type of Aphasia	*Repetition*	*Comprehension*	*Speech*
Global	Impaired	Impaired	Non-fluent
Wernicke	Impaired	Impaired	Fluent
Broca	Impaired	Intact	Non-fluent
Conduction	Impaired	Intact	Fluent
Transcortical			
Motor	Intact	Intact	Non-fluent
Sensory	Intact	Impaired	Fluent

5. **Visuospatial skill. Drawing intersecting geometric figures or drawing a clock (with hands indicating, for example, "10 to 2") are simple tests of visuospatial skills.** Demented or confused patients or those with lesions of the association cortex in the parietal, temporal, and frontal lobes typically show significant impairment. However, damage of the visual pathways from the retina to primary visual cortex can also result in impairment. **Damage to the parietal lobe of the non-dominant hemisphere is especially prone to produce visuospatial deficits.** Such patients might also show dyspraxia (i.e., a difficulty in executing purposeful movements, such as brushing teeth, combing hair, or dressing).

H. Abstracting Abilities

Testing for abstract similarities (What do a plane and a car have in common?), interpretation of proverbs, or assessing practical judgment (How many slices are in a loaf of bread?) **is a helpful probe for abstracting abilities, affiliated with the dorsolateral frontal cortex.** Patients with frontal lobe damage also tend to perseverate, often adhere concretely to the material presented, and have difficulties shifting attention. However, frontal lobe deficits might not be apparent during formal testing in the office but more so by assessing the patient's level of functioning at home. Bilateral frontal lobe damage may lead to **abulia,** the lack of motivation to speak, move, or act. Other syndromes associated with frontal lobe damage are **reduplicative paramnesia** (**Capgras syndrome;** i.e., the delusion that a person is replaced by an imposter) and echopraxia (the involuntary imitation of movements made by another person).

I. Insight/Judgment

Neurologic insults leading to **unilateral neglect or anosognosia** typically cause impaired awareness and insight. Moreover, psychiatric conditions, such as mood disorders, schizophrenia, dementia, and amnestic disorders, also produce poor insight. **To assess the quality of the patient's insight, ask the patient how much the observed deficits affect him or others around him.**

IV. Summary

Patients with neuropsychiatric dysfunction present a complex diagnostic and management challenge. At times, the diagnosis can easily and quickly be made with an abnormal blood test or a very specific clinical finding. **With a good foundation in the general principles of neuropsychiatry the physician can streamline and optimize the evaluation and consultation process.**

Suggested Readings

Crum, R.M., Anthony, J.C., Bassett, S.S., & Folstein, M.F. (1993). Population-based norms for the Mini-Mental State Examination by age and education level. *Journal of the American Medical Association, 269,* 2386–2391.

Damasio, A.R. (1992). Aphasia. *New England Journal of Medicine, 326,* 531–539.

Fogel, B.S., & Schiffer, R.B. (1996). *Neuropsychiatry.* Baltimore, MD: Williams and Wilkins.

Folstein, M.F., Folstein, S.E., & McHugh, P.R. (1975). "Mini-Mental State": A practical method of grading the cognitive state of patients for the clinician. *Journal of Psychiatric Research, 12,* 189–198.

Hier, D.B., Gorelick, P.B., Shindler, A.G. (1987). *Topics in behavioral neurology and neuropsychology.* Boston, MA: Butterworths.

Mesulam, M-M. (2000). *Principles of behavioral and cognitive neurology.* New York: Oxford University Press.

Chapter 37

Clinical Neurophysiology and Electroencephalography

Shahram Khoshbin

I. Overview

A. The Electroencephalogram

1. Characteristics of recordings

a. **The electroencephalogram (EEG) records low-voltage electrical activity produced by the brain.** Recordings are often characteristic of certain ages and states of consciousness; in addition, it is possible to recognize generalized malfunction of the brain, as well as localized or paroxysmal abnormalities. **Ordinarily, the EEG is recorded from the scalp with small surface electrodes.** Although the precise origin of the electrical activity is unknown, most investigators believe that most of the activity represents dendritic synaptic potentials in the cortical pyramidal cells.

b. **Electrical activity is recorded from a variety of standard sites on the scalp, according to the international electrode placement system.** The nasopharyngeal lead may also be employed; this is a long electrode that is passed through the nose and which rests on the back of the throat near the medial aspect of the temporal lobe.

c. **Recording electrical activity requires the measurement of the voltage between two electrodes.** It is impossible to record from all pairs of electrodes at the same time. The typical EEG machine has eight or 16 channels. Thus, a series of electrode pairs are evaluated.

d. **Two different styles of recording exist.** In **the referential (or monopolar) method,** a series of different electrodes are referred to the same reference electrode, which is presumed to be relatively electrically inactive. Commonly used reference points are the ears, the vertex, or a non-cephalic reference. In another method, **the bipolar method,** electrodes placed in a line are recorded serially as successive pairs. (The first recording would be from the first and second electrodes, the second recording would be from the second and third electrodes, and so on.) Creation of different montages gives various views of the electrical activity at different parts of the brain.

e. **The electrical activity from any electrode pair can be described in terms of amplitude and frequency.** Amplitude ranges from 5 μV to 200 μV. Frequency of EEG activity ranges from 0 Hz to about 20 Hz. **The frequencies are described by Greek letters: delta (0–4 Hz), theta (4–8 Hz), alpha (8–12 Hz), and beta (more than 12 Hz).**

2. Recordings during sleep

a. **In the normal awake adult (with eyes closed), alpha rhythm seen in the posterior part of the head predominates.** The amplitude of the alpha waves falls off anteriorly and it is often replaced by low-voltage beta activity. Often, some low-voltage theta activity can be seen in frontocentral or temporal regions. **The alpha rhythm, which is prominent posteriorly, disappears (or is blocked) when the eyes open.**

b. **When a normal adult becomes drowsy, the alpha rhythm gradually disappears, frontocentral beta activity may become more prominent, and frontocentral-temporal theta activity becomes predominant.**

c. **Drowsiness is stage I sleep.** As sleep becomes deeper, high-voltage single or complex theta or delta waves, called vertex sharp waves, appear centrally.

d. **Stage II sleep is characterized by increased numbers of vertex sharp waves, and centrally predominant runs of sinusoidal 12–14 Hz activity, called sleep spindles, occur.**

e. Deeper sleep, characterized by progressively more and higher-voltage theta and delta activity, is not usually seen in routine EEG recordings.

f. In routine EEG studies, some **"activations" (3 minutes of hyperventilation and a flashing strobe light at different frequencies) are employed to try to bring out abnormalities** not apparent in the record without the activations. Drugs can be used in certain circumstances to activate epileptic activity. Convulsants (such as pentylenetetrazol) could be used for this purpose.

3. EEG abnormalities

a. **Abnormalities of the EEG are either focal (only one area of the brain), or generalized (whole brain).** Additionally, abnormalities are **either continuous or intermittent. An abnormality which appears and disappears suddenly is called paroxysmal.**

b. **Increased "slow activity"** (i.e., theta and delta activity in a waking record) **is nearly always abnormal.**

c. Focal delta activity is usually irregular in configuration and is termed polymorphic delta activity (PDA). PDA is usually indicative of a focal lesion of brain. Another type of delta activity is called **FIRDA (frontal intermittent rhythmic delta activity);** this is indicative of increased intracranial pressure in young people and is a less specific sign of some brain abnormality in the elderly. Generalized theta and delta activity is a sign of an encephalopathy. As a general rule, the EEG is a sensitive test for abnormalities, but it is not specific.

d. Increased beta activity is often a sign that the patient is taking some kind of sedative.

4. Seizure disorders

a. **The EEG has been particularly useful in the analysis of patients with seizure disorders. Paroxysmal abnormalities are common between overt seizures (interictally) as well as during seizures (ictally).** Paroxysmal abnormalities include the spike and the sharp wave.

b. A **spike** is a single wave which stands out from the background activity and has a duration of less than 80 milliseconds. A **sharp wave** is similar with a duration of more than 80 milliseconds. A spike or sharp wave is often followed by a slow wave and spikes and slow waves can alternate at frequencies from 2 Hz to 5 Hz.

c. **Epileptic paroxysmal abnormalities can be generalized or focal.** The classic generalized abnormality is the 3 Hz spike and wave pattern which underlies the petit mal absence attack. A typical focal abnormality is a focal single spike followed by a slow wave. This abnormality can be seen in focal epilepsy or in grand mal epilepsy if the abnormal electric activity spreads rapidly to the entire brain.

d. **Activations, such as hyperventilation, photic stimulation, sleep, sleep deprivation, and use of drugs, are useful in bringing out epileptic activity.** On any one record, it is possible to miss epileptic activity that is infrequent; for this reason multiple recordings are useful.

e. The relationship of any of these abnormalities to the particular patient is complex. For example, **paroxysmal activity on an EEG may or may not mean that the patient's problem is related to epilepsy;** the final determination typically rests on the overall clinical picture and on the results of a therapeutic trial. One should resist the temptation to consider the EEG independently. In particular, a normal EEG does not exclude epilepsy, since (to cite an extreme case) the EEG may be normal during a focal seizure which is observed clinically. Reading EEGs is tricky; it takes experience since there are a wide variety of normal variant wave forms and artifacts that must be recognized.

II. Evoked Potentials

A. Overview

1. **A sensory stimulus in any modality (visual, auditory, or somatosensory) will produce a change in the EEG.** The change is usually small in magnitude compared with the background EEG; **the exact configuration of the change depends on the nature of the stimulus and the site of recording on the scalp.**
2. **The evoked potential is the change in the EEG which is dependent on and time-locked to the stimulus; to see it, the stimulus must be repeated many times and the EEG averaged.**
3. **Evoked potentials can be used to test the integrity of a pathway in the central nervous system (CNS). The most common use of evoked potentials at present is to test the speed of conduction in a particular pathway.** Multiple sclerosis is a disease of central myelin; if myelin is damaged, conduction is slowed and the evoked potentials will be delayed. Although many multiple sclerosis plaques are clinically silent they show themselves with this electrical test. Hence, evoked potentials are quite useful in making the diagnosis of multiple sclerosis.

B. Visual Evoked Potentials

1. Visual evoked potentials (VEPs) were the first to become popular. They **are ordinarily obtained with a checker-board stimulus that alternates black and white squares repetitively. Each eye is stimulated individually and then responses are measured from the occipital area of the scalp.** The major wave measured is a large positive wave at a latency of about 100 milliseconds. In multiple sclerosis or optic neuritis, the wave is delayed. Delayed or absent VEPs can be seen in many other conditions, including ocular conditions (e.g., glaucoma), compressive lesions of the optic nerve (e.g., pituitary lesions), and pathological conditions of the optic radiations or the occipital cortex.

C. Auditory Evoked Potentials

1. **Auditory stimulation produces complex waveforms.** Stimulation with brief clicks produces six small waves in the first 10 milliseconds. Quite surprisingly, **the sources of this electrical activity are in serial ascending structures in the brainstem.** It becomes possible to study the integrity of the brainstem with these waves, and the test has also been used to assess "brainstem death" in cases suspected of "brain death." The waves are also delayed in multiple sclerosis.

D. Somatosensory Evoked Potentials

1. Somatosensory evoked potentials (SEPs) **are the averaged electrical responses in the CNS to somatosensory stimulation.** Like sensory action potentials (SAPs) in the peripheral nervous system, **most components of SEPs represent activity carried in the large sensory fibers of the dorsal column** (medial lemniscus primary sensorimotor cortex pathway). SEPs can be used to test the integrity of the pathway and to test the speed of conduction in the pathway.
2. SEPs from the upper extremity are commonly produced by stimulation of the median nerve at the wrist. The cerebral SEP to this type of stimulation was the first EP to be discovered (by Dawson in 1947). The cerebral SEP to median nerve stimulation is best recorded from a site approximately 2 cm posterior to the contralateral central electrode. SEPs from the lower extremity are produced by stimulation of the posterior tibial nerve at the ankle or the peroneal nerve at the fibular head.
3. **It is possible to localize a lesion in the somatosensory pathway by using short latency SEPs from sub-cortical structures.** Several systems of electrode placement can be used, but the one which seems to produce potentials of greatest amplitude is where the active electrode is placed over the cervical spine and referred to an "inactive" site. By stimulating leg

nerves, it is possible to obtain EPs at all levels of the neuraxis, including over the spinal cord.

III. Nerve Conduction

A. Sensory Nerve Conduction

1. **The cell bodies of sensory neurons are located in the dorsal root ganglia.** Each neuron has a central process entering the spinal cord through the dorsal horn and a peripheral process connecting to a sensory receptor in the skin or deep tissues of the limb. **The receptors transduce somatosensory stimuli into electrical potentials, which eventually give rise to action potentials in the axons which are transmitted along the peripheral process to the central process.** There are a variety of sensory neurons, each with a characteristic spectrum of axonal diameters. Some neurons are myelinated while some are unmyelinated; in routine studies the unmyelinated fibers cannot be measured. **Many sensory axons with differing function and size run together with motor axons.**
2. **The goals of sensory nerve conduction studies are:**
   a. To assess the number of functioning axons
   b. To assess the state of the myelin of these axons
3. Nerve conduction studies
   a. **In the usual sensory nerve conduction study, all of the axons in a sensory nerve are activated with a pulse of electric current.** Action potentials travel along the nerve and the electric field produced by these action potentials is recorded at a site distant from the site of stimulation. **Each axon makes a contribution to the magnitude of the electrical field and thus the amplitude of the recorded sensory action potential is a measure of the number of functioning axons.**
   b. **Utilizing the distance between the site of stimulation and the site of recording and the time between stimulation and the arrival of the action potentials at the recording site, it is possible to calculate a conduction velocity which reflects the quality of myelin of the axons.**
   c. **In axonal degeneration neuropathies, the primary feature is reduced sensory action potential amplitudes.** The conduction velocity may be slightly slowed, but only to the extent that the normally largest axons are gone and the measured conduction velocity reflects the velocity of the largest remaining axons. **In demyelinating neuropathies, the primary feature is slowing of conduction. In radiculopathies, sensory action potential amplitudes and conduction velocities are fully normal.** This is because the lesion is virtually always proximal to the dorsal root ganglion and the cell body and its peripheral process remain normal. Sensory action potential similarly remains normal with lesions of the CNS.

B. Motor Nerve Conduction

1. **There are significant differences between sensory and motor nerve conduction which depend in large part on the differences of the anatomy in the two situations.** Motor neurons have cell bodies in the anterior horn of the spinal cord and send their axons to innervate muscle fibers. **Motor axons are always intertwined with sensory axons; there are no nerves that are pure motor nerves. Hence, the electrically stimulated compound action potential of any nerve with motor fibers in it is really a mixed nerve action potential.** Consequently, it is not possible to deduce the number of functioning motor axons by looking at the amplitude of a nerve action potential.
2. It is possible to study motor nerve axons separately from sensory axons by electrically stimulating a nerve and by recording from the muscle fibers innervated by the motor axons in that nerve. Since each motor axon typically innervates hundreds of muscle fibers, the compound muscle action potential is very much larger than the nerve action potential.
3. The number of axons can be diminished and the action potential normal if the process of collateral re-innervation by the remaining axons has been complete. The number of axons can be normal and the action potential diminished if there is a neuromuscular junction deficit or if there is loss of muscle fibers. As a neuropathy progresses and collateral re-innervation fails to keep pace, then the muscle action potential will decline.
4. **The time interval between delivery of the electrical stimulus and the onset of the muscle action potential may be difficult to interpret.** This time period is composed of the time it takes for the motor nerve action potential to travel down the terminal branches of the axon, the time for the release of acetylcholine into the neuromuscular junction, the time for the acetylcholine to produce an endplate potential, the time for generation of a muscle action potential, and, depending on the position of the recording electrodes, the time for the muscle action potential to propagate to the recording electrodes. Calculation of a conduction velocity for these neurons is not as straightforward as it is for the sensory nerve. The time period itself, if obtained under standard conditions, can be a useful measure of the conduction time in the terminal part of the axon; it is called the distal motor latency.
5. The conduction velocity of motor axons can be determined for parts of the axon proximal to the distal portion. If the nerve is stimulated supramaximally in two places, then virtually identical muscle action potentials will result; the major difference will be the different latencies from the time of stimulation. The difference in the latencies is due to the difference in the distances

from the sites of stimulation to the muscle. Dividing the difference in the distances by the difference in the times produces a conduction velocity for the segment of nerve between the two sites of stimulation. Similar to the measurement of the sensory action potential, measurements of the muscle action potential are ordinarily made to the time of onset; hence, the calculated conduction velocity refers to the fastest (and largest) axons in the nerve.

6. **In axonal degeneration neuropathies, motor nerve conduction studies are not significantly abnormal until the process is moderately advanced.** Total reliance on motor nerve conduction would result in failure to detect many significant neuropathies. Typically, there will be a slight slowing of conduction velocity and prolongation of the distal motor latency since the largest axons are lost. There may be loss of action potential amplitude when the process is advanced. In demyelinating neuropathies, there will be slowing of conduction velocity and prolongation of distal motor latency.
7. **A focal lesion of a nerve will lead to slowing of conduction and to a decrement of amplitude across the segment, including the area of the lesion, but studies of the nerve distal to the lesion will be fully normal.** Studies of nerve segments proximal to the lesion will show normal conduction velocity with an unchanging and reduced action potential amplitude. Quite dramatic nerve conduction findings are seen with a focal, total lesion. The nerve is fully normal below the lesion but electrical stimulation proximal to the lesion produces no response (similar to the patient's attempts to activate the muscle).
8. **In radiculopathy, motor nerve conduction studies will ordinarily be normal.** There may be slight slowing of conduction velocity in direct relation to the amount of loss of large fibers. In CNS disease, there will ordinarily be no change in motor nerve conduction unless there is involvement of anterior horn cells.

C. Late Responses

1. **Studying the most proximal segments of nerves is difficult, because they are deep and not easily accessible as they leave the spinal column.** However, it is useful to study the proximal segments of nerves since processes, such as radiculopathies from disc protrusion and certain neuropathies (e.g., Guillain-Barré), affect this segment predominantly. **The so-called late responses (the E-reflex and the F-response) provide a relatively easy technique for study of the proximal segments of nerves. These responses are produced in certain circumstances after an electrical stimulus to a peripheral nerve, and are late with respect to the muscle response (the M-response) produced by the orthodromic volley of action potentials traveling to the muscle directly from the electrical stimulus.**
2. **The H-reflex is a monosynaptic reflex response similar in its pathway to that of the tendon jerk.** The electrical stimulus activates the I-a afferents (coming from the muscle spindles) and action potentials travel orthodromically to the spinal cord. In the cord, the I-a afferents make excitatory monosynaptic connections to the alpha motor neurons; a volley of action potentials is set up in the motor nerve which runs orthodromically the entire length of the nerve from the cell bodies to the muscle. Hence, action potentials travel through the proximal segment of the nerve twice during the production of the H-reflex (once in the sensory portion of the nerve and once in the motor portion). **Obtaining an H-reflex depends on the ability to stimulate the I-a afferents.** If a motor axon is electrically stimulated, then an action potential will travel along the axon antidromically toward the spinal cord as well as orthodromically toward the muscle. The antidromic action potential will collide either in the proximal motor axon or in cell body with the developing H-reflex in that axon and nullify it. In routine clinical practice, it is possible to get this differential stimulation and to produce E-reflexes only in the posterior tibial division of the sciatic nerve while recording from the triceps surae.
3. **The F-response or F-wave has an advantage over the H-reflex in that it can be found in most muscles. It is a manifestation of recurrent firing of an anterior horn cell after it has been invaded by an antidromic action potential.** After a motor nerve is stimulated, an action potential runs antidromically as well as orthodromically; a small percentage of anterior horn cells that have been invaded antidromically will produce an orthodromic action potential that is responsible for the F-response. Thus, to produce an F-response, action potentials must travel twice through the proximal segment of the motor nerve.

IV. Electromyography

A. The Physiology Underlying EMG

1. Understanding the concept of the motor unit is central to the understanding of the physiology of electromyography (EMG). **A motor unit is composed of all the muscle fibers innervated by a single anterior horn cell. In most proximal limb muscles, there are hundreds of fibers in each motor unit. In the normal situation, the muscle fibers from the same unit are not clumped together, but are intermingled with fibers from other motor units. When a motor axon fires, each muscle fiber in its motor unit is activated in a constant time relationship to the other fibers in the unit.**
2. **EMG activity is ordinarily recorded with a needle placed into the muscle.** Because the muscle fibers of

a single motor unit are not packed closely together, the **EMG needle records from only about ten fibers from each motor unit. The amplitude, duration, and configuration of the electrical activity recorded from a motor unit varies as the needle changes its orientation to the muscle fibers.** Despite its variability it is possible to specify a normal range for the amplitude, duration, and configuration of motor unit action potentials (MUAPs) for each muscle and each age.

3. **When an EMG needle is placed in a normal muscle at rest, there is no electrical activity. With weak effort, first one and then several motor units are activated.** At this low level of activation, it is possible to see the individual MUAPs and evaluate their parameters. With maximal effort so many units are brought into action that individual MUAPs cannot be discerned; all that can be seen is a dense electrical pattern, called an interference pattern, which can be characterized by its density and peak-to-peak amplitude. The normal density would be either "full," if there are no gaps, or "highly mixed," if there are a few, short gaps. Some people are not willing or able to exert a maximal effort and the pattern will be less dense as a result. Hence, the degree of effort has to be taken into account when assessing the interference pattern.

B. Findings on the EMG

1. **Acute partial injury (e.g., a partial laceration of a nerve).** Motor axons that are injured undergo Wallerian degeneration over the course of about 5 days, leaving muscle fibers previously innervated by those axons in a denervated state. **Within approximately 10–14 days, denervated muscle fiber action potentials are recorded by the EMG needle as fibrillations and positive sharp waves.** There is nothing different about fibrillations and positive sharp waves other than a slight difference in the particulars of the recording; both are simply small, diphasic potentials beginning with a positive phase. The motor units that can be activated will be normal; it will not be possible to activate voluntarily the denervated muscle fibers. Descriptive terminology for these patterns is "high mixed," "mixed," "low mixed," and "single unit," in order of decreasing density.
2. **Chronic partial injury. After weeks to months, there will be collateral sprouting from surviving motor axons to innervate denervated muscle fibers.** Spontaneous activity will cease. Motor units will now contain more muscle fibers than normal; hence, MUAPs will be long in duration, high in amplitude, and more complex in shape or polyphasic. The interference pattern may improve in density, but probably will remain less than full although the amplitude will increase.
3. **Complete injury. In this circumstance no voluntarily initiated motor nerve action potentials can reach the muscle due to a focal demyelinating injury. Muscle fibers will not be denervated so they will not fibrillate.** EMG examination will reveal no spontaneous activity, no MUAPs, and no interference pattern. This is no different from the first few days of a total injury; after these first days the denervated muscle fibers begin to fibrillate.
4. **Myopathy. The simple model of myopathy is characterized by dropout of individual muscle fibers from their motor units. In active myopathies, especially polymyositis, there may be some segmental muscle necrosis.** This process divides a muscle fiber into an innervated segment and an uninnervated segment. The uninnervated segment might fibrillate and, hence, result in active myopathies, some fibrillation, and positive sharp waves; most commonly spontaneous activity is lacking.

Suggested Readings

Aminoff, M.J. (1980). *Electrodiagnosis in clinical neurology.* New York: Churchill Livingstone.

Asselman, P., Chadwick, D.W., & Marsden, C.D. (1975). Visual evoked responses in the diagnosis and management of patients suspected of multiple sclerosis. *Brain, 98,* 261–282.

Goodgold, J. (1974). *Anatomical correlates of clinical electromyography.* Baltimore, MD: Williams and Wilkins.

Halliday, A.M., McDonald, W.I., & Mushin, J. (1972). Delayed visual evoked response in optic neuritis. *Lancet, i,* 982–985.

Johnson, E.W. (Ed.). (1980). *Practical electromyography.* Baltimore, MD: Williams and Wilkins.

Jones, S.J. (1977). Short latency potentials recorded from neck and scalp following median nerve stimulation in man. *Electroencephalography and Clinical Neurophysiology, 43,* 853–863.

Khoshbin, S., & Hallet, M. (1978). Somatosensory evoked potentials in the diagnosis of MS: Comparison with other evoked potentials and blink reflex. *Neurology, 28,* 388.

Khoshbin, S., & Hallet, M. (1980). Pattern reversal visual evoked potentials in patients with multiple sclerosis. In J.L. Smith (Ed.), *Neuro ophthalmology-focus,* pp. 229–235.

Khoshbin, S., & Hallet, M. (1981). Multimodality evoked potentials and blink reflex in multiple sclerosis. *Neurology, 31,* 138–144.

Kiloh, L.G., McComas, A.J., & Osselton, J.W. (1972). *Clinical electroencephalography* (3rd ed.). London: Butterworths.

Klass, D.W., & Daly, D.D. (1979). *Current practice of clinical electroencephalography.* New York: Raven Press.

Kosi, K.A., Tucker, R.P., & Marshall, R.E. (1978). *Fundamentals of electro-encephalography* (2nd ed.). Hagerstrom, MD: Harper and Row.

Picton, T.W., & Hink, R.F. (1974). Evoked potentials, how? what? and why? *American Journal of EEG Technology, 14,* 9–44.

Robinson, J., & Rudge, P. (1977). Abnormalities of auditory evoked potentials in patients with multiple sclerosis. *Brain, 100,* 19–40.

Shahrokhi, F., Chiappa, K., & Young, R. (1978). Pattern shift visual evoked responses. *Archives of Neurology, 35,* 65–71.

Shibasaki, H., Yamashita, Y., & Tsuji, S. (1977). Somatosensory evoked potentials: Diagnostic criteria and abnormalities in cerebral lesions. *Journal of Neurological Science, 34,* 427–439.

Starr, A. (1978). Sensory evoked potentials in clinical disorders of the nervous system. *Annual Review of Neuroscience, 1,* 103–137.

Starr, A., & Joseph, A. (1979). Auditory brain responses in neurologic disease. *Archives of Neurology, 29,* 827–834.

Stockard, J., Stockard, J., & Sharbrough, F.W. (1977). Detection and localization of occult lesions with brainstem auditory responses. *Mayo Clinical Procedures, 52,* 761–769.

Chapter 38

Seizure Disorders (Epilepsy)

SHAHRAM KHOSHBIN

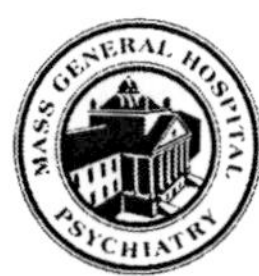

I. Overview

Psychiatrists often play an important role in the diagnosis, initiation of therapy, and long-term management of seizure disorders. Frequently, one must rely on behavioral manifestations to make the diagnosis, yet epileptic behavior is often difficult to distinguish from non-epileptic behavior. **A seizure is defined as an episodic and paroxysmal change in behavior, usually associated with an alteration in, or loss of, consciousness.** It can be precipitated by a variety of systemic pathophysiological processes (e.g., fever), or by metabolic derangements (e.g., hypoglycemia), or by toxic reactions. **Epilepsy is characterized by recurrent paroxysmal abnormalities in brain function associated with abnormal electrical discharges from neuronal aggregates.** Epileptic seizures are usually brief and self-limited.

Both in terms of its physical and psychological effects, and its associated social stigma, epilepsy can be disabling (e.g., seizures may prevent an epileptic patient from driving a car or piloting an aircraft); epilepsy also presents special problems during pregnancy. Management is often challenging, because an individual patient may require different types of treatment at different times and because inappropriate therapy may actually *worsen* the patient's condition.

II. Models for Classifying Epilepsy

A. Focal Models

In the mid-nineteenth century, **John Hughlings Jackson,** the father of the British school of neurology, proposed **the focal model of epilepsy.** Jackson hypothesized that, when a lesion developed in a particular part of the brain, function of that area would be affected during a seizure. In 1860, Jackson described the case of Dr. Z (the pseudonym of a British physician who often corresponded with Jackson). Dr. Z had written that he had spells during which he smelled a noxious odor. On the basis of this description, Jackson suggested that these spells were epileptic seizures, a revolutionary idea, since Jackson's contemporaries viewed epilepsy as a disorder that caused a person to fall on the ground, jerk uncontrollably, and foam at the mouth. Jackson also guessed that Dr. Z must have had a lesion in the uncinate region of the temporal lobe, a portion of the brain associated with the sense of smell. His hypothesis was later confirmed on autopsy.

B. The Centrencephalic Model

In the 1950s, the prominent **Canadian neurosurgeon, Wilder Penfield,** proposed **the centrencephalic model of epilepsy.** Working with the **American electroencephalographer, Jasper,** Penfield found that **some of his epileptic patients had seizures in which the electroencephalographic (EEG) manifestations were bilateral and symmetrical.** He postulated that these seizures originated in the central area of the brainstem, a region Penfield named the centrencephalon.

C. The International Classification of Epilepsy

These two models (focal and centrencephalic) provide the basis for the current international classification of epilepsy adopted by epileptologists in 1971, which has since been modified twice. According to this classification (Table 38-1), **epileptic seizures are considered as either partial (consistent with the focal model) or generalized (consistent with the centrencephalic model).** In persons with partial seizures, neuroimaging techniques, such as magnetic resonance imaging (MRI), have made it relatively easy to detect brain lesions (e.g., tumors, stroke, and vascular malformations), and even ventricular asymmetries or very small lesions that previously could be detected only on biopsy. **In contrast, findings on neuroimaging in patients with generalized seizures are usually unremarkable. In most cases of generalized seizures, the etiology is either metabolic or unknown.**

D. Seizure Symptoms

1. **Changes in consciousness provide important clues to the nature of the seizure. Patients invariably lose consciousness during generalized seizures, or when a partial seizure spreads to the centrencephalon and becomes secondarily generalized. The important difference, however, is that in partial seizures the loss of consciousness is preceded by a sensation known as an "aura"** (from the Greek word for "cold breeze"). In A.D. 175, the Greek physician Galen first used the term aura to describe the case of a young boy who mentioned that prior to his seizure he felt a "breeze blowing upon him," referring to what we now know to be a partial seizure that becomes secondarily generalized. Patients with temporal lobe epilepsy (complex partial seizures) often describe the feeling that something is rising over the chest towards their throat. An aura may take one of several forms, from sensations of dizziness to attacks of fear and depression. As in the case of Dr. Z, the type of aura may offer a clue to the location of the lesion.
2. In order to classify seizure disorders, the physician should carefully question the patient about his or her state of consciousness at the time of the seizure. **If the patient remains conscious during the episode, the seizure is classified as "partial;" if the patient loses**

Table 38-1. Classification of Epileptic Seizures

Generalized seizures (convulsive or non-convulsive)
• Tonic-clonic seizures (grand mal)
• Absence seizures (petit mal)
• Minor motor seizures (myoclonic and atonic)
Partial seizures (focal, local)
• Simple partial (without impairment of consciousness)
Focal motor seizures (Jacksonian)
Somatosensory and special sensory
Autonomic
Psychic
• Complex partial (with impairment of consciousness)
Motor symptoms (automatisms)
Sensory symptoms
Affective symptoms
Psychic (cognitive) symptoms

consciousness with no warning, the seizure is "generalized," or "secondarily generalized" if an aura precedes the loss of consciousness.

3. Once the seizure has been classified, appropriate additional tests can be selected. For strictly generalized seizures, the physician should evaluate the patient for metabolic disorders, including hyponatremia, hypokalemia, hypocalcemia, and hypoglycemia, as well as withdrawal from alcohol or other drugs. In the adult population, *de novo* generalized seizures nearly always have a metabolic origin. **Since some apparently generalized seizures are actually secondarily generalized, all adult patients should be evaluated for brain lesions.**
4. The incidence of partial seizures is very high in adults. In such cases the physician should rely on computed tomography (CT) or MRI to detect the associated scar, tumor, or other lesion.
5. Although it was once believed that patients should not be examined immediately after a seizure because the findings would be meaningless, in fact the opposite is true. **Patients should always be examined after a seizure to detect any evidence of asymmetry** (e.g., weakness or twitching that is more pronounced in one arm than in the other). Such evidence would indicate a focal, rather than a generalized, seizure.
6. **Since patients often have preconceived notions about the type of epilepsy they have, the physician should always ask for a detailed description of the seizures rather than accepting the patient's reported "diagnosis" or accepting it at face value.** Patients often mistakenly assume that "petit mal" simply means a relatively minor seizure and that "grand mal" means a major seizure. However, the distinction between the different types of epilepsy is considerably more complex. Nearly half of all adult patients will claim they have petit mal epilepsy, but this condition usually occurs in children between the ages of 2 and 9 years and is almost never seen in adult patients.

III. Generalized Seizures

Although there are seven distinct types of generalized seizures, the events are usually classified into three major groups: major motor seizures, absence seizures, and minor motor seizures.

A. Grand Mal (Tonic-Clonic or Major Motor) Seizures

1. **Grand mal seizures are the most common type of generalized seizure;** they also occur when a partial seizure becomes secondarily generalized.
2. **In a purely generalized grand mal seizure, the first event is loss of consciousness; the patient will be unaware of what has happened.**
3. **The second event is the tonic stage, characterized by contraction of the skeletal muscles, extension of the axial musculature, upward deviation of the eyes, and paralysis of the respiratory muscles** due to thoracoabdominal contractions. This stage is brief, ranging from only about 3 seconds to a maximum of 30 seconds, although it may seem longer because of its dramatic appearance.
4. **The most striking feature is extension of the upper and lower extremities into a semi-opisthotonic posture.** Sudden spasm of the respiratory muscles results in forced exhalation that may sound like a scream, the so-called epileptic cry. **Although contraction of the respiratory muscles causes the patient to stop breathing, it is not a cause for concern, since the tonic stage lasts only a few seconds.**
5. As the muscles of mastication go into spasm, the patient may bite down hard. Contrary to popular belief, the patient will not swallow his or her tongue, so objects such as a spoon or tongue depressor should not be inserted forcefully into the patient's mouth. In the young patient, this action could also dislodge a loose tooth, which could later be aspirated. Once the tonic phase is over, insertion of a short, plastic airway will prevent injury.
6. **Eye movements that occur during the tonic stage can provide clues as to the nature of the seizure. In a generalized seizure, the eyes deviate directly upward, whereas in focal seizures, particularly those involving the frontal lobe, the eyes deviate to either the right or the left.** Even inexperienced observers tend to notice whether the patient's eyes moved straight up or to one side.

7. The best approach to the tonic stage is to observe the patient and to take any necessary measures to prevent inadvertent injury.
8. **Once the tonic stage ends, the patient enters the clonic stage, which is characterized by rhythmic jerking movements.** Clonic movements have a high amplitude and low frequency, unlike myoclonic movements, which are very brief, or tremors, which have a low amplitude and high frequency. **In a generalized seizure, clonic movements are symmetrical, with the arms and legs moving in unison.** Clonic arm movements generally have greater amplitude than clonic leg movements, and the trunk is usually not involved. You may recall that, on drawings of the homunculus which is used to represent parts of the body and the corresponding areas of the brain that govern them, the face and hands are large but the body is very small. (**This relative lack of trunk movement is an important point to recognize because it may help distinguish a grand mal seizure from a pseudoseizure.** When patients experiencing pseudoseizures are attempting to move, they will often move their trunk.)
9. The clonic stage generally lasts between 3 and 7 minutes, after which time the patient is usually conscious but confused. **If after 7 minutes the patient either does not wake up or has another seizure, the diagnosis is status epilepticus.**
10. Grand mal seizures are also characterized by symptoms (some of which may alarm the inexperienced physician) involving the autonomic nervous system. **Hippus, in which the pupils alternately contract and dilate in a rhythmic pattern, is common, but occasionally the pupils may either contract or dilate.** It is often useful to examine the pupils during a seizure, even in patients on a respirator, since hippus can be a sign of seizures. Other common autonomic signs include changes in facial color to either pallid or flushed, excessive salivation to the point of drooling, increased heart rate and blood pressure, increasing intravesicular pressure, and relaxation of the urinary and anal sphincters (resulting in incontinence or defecation).
11. **Once patients regain consciousness after a grand mal seizure, they enter the post-ictal period in which they typically fall asleep for about 2 hours and wake up with headache.**
12. Physicians rarely see their epileptic patients in the throes of a grand mal seizure because the 3–7-minute event is usually over by the time they arrive. Because the event ends naturally within a few minutes, it may not be necessary to administer medication unless the patient has repeated seizures.

B. Absence Seizures

1. **The second group of generalized seizures, which includes petit mal, are referred to as absence seizures. Absence seizures occur mainly during childhood and are rare after puberty. They are characterized by the arrest or suspension of consciousness for 5–10 seconds.** Although a mother might say that her son appears healthy, and may not notice the typically brief seizures, his teacher will report that the boy stares absently for short intervals throughout the day. **Without treatment, petit mal seizures occur about 70–100 times a day,** and such frequent blackouts can seriously impair a child's school performance.
2. **If petit mal epilepsy is suspected, the physician can usually confirm the diagnosis by asking the child to hyperventilate, since this maneuver will precipitate an attack.**

Table 38-2. Management of Status Epilepticus

Immediate

- Insert short oral airway/suction
- Establish continuous EKG and monitor blood pressure every 2–3 minutes
- Sample venous blood for glucose, electrolytes, BUN, and levels of anticonvulsant drugs
- Measure arterial pO_2, pCO_2, and pH

Within 5 minutes

- Administer normal saline and thiamine IV
- Administer 50 ml 50% normal glucose
- Administer a benzodiazepine IV
  - EITHER diazepam (2 mg/minute, maximum 10 mg), for short action
  - OR lorazepam (2 mg/minute, maximum 8 mg), for longer action
- Start phenytoin IV in normal saline, no faster than 50 mg/minute, to a total dose of 15–20 mg/kg
- Watch for hypotension!

Within 30 minutes (if seizures have not stopped)

- Intubate
- Add
  - EITHER phenobarbital IV, no faster than 100 mg/minute, for a total dose of 10–20 mg/kg
  - OR benzodiazepine-diazepam (50 mg in 500 ml D5W at 40 ml/hour)
  - OR midazolam (0.1–0.4 mg/kg/hour)
  - OR paraldehyde (0.1–0.2 ml/kg rectally)
  - OR lidocaine (50–100 mg IV push)

Within 1 hour (if seizure persists)

- General anesthesia with halothane and neuromuscular blockade

3. **Once you have seen a petit mal attack, you will never forget it. The child will seem to be looking straight through you.** Other signs include **rhythmic blinking** (at a rate of 3 blinks/second), and **rudimentary motor behaviors called automatisms,** which also occur in adult temporal lobe epilepsy. Petit mal epilepsy is the easiest seizure disorder to diagnose because of its pathognomonic EEG (a spike-and-wave pattern that occurs at a frequency of 3 cycles/second), especially when the child hyperventilates.

C. Minor Motor Seizures

The most common types of minor motor seizures are myoclonic and akinetic seizures. Although these seizures usually occur in childhood, adults may sometimes experience them.

1. **Myoclonic seizures are characterized by sudden, brief muscular contractions that may occur singly or repetitively.** One type of myoclonic epilepsy of childhood is **West syndrome or infantile spasms,** which typically appear at about 6 months of age and consist of sudden abduction of the upper extremity and flexion of the hip and knees. This disorder has a poor prognosis in terms of both intellectual development and long-term survival. Myoclonic seizures may also occur in adolescents with gray matter disease and in adults with viral infections, such as encephalitis. Unfortunately, these seizures will probably become more common in the years ahead as a result of the increasing prevalence of infections due to the human immunodeficiency virus (HIV); they may also occur in association with dialysis dementia.
2. Unlike myoclonic seizures, **akinetic seizures are characterized by a loss of muscle tone.** The appearance depends on the muscles affected. "Head bobbing" occurs if the neck loses muscle tone, "bending seizures" occur if the upper extremities are affected, and "drop attacks" occur if the lower extremities are involved. However, it is much more common for children to faint than to have akinetic seizures. Although not diagnostic, the EEG is often helpful in identifying akinetic seizures. **A typical pattern consists of slow spikes and waves (or polyspikes and waves), even during the periods between seizures.** In contrast, patients with syncope have a normal EEG.

IV. Partial Seizures

As described above, partial seizures follow Jackson's focal model of epilepsy and are associated with brain lesions. **These disorders are usually classified as either simple or complex, depending on whether consciousness is affected.**

A. Simple Partial Seizures

1. **In a simple partial seizure, consciousness is maintained.** Since much of the motor cortex is devoted to controlling the face and hands, focal motor seizures most commonly affect these parts of the body. **Motor movements may spread along the body, usually starting in the hands and then affecting other areas, such as the face and the upper half of the body. This is known as the "Jacksonian march."** (There is almost never movement of the hip or trunk.) Motor seizures may also occur when the lesion (particularly a tumor) affects the frontal lobe. Turning of the head and eyes away from the side of the focus is an adversive seizure. In what is sometimes called a **fencing seizure,** the arm also flexes ipsilateral to the focus and extends contralateral to the focus. These signs indicate frontal lobe lesions affecting areas 6 and 8.
2. **Sylvian seizures are benign motor seizures that involve the tongue and may lead to aspiration.** They are seen in adolescents, usually at night, and generally disappear once the child reaches adulthood. Although the seizure itself is benign, the potential for fatal aspiration makes it essential to diagnose and treat this condition appropriately. Fortunately, sylvian seizures are easily controlled with phenytoin.
3. **Simple partial seizures also include a large subgroup of sensory seizures that can sometimes be difficult to diagnose. The vertiginous seizure, originating in the temporal lobe, is probably the most common type of sensory seizure;** unfortunately, dizziness has a broad differential diagnosis. Somatosensory seizures are usually described as a tingling feeling (paresthesia) or by a sensation of heat or water running over the affected area; this sensation may spread rapidly from one body part to another. Rarely, a patient will report pain or a burning sensation as well as various auras. When a somatosensory seizure causes tingling of the hands and face the physician may attribute this finding to a transient ischemic attack (TIA) involving the middle cerebral artery. **Unlike TIAs, which may start abruptly but end gradually, somatosensory seizures both begin and end abruptly.** Although the differential diagnosis of tingling of the hands and face should also include migraines, which begin gradually and spread slowly to other parts of the body, these differ from somatosensory seizures, in which spread is rapid.
4. **Auditory seizures are produced by discharges in the anterior transverse temporal gyrus (Heschl's convolution) and the superior temporal convolution. The patient reports tinnitus typically in the form of hissing, buzzing, or roaring sounds. Visual seizures, produced by discharges from the occipital focus, take the form of flickering lights or flashing colors (usually red or white), and are distinct from the "zig-zag" pattern of light sometimes reported by patients experiencing migraine. It is worth noting that nearly all epileptic patients have migrainous headaches and many migraine sufferers have abnormal EEGs.** Despite the overlap between these two conditions, the visual features just described can

help one distinguish migraine from simple partial seizures due to epilepsy.

B. Complex Partial Seizures

These are the most common type of seizures seen in adult medicine. They are characterized by an alteration of consciousness as well as by other complex manifestations; they are also the most difficult to diagnose and to treat. **Patients *may* experience any or all of four symptom types: psychomotor, psychosensory, cognitive, and affective.**

1. **Psychomotor symptoms or "automatisms" may take the form of simple vegetative movements, or complex actions, such as disrobing. The most common automatisms are oral and buccal movements (e.g., lip smacking, licking, or chewing), and the picking behavior sometimes seen in patients with dementia.** In some cases, these individuals may pick at their skin to the point of maceration. Walking is one of the most interesting automatisms that may occur during a complex partial seizure. The physician should not attempt to prevent such behavior during a seizure because the patient may become violent if restrained. When questioned about their behavior, patients often say they have the urge to leave their present location, and some may drive off or go to the bus station or airport out of a desire to travel. **Psychomotor symptomatology also includes staring behavior similar to that seen in petit mal epilepsy. However, unlike petit mal seizures, which last only about 6 seconds, staring episodes in complex partial seizures typically last about 1–3 minutes (i.e., long enough to be recognized).**
2. **Psychosensory symptoms include visual, auditory, and other sensory symptoms.** Although **psychosensory symptoms are most often due to a lesion in the temporal lobe, they may also be caused by a parietal lobe lesion. Patients generally describe their psychosensory symptoms as being similar to some other sensation or experience.** For example, the patient may describe the sensation of insects crawling under the skin—a common paresthesia called formication (from *formica,* the Latin word for "ant"). This may at least partially explain the scratching or picking automatisms seen in some patients. The visual phenomenon is not merely flashes of lights, but true hallucinations, such as the detonation of a bomb or "fireworks." **Olfactory or uncinate fits are also common and usually take the form of a noxious smell** (e.g., burning rubber) or a metallic taste. It is important to question patients about olfactory or gustatory symptoms, because they generally do not mention these sensations unless asked directly.
3. **Cognitive symptoms may be simple or take the form of hallucinatory experiences similar to those reported by patients with psychosis. Unlike psychotic hallucinations, which may take various forms in the individual patient, the hallucinations that occur as part of a complex partial seizure are stereotypical and repetitive.** Patients commonly envision scenes involving water.
   a. **Visual distortions.** The perception that objects are getting bigger (macropsia) or smaller (micropsia) may also be reported. The British mathematician and author Lewis Carroll had temporal lobe epilepsy. In a sense, Carroll's *Alice in Wonderland* may be considered a long description of visual phenomena, such as those experienced in temporal lobe epilepsy—things shrinking and growing, passing through mirrors, and so forth.
   b. **Other cognitive symptoms include the feeling of familiarity known as *déjà vu*** (French for "already seen") **and, more commonly, the feeling of unfamiliarity referred to as *jamais vu*** (French for "never seen"). Children generally find it easy to describe jamais vu, whereas adults find the sensation confusing and disturbing.
4. **Affective symptoms, or ictal emotions, are another characteristic of complex partial seizures.** In some cases patients with affective symptoms do not realize they are having a seizure. **Since fear and anxiety are the most common affective symptoms reported in temporal lobe epilepsy, it is always important to rule out this possibility during the differential diagnosis of panic disorders.** The diagnosis of complex partial seizures is further complicated by the fact that depression is such a common affective symptom in the general population. However, unlike other types of depression, depression related to seizures begins and ends abruptly. Pleasant ictal feelings may also occur, but they are very rare. Some females may experience orgasms; the only corresponding feeling in the male genitalia is an uncomfortable penile sensation.
   a. Although rage reactions and aggression are sometimes reported in temporal lobe epilepsy, these behaviors are extremely rare.
   b. Aggressive behavior generally occurs late in a seizure and is usually undirected. For instance, a patient might punch into the air, but he is unlikely to attack his mother-in-law.

V. Evaluation of Seizure Disorders

A. Obtaining a Description of the Seizure

As described earlier, the physician should begin by obtaining a detailed description of the patient's seizures. Although the physical examination is almost always normal, a few signs may provide clues to the diagnosis. Since patients with epilepsy often have a history of brain lesions at an early age, the physician should **look for evidence of hemiatrophy.** For example, if a patient is asked to place his hands palm to palm, you may find that one hand is smaller than the other. In partial complex seizures, the physical expression of an emotional response may be asymmetrical (e.g., a smile is almost always one-sided). **In about 80% of patients with asymmetrical emotional responses or reflexes, the responsible brain lesion is in the hemisphere opposite the weaker side of the body.**

B. Obtain an EEG

Although the EEG is a valuable tool for diagnosing seizure disorders in pediatric patients, it has only limited value in adults. Nevertheless, **physicians should obtain an EEG if they suspect a seizure disorder. It is often possible to increase the yield of an EEG by asking the patient what events or stimuli seem to trigger a seizure and then trying to reproduce these in a controlled setting.** For instance, if a patient says he has seizures after a sleepless night, you might ask him to remain awake one night and then come in for an EEG the following day. In other patients, you might be able to induce abnormal brain activity by asking them to hyperventilate or by exposing them to a flashing light. To detect EEG abnormalities one must be careful to place the electrodes in the proper positions. Most temporal lobe lesions are on the mesial aspect of the lobe, so the physician should ask the EEG technician to place nasopharyngeal electrodes or surface electrodes on the zygoma or to use special sphenoidal electrodes.

For patients with focal seizures, MRI is better than CT, in which bone artifact can obscure the temporal lobe. If a patient has a lesion on the temporal lobe, a coronal MRI section will usually reveal that the entire lobe is smaller, the ventricle is dilated, or the hippocampus is smaller. MRI scans may also reveal gliosis, which cannot be detected on CT scans. CT should be used only if MRI is not available or if there is no time to arrange for an MRI evaluation.

VI. Behavioral Changes in Epilepsy

A. Inter-ictal Personality Changes

Geschwind described the following five interesting types of personality changes associated with partial complex epilepsy: hypergraphia, hyperreligiosity, hyposexuality, aggressivity, and viscosity. The Russian author Fyodor Dostoyevsky is perhaps the best-known example of an epileptic with hypergraphia, which is the tendency to write prolifically.

Some patients with epilepsy are **deeply interested in religion,** although not necessarily one of the world's major religions.

In some adult patients, the onset of seizures coincides with a **sudden loss of interest in sex.** Since patients rarely volunteer this information, the physician should make a point of asking whether they have noticed any change in their sexual desire. Some patients with temporal lobe epilepsy also report a change in their sexual preference.

Aggressivity, the fourth type of personality change associated with epilepsy, **is distinct from the automatic aggressive behavior occasionally seen during seizures.** Again, patients often do not volunteer information about this type of personality change. If patients are asked about their temper, they may become defensive or evasive. Upon further questioning, you might learn that they engage in aggressive behavior, such as breaking dishes or throwing objects out of a window.

Finally, some epileptic patients develop a personality trait Geschwind called viscosity, meaning that the patients tend to be "sticky." For example, some patients with temporal lobe epilepsy may call you every night, and, once they start talking, they won't stop.

These five characteristic personality disturbances provide evidence that brain lesions can cause long-term changes in behavior.

VII. Therapy of Seizure Disorders

A. Historical Notes

1. Perhaps the first description of an authentic treatment for epilepsy appeared in the Book of Mark in the New Testament. Mark described how Jesus advised a man with falling sickness (epilepsy) to pray for 3 days. For Jesus (who was still Jewish at the time), prayer also implied fasting. When the man prayed and fasted for 3 days, he naturally developed ketosis, which stopped his seizures. Physicians now recognize that **a "ketogenic diet"** (i.e., **a diet high in saturated fats,** such as butter and cream) is one of the most effective ways to halt myoclonic and akinetic seizures. Thus, Jesus might be considered the world's first epileptologist.
2. Despite this promising beginning nearly 2,000 years ago, the treatment of seizure disorders remained in the "Dark Ages" until relatively recently. The dramatic seizures and inter-ictal behavioral changes, which are seen particularly in patients with complex partial seizures, may account for the fear and superstitions that have impeded the scientific study of epilepsy.
3. **Initially, bromides were used by Sir Charles Lockock to treat catamenial disorders, including epilepsy. In the early twentieth century, physicians first recognized the anticonvulsant effects of phenobarbital,** and, later, of other barbiturates. Today, phenobarbital is reserved for those epileptic patients who cannot take drugs orally, other than phenytoin and the benzodiazepines. Phenobarbital and phenytoin are the only antiepileptic agents that may be given intravenously. Only one other barbiturate, primidone, is still used because it is effective in treating complex partial seizures.

B. Phenytoin

1. **Oral and intravenous phenytoin has been the mainstay of epilepsy treatment since it was first used in the 1930s by two Boston physicians, Houston Merritt and Hillary Putnam. Although the usual oral dosage for adults is 100 mg three times a day, the**

dose prescribed should actually be based on serum levels, which should be in the range of 10–20 μg/mL which is easy to achieve in the oral form. If phenytoin is given intravenously, it must be delivered in a normal saline solution; if a 5% dextrose solution is used, the drug will precipitate out and be ineffective. One can determine when the drug has reached therapeutic levels by measuring the serum concentration or looking for nystagmus. If the concentration reaches toxic levels, ataxia will develop.

2. **The main side effect of phenytoin is drowsiness,** which may be a major concern to many patients. To ensure compliance, the physician should warn patients about this potential effect and assure them that it is only temporary. Phenytoin is generally not prescribed during adolescence since it may induce hirsutism, acne, and gingival hyperplasia.
3. **Some patients may develop important medical complications, including megaloblastic anemia and osteopenia.** In general, the anemia will develop quickly and should be treated with vitamin B_{12} and folate. Osteopenia may develop over a long time in female patients and may lead to pathologic fractures. Some patients are allergic to phenytoin and develop erythema multiforme and Stevens-Johnson syndrome up to 2 months after the start of therapy. It is important to inform patients about the manifestations of Stevens-Johnson syndrome and emphasize that they should seek immediate medical attention at the first sign of this potentially fatal condition.

C. Carbamazepine

The anticonvulsant carbamazepine is the drug of choice for temporal lobe epilepsy. The typical dosage for adults is 200 mg three times a day, with **serum levels in the range of 4–12 μg/mL. The major side effects of this agent are bone marrow suppression and hepatic toxicity.** Like the related drug imipramine, carbamazepine can also act as an antidepressant.

D. Valproate

Although valproate is considered the drug of choice for generalized seizures in children, it is now widely used in adult epilepsy. The usual adult dosage is 250 mg three times a day, with **serum levels in the range of 50–100 μg/mL.** The most significant side effects of valproate are alopecia and hepatotoxicity.

E. Other Anticonvulsants

For more detailed information on newer anticonvulsants (e.g., lamotrigine, gabapentin, topiramate, tigabine, and vigabatrin) see chapter 49 (Anticonvulsants).

Suggested Readings

Bear, D.M., & Fedio, P. (1977). Quantitative analysis of interictal behavior in temporal lobe epilepsy. *Archives of Neurology, 34,* 454–467.

Blumer, D. (1975). Temporal lobe epilepsy and its psychiatric significance. In D. Benson, & D. Blumer (Eds.), *Psychiatric aspects of neurological disease.* New York: Grune and Stratton.

Britton, J.W., & So, E.L. (1996). Selection of antiepileptic drugs: A practical approach. *Mayo Clinical Procedures, 71,* 778–786.

Delgado-Escuela, A.V., et al. (1982). Current concepts in neurology. Management of status epilepticus. *New England Journal of Medicine, 306,* 1337.

Furkenstein, H., & Khoshbin, S. (1987). Seizure disorders. In W.T. Branch (Ed.), *Office practice of internal medicine.* Philadelphia, PA: W.B. Saunders.

Gastaut, H. (1969). Clinical and electroencephalographical classification of epileptic seizures. *Epilepsia, 10*(suppl), 1–28.

Geschwind, N. (1977). Behavioral change in temporal lobe epilepsy. *Archives of Neurology, 34,* 453.

Heckers, S., & Cole, A.J. (1998). Approach to the patient with seizures. In T.A. Stern, J.B. Herman, & P.L. Slavin (Eds.), *The MGH guide to psychiatry in primary care.* New York: McGraw-Hill.

Hughes, J.R., & Olson, S.F. (1981). An investigation of eight different types of temporal lobe discharges. *Epilepsia, 22,* 421–435.

Khoshbin, S. (1986). Van Gogh's malady and other cases of Geschwind's syndrome. *Neurology, 36*(suppl), 213–214.

Khoshbin, S. (1989). Clinical neurophysiology of aggressive behavior. *Clinical Electroencephalography, 1,* 74–75.

Khoshbin, S., & Dawson, D.M. (1979). Epilepsy. An update. In H.R. Tyler, & D.M. Dawson (Eds.), *Current neurology* (Vol. 2, pp. 219–229). Boston, MA: Houghton-Mifflin.

Khoshbin, S., Levin, L., Milrod, L., Carlson, L., & Hallett, M. (1984). Cortical evoked potential mapping in complex partial seizures. *Neurology, 34*(suppl), 219.

Mayeux, R., Brandt, J., Rosen, J., & Benson, D.F. (1980). Interictal memory and language impairment in temporal lobe epilepsy. *Neurology, 30,* 120–125.

Penfield, W., & Jasper, M. (1954). *Epilepsy and functional anatomy of the human brain.* Boston, MA: Little, Brown.

Slater, E., & Beard, A.W. (1963). Schizophrenia-like psychoses of epilepsy. *British Journal of Psychiatry, 209,* 95–150.

Stevens, J.R. (1975). Interictal clinical manifestations of complex partial seizures. *Advances in Neurology, 11,* 85–107.

Tisher, P.W., Holzer, J.C., Greenberg, M., et al. (1993). Psychiatric presentations of epilepsy. *Harvard Review of Psychiatry, 1,* 219–228.

Waxman, S.G., & Geschwind, N. (1974). Hypergraphia in temporal lobe epilepsy. *Neurology, 24,* 629–634.

Woodbury, D.M., et al. (Eds.). (1982). *Antiepileptic drugs* (2nd ed.). New York: Raven Press.

Chapter 39

Headache

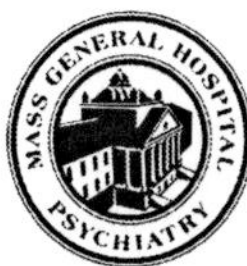

John W. Denninger, Edward R. Norris, and Martin A. Samuels

I. Introduction

Headache is one of the most frequent complaints heard in medical practice, and it is the most common reason for referral to a neurologist. Headache is so common that almost everyone has had at least one headache, and 90% of Americans have at least occasional headaches. The majority of these are migraine, tension-type, or cluster headaches. **While most headache sufferers treat themselves, patients who do see a doctor are always in pain and are often worried about a serious underlying disease, often brain tumor, aneurysm, or stroke.** The International Headache Society has developed a classification of, and diagnostic criteria for, headache analogous to the *Diagnostic and Statistical Manual of Mental Disorders.*

II. Evaluation of the Patient with a Headache

A. Medical History

Taking a good headache history is the most important step in the diagnosis of the patient. Typically, an accurate diagnosis can be made with the information derived from the history and the physical examination.

1. The optimal history begins with the asking of open-ended questions in a supportive environment.
2. The history should identify:
   a. The severity, character, and location of the headache
   b. The onset, duration, frequency, and timing of the headache
   c. Precipitating and ameliorating factors
   d. The effect of medications
   e. Other associated symptoms
   f. Past headache history and family history
3. Sudden-onset, accelerating, or progressive headaches can be signs of serious or life-threatening diseases of the brain, including temporal arteritis, intracranial mass lesions, idiopathic intracranial hypertension (pseudotumor cerebri), meningitis, and subarachnoid hemorrhage.

B. Examination

The examination of a headache patient must include a neurological examination, a funduscopic examination, and a physical examination of the head.

1. The neurological examination is aimed at excluding lateralized or focal findings, especially on visual field confrontation and testing of strength and gait.
2. A funduscopic examination searches for papilledema.
3. A physical examination of the head includes observing, palpating for tenderness or masses, and listening over the temples and eyes for bruits.

C. Ancillary Tests

It is unusual for any test to demonstrate an abnormality not suggested by the history and the physical examination. A test is indicated when the history suggests a specific diagnosis (e.g., epilepsy or tumor), **the headaches develop a new quality or become intractable, the history is atypical** (e.g., trigeminal neuralgia in a young patient that may suggest multiple sclerosis), **or when the neurological examination is abnormal.**

1. Imaging with a non-contrast, computed tomography (CT) scan of the head carries little risk and will pick up many ominous causes of headache; magnetic resonance imaging (MRI) of the head is more sensitive and expensive.
2. A lumbar puncture is indicated when elevation of intracranial pressure or infection is suspected or if neuroimaging is negative and subarachnoid hemorrhage is suspected.
3. An elevated erythrocyte sedimentation rate (e.g., 70–80 mm/hour) suggests giant cell arteritis in an elderly person with new-onset headache.
4. An electroencephalogram (EEG), evoked responses, and an angiogram are rarely indicated in the evaluation of headache.

III. Primary Headache Disorders

A. Migraine

Migraine headaches are a type of vascular headache. The term vascular headache is somewhat of a misnomer because the name implies that the cause is entirely related to blood vessels, **whereas most evidence indicates that the cause is an abnormality in neurotransmitters** (e.g., substance P), which deal with pain perceptions, with inconsistent secondary vascular phenomena. **The term vascular is meant to emphasize the pulsating nature of the pain.** The frequency and severity of vascular headaches occur on a spectrum from infrequent brief pains to daily severe migraine headaches.

1. Migraine headaches are common and **prevalence in females is estimated at 20%. The ratio of females to males is 3:2. There is a family history in 90% of patients.**
2. **Individual migraine symptoms are usually stereotypic** and recurrent for every patient. Migraine headaches present with a **unilateral pulsating headache,** often in the frontotemporal region. **Photophobia and phonophobia are common features,** indicative of sensory hypersensitivity (allodynia). Autonomic

dysfunction and disability often accompany the migraine and can cause nausea, vomiting, and slow gastric emptying. Personality changes can also occur.

3. Migraine patients usually have a life history that varies with age. The history starts early with infants who have colic, and young children who have episodic abdominal pain. The headaches begin in puberty and wax and wane throughout life, often with long headache-free intervals. Vascular headaches often improve in middle age. **The headache can last from seconds to days, but usually lasts from 4 to 24 hours.**
4. Patients are usually the best informants on what precipitates their headaches. Many foods, such as **aged cheese, red wine, chocolate, and peanuts,** can precipitate migraines. **Skipping meals, too little or too much sleep,** and other **psychological stresses can aggravate vascular headaches.** Birth control pills can make headache better or worse, and pregnancy may ameliorate the vascular headache.
5. Common migraines (migraine without aura) are more frequent. However, **migraine headaches can be preceded by an aura** (migraine with aura). Auras can be moving visual lights, but can include visual field cuts (**scotoma**) and flashing zigzag lines (**scintillations**). The aura usually lasts 20 minutes. **The aura can consist of any particular transient alteration in any neurological function.**
6. There are a range of treatments available for the migraine patient. Reduction of aggravating factors (e.g., caffeine intake, alcohol [especially red wine], chocolate, and peanuts) can reduce headache frequency.

   Acute or abortive treatment is effective for patients who have infrequent headaches. It is important to treat at the onset of headache or aura. The most common reason for ineffective treatment is the time delay between when the headache begins and when the patient takes the medication. **Effective treatments for mild to moderate headaches include analgesics, NSAIDs, or caffeine adjuvant combinations. For more severe headaches, ergotamine and dihydroergotamine, or the selective 5-HT$_1$ agonists (e.g., sumatriptan, naratriptan, zolmitriptan, rizatriptan, almotriptan, eletriptan, and frovatriptan) are most effective.** Suppositories, nasal sprays, and injections can be used when oral medication is ineffective or contraindicated because of nausea and vomiting. Adjunctive antiemetic and prokinetic medications (e.g., metoclopramide) can be used to increase gastric absorption of oral medications and to treat nausea and vomiting.

   Prophylactic treatment is necessary for patients with frequent headaches. Beta-blockers, calcium-channel blockers, antidepressants, serotonin antagonists, anticonvulsants, and NSAIDs have all been used effectively for preventive migraine treatment. Lipophilic beta-blockers are the most effective (e.g., propranolol, atenolol, or nadolol). The calcium-channel blocker verapamil may be useful in patients who cannot tolerate a beta-blocker, but is generally more effective for cluster-like headaches. Valproic acid has also demonstrated efficacy. Ciproheptadine (Periactin), a weak serotonergic blocking drug, is effective in some patients. Anticholinergic tricyclics (e.g., amitriptyline) are also beneficial.

   Status migrainosis is diagnosed when a migraine lasts longer than 72 hours. Steroids can abort longer migraine headaches. When this is ineffective, intravenous barbiturates can be used to induce sleep.

B. Tension-Type Headache

1. **Tension-type headache (formerly "tension headache") has not been shown to be associated with increased pericranial muscle contraction; instead, the mechanism is thought to be related to increased pain sensitivity.** A family history is common, and the prevalence is higher in women than in men.
2. **The pain is band-like around the head.** It can be generalized or located in the frontal, occipital, or cervical areas. It is not associated with photophobia or phonophobia.
3. The onset is usually brief, and the pain is worse during the day.
4. **Tension-type headaches can be precipitated by stress.** They are **often relieved by alcohol.** Exercise, jogging, neck massage, hot bath, or other stress-relieving activity can often ameliorate symptoms.
5. Many **non-medical treatments,** including biofeedback, relaxation techniques, physical therapy, and stress reduction, are effective. Patients should avoid expensive or potentially harmful strategies. Benzodiazepines and narcotics, although effective, should be avoided. **Effective pharmacological treatments include simple analgesics with and without caffeine and NSAIDs;** however, these medications should be limited to fewer than 3–4 days per week to prevent medication overuse headache (see below).

C. Cluster Headache

1. **The prevalence of cluster headache is estimated at less than 0.4%. The ratio of males to females is 5:1.**
2. The aptly named **cluster headache occurs in clusters of one to eight times daily for several weeks.** The headache **pain is often sharp and orbital, suborbital, or temporal. Autonomic dysfunction is present,** with injected conjunctiva, nasal blockage, profuse sweating, facial flushing, ptosis, or miosis.
3. The onset is usually in middle-aged men and may have a cyclical pattern that occurs in the spring. **The cluster headache pain peaks in 5–10 minutes and can last up to 3 hours.**
4. Persons with cluster headaches are sensitive to alcohol. Cluster headaches often occur several hours after going to sleep and are not relieved by sleep. Tobacco smoking can also precipitate headache.

5. **Treatments to abort headaches include 100% oxygen by mask for 15 minutes or vasoconstrictive medications and sumatriptan.** Prophylactic treatment includes use of calcium-channel blockers (e.g., verapamil) or lithium carbonate (with target blood levels of 0.6–1.0 mmol/L).

IV. Secondary Headache Disorders

These headaches typically do not follow the characteristic patterns of migraine, tension-type, or cluster headache. Structural causes should be suspected with an abnormal neurological examination or when the headache is acute or progressive.

A. Post-traumatic Headache

1. **Up to half of all people with concussions can have headaches for 2 months after the incident.** Acceleration and deceleration forces of the injury can cause shear injury to neurons. The extent of the contribution of psychosocial and medicolegal factors to this syndrome is unclear.
2. **Post-traumatic headaches usually occur within 14 days of head injury and resemble migraine or tension headaches.** Nausea, vomiting, dizziness, vertigo, and mood symptoms can occur.
3. Treatment is the same as for tension and migraine headaches. Benzodiazepines and narcotics should be avoided.

B. Subarachnoid Hemorrhage

1. **The cause of subarachnoid hemorrhage is rupture of a cerebral artery, usually from the circle of Willis or from rupture of a vascular malformation.** Head trauma and a bleeding diathesis (e.g., thrombocytopenia or factor deficiency) may also result in subarachnoid hemorrhage.
2. Hypertensive crises by ingestion of tyramine by patients on monoamine oxidase inhibitor (MAOI) antidepressants or the use of cocaine can also cause subarachnoid hemorrhage.
3. **A severe headache with nuchal rigidity is the most common symptom. A sentinel bleed or leak with milder headache can occur during exercise, with straining, or during sexual intercourse.**
4. **Diagnosis is made by lumbar puncture or a head scan.**
5. **Treatment is the repair of the leaking or ruptured blood vessel.** Intravanous phentolamine (Regitine), an alpha-adrenergic blocking agent, should be used in patients with MAOI-related hypertensive headaches.

C. Giant Cell (Temporal) Arteritis

1. **Patients with temporal arteritis are usually older than 55 years.** Although the etiology is unknown, **histology reveals a focal granulomatous arteritis containing giant cells.** The erythrocyte sedimentation rate (ESR) is usually greater than 40 mm/hour.
2. The pain is typically a dull, continuous headache in the temples; in advanced stages, the temporal arteries appear inflamed. **The headache may be accompanied by dysphoric mood, pain and joint stiffness, fever, weight loss, night sweats, and visual loss (including amaurosis fugax).**
3. Chewing can precipitate the pain (**jaw claudication**).
4. Treatment with high-dose steroids is standard; untreated arteries can occlude, causing blindness or stroke.

D. Idiopathic Intracranial Hypertension (Pseudotumor Cerebri)

1. **These headaches usually occur in young obese women,** sometimes with menstrual abnormalities. **Although the pathophysiology is unknown, interstitial brain edema and decreased CSF absorption at the arachnoid villi are the hypothesized mechanisms.**
2. The headache is a dull, generalized pain. Papilledema is usually present. Unlike mass-lesion headache, there is no alteration in personality or cognitive function.
3. **Treatment includes serial lumbar punctures to relieve symptoms.** Diuretics are helpful, as is a steroid taper. Dieting can also reduce headache severity. Surgical placement of a shunt may be used in refractory cases.

E. Low Cerebrospinal Fluid (CSF) Pressure Headaches

1. Post-lumbar puncture headaches are the most common of this type, but headaches can occur following trauma, an operation, or with idiopathic CSF leaks.
2. **Pain is bilateral, and nausea, blurred vision, photophobia, and postural syncope are often present.** They usually last several days and rarely persist for weeks.
3. **The pain is worse within 15 minutes of the patient sitting or standing, and worsened by cough, strain, or head movement. It is relieved within 30 minutes of lying flat.**
4. Remaining flat in bed and taking analgesics are the most effective treatments. Injection of sterile autologous blood (blood patch) in the epidural space can seal the leak.

F. Headaches Secondary to Infections

1. **Acute meningitis is usually caused by *Meningococcus* or *Pneumococcus;*** it often occurs in small epidemics in confined areas. **Acute meningitis is associated with a rapid onset of a severe headache with photophobia, fever, nuchal rigidity, and malaise.**
2. **Chronic meningitis occurs most frequently in people with compromised immune systems,** especially people with acquired immunodeficiency syndrome (AIDS), those on steroids, or the elderly. Chronic meningitis is associated with a continuous dull headache, with symptoms of systemic illness and cognitive decline.
3. **Herpes simplex encephalitis has a predilection for the inferior surface of the frontal and temporal lobes. It causes fever, somnolence, delirium, and complex partial seizures with amnesia.**

4. **Diagnosis is facilitated by lumbar puncture and a head scan. Treatment with appropriate antibiotics is the cure.**

G. Intracranial Mass Lesions

1. **Headaches from mass lesions are caused by an increase in intracranial pressure.**
2. **The pain is often bilateral, dull, and mild.** Papilledema is often absent. Subtle personality and cognitive changes are usually present. **Lateralized neurological signs often occur** within weeks of the onset of symptoms.
3. An increase in intracranial pressure by bending or coughing can worsen headaches.
4. Treatment is the removal of the mass-causing lesion.

H. Headaches Due to Substances and/or Their Withdrawal

1. **Iatrogenic headaches are caused by medicines.** The addition or withdrawal of a medication or substance can precipitate headaches. People who have migraine or other headaches and who use medications to treat their original headache encounter these headaches. The diagnosis is confirmed after exclusion of other causes.
2. These headaches are not usually associated with nausea, a throbbing sensation, or hypersensitivity. They can mirror the symptoms of tension headaches.
3. **The onset occurs after the discontinuation or addition of a substance.** This type of headache can last many weeks without treatment.
4. These headaches are precipitated by the addition of nitroglycerin or isosorbide. The withdrawal of external substances, including caffeine, can cause headache. The withdrawal of any substance used to treat headaches, including aspirin, acetaminophen, NSAIDs, and narcotics, can precipitate headaches.
5. **Discontinuation of the causative substance or reintroduction of the substance that was withdrawn effectively stops the headache.** A brief course and taper of steroids (e.g., prednisone 30 mg/day, 20 mg/day, and 10 mg/day) can help break the cycle.
6. Medication overuse headache or "painkiller headache" describes a syndrome in which escalating doses of medication (e.g., NSAIDs, ergots, or triptans) are used to control headache, leading to the development of chronic daily headaches. It is thought that disruption of the normal pain modulation system perpetuates the syndrome. **Discontinuation of the medication during an inpatient or outpatient "detox" eliminates or reduces the frequency of the headaches.**

I. Trigeminal Neuralgia (Tic Douloureux)

1. **This type of headache is common in patients over the age of 60 years. One possible cause is compression of the trigeminal nerve root by a cerebral blood vessel** at its origin from the brainstem. Occurrence in young people may suggest multiple sclerosis with a plaque involving the trigeminal nerve root.
2. **Trigeminal neuralgia is manifested by brief (20–30 second) jabs of sharp pain that extend along the three divisions of the fifth cranial nerve.** The pain usually subsides at night.
3. Unlike other headaches, **stimulation of affected areas by touch, eating, or drinking cold liquids results in a sharp pain.**
4. Injection of an anesthetic in the nerve root can stop the pain. Use of carbamazepine is often helpful. In refractory cases, surgical placement of a barrier between the vessel and the trigeminal nerve may be necessary.

V. Conclusions

A. **Headache is common; 90% of Americans have at least occasional headache.** Patients who are seen for evaluation of headache are always in pain and worried about a serious underlying disease.

B. Evaluation of headache involves taking a careful history with identification of the severity and character of the pain, the onset and duration of the pain, the precipitating and ameliorating factors, the effect of medications, and other associated symptoms.

C. **Examination of the patient must include a neurological examination** focused on excluding lateralized or focal findings, **a funduscopic examination, and a physical examination of the head.**

D. **Migraine, cluster, and tension-type headaches account for the majority of headache syndromes.**

E. Patients with headaches that do not have a pattern clearly characteristic of one of the primary headache disorders or who have an abnormal neurological examination require a thorough work-up for organic etiologies.

Suggested Readings

Baldassano, C. (1998). Approach to the patient with headache. In T.A. Stern, J.B. Herman, & P.L. Slavin (Eds.), *The MGH guide to psychiatry in primary care,* pp. 61–65. New York: McGraw-Hill.

Kaufman, D.M. (1995). *Clinical neurology for psychiatrists* (4th ed., pp. 197–220). Philadelphia, PA: W.B. Saunders.

Merikangas, K.R., & Merikangas, J.R. (2000). Neuropsychiatric aspects of headache. In B.J. Sadock, & V.A. Sadock (Eds.), *Kaplan and Sadock's comprehensive textbook of psychiatry VII* (7th ed., pp. 345–350). Philadelphia, PA: Lippincott, William & Wilkins.

Samuels, M.A. (1997). *Video textbook of neurology for the practicing physician.* Boston, MA: Butterworth-Heinemann (Elsevier).

Samuels, M.A. (1999). *Manual of neurologic therapeutics* (6th ed.). Philadelphia, PA: Lippincott, Williams and Wilkins.

Samuels, M.A., & Feske, S. (2003). *Office practice of neurology* (2nd ed.). Philadelphia, PA: Churchill-Livingstone (Elsevier).

Silberstein, S.D., Lipton, R.B., & Goadsby, P.J. (1998). *Headache in clinical practice.* Oxford, UK: Isis Medical Media.

Chapter 40

Pain

MENEKSE ALPAY AND NED H. CASSEM

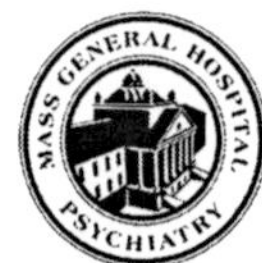

I. Introduction

Pain is a common, yet complex and challenging, symptom. It is defined by the International Association for the Study of Pain as "an unpleasant sensory and emotional experience arising from the actual or potential tissue damage or described in terms of such damage." An individual's affective state, previous conditioning, and endogenous system of analgesia all affect the experience of pain. Frequently, a multidisciplinary approach is effective in controlling pain and restoring function. To manage pain in a timely and effective manner a variety of terms and mechanisms need to be understood.

II. Pathophysiology of Pain

A. Nociception

Nociception is the neural mechnism of detection of noxious stimuli; it is not synonymous with pain. Differentiation of somatic pain (involving activation of nociceptors in peripheral tissues) and visceral pain (involving activation of nociceptors in bodily organs) can be problematic. Somatic pain is usually well localized, attributable to certain anatomical structures or areas, **and is characteristically described as stabbing, aching, or throbbing. Visceral pain is typically poorly localized,** not necessarily attributable to the involved organ (i.e., referred pain), **and is characteristically described as dull and crampy.**

B. Peripheral conduction of nociception

Pain originating from the skin is often used as the model for nociception. Nociceptors in the skin transduce mechanical, thermal, and chemical stimuli into action potentials. **When tissue is injured, nociceptors are stimulated by the liberation of prostaglandins, arachidonic acid, histamine, and bradykinin.** Aspirin, acetaminophen, steroids, and non-steroidal antiinflammatory agents (NSAIDs) act at this stage of the pain pathway.

Subsequently, axons transmit the pain to the spinal cord (to cell bodies in the dorsal root ganglia). **Three different types of axons are involved in transmission of painful stimuli from skin to the dorsal horn. They are classified by their diameters; the velocity of their conduction increases as the diameter and thickness of the myelin sheath increase** (see Figure 40-1).

1. **A-β fibers** are the largest and most heavily myelinated fibers that transmit light touch.
2. **A-Δ fibers** and **C fibers** are the primary nociceptive afferents.
   a. A-Δ fibers are 2–5 micrometers in diameter and are thinly myelinated. They conduct immediate, rapid, sharp, and brief pain (first pain) with a velocity of 20 m/second.
   b. C fibers are 0.2–1.5 micrometers in diameter and are unmyelinated. They conduct prolonged, burning, and unpleasant pain (second pain) at a speed of 0.5 m/second.

C. Central conduction of nociception

1. **The dorsal horn of the spinal cord**
   a. **A-Δ and C fibers enter the dorsal root and ascend or descend one to three segments before synapsing with neurons in the lateral spinothalamic tract** (laminae I, II, and V of the substantia gelatinosa in the gray matter).
   b. **Substance P, an 11-aminoacid polypeptide, is released from the fibers at many of these synapses.** It is the major pain neurotransmitter. Capsaicin, which is extracted from red-hot pepper, inhibits nociception by inhibiting substance P.
   c. Inhibition of nociception in the dorsal horn is functionally quite important. Stimulation of the A-Δ fibers not only excites some neurons but also inhibits others. This inhibition of nociception through A-Δ fiber stimulation may explain effects of acupuncture and transcutaneous nerve stimulation (TENS).

D. Spinothalamic tract

The lateral spinothalamic tract crosses the midline and ascends towards the thalamus. At the level of the brainstem more than half of this tract synapses in the reticular activating system (in an area called the spinoreticular tract), in the limbic system, and in other brain stem regions. The close relationship of pain, affect, and sleep may be explained by these synapses. Another site of projections is the periaqueductal gray (PAG) (see Figure 40-1), which plays an important role in the brain's endogenous analgesia system.

The lateral spinothalamic tract has two parts:

1. **The neospinothalamic tract, which serves to localize pain,** is phylogenetically recent in evolutionary terms, **ends in the ventroposterolateral (VPL) and ventroposteromedial (VPM) nuclei of the thalamus.** These nuclei project to the primary somatic sensory cortex in the parietal lobe.
2. **The paleospinothalamic tract** is a phylogenetically older pain system; it **projects to the intralaminar nucleus of the thalamus,** which has widespread cortical projections. These projections, which are involved in the affective nature of pain (in addition to the reticular activating system and limbic system projections), serve to alert to, rather than to localize pain.

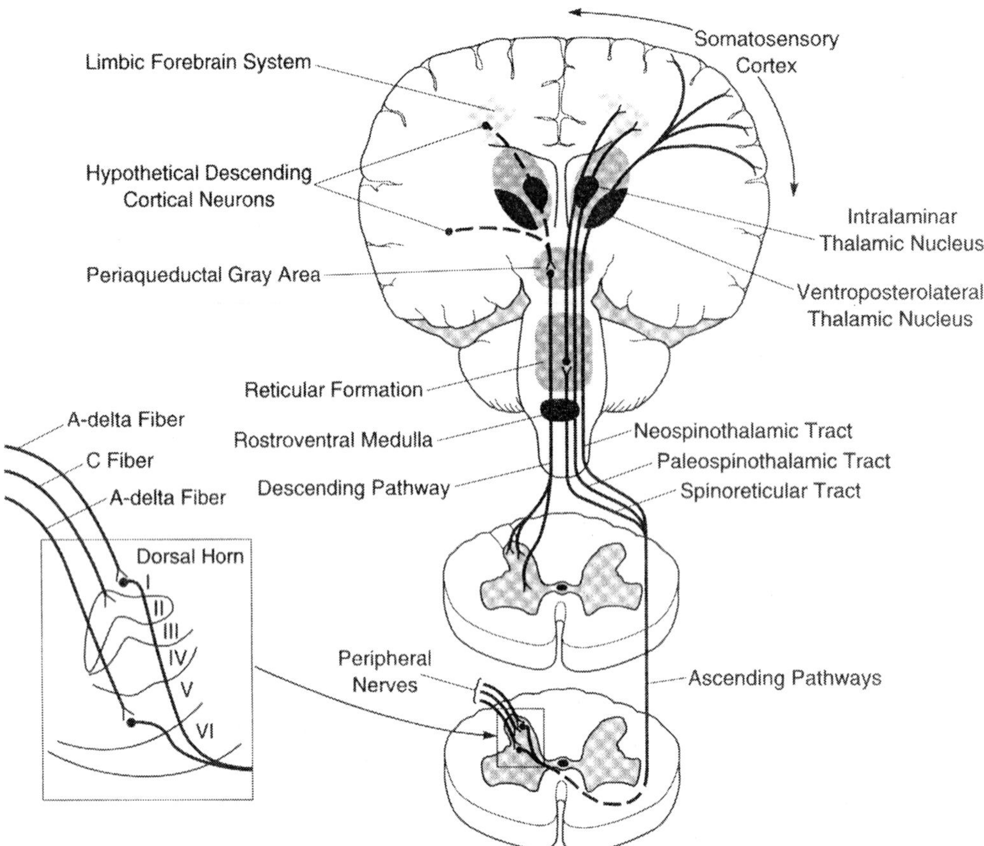

Figure 40-1. Schematic diagram of neurologic pathways for pain perception. (Source: Hyman, S.H., Cassem, N.H., *Pain,* 1989.)

E. Cortex

After synapsing in the thalamic nuclei, pain fibers project to the somatosensory cortex, located posterior to the sylvian fissure in the parietal lobe (Brodmann areas 1, 2, 3).

III. Endogenous Analgesic System

A. Overview

There at least 18 endogenous peptides with opiate-like activity in the CNS. They are the products of three precursor proteins:

1. **Pro-opiomelanocortin** is the precursor of beta-endorphin and adrenocorticotropic hormone.
2. **Pro-enkephalin** is the precursor of met-enkephalin and leu-enkephalin.
3. **Pro-dynorphin** is the precursor of dynorphin and related peptides.

B. Central Opiate Receptors

1. **μ-receptors** are **involved in the regulation of analgesia, respiratory depression, constipation, and miosis.** They are the receptors (located in the periaqueductal gray, rostraventral medulla, medial thalamus, and dorsal horn of the spinal cord) mainly responsible for supraspinal analgesia.
2. **κ-receptors** are **involved in spinal analgesia, sedation, and miosis.** They are located in the dorsal horn (spinal analgesia), deep cortical areas, and other locations; pentazocine preferentially acts on these receptors.
3. **Δ-receptors,** like κ-receptors **mediate spinal analgesia, hypotension, and miosis.** Enkephalins have a higher affinity for these receptors than do opiates. They are located in the limbic system, the dorsal horn, and in other locations unrelated to pain. **Δ-receptors also mediate psychotomimetic effects** (i.e., psychosis) in the CNS. Their effects are not reversed by naloxone, an opiate antagonist.

IV. Descending Analgesic Pain Pathway

The descending analgesic pain pathway starts in the PAG (rich in endogenous opiates), projects to the rostroventral medulla, and from there descends through the dorsolateral funiculus of the spinal cord to the dorsal horn. The neurons in the rostroventral medulla use serotonin to activate endogenous analgesics (enkephalins) in the dorsal horn. This effect inhibits nociception at the level of the dorsal horn since neurons containing enkephalins synapse with spinothalamic neurons.

Additionally, there are noradrenergic neurons that project from the locus coeruleus (the main noradrenergic center in the CNS) to the dorsal horn, thereby inhibiting the response of dorsal horn neurons to nociceptive stimuli. The effect of tricyclic antidepressants (TCAs) and other newer antidepressants (thought to increase serotonin and norepinephrine) inhibits nociception at the level of the dorsal horn.

V. Categories of Pain

A. **Acute pain is usually related to an identifiable injury or to a disease;** it is self-limited, and resolves over hours to days or in a time frame that is associated with healing. Acute pain is usually associated with objective autonomic features (e.g., tachycardia, hypertension, diaphoresis, mydriasis, or pallor).

B. **Chronic pain is pain that persists beyond the normal time of healing or lasts longer than six months.** Characteristic features include vague descriptions of pain and an inability to describe the pain's timing and localization. Unlike acute pain, chronic pain lacks signs of heightened sympathetic activity. Depression, anxiety, and pre-morbid personality problems are common in those with chronic pain. Usually the major problem is a lack of motivation and an incentive to get better. It is usually helpful to:

1. **Determine the presence of dermatomal pattern**
2. **Determine the presence of neuropathic pain**
3. **Assess pain behavior**

C. **Continuous pain in the terminally ill** originates from well-defined tissue damage due to the terminal illness (e.g., cancer). It is a variant of nociceptive pain. Stress, sleep deprivation, depression, and pre-morbid personality problems may exacerbate this type of pain.

D. **Neuropathic pain is caused by an injured or dysfunctional central or peripheral nervous system; it is manifest by spontaneous, sharp, shooting, or burning pain that is usually distributed along dermatomes** (see Figure 40-2). Neuropathic pain is often referred to as deafferentation syndrome, reflex

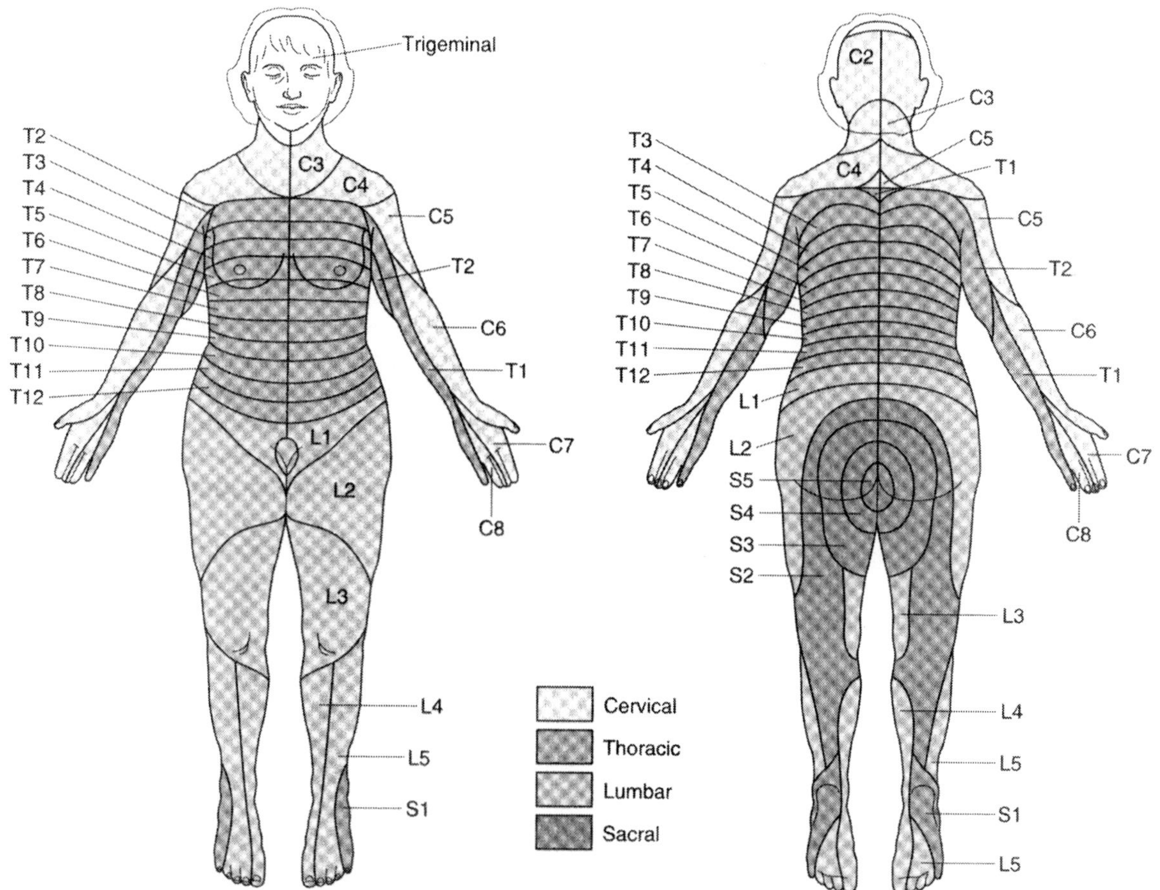

Figure 40-2. Schematic diagram of segmental neuronal innervation by dermatomes. (Source: Hyman, S.H., Cassem, N.H., *Pain*, 1989.)

sympathetic dystrophy (RSD), diabetic neuropathy, central pain syndrome, trigeminal neuralgia, or post-herpetic neuralgia.

Terms commonly used to describe neuropathic pain include:

1. **Hyperalgesia:** an increased response to a stimulus that is normally painful.
2. **Hyperesthesia:** an exaggerated pain response to a noxious stimulus (pressor or heat).
3. **Allodynia:** pain from a stimulus that is not normally painful (e.g., light touch or cool air).
4. **Hyperpathia:** pain from a painful stimulus with a delay, and a persistence that is distributed beyond the area of stimulation.

E. Reflex sympathetic dystrophy (RSD) is a syndrome of sympathetically maintained pain, or a complex regional pain syndrome in an extremity that is mediated by sympathetic overactivity; it does not involve a major nerve or involve sensory, autonomic, motor, or trophic changes. The syndrome is usually caused by injury; however, the cause is unknown in approximately 10% of cases. It may be caused by either microtrauma or macrotrauma, such as a sprain, a fracture, or a contusion; iatrogenic causes include amputation, lesion resection, myelography, and IM injections. RSD may be disease-related (e.g., due to myocardial infarction, shoulder-hand syndrome, herpes zoster, cerebrovascular accidents, diabetic neuropathy, a disc herniation, degenerative disc disease, neuraxial tumors or metastases, multiple sclerosis, or poliomyelitis).

1. **A sensory component includes spontaneous pain** and evoked pain in the affected extremity.
2. **Autonomic changes** occur (marbled, hyperemic to cyanotic skin color, edema), as well as changes in blood flow, asymmetrical skin temperatures, and perspiration in the affected limbs.
3. **Motor changes** involve decreased strength and range of motion, tremor, hypotonia, atrophy, and dystonias.
4. **Trophic changes** are seen in approximately 30% of cases and rarely occur within first 10 days of initial symptoms. These changes include disturbed nail growth, increased hair growth, palmar/planter fibrosis, thin glossy skin, hyperkeratosis, and distal osteoporosis.

The clinical course (which may last up to 6 months) starts with an acute phase involving pain, edema, and warm skin. Subsequently dystrophic changes dominate the picture with cold skin and trophic changes (3–6 months after the onset of the untreated acute phase). Irreversible atrophic changes (atrophy and contractures) eventually occur.

There may be symptom improvement with inhibition of sympathetic output; sympathetic blockade may be both diagnostic and therapeutic.

F. Idiopathic pain, previously referred to as "psychogenic pain," is poorly understood. The presence of pain does not imply or exclude a psychological component. Typically, there is no evidence of an associated organic etiology or anatomical pattern of symptoms. Symptoms are often grossly out of proportion to identifiable organic pathology.

Jurisigenic pain results from perceived physical or emotional damage related to medical, personal, work, or product injury. Patients with this pain syndrome usually maintain the sick role for as long as possible to maximize financial return. It is important to recognize the existence of a conflict and to educate patients and attorneys; maintenance of a helping and neutral posture is critical.

G. Phantom pain refers to severe and excrutiating pain after amputation, presenting a major obstacle to the treatment of the amputee. It is usually localized to the distal amputated limb and tends to vanish 2–3 years after the amputation. The pathophysiology of this pain is poorly understood. The chaotic innervation of the amputation site and supraspinal mechanisms (e.g., attention and stress) may contribute to this pain syndrome.

VI. Psychopathology and Pain

A wide variety of psychotropics (e.g., antidepressants, anticonvulsants, benzodiazepines, neuroleptics, stimulants, alpha-2 agonists) can treat pain syndromes.

A. Mood disorders are commonly co-morbid with pain

1. Depressive disorders have been found in 30–87% of pain patients.
   a. Major depression develops in 8–50% of pain patients.
   b. Dysthymia is seen in more then three-fourths of patients with chronic pain.
2. Anxiety disorders (including panic disorder, generalized anxiety disorder, and post-traumatic stress disorder) are found in more than a half of patients with chronic pain.

B. Somatoform disorders, including body dysmorphic disorder, conversion disorder, hypochondriasis, somatization disorder, and pain disorder, are detected in patients with chronic pain. In somatoform pain disorder, pain is a major part of clinical presentation, and it causes significant impairment in function.

C. Other psychiatric states may also be co-morbid with pain:

1. **Factitious disorders** involve the intentional production or feigning of physical or psychological symptoms (unconscious motivation, conscious production).
2. **Malingering** involves the intentional production or feigning of physical or psychological symptoms moti-

vated by clear external incentives (conscious motivation, conscious production).

3. **Psychoactive Substance Use Disorders:** Dependence and abuse may develop as a result of chronic pain.
   a. Oxycodone is a controversial medication. It is superior to morphine in its oral absorption and bioavailibility but is similar in its potential for abuse. Both its analgesic benefits and its side effects are similar to those of morphine. Deaths attributable to this agent are usually associated with polysubstance abuse.
4. **Personality disorders**
5. **Adjustment disorders**

VII. Analgesic Therapies

A. Overview

1. **The initiation of analgesic therapy involves a multifactorial decision process.**
   a. At times analgesia may be delayed until psychopathology can be identified and managed.
   b. Efficiency of analgesia needs to be monitored. Function needs to be assessed to guide treatment.
2. **Pharmacological approaches**
   a. Pharmacological approaches (including opioids and non-opioids) vary depending on whether pain is acute or chronic (see Tables 40-1 and 40-2 for the various agents and dosing details).
3. **Non-pharmacological approaches include:**
   a. Invasive techniques (e.g., nerve blocks, implantable devices, neurosurgery)
   b. Non-invasive (e.g., physical therapy, acupuncture, massage, biofeedback, cognitive-behavioral therapy, relaxation techniques, and hypnosis) approaches

B. Acute Pain

1. **Acute pain is usually treated medically via treatment of the underlying disorder.**
2. **Management follows the analgesic ladder of the World Health Organization (WHO)** (see Figure 40-3).
3. **Severe acute pain typically requires use of strong opioids** (e.g., hydromorphone, levorphanol, or morphine). These may be delivered by patient-controlled analgesia (PCA) or by an epidural route either with or without local anesthetics (see Table 40-1 for prescription guidelines).

Table 40-1. Non-steroidal Anti-Inflammatory Drugs

Drug	*Dose (mg)*	*Dosage Interval (hours)*	*Daily Dose (mg)*	*Peak Effect (hours)*	*Half-Life (hours)*
Diclofenac	25–75	6–8	200	2	1–2
Etodolac acid	200–400	6–8	1,200	1–2	7
Fenoprofen	200	4–6	3,200	1–2	2–3
Flurbiprofen	50–100	6–8	300	1.5–3.0	3–4
Ibuprofen	200–400	6–8	3,200	1–2	2
Indomethacin	25–75	6–8	200	0.5–1.0	2–3
Ketoprofen	25–75	6–8	300	1–2	1.5–2.0
Ketorolac[a]					
Oral	10	6–8	40	0.5–1.0	6
Parenteral	60 load, then 30	6–8	120		
Meclofenamic acid	500 load, then 275	6–8	400		
Mefenamic acid	500 load, then 250	6	1,250	2–4	3–4
Nabumetone	1,000–2,000	12–24	2,000	3–5	22–30
Naproxen	500 load, then 250	6–8	1,250	2–4	12–15
Naproxen sodium	550 load, then 275	6–8	1,375	1–2	13
Oxaprozin	60–1200	Every day	1,800	2	3–3.5
Phenylbutazone	100	6–8	400	2	50–100
Piroxicam	40 load, then 20	24	20	2–4	36–45
Sulindac	150–200	12	400	1–2	7–18
Tolmetin	200–400	8	1,800	4–6	2

SOURCE: Borsook, D., Lebel, A.A., & McPeek, B. (1995). *MGH handbook of pain management*. Boston, MA: Little, Brown.

[a]Use no longer than 5 days.

Table 40-2. Pharmacological Treatment of Acute Pain with Opiates

Drug	Approximate Equianalgesic Oral Dose	Approximate Equianalgesic Parenteral Dose	Recommended Starting Dose (adults more than 50 kg body weight)	
			Oral	Parenteral
Opiate agonist				
Morphine	30 mg q 3–4 h	10 mg q 3–4 h	30 mg q 3–4 h	10 mg q3–4 h
Codeine	130 mg q 3–4 h	75 mg q 3–4 h	60 mg q 3–4 h	60 mg q 2 h
Hydromorphone (Dilaudid)	7.5 mg q 3–4 h	1.5 mg q 3–4 h	6 mg q 3–4 h	1.5 mg q 3–4 h
Levorphanol (Levo-Dromoran)	4 mg q 6–8 h	2 mg q 6–8 h	4 mg q 6–8 h	2 mg q 6–8 h
Meperidine (Demerol)	300 mg q 2–3 h	100 mg q 3 h	Not recommended	100 mg q 3 h
Methadone (Dolophine, others)	20 mg q 6–8 h	10 mg q 6–8 h	20 mg q 6–8 h	10 mg q 6–8 h
Oxycodone (Roxicodone, also in Percocet, Percodan, Tylox, others)	30 mg q 3–4 h	Not available	10 mg q 3–4 h	Not available
Oxymorphone (Numorphan)	Not available	1 mg q 3–4 h	Not available	1 mg q 3–4 h
Opioid agonist-antagonist and partial agonist				
Buprenorphine (Buprenex)	Not available	0.3–0.4 mg q 6–8 h	Not available	0.4 mg q 6–8 h
Butorphanol (Stadol)	Not available	2 mg q 3–4 h	Not available	2 mg q 3–4 h
Nalbuphine (Nubain)	Not available	10 mg q 3–4 h	Not available	10 mg q 3–4 h
Pentazocine (Talwin, others)	150 mg q 3–4 h	60 mg q 3–4 h	50 mg q 4–6 h	Not recommended

NOTE: Published tables vary in the suggested doses that are equianalgesic to morphine. Clinical response is the criterion that must be applied for each patient; titration to clinical response is necessary. Because there is not complete cross-tolerance among these drugs, it is usually necessary to use a lower than equianalgesic dose when changing drugs and to retitrate to response.

CAUTION: Recommended doses do not apply to patients with renal or hepatic insufficiency or other conditions affecting drug metabolism and kinetics.

CAUTION: Doses listed for patients with body weight > 50 kg cannot be used as initial starting doses in children and patients < 50 kg. Consult the *Clinical Practice Guideline for Acute Pain Management: Operative or Medical Procedures and Trauma* (section on management of pain in neonates) for recommendations. For morphine, hydromorphone, and oxymorphone, rectal administration is an alternate route for patients unable to take oral medications, but equianalgesic doses may differ from oral and parenteral doses because of pharmacokinetic differences.

CAUTION: Codeine doses > 65 mg often are not appropriate due to diminishing incremental analgesia with increasing doses but continually increasing constipation and other side effects.

CAUTION: Doses of aspirin and acetaminophen in combination with opiate/nonsteroidal anti-inflammatory drug preparations must also be adjusted to the patient's body weight.

SOURCE: Borsook, D., Lebel, A.A., & McPeek, B. (1995). *MGH handbook of pain management.* Boston, MA: Little, Brown.

C. **Chronic pain is usually treated with a multidisciplinary approach,** since long-standing pain has far-reaching effects on many physical and psychological systems.

1. **Neuropathic pain is typically treated with anticonvulsants** (e.g., carbamazepine, phenytoin, gabapentin, and clonazepam) or antiarrhythmics (e.g., lidocaine, mexiletine, and TCAs). Response may also be seen with other analgesics (e.g., opioids or NSAIDs). Nerve blockade and nerve transection rarely offer persistent relief.
2. **Chronic regional pain syndromes (e.g., RSD) involve initial treatment with conservative therapy**

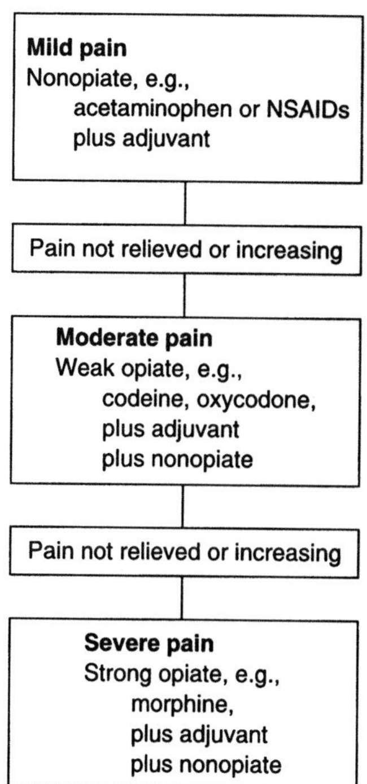

Figure 40-3. The analgesic ladder. (Source: Borsook D., Lebel, A.A., & McPeek, B. (1995). *MGH handbook of pain management.* Boston, MA: Little, Brown.)

(e.g., mild analgesics and physical therapy). Sympathetic interruption may be both diagnostic and therapeutic. Direct sympatholysis usually involves lumbar sympathetic or stellate ganglion block, or a systemic drug challenge with sympatholytic agents (e.g., phentolamine or phenoxybenzamine).

3. **Idiopathic pain or pain that fails conventional therapy**
   a. This type of pain requires a multi-disciplinary approach including anesthesia, psychiatry, behavioral medicine, surgery/neurosurgery, physiatry, physical therapy, occupational therapy, nursing, pharmacy, social work, and case management.
   b. Invasive interventions are of unclear value.
   c. Some severe cases may warrant use of opioids.

D. The Use of Opioids

Opioids are the gold standard for severe or unremitting pain.

1. **The basic principles of opioid use follow the guidelines put forth in the WHO analgesic ladder.** Physicians should explain to patients that opioids are not curative, may be addictive, and have no prophylactic value. When used chronically, function rather than pain, should be followed (see Table 40-2 for agents and doses).
2. **Efficacy: Opioids are equally efficacious when used in equianalgesic dosages;** however, for unknown reasons one individual may respond better to one agent than to another.
3. **Synergy: Analgesia may be potentiated by other drugs** (e.g., NSAIDs, antihistamines, clonidine, neuroleptics, or TCAs).
4. **Administration:** An as-needed (p.r.n.) dosing may reinforce the pain cycle, whereas long-acting agents may be preferable for long-term use.
5. **Routes of administration:** Oral (PO), per rectum (PR), sublingual (SL), intramuscular (IM), intravenous (IV), patient-controlled analgesic (PCA), epidural, or spinal routes are available.
6. **Adverse effects** are common and often limit the use of a drug. Such effects are usually idiosyncratic; it is unclear why some patients are more sensitive than others. Predictors as to which patients will experience which side effects and which narcotics will produce them are lacking. Thus, one should expect side effects and take preventive actions. Tolerance to the adverse effects of opiates, except constipation, occurs.
   a. Common adverse effects from opioids include
      i. **Constipation,** which is the most common side effect of opioids; it persists over time, requires use of a daily stimulating cathartic, and may respond to oral dosages of naloxone.
      ii. **Respiratory depression** is a potentially serious complication. However, tolerance occurs early in chronic therapy and significant respiratory depression can be managed with naloxone.
      iii. **Severe nausea and vomiting** caused by opioids is rare; it is usually mild.
      iv. **Pruritus,** which probably occurs through a central mechanism, is rare with oral agents but is very common with spinal and epidural opioids. If tolerance to pruritus does occur, it can be treated with naloxone, antihistamines (except when caused by spinal opioids), and by propofol (10 mg IV q 10 minutes given in two to three doses).
7. **Tolerance** to analgesia may require dose escalation. Changing agents may allow dosing at lower than equianalgesic dose, as cross-tolerance between opioids may be incomplete. Tolerance impairs the ability to assess the appropriate opioid dosage.
8. **Opioids for chronic non-malignant pain are highly controversial,** but there is growing acceptance in well-selected cases. Such management has been avoided owing to high abuse potential, tolerance, dependence, and other adverse effects. However, opioids may be a reasonable option for patients with chronic non-malignant pain who have failed other reasonable conventional non-opioid interventions.
   a. **Guidelines for using opioids in chronic non-malignant pain include:**
      i. Individualize therapy with opioids.
      ii. Use a single opioid agent, if possible.
         - Use long-acting preparations.
         - Mix a single short-acting agent and a single long-acting agent.

Table 40-3. DEA Guidelines for the Prescription of Controlled Substances

1. A prescription for a controlled substance is lawful only if issued for a legitimate medical purpose by an individual practitioner acting in the usual course of professional practice. Prescriptions under the law may not be issued for narcotic drugs for the purpose of detoxification or maintenance of narcotics addicts.
2. All prescriptions for controlled substances must bear the following information:
   a. Name of patient
   b. Home address of patient
   c. Name of practitioner
   d. Address of practitioner
   e. Registration number of practitioner
   f. Name of the drug, strength, and quantity of the medicine to be dispensed
   g. Directions for use
3. All prescriptions must be dated with the day when issued to the patient and must be signed manually on that day by the practitioner.
4. It is illegal under both federal and state law to issue a prescription for other than a legitimate *bona fide* medical need or to date a prescription other than the date when it is issued to the patient and signed by the practitioner.
5. Schedule II controlled substances require written prescriptions prior to dispensing. They may not be refilled. A schedule II drug may be dispensed in an emergency by a pharmacist upon oral prescription of a practitioner if the quantity is limited to the emergency period, if the prescription is reduced immediately to writing by the pharmacist and contains all the information required of written prescriptions except the signature of the prescriber, if the pharmacist knows the prescriber, or makes a reasonable effort to verify the order's validity, and if the prescriber issues to the pharmacist a written prescription within 48 hours of the oral order. If the pharmacist does not receive a written prescription from the prescriber within 72 hours, he or she must by law notify the DEA regional office.
6. A controlled substance prescription must be for no more than 30 days of medicine.

SOURCE: Borsook, D., Lebel, A.A., & McPeek, B. (1995). *MGH handbook of pain management.* Boston, MA: Little, Brown.

- For daily usage, use around-the-clock dosing rather than p.r.n. dosing.

iii. Document the efficacy of opioid analgesia.
- Function is of greater interest than analgesia.

iv. Use opioid contracts and provide informed consent.
v. Discuss side effects and risks of addiction, dependence, tolerance, cognitive impairment, fetal dependency in pregnancy, rules of usage and prescribing, and consequences of breaking the contract.
vi. Designate a single prescriber for all opioids.
vii. Designate a single pharmacy for distribution of all opioids.
viii. Maintain a symptom diary.
ix. Do not provide over-the-phone prescriptions.
x. Maintain close follow-up.
xi. Maintain a high level of suspicion of toxicity and addictive tendencies.
- Watch for evidence of drug hoarding, acquisition of opioids by multiple physicians, uncontrolled dose escalations, or other aberrant behaviors.

xii. Follow usage guidelines.
xiii. Consult with an addictions specialist.
xiv. Periodically review the case with a multi-disciplinary team.
xv. Be aware of relative contraindications (e.g., a history of substance abuse, a severe character disorder, an inability to follow rules, and for those with a substance abuse history, the relative nature of these contraindications must yield to compassionate use of narcotics for pharmacological treatment.

E. Analgesic Adjuvants

1. Use of adjuvants, such as NSAIDs, antihistamines, clonidine, corticosteroids, neuroleptics, psychostimulants, and tricyclics can be effective.
2. Partial analgesic effects may be achieved with tricyclics, clonidine, baclofen, muscle relaxants, corticosteroids, antiarrhythmics, and anticonvulsants
3. Antidepressants: TCAs but not SSRIs are well established as having independent analgesic properties.
   a. Efficacy of specific TCAs
      i. TCAs that are supported as analgesics by controlled studies include amitriptyline (Elavil), nortriptyline (Pamelor), desipramine (Norpramin), imipramine (Tofranil), and maprotiline (Ludiomil).

ii. TCAs that are supported as analgesics by anecdotal reports include doxepin, trazodone, and clomipramine.

b. TCA analgesia strategy: Complete analgesia is rare and side effects are common with the use of TCAs, so usually one must accept mild side effects in exchange for analgesia. Use of TCAs is particularly compelling when pain is accompanied by co-morbid depression or by insomnia. Reasonable goals of therapy include decreasing pain intensity by 10–50% or by decreasing pain from unbearable to bearable levels.

c. Analgesic TCA dosages may be lower than antidepressant dosages; some patients require higher dosages.
   i. Start at a dose of 10 to 25 mg; very low doses should be used for those > 65 years of age.
   ii. Slowly increase the dosage to minimize side effects and avoid overshooting the minimal analgesic dose.
   iii. Intolerable side effects may be alleviated by changing to desipramine or nortriptyline
   iv. Relief may be experienced in 1 to 7 days to several weeks (maximal analgesia may require 2 to 4 weeks).
   v. TCA-induced analgesic effects persist over time.

F. Non-pharmacological Approaches

1. **Invasive**
   a. **Nerve blocks and implantable devices:** trigger point injections, epidural injections, selective nerve root injections, stellate ganglion, and lumbar sympathetic nerve blockade can be employed
   b. **Neurosurgery**
      i. **Augmentative**
         - An intrathecal pump, typically delivers an opioid but may involve baclofen (for spasticity) or a local anesthetic (less common).
         - A spinal cord stimulator (dorsal column stimulator) is a catheter device placed in the epidural space that electrically stimulates the spinal cord. It is used in neuropathic pain and in sympathetically maintained pain states.

      ii. **Ablative therapy**
         - Radiofrequency lesions are used in peripheral pain (e.g., trigeminal and glossopharyngeal neuralgia)
         - Treatments for spinal cord lesions include ganglionectomy (with ablation of the dorsal ganglia), dorsal rhizotomy (with sensory loss in lesioned distribution) with dorsal root entry zone (DREZ), phantom limb pain, and with midline myelotomy (for bilateral pain).
         - Central techniques include mesencephalotomy (for lesions of midbrain spinothalamic and secondary trigeminal tracts—for unilateral head and neck pain), thalamotomy (which is sometimes used with bilateral analgesia), and **cingulotomy (for diffuse chronic pain associated with affective disorders).**

2. **Non-invasive techniques** include physical therapy, transcutaneous electrical stimulation (TENS), acupuncture (relatively non-invasive), massage, cognitive or behavioral therapy, and distraction (e.g., hypnosis or biofeedback).

G. The Multi-disciplinary Approach

1. Goals of the multi-disciplinary approach include improvements in coping, plans for focus on function rather than on analgesia, and a decrease in addictive behaviors. This approach offers alternatives to drugs, to injections, or to surgery for pain control, and it improves overall physical and psychological well-being. It strives to improve social supports, to decrease social isolation, and to decrease dependence on the health-care system.
2. Multi-disciplinary team meetings involve practitioners from medicine, neurology, pediatrics, physiatry, psychiatry, surgery, anesthesia, neurosurgery, and physical therapy.
3. **Alternative therapies** (e.g., acupuncture, yoga, tai chi, massage, and herbal remedies) are of unknown efficacy.

Suggested Readings

Acute Pain Management Guideline Panel. (1992). *Acute pain management: Operative or medical procedures and trauma. Clinical practice guideline.* Rockville, MD: Agency for Health Care Policy and Research, Public Health Service, U.S. Department of Health and Human Services, AHCPR Pub. No. 92-0032.

Arash, A. (2000). The efficacy of newer antidepressants in the treatment of chronic pain: A review of current literature. *Harvard Review of Psychiatry, 7,* 257–277.

Bonica, J.J. (Ed.). (1990). *The management of pain* (2nd ed.). Philadelphia: Lea & Febiger.

Borsook, D., Lebel, A.A., & McPeek, B. (1995). *MGH handbook of pain management.* Boston, MA: Little, Brown.

Breitbart, W. (1989). Psychiatric management of cancer pain. *Cancer, 63,* 2336–2342.

Davis, M.P., Varga, J., Dickerson, D., et al. (2003). Normal release and controlled-release oxycodone: Pharmacokinetics, pharmacodynamics, and controversy. *Support Care Cancer, 11,* 84–92

Fields, H.L. (1987). *Pain.* New York: McGraw-Hill.

Foley, K.M. (1983). The practical use of narcotic analgesics. *Medical Clinics of North America, 66,* 1091–1104.

Hyman, S.H., & Cassem, N.H. (1989). Pain. In E. Rubenstein, & D.D. Fedeman (Eds.), *Scientific American medicine: Current topics in medicine. Subsection II,* pp. 1–7. New York: Scientific American.

NIH Consensus Development Conference. (1987). The integrated approach to the management of pain. *Journal of Pain Symptom Management, 2,* 35–41.

Portnoy, R.Y. (1990). Chronic opioid therapy in nonmalignant pain. *Journal of Pain Symptom Management, 5,* S46–S62.

Sternbach, R. (1974). *Pain patients: Traits and treatments.* New York: Academic Press.

Taber, K.H., Rashid, A., & Hurley, R.A. (2001). Functional anatomy of central pain. *Journal of Neuropsychiatry and Clinical Neuroscience, 13,* 437–440.

Wall, P.D., & Melzack, R. (Eds.). (1995). *Textbook of pain* (3rd ed.). New York: Churchill-Livingstone.

Chapter 41

Stroke

ALICE W. FLAHERTY, SCHAHRAM AKBARIAN, AND MARTIN A. SAMUELS

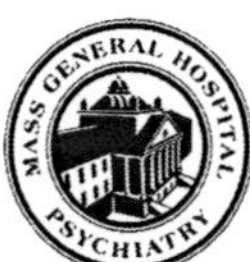

I. Introduction

Stroke is the third leading cause of mortality and morbidity in the United States. Advances in acute stroke management now make rapid diagnosis and referral important. Because treatment strategies may be opposite for strokes of different types (e.g., an aspirin given for an ischemic stroke will worsen a hemorrhagic stroke), practitioners should know how to identify the major stroke syndromes. Many strokes present with, or are followed by, neuropsychiatric symptoms, and knowledge about stroke is thus important in the differential diagnosis of mood disorders, delirium, dementia, and other psychiatric diseases.

II. Stroke Classification and Pathophysiology

A. Definitions

1. **Stroke** is the rapid onset of a neurological deficit caused by cerebrovascular disease, either ischemic or hemorrhagic. Neurologists usually use the word stroke to mean ischemic stroke, and they will speak of hemorrhages separately. Patients will use the term stroke to refer to either ischemic strokes or bleeds. Until recently, the neurological deficit was required to last more than 24 hours to qualify as a stroke. Now, however, if there is evidence of permanent tissue damage by MRI, an event is considered a stroke even if the symptoms or deficit lasted only a few hours.
2. **Transient ischemic attack (TIA)** (formerly defined as cerebrovascular ischemia causing a deficit lasting less than 24 hours) is more recently used to cover only ischemic episodes with no permanent tissue damage. In practice, this means that most TIAs are symptomatic for five minutes or less. TIAs should generally be investigated as seriously as strokes. Because the deficits associated with TIAs have resolved by the time most patients are evaluated, the history is crucial. Be careful: many patients will say that their arm felt "numb" to describe one that was in fact paralyzed, a much more ominous symptom. Similarly, an arm that was "numb" (pins and needles, or paresthesias) is of less concern than an arm that was "numb" (insensate).

B. Ischemic Stroke

1. **Diagnosis**
   a. **History and exam.** If an acute/interventional stroke service is available in your area, page them as soon as a stroke is suspected, not when it is confirmed. The sudden painless onset of a focal deficit is typical. Headache or coma usually suggests a bleed rather than an ischemic stroke. Stroke syndromes are listed below.
   b. **Imaging.** CT scans are useful only to rule out bleeds or to detect large old strokes. Diffusion-weighted MRI can detect ischemic strokes within 30 minutes of their onset. Obtaining CTs and MRIs may waste precious time if the patient is to be transferred to a stroke center for possible intervention. CT angiograms, MR angiograms, and vascular ultrasounds all help assess arterial stenosis, and often determine whether intra-arterial clot lysis or disruption is attempted. They have largely replaced conventional angiograms.
2. **Management**
   a. **Treatment.** Acutely, do not aggressively lower blood pressure. Intravenous and intraarterial thrombolysis, and mechanical clot disruption (e.g., intraarterial coils or balloons) are now done at some centers. These procedures must usually be done within 4–6 hours. In other cases, heparin may be used to decrease stroke extension. It can, however, cause hemorrhagic conversion of the dead tissue. Avoid neuroleptics, benzodiazepines, and alpha-antagonists. Early aggressive physical therapy may help brain remodeling.
   b. **Primary prevention.** Lipid-lowering drugs decrease the risk of stroke. Nearly all patients with atrial fibrillation should be on warfarin even if they have never had a stroke. This is a problem for the relatively many alcoholics with atrial fibrillation, who are at risk for head injuries, and whose psychiatric medications may interact with their warfarin.
   c. **Secondary prevention.** Whether to use anti-clotting agents (e.g. warfarin, heparin) or anti-platelet agents (e.g., aspirin, clopidogrel) for secondary prevention depends on the cause of the stroke, and on co-morbid illnesses. Carotid endarterectomy is indicated for symptomatic stenoses greater than 70%.
3. **Causes of ischemic strokes**
   a. **Thrombosis.** About 50% of strokes are caused by atherosclerosis and gradual narrowing of the carotids, the vertebrals, or the circle of Willis.
   c. **Emboli.** About 20% of strokes come from cardiac or artery-to-artery emboli. Patients with atrial fibrillation should be on warfarin prophylaxis. Other types of heart disease, especially patent foramen ovale and a low ejection fraction can also increase one's embolic risk.
   b. **Lacunes.** About 20% of strokes stem from lipohyalinosis and narrowing of tiny end-arteries. Associated with hypertension and smoking, lacunar strokes are white-matter strokes, unlike the gray-matter large-vessel strokes described earlier.
   d. **Arterial dissections.** Head or neck injury can cause immediate or delayed stroke in young patients. Usually there

is a history of neck pain. One must have a high suspicion for this.

e. **Hypercoaguability** may be induced by pregnancy, use of oral contraceptives, the antiphospholipid antibody syndrome, and a sickle cell crisis.

C. Hemorrhagic Stroke

1. Diagnosis

a. **History and exam.** Thunderclap headache, altered consciousness, and progressive deterioration may help distinguish bleeds from ischemic strokes. The neurological deficits are often less focal and may cross vascular territories.

b. **Imaging.** CT is generally all that is needed to make the diagnosis, except for very small posterior fossa bleeds. MRI with iron susceptibility sequencing gives evidence about prior bleeds. In subarachnoid hemorrhage, a sentinel bleed may be missed on CT and be seen only through lumbar puncture red blood cell counts or xanthochromia.

2. Management

a. **Neurosurgery.** A neurosurgeon should be consulted immediately for all subarachnoid and epidural bleeds, and for intracerebral and subdural bleeds where there is altered consciousness, progressive deterioration, hydrocephalus, blood in the ventricles, or a posterior fossa clot greater than 3 cm wide.

b. **Conservative management.** The chief concerns are continued bleeding and mass effect. Keeping the patient's blood pressure less than 150 mmHg and giving vitamin K to patients on warfarin are simple but important things to do while waiting for the neurologist or neurosurgeon. As secondary prevention, most patients should avoid anticoagulants and aspirin in the future.

3. Causes of hemorrhagic strokes

a. **Intracerebral hemorrhage.** Although a patient's deficits from an intracerebral hemmorhage are initially worse than those from an ischemic stroke of the same size, he or she will eventually have a greater recovery—much of the deficit was a result of mass effect, not cell death.

i. **Basal ganglia and intraventricular bleeds** are often associated with hypertension.

ii. **Lobar or cerebellar bleeds** are often due to amyloid angiopathy.

iii. **Arteriovenous malformations** can cause both lobar and subarachnoid bleeding. They may also present with seizures or focal deficits.

b. **Subarachnoid hemorrhage.** Spontaneous subarachnoid bleeds are much more dangerous than traumatic ones, as they indicate the likelihood of a Berry (saccular) aneurysm that has a high likelihood of re-bleeding. Ruptured aneurysms are associated with a 30% mortality rate. Aneurysms are usually found around the circle of Willis; they sometimes press on cranial nerves and cause chronic focal deficits. They may be repaired by neurosurgical clipping or intra-arterial coiling. Incidentally detected aneurysms less than 5 mm are usually monitored by MR or CT angiography.

c. **Subdural and epidural hematomas** usually stem from trauma, and are not generally called strokes except by patients. Epidural hematomas are neurosurgical emergencies. Chronic subdural hematomas, are common in the elderly. They are often discovered incidentally and may not need treatment. Sometimes they cause headache, focal signs, or altered consciousness.

III. Stroke Syndromes

A. General Rules

Of the many stroke syndromes, only those which affect management will be discussed here. Syndromes are organized by vascular territory.

1. **Anterior (carotid) vs. posterior (basilar) circulation strokes**. The distinction is crucial: the latter are generally more dangerous, although there is less danger of secondary bleeding and thus a longer time window for invasive treatment. Evidence for posterior circulation ischemia includes altered consciousness, cerebellar signs, lower cranial nerve deficits, and crossed (e.g., right face and left body) or bilateral deficits.
2. **Large artery vs. lacunar strokes.** This is essentially the difference between gray matter and white matter strokes. The latter are less dangerous and less treatable.
3. **Left (dominant) hemisphere strokes are more disabling**, primarily because of language deficits and depression.
4. **Pure sensory deficits in young people are rarely secondary to stroke.** The classic example is hemibody numbness associated with conversion disorder.

B. Anterior Circulation Strokes

1. **Internal carotid artery syndromes.** Clinical manifestations vary with the efficacy of collateral vessels. A complete infarct, however, destroys the entire anterior two-thirds of that cerebral hemisphere, and may be fatal due to secondary swelling. Occlusion of the internal carotid artery can present with some or all of the clinical symptoms that occur after occlusion of its three major branches (the anterior cerebral, the middle cerebral, and the ophthalmic arteries).
2. **Anterior cerebral artery (ACA) syndromes** cause contralateral leg weakness, a grasp reflex, and frontal signs, including apathy or disinhibition, depression, poor judgment, shuffling gait, perseveration, and urinary incontinence. The leg weakness may be bilateral: some right and left ACAs have a common origin.
3. **Middle cerebral artery syndromes**

a. **Superior division strokes** cause contralateral arm and face weakness with sensory loss. Severe leg weakness implies a full internal carotid stroke, or a lacunar pure motor stroke. Dominant hemisphere strokes cause a Broca's (expressive) aphasia, with non-fluent speech and relatively retained comprehension. Of note, though, many aphasias appear global (no comprehension or expression) during the first few hours after the stroke. It is important to distinguish this muteness, in which gestural imitation may be preserved, from delirium (altered attention, dreamy nonsense speech), dementia (anomia), and psychiatric language disorders. Non-dominant strokes cause left-sided neglect and indifference to one's disability.

b. **Inferior division strokes** cause mild or transient sensorimotor deficit. Dominant hemisphere lesions usually cause a Wernicke's (receptive) aphasia, with fluent, contentless speech (politician speech). Non-dominant lesions result in an inability to recognize the emotional inflections of speech, as well as left neglect. There may sometimes be a contralateral field cut.

4. **Ophthalmic artery syndrome** causes transient (amaurosis fugax) or permanent sudden monocular blindness due to optic nerve and retinal ischemia. This deficit is ipsilateral, and thus you may see left blindness with a right facial droop from middle cerebral ischemia. Pressing the eyeball firmly (4 seconds on, 4 seconds off) can occasionally move the clot through the circulation. The differential diagnosis includes temporal arteritis: give 60 mg of prednisone presumptively, and draw an erythrocyte sedimentation rate.

C. Posterior Circulation Strokes

1. **Posterior cerebral artery (PCA) strokes.** Most blood to the PCAs comes from the basilar artery, and PCA strokes can signal the life-threatening "top of the basilar" syndrome (see below). Strokes in the occipital lobe usually cause a contralateral field cut (homonymous hemianopsia). Medial temporal lobe strokes can damage the hippocampus and cause anterograde amnesia. Thalamic strokes can cause amnesia as well as contralateral sensory disturbances and, sometimes, tremor. Rostral midbrain lesions can paralyze vertical eye movements.
2. **Basilar artery strokes.** The basilar artery supplies the occipital lobe, midbrain, the pons, much of the cerebellar hemispheres, and the nuclei of cranial nerves III, IV, V, VI, VII, and VIII. Strokes in this territory therefore cause complicated combinations of visual loss, double vision, nystagmus, ataxia, hearing loss, weakness, and numbness.
   a. **Top of the basilar syndrome** occurs when a clot lodges at the origins of the posterior cerebral arteries and fragments fly off over a period of hours or days. The resulting protean change in exam and focal deficits may be dismissed as conversion disorder, but this syndrome is often fatal. Immediate treatments include raising the blood pressure, and often anticoagulation or thrombolysis.
   b. **A complete basilar territory stroke** results either in a comatose patient (due to lesions of the reticular activating system), or a conscious but paralyzed ("locked-in") patient. Vertical eye movements and blinking are often spared.
3. **Vertebral artery syndromes.** The vertebral arteries supply the medulla and the inferior cerebellum. They then fuse to form the basilar artery.
   a. **Cerebellar strokes** cause severe ataxia, dysmetria, vertigo, nausea, and nystagmus. While it is unusual for strokes to cause headache, these strokes do. Have a high suspicion for a cerebellar stroke or bleed in any older patient who presents with sudden vomiting and incoordination from "labyrinthitis" or "gastroenteritis." Large cerebellar strokes can cause rapid herniation and death if not detected quickly.
   b. **The lateral medullary syndrome** (Wallenberg's syndrome), despite its bizarre array of crossed symptoms, is relatively common. Prognosis is good, although there is a risk of silent aspiration from the associated dysphagia. Symptoms include ipsilateral ataxia, vertigo, and nystagmus, ipsilateral Horner's syndrome (drooping lid and small pupil), ipsilateral face and contralateral body loss of pain and temperature sense, and hoarseness.

D. Lacunar Syndromes

These are usually subcortical in location, most often in the putamen, caudate nucleus, thalamus, internal capsule, and pons. The most common kinds include:

1. **Pure motor strokes.** These have face, arm, and leg weakness, but no cortical signs, such as aphasia. They are most often from lacunes in the internal capsule, the base of the pons, or the cerebral peduncle.
2. **Pure sensory strokes.** These have face, arm, and leg numbness, but no cortical signs. They are most often from sensory lesions.

IV. Psychiatric Sequelae of Stroke

Certain stroke syndromes may produce neuropsychiatric symptoms that can be mistaken for symptoms of primary psychiatric disease, especially in the acute setting (e.g., the emergency department). It is good clinical practice to carefully rule out neurological factors—including metabolic and toxic causes as well as focal brain lesions—in a patient with suspected primary psychiatric disease.

A. Aphasia can be mistaken for psychiatric disorders or delirium. The laconic speech of Broca's (expressive) aphasia may be misinterpreted as depression or psychotic withdrawal, or its agrammatisms interpreted as mental retardation. Wernicke's (receptive) aphasia, with its pressured speech and clang associations, may be misinterpreted as mania. Semantic paraphasias ("hotel" for "hospital") may incorrectly be taken as signs of a formal thought disorder.

B. Frontal lobe lesions can be mistaken for depression and personality disorders. Akinetic mutism may resemble psychotic withdrawal, but it lacks negativism and catatonic waxy flexibility.

1. **Orbitofrontal lesions** cause disinhibition, indifference, and sophomoric humor (*Witzelsucht*). It is more often caused by right hemisphere lesions, and is accompanied by left neglect with minimization of one's deficits.
2. **Frontal convexity lesions** cause apathy, poor sequencing, and perseveration.
3. **Medial frontal lesions**, which can look like normal pressure hydrocephalus or atypical parkinsonism, cause leg weakness or incoordination, incontinence, akinesia, and abulia.

C. Dementia

Vascular or multi-infarct dementia is a very common cause of dementia. It usually stems from multiple tiny subcortical strokes (periventricular white matter disease) associated with hypertension, smoking, diabetes, and other vascular risk factors. Less often, multiple emboli to cortical gray matter can produce dementia.

1. **Subcortical dementia** has normal language, slowed but normal cognition, normal memory encoding with poor retrieval, depression or atrophy, and hypophonia, bradykinesia, or a gait abnormality.
2. **Cortical dementia** has anomia, abnormal cognition with normal processing speed, poor memory encoding but normal retrieval, normal or disinhibited affect, and no hypophonia, bradykinesia, or gait problems.
3. **Mixed types**

D. Delirium

D. Delirium can rarely be seen during the acute phase of strokes involving the thalamus or midbrain, or occasionally of strokes of the right temporal lobe. However, the presence of delirium is rare enough in ischemic stroke that it should be a strong clue that metabolic or toxic factors are involved.

E. Mood Disorders

1. **Post-Stroke Depression**
   a. **Major depression may occur after about 20% of strokes.** Three-fourths of patients with post-stroke depression develop a mood disorder within the first 6 months following stroke. In contrast to "endogenous" major depressive disorder, post-stroke depression appears to have no gender bias. Full-blown major depression secondary to a stroke has an average duration, if left untreated, of 12 months. In the DSM-IV, post-stroke depression is listed under mood disorder with depressive features due to a general medical condition.
   b. **Differential diagnosis** includes abulia from frontal lesions, flattened prosody from lesions in the right hemisphere equivalents of Broca's area, and benzodiazepine dependence.
   c. **Pathology.** There seems to be a tendency for infarction of the left hemisphere, in particular of the left prefrontal cortex and rostral caudate, to carry the highest risk for post-stroke depression.
   d. **Treatment of post-stroke depression is similar to that of other types of depression.** SSRIs, stimulants, tricyclic antidepressants (TCAs), and electroconvulsive therapy (ECT) may all treat post-stroke depression. Stimulants have the advantage of inducing an antidepressant response within days of initiation of treatment, and are more effective for frontal abulia than are traditional antidepressants or ECT. This could be a critical factor for mental well-being, early rehabilitation, and avoidance of the serious medical sequelae associated with prolonged immobility.
   e. **A catastrophic reaction** with restlessness and lability are part of a syndrome associated predominantly with left hemispheric lesions and with Broca's aphasia. The response to the sudden experience of disability may play an important role. Some believe that the catastrophic reaction is a special subtype of post-stroke depression.
2. **Post-stroke mania** occurs after about 1% of strokes. The first onset of mania in an elderly patient should be considered as having a neurological origin until proven otherwise. Right hemisphere strokes are more likely to cause mania and hypomania than are left hemisphere ones.
3. **Pseudobulbar affect** is manifest by disinhibition of emotional expression without a significant underlying mood disorder. Affect may be scrambled, so that the patient cries at any strong emotion, but realizes it is incongruent. Because the behavior is usually caused by brainstem damage, pseudobulbar affect is usually found along with spasticity and dysphagia. Use of baclofen or antidepressants may help.
4. **Hallucinations** are very occasionally signs of stroke.
   a. **Simple auditory hallucinations** (i.e., sounds rather than voices), without confusion, have been described after temporal lobe and pontine lesions.
   b. **Simple visual hallucinations** usually stem from occipital cortex lesions.
   c. **Complex hallucinations** (e.g. voices, dreamlike images) typically occur with temporal lobe lesions or lesions of the cerebral peduncle causing "peduncular hallucinosis."

Suggested Readings

Birkett, P.B. (Ed.). (1996). *The psychiatry of stroke.* Washington, DC: American Psychiatric Press.

Bradley, W.B., Daroff, R.B., Fenichel, G.M. (Eds.). (2000). *Neurology in clinical practice* (3rd ed.). Boston, MA: Butterworth Heinemann.

Flaherty, A.W. (2000). *The Massachusetts General handbook of neurology.* Philadelphia, PA: Lippincott, Williams and Wilkins.

Fricchione, G., Weilburg, J.B., & Murray, G.B. (1996). Neurology and neurosurgery. In J.R. Rundell, & M.G. Wise (Eds.), *Textbook of consultation-liaison psychiatry*, pp. 697–719. Washington, DC: American Psychiatric Press.

Samuels, M.A. (1997). Stroke. *Video textbook of neurology for the practicing physician.* Boston, MA: Butterworth-Heinemann.

Chapter 42

Movement Disorders

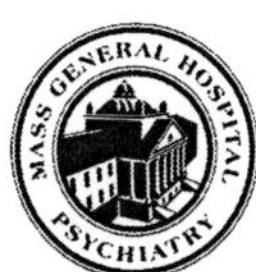

ALICE W. FLAHERTY, SCHAHRAM AKBARIAN, AND MARTIN A. SAMUELS

I. Introduction

A. **Movement disorders are particularly important for psychiatry,** as they often cause or are caused by major psychiatric diseases including major depression, psychosis, dementia, and conversion disorder. Abnormalities of movement are frequent and sometimes devastating side effects of psychotropics. Of these neuroleptic malignant syndrome is immediately life-threatening.

B. **Evaluation.** Nearly all movement disorders are diagnosed by exam and history, not tests. Textbook knowledge helps little in telling a Tourette patient's facial tics from his pimozide-induced tardive dyskinesia. Observing real patients or videotapes is the only way to learn this crucial distinction. In evaluating a patient, ask about falling, drug use, memory loss, hallucinations, incontinence, and what daily tasks are difficult. Watch for involuntary movements and excessive "normal" gestures, weakness, muscle tone, movement speed, postural reflexes, festination, freezing, and ataxia.

C. **Pathophysiology.** Although movement disorders are usually classified as hypokinetic (too little movement) and hyperkinetic (too much), most contain complicated combinations of the two. For instance, a person with Parkinson's disease can have bradykinesia and a tremor simultaneously. By convention, most neurologists consider as movement disorders only symptoms with a presumed basal ganglia origin.

1. **Basal ganglia circuitry.** The basal ganglia include the striatum (caudate nucleus and putamen), globus pallidus, substantia nigra, parts of the thalamus, and the subthalamic nucleus. Hypokinetic disorders usually stem from damage to the direct pathway through the internal globus pallidus; hyperkinetic movements from damage to the indirect pathway through external globus pallidus and subthalamic nucleus. These pathways control affect and cognition as well as movement. **Extrapyramidal symptoms (EPS) is an anatomically inaccurate term** for problems with this network, but it is entrenched in clinical usage.
2. **Other systems.** Paralysis (complete inability to voluntarily use a muscle), paresis (partial paralysis), fasciculations, and ataxia are not, by convention, movement disorders, because they stem from damage to motor neurons or the cerebellum. However, they will be covered briefly below, because they are often an important part of the differential diagnosis.

II. Hypokinetic Signs

A. **Akinesia** is the tendency not to move and bradykinesia is the presence of abnormally slow movements. They are characteristic of parkinsonism, whether idiopathic, drug-induced or from other causes. Balance is often impaired.

B. **Catatonia.** Motor immobility including waxy rigidity, with mutism or echolalia. There is sometimes excess motor activity or unusual voluntary movements. It can be seen in psychiatric disease, parkinsonism, and neuroleptic malignant syndrome (see chapter 28).

C. **Freezing.** Sudden inability to move, often triggered by doorways or rising from a chair. It is seen in parkinsonism.

D. **Rigidity** is increased tone in a muscle group. It probably contributes to akinesia. There is constant "lead pipe" resistance to movement along the whole range of the joint. **"Cogwheel rigidity"** is simply a superimposed tremor, although the tremor is not always apparent visually. Rigidity is characteristic of parkinsonism, with cogwheeling a sign of idiopathic Parkinson's disease. The differential diagnosis of rigidity includes:

1. **Spasticity** is a jerky "clasp-knife" rigidity seen after strokes. The presence of hyperreflexia and spasms helps distinguish this from rigidity. Spasticity is often treated by baclofen, a $GABA_B$ antagonist, or tizanidine, an α_2 noradrenergic agonist.
2. **Paratonia ("Gegenhalten") is a progressive resistance to the examiner's force.** The harder the examiner pushes, the more the limb resists, despite all efforts of the patient to relax. This is common in prefrontal damage as in dementia or some strokes.
3. **"Give-way weakness,"** jerky lapses of tone in testing the strength of a supposedly paretic limb, are most often a sign of a patient who is feigning weakness. However, they are also often present in patients who are elaborating real weakness, in those with proprioceptive deficits, and in those with multiple sclerosis.

E. **Paralysis and paresis** stem not from basal ganglia damage but from interruption of the corticospinal (pyramidal) motor system. This includes upper motor neurons, such as the giant Betz pyramidal cells in layer V of the primary motor cortex (as in stroke), lower motor neurons (as in amyotrophic lateral sclerosis [ALS or Lou Gehrig's disease]), or peripheral nerve injury (as in severe alcoholic neuropathy). Upper and lower motor neuron lesions can be distinguished by spasticity in the former and flaccidity in the latter. ALS is unique in that it usually has both.

III. Hyperkinetic Signs

A. **Akathisia is motor fidgetiness.** It is of lower amplitude than chorea or dyskinesia, more natural looking, and, crucially, accompanied by an often severe inner restlessness and desire to move. It can be caused by dopamine antagonists or boredom.

B. **Chorea and athetosis** are two ends of a spectrum, differing only in speed of movement. Both are involuntary and dance-like, but chorea is jerky and athetosis more writhing. Both come from basal ganglia injury. Causes include use of neuroleptics or oral conctraceptives, lupus, pregnancy, Huntington's disease, or Wilson's disease. Choreoathetosis is best treated with typical neuroleptics, such as haloperidol, but these can cause a tardive worsening of the syndrome.

C. **Dyskinesia** looks a lot like chorea; the distinction is to a large extent a matter of convention. The two major types are tardive dyskinesia, from long-term exposure to dopamine antagonists, and parkinsonian dyskinesia, from long-term exposure to dopamine agonists (see below).

D. **Dystonia** is marked by slow, tonic muscle contractions. It is the slowest end of the spectrum that includes chorea and athetosis, and it is on the border between hyperkinetic and hypokinetic movement. Focal dystonias are best treated with botulinum toxin injections; acute or generalized dystonias respond to anticholinergics.

1. **Acute dystonia** is usually drug-induced (see below).
2. **Meige's syndrome** (orofacial dystonia) involves tonic and clonic grimacing. Usually idiopathic, it is sometimes the result of a dopaminergic drug side effect.
3. **Blepharospasm** resembles Meige's syndrome but it affects only the muscles around the eye.
4. **Torticollis** (cervical dystonia) affects the neck. It is the most common cause of dystonia.
5. **Writer's cramp** and other occupational cramps are task-specific. They are not psychogenic despite the oddness of being able to, say, play the piano but not write.
6. **Progressive generalized dystonia** is usually congenital and results from the DYT-1 mutation; however, it can be from drugs, as in tardive dystonia.

E. **Festination.** Tiny, accelerating steps associated with a difficulty stopping—may cause the patient to run into a wall. Festination is characteristic of parkinsonism.

F. **Hemiballism** is manifest by sudden flinging movements of a limb. A subthalamic nucleus stroke is usually the underlying cause.

G. **Myoclonus** consists of quick, non-rhythmic jerks. Asterixis is negative myoclonus, i.e., sudden lapses of tone. Both can be seen in encephalopathy, drug intoxication (especially from opiates) and neurodegenerative diseases. Unlike tics, myoclonus is completely involuntary. Use of clonazepam or valproate may be helpful. Myoclonus during sleep is normal. Clonazepam is frequently the drug of choice for the treatment of myoclonus.

H. **Restless legs syndrome** is akathisia, triggered by relaxation; it is seen predominantly in the legs. It is sometimes associated with Parkinson's disease, iron-deficiency anemia, pregnancy, dopamine antagonists, and lithium. Levodopa is the main treatment; clonazepam, and low-dose opiates can also help.

I. **Tics** are brief, multi-focal, repetitive, and stereotyped muscle contractions. They most often affect the face, giving rise to blinking, sniffing, facial grimacing, or coughing. Most tics can be distinguished from myoclonus by their complexity (they may look like complex gestures) and by tics' subjective sensations: there is an urge to perform the tic and it can be temporarily suppressed by will power. Tics are common in children between 5 and 10 years of age. Tourette's syndrome (see below) is a subtype of tic disorder.

J. **Tremor is an involuntary oscillatory movement.** The differential diagnosis includes focal seizure, frequent segmental myoclonus or tics, chorea, and dysmetria.

1. **Rest tremors.** These tremors are worst when the patient relaxes—but, like all tremors, they disappear during sleep.
   a. **Parkinsonian tremor** typically improves with action; it is often asymmetric. Classically it is manifest by a 3–5 Hz large-amplitude "pill-rolling" hand movement, associated with other signs of Parkinsonism. There may occasionally be a smaller action component. They are associated with tiny handwriting.
   b. **Rubral tremor,** from lesions in the cerebellar outflow tract, is alternating and rhythmic when the patient is in repose and becomes ataxic on goal-directed action. It is not common.
2. **Action tremors.** These tremors can cause significant disability even if they are apparently minor during office visits. They are typically 8–15 Hz and cause large sloppy handwriting. It is important to distinguish them from cerebellar dysmetria. Propranolol is generally the first-line treatment for action tremor.
   a. **Enhanced physiological tremors** are caused by catecholamine release during anxiety, illness (such as hyperthyroidism), or after drugs, such as caffeine or cocaine.
   b. **Drug-induced tremors.** (See below).
   c. **Familial essential tremors** are often treated with primidone.

K. Hyperkinetic movements not of basal ganglia origin.

1. **Ataxia and dysmetria are of cerebellar origin.** They cause difficulty reaching targets, often with wild oscillations. The gait may be remarkable (e.g., swaying without falls). Cerebellar deficits are common in alcoholism.
2. **Fasciculations** are tiny twitches of the skin surface caused by spontaneous activation of motor units. They are of neuromuscular, not basal ganglia, origin, and are often due merely to exercise, anxiety, or drugs (such as opiates). However, lower motor neuron disease can cause fasciculations.

IV. Movement Disorders with Psychiatric Symptoms

A. Parkinsonism. Terminology: Parkinsonism is a set of symptoms, which can be caused by a number of different disorders, such as idiopathic Parkinson's disease (IPD). Classically, IPD involves the triad of tremor, bradykinesia, and rigidity. Additional features, such as poor levodopa response, early falling, early dementia, or early autonomic signs, suggest one of the "parkinson's plus" syndromes (see below). One should not prescribe dopamine antagonists, with the exception of clozapine and quetiapine, to any patient with parkinsonism. This prohibition includes use of antiemetics, and such nominal atypicals as risperidone and ziprasidone. These drugs will greatly worsen the patient's motor symptoms, sometimes for many days.

1. **Idiopathic Parkinson's disease.** Parkinson's disease affects 3% of people over the age of 65 years, and it is sometimes seen below the age of 40. It results from dopaminergic cell death in the substantia nigra. Levodopa is the treatment of choice for older patients because it has the fewest side effects. Dopamine agonists, such as pramipexiole and ropinrole, are also helpful, although claims that they are relatively neuroprotective are still controversial. Lesions in the globus pallidus, and, more recently, electrical stimulation in the subthalamic nucleus, are increasingly popular treatments.
   a. **About 30% of Parkinson's patients are depressed.** However, the masked face, fatigue, and psychomotor slowing of Parkinson's disease can cause overdiagnosis of depression. Treatment is similar to that of the general population, but SSRIs can in a few cases worsen parkinsonian symptoms. Bupropion, mirtazapine, and selegiline are better first-line choices, with bupropion also being helpful for parkinsonian fatigue, mirtazapine being helpful for tremor, and selegiline possibly being neuroprotective. Modafinil or stimulants can help fatigue from both the disease itself and from dopamine agonists. ECT can help both parkinsonian motor symptoms and depression.
   b. **30% of patients with Parkinson's eventually have some dementia.** The dementia is usually a subcortical dementia, with bradyphrenia (slowed responses) parallelling bradykinesia. Frontal and executive deficits are also present. Donepezil and levodopa can help cognitive performance. In some cases, concomitant Alzheimer's disease is found on autopsy. Early or severe dementia is evidence against idiopathic Parkinson's disease.
   c. **Psychosis and "on-off phenomena."** In advanced Parkinson's disease, levodopa wears off precipitously, and some patients alternate in two- or three-hour blocks between being immobile and being wildly dyskinetic. During their off phases, they may have panic attacks. Benzodiazepines can help. On-phase dyskinesia can be associated with mania or psychosis. Amantidine may greatly help dyskinesias but sometimes worsens psychosis. If giving smaller, more frequent doses of levodopa does not help, psychosis may benefit from very low doses of quetiapine or clozapine.
2. **"Parkinson's plus" syndromes.**
   a. **Dementia with Lewy bodies** usually presents with dementia, and then parkinsonism. It is the second leading cause of neurodegenerative (non-vascular) dementia after Alzheimer's disease. Spontaneous hallucinations and fluctuating levels of cognition are also characteristic. Dopaminergic agonists may worsen the hallucinations more than they help the movement disorder, creating a more mobile but more psychotic patient who is better able to injure himself. As with all parkinsonism, one should avoid use of all dopamine antagonists except clozapine and quetiapine.
   b. **Progressive supranuclear palsy** presents with early down-gaze palsy and falls, as well as parkinsonism. Dementia and pseudobulbar affect soon follow. Levodopa helps little.
   c. **The multiple system atrophies include Shy-Drager syndrome, striatonigral degeneration, and olivopontocerebellar atrophy.** Early signs of dysautonomia (e.g., orthostatic hypotension), cerebellar dysfunction, and spasticity may be present as well as parkinsonism. Levodopa helps little.
   d. **Dementia pugilistica** results from repeated head injuries. There is greater dementia and less levodopa responsiveness than in idiopathic Parkinson's disease.
3. **Normal pressure hydrocephalus.** Symptoms include the triad of frontal gait (feet stuck to floor, falling backward), frontal or abulic dementia, and incontinence. CT shows ventricular dilation out of proportion to gyral atrophy. If a large-volume lumbar puncture relieves a gait disturbance, one should consider a ventriculoperitoneal shunt as treatment.
4. **Huntington's disease** is an autosomal dominant disorder characterized by chorea, and by psychiatric and

cognitive changes. It affects about 8/100,000 of the population. Psychiatric changes are often the presenting symptoms; dementia is a late phenomenon.

a. **Treatment of the psychiatric disturbances is symptomatic,** using conventional antipsychotics (which also help the chorea) and antidepressant drugs. Cell death is prominent in the striatum and cortex.

b. **The Huntington's gene defect** is a CAG triplet repeat expansion. Other such expansions have been found in other neuropsychiatric genetic disorders, such as fragile X syndrome and some spinocerebellar atrophies. The longer the expansion, the earlier and worse the symptoms. Huntington's disease is treated symptomatically, often with neuroleptics for the chorea and thought disorder.

5. **Wilson's disease** is an autosomal recessive disorder causing copper deposition. Symptoms are related to dysfunction of the liver and brain; they include dystonia, chorea, ataxia, tremor, mood disorder, psychosis, and intellectual decline. Although Wilson's disease is rare (prevalence 0.25/100,000), one should have a high index of suspicion, because it is highly treatable with chelation therapy (e.g., D-penicillamine) and dietary copper restriction. Diagnosis is made by way of a low serum ceruloplasmin, by high 24-hour urinary copper, a liver biopsy, or a slit-lamp ophthalmic examination looking for Kayser-Fleischer rings.

6. **Tourette's syndrome** is defined as multiple motor tics and at least one vocal tic, lasting more than a year, starting before 18 years of age. Its prevalence is 70/100,000, with a male:female predominance of 3:1. There is a waxing and waning course, but no progressive deterioration. Spontaneous remissions lasting as long as two decades have been described.

a. **Co-morbidity.** Tourette's is very often accompanied by obsessive-compulsive disorder (OCD) and depression, as well as by hyperactivity, impulsivity, and mild learning disabilities.

b. **Treatment.** Tics should be treated only if they significantly bother the patient. Clonidine is often the first-line agent because it has few side effects, but it is not especially effective either. Low doses of conventional antipsychotics, especially pimozide, are the mainstay of treatment. Beware antipsychotic-induced tardive dyskinesia that may then be mistaken for more tics. Withdrawal can worsen tics; do it slowly. SSRIs help OCD and the social phobia caused by having tics in public. Stimulants can help attention deficit, but stimulants sometimes worsen tics.

7. **Basal ganglia calcifications** are usually incidental, but in hypopararathyroidism and Fahr's disease it may be associated with movement and psychiatric disorders.

V. Drug-Induced Movement Disorders

A. Acute Drug Reactions

1. **Neuroleptic malignant syndrome (NMS) is the most serious psychiatric drug reaction.** It has a fatality rate of 25%. It shares many features with catatonia.

a. **Diagnosis.** The cardinal features of NMS are hyperthermia, rigidity, altered consciousness, autonomic instability, and high creatine kinase (from rhabdomyolysis). The differential diagnosis includes phenothiazine-related heat stroke, anesthesia-induced malignant hyperthermia, lethal catatonia, drug interactions with MAOIs, serotonin syndrome, and central anticholinergic syndromes. NMS can be caused not only by dopamine antagonists, but by significantly lowering dopamine agonists in parkinsonian patients. (Therefore, always taper rather than suddenly stop such medications.)

b. **Treatment.** Typically, one discontinues the neuroleptic and admits the patient to an ICU for cooling, hydration, and IV dantrolene. Dantrolene or bromocriptine can also be given PO to relatively stable patients.

2. **Akathisia** is the most common psychiatric drug reaction. Less dramatic in appearance than the others, it can nonetheless be extremely uncomfortable. It is caused by a variety of drugs, including neuroleptics, TCAs, lithium, and the more stimulating antidepressants. Relatively high doses of propranolol are the first-line treatment. Benzodiazepines and selegiline may sometimes help.

3. **Acute dystonia** is experienced by roughly 10% of neuroleptic-treated patients within the first hours and days of treatment. They can be agonizing. Acute dystonias respond quickly to IV or PO anticholinergic drugs, such as diphenhydramine or benztropine. These drugs may be started concurrently with conventional neuroleptics, in order to prevent acute dystonia. Anticholinergics should be used with caution in patients at risk for delirium, cardiac arrhythmia, glaucoma, ileus, urinary retention, or prostatic hypertrophy.

4. **Ataxia** is seen with initiation of therapy or in association with supratherapeutic blood levels of many drugs. It is especially common with mood stabilizers, but an apparent ataxia is sometimes produced simply by the sedative effects of some neuroleptics or antidepressants. Ataxia can cause dangerous falls in the elderly.

5. **Parkinsonism** may begin 5–30 days after starting a dopamine antagonist. It is dose-dependent. It cannot be treated with dopamine agonists without worsening the symptoms for which the antagonist was prescribed. Thus, anticholinergics are the mainstay of treatment. It is controversial whether drug-induced parkinsonism always resolves once the offending medication is stopped—in some cases the parkinsonism may eventually develop over time.

6. **Tremor.** Drug-induced action tremor, of which lithium and valproic acid are the most common offenders, must be distinguished from the rest tremor of drug-induced parkinsonism because the treatment is so different. Adding propranolol, mysoline, or substituting carbamazepine or clozaril for lithium or valproate can help action tremors. Because patients often use caffeine heavily to combat the sedation from mood stabi-

lizers, replacing caffeine with modafinil can alleviate tremor.

B. Delayed Drug Reactions

Tardive dyskinesia (TD) and tardive dystonia, are most often caused by the long-term administration of dopamine blockers, but they can occur after use of other drugs as well.

1. **Diagnosis.** TD most often affects the mouth and tongue (e.g., with lip smacking, sucking, or facial grimacing), or causes limb choreoathetosis or dystonia. TD often develops rapidly, then stabilizes. Because the movements decrease during voluntary movements, they usually do not interfere with eating or hand use. TD is seen in 10–20% of patients treated with an antipsychotic for more than 1 year, but it can be seen after only three months of exposure. After the first year, the risk appears to be about 5% per patient per year. Patients at highest risk for TD appear to be mood-disordered patients, elderly women, children, and African-Americans. TD-like symptoms are also seen in some never-medicated schizophrenics. The differential diagnosis for TD includes other causes of chorea. Increased sensitivity to dopamine receptors may underly the pathophysiology of TD.
2. **Treatment.** The management of TD includes a dose reduction of the dopamine receptor blocker, although this may cause a transient worsening of symptoms. Switching to clozapine sometimes helps existing TD, as it is the least likely of the atypical antipsychotics to cause TD. Quetiapine may also be of some use. Risperidone and probably zisprasidone are the *most* likely of the atypical neuroleptics to cause TD. Increasing the dose of the dopamine receptor blocker may help in the short-term, but it may worsen the TD in the long-term. Documentation of movement disorders should include use of scales, such as the Abnormal Involuntary Movement Scale (AIMS).

VI. Psychogenic Movement Disorders

A. Movement disorders are a very common manifestation of conversion disorder; malingering and factitious disorder are less common.

The diagnosis of psychogenic movement disorder is very difficult to make because so many movement disorders thought to be purely neurological have such odd features—e.g., a boy with DYT-1 hereditary dystonia whose dystonia disappears when he tap-dances, or a Parkinson's patient whose feet are frozen unless you put a pencil on the ground for her to step over. Many patients have both neurological illness and conversion symptoms.

1. **Clues to the presence of a psychogenic movement disorder** include abrupt onset with a normal MRI, varying body distribution, not fitting typical movement disorder phenotypes, movements disappearing with distraction, response to placebo, paroxysmal symptoms, bursts of gibberish, excessive startle, and no real falls or self-injury. Unfortunately, all of these are sometimes seen in those with basal ganglia movement disorders.
2. **Hysterical paralysis** can be distinguished from true paralysis by the following tests:
   a. **The face-drop test.** Lift the patient's flaccid hand above his face and drop it. In hysterical paralysis, the hand will drop next to the face, not on it.
   b. **Babinski's plantar reflex.** The classic. It was used to tell corticospinal injury from shell-shock conversion in WWI. Firmly stroking the outer edge of the sole towards the toes makes the big toe dorsiflex in the former case; in normal or hysterical subjects, all toes will curl.
   c. **Dragging leg.** Patients with hysterical leg weakness will drag the leg semi-uselessly, in distinction to the circumduction of upper motor neuron damage or the foot drop of lower motor neuron damage.
   d. **Hoover's sign.** With the patient lying down, place your hands under each of the heels of the patient. Ask them to raise the affected leg. If they are truly making effort, there should be a compensatory downward pressure of the good leg.
3. **Hysterical tremor** tends to be low frequency, high amplitude, and paroxysmal, in part because it takes too much energy to sustain it for long. A tremor that moves to another body part, if the originally affected limb is restrained by the examiner, and that disappears rather than worsens with such distractions (as anger at the examiner), may be a hysterical tremor.

Suggested Readings

Bradley, W.G., Daroff, R.B., Fenichel, G.M., & Marsden, C.D. (Eds.). (2000). *Neurology in clinical practice* (3rd ed.). Boston, MA: Butterworth Heinemann.

Flaherty, A.W. (2000). *The Massachusetts General Hospital handbook of neurology.* Philadelphia, PA: Lippincott Williams and Wilkins.

Fricchione, G., Bush, G., Fozdar, M., et al. (1997). Recognition and treatment of the catatonic syndrome. *Journal of Intensive Care Medicine, 12,* 135–147.

Kaplan, H.I., & Sadock, B.J. (Eds.). (2000). *Comprehensive textbook of psychiatry* (7th ed.). Baltimore, MD: Williams and Wilkins.

Lang, A.E., Lozano, A. (1998). Parkinson's disease. *New England Journal of Medicine, 339,* 1044–1053.

Marsh, L. (2000). Neuropsychiatric aspects of Parkinson's disease. *Psychosomatics, 41,* 15–23.

Prager, L.K., Millham, F.H., & Stern, T.A. (1994). Neuroleptic malignant syndrome: A review for intensivists. *Journal of Intensive Care Medicine, 9,* 227–234.

Samuels, M.A. (1997). *Movement disorders. Video textbook for the practicing physician.* Boston, MA: Butterworth-Heinemann (Elsevier).

Samuels, M.A., & Feske, S. (1997). *Office practice of neurology* (2nd ed.). Philadelphia, PA: Churchill-Livingstone (Elsevier).

SECTION IV

Treatment Approaches

Chapter 43

Basic Psychopharmacology

STEPHAN HECKERS

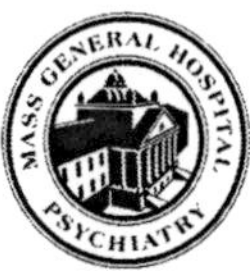

I. Overview

Modulation of neuronal activity via neurotransmitters is a fundamental mechanism of brain function. The premier therapeutic avenue of psychiatry is, arguably, the facilitation or inhibition of neurotransmitter systems in the brain, either through the administration of drugs or through psychotherapy. The release of neurotransmitters, their mechanisms of action, and their effect on target neurons are complex and still poorly understood. **However, despite the diversity of neurotransmitters and receptors in the human brain, they have one common goal: to modulate neuronal activity. This is achieved by changing either the electrical or the chemical properties of the cell.** A balance of intracellular and extracellular ions maintains the electrical properties of a neuron. At rest, this balance is called the resting membrane potential. Decreasing the resting potential leads to excitation, increasing it leads to inhibition. The expression of specific genes, the production of proteins, and the creation of a distinct metabolism characterize the chemical properties of a neuron. Regulation of gene expression and protein function determines the biochemical status quo of the cell.

II. Basic Principles

A. Anatomy of the Neuron

Neurons have three compartments: dendrites, cell body (perikaryon), and axon. The cell body integrates the different inputs provided by the dendrites. This integration can occur through modulation of the membrane potential or at the level of the nucleus (regulation of gene expression). **The axon is the output station of the neuron.** The axon can be short (local circuit neuron) or long (projection neuron). If a deviation from the resting membrane potential is above a certain threshold, an action potential is created and travels downstream rapidly. **The nerve terminal is the widened terminal part of the axon. It provides a small area of close contact with dendrites of neighboring cells: a synapse** (see Figure 43-1).

B. The Synapse

1. **The presynaptic neuron, which releases the neurotransmitter into the synapse, can express two proteins that affect synaptic communication:**
   a. **Membrane-bound receptors bind the intrinsic neurotransmitter (autoreceptor) or transmitters of neighboring neurons (heteroreceptor) and affect the cell via intracellular messengers.** One response, e.g., is the modulation of neurotransmitter release.
   b. **Membrane-bound reuptake transporters pump the released neurotransmitter back into the cell.**
2. **The neuron receiving the input (post-synaptic cell) can be modulated via two different types of receptors:**
   a. **Fast-acting, class I (ionotropic) receptors.** The neurotransmitter binds to the receptor protein and within milliseconds a change in the permeability of the associated ion channel occurs, allowing the influx of ions, such as Ca^{2+}, Na^{+}, K^{+}, or Cl^{-}.
   b. **Slow-acting, class II (G-protein-coupled) receptors.** The neurotransmitter binds to the receptor protein and thereby changes the protein conformation. This change is relayed to an associated G-protein, so called because it binds guanidine triphosphate (GTP) in order to be activated. G-proteins regulate two major classes of effector molecules: ion channels and second messenger-generating enzymes.

C. Intracellular Information-processing

1. **The activity of receptors and ion channels influences gene and protein expression in neurons. Gene expression is regulated by transcription factors that bind to specific sequences of the DNA in the nucleus.** Therefore, membrane-bound receptors or ion channels in distal parts of the neuron must be able to activate intraneuronal signal transduction pathways that can span long distances and translocate to the nucleus. Since proteins assemble the neuron and determine neuronal properties, gene expression regulates neuronal function and may cause malfunction. Many psychopharmacological agents with delayed therapeutic effects are thought to produce their therapeutic benefits through modulation of gene expression.
2. **Release of neurotransmitters from the pre-synaptic neuron into the synapse activates receptors on the post-synaptic neuron.** Upon activation of ionotropic receptors, ions such as Ca^{2+} enter the cell and act as second messengers. **Activation of G-protein-coupled receptors facilitates the opening of neighboring ion channels, or the synthesis of second messengers,** such as cyclic AMP (cAMP). **Second messengers** (Ca^{2+}, cAMP) **regulate the activity of protein kinases** (proteins that transfer phosphate groups to a substrate protein) **and phosphatases** (proteins that remove phosphate groups from a substrate protein). In all cases investigated to date, the activation of neurotransmitter receptors changes the state of phosphorylation of neuronal proteins.
3. Since neurotransmitters and receptors influence gene and protein expression in the brain, small but persistent abnormalities in neurotransmission can have

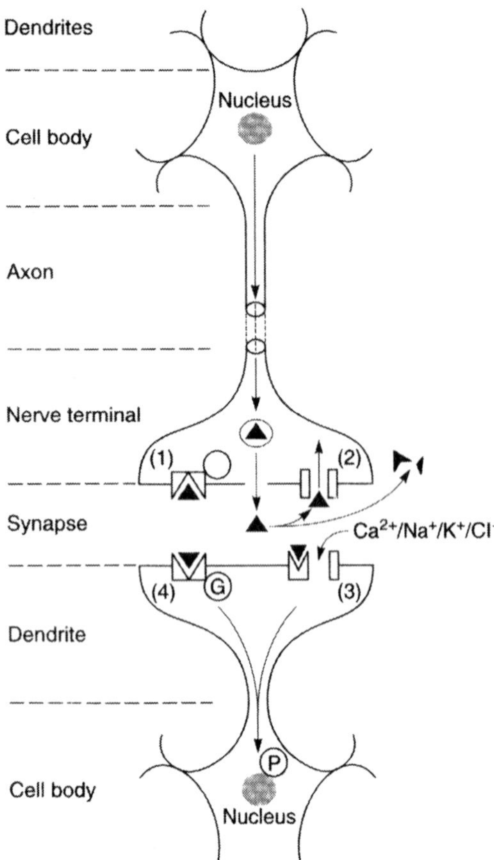

Figure 43-1. A neurotransmitter released into the synapse may affect the pre-synaptic neuron (top) via membrane-bound receptors (1) and re-uptake transporters (2) and the post-synaptic neuron (bottom) via ion-channel-coupled receptors (3) and G-protein-coupled receptors (4).

far-reaching consequences. An understanding of signal transduction pathways and of transcription factors will be instrumental in providing us with new therapeutic avenues in psychopharmacology.

D. Neuronal Circuitry

How are neurons arranged to process information? **There are about 10^{11} neurons in the central nervous system (CNS) and each neuron establishes about 10^3–10^4 connections to other neurons.** Here we focus on **four major anatomical systems: the cortex, the thalamus, the basal ganglia, and the medial temporal lobe.** The function of these four systems is modulated by several groups of neurons that are characterized by their use of a specific neurotransmitter. **Most of psychopharmacology is aimed at strengthening or inhibiting these modulatory systems.**

1. **The thalamus is the gateway to cortical processing of all incoming sensory information.** Primary sensory cortices receive information from the appropriate input modules (sensory organ + thalamus).
2. **The association cortex integrates information from primary cortices, from sub-cortical structures, and from brain areas affiliated with memory.**
3. **The medial temporal lobe** (i.e., hippocampus, amygdala) **serves** two major functions in the brain: **to integrate multi-modal sensory information** for storage into and retrieval from memory, **and to attach limbic valence to sensory information** (e.g., pleasant or unpleasant, fight or flight).
4. **The basal ganglia are primarily involved in the integration of input from cortical areas.** The basal ganglia modulate cortical activity via a cortico-striato-pallido-thalamo-cortical loop. The most prominent projections to the striatum arise from the motor cortex.
5. **Four groups of densely packed neurons provide diffuse projections to all areas of the brain** to modulate their functions: **cholinergic neurons** in the basal forebrain and brainstem, **dopaminergic neurons** in the substantia nigra and ventral tegmental area, **noradrenergic neurons** in the locus coeruleus, and **serotonergic neurons** in the raphe nuclei. Although there are many more neurotransmitter systems in the brain, in clinical psychopharmacology **we have to be primarily concerned with six systems: the glutamatergic, GABAergic, cholinergic, serotonergic, noradrenergic, and dopaminergic systems.** These six systems can be divided into two groups based on their anatomical characteristics.
   a. **The first group includes the glutamatergic and GABAergic systems.** Their neurons are by far **the two most prevalent and most widely distributed types in the human brain.** The widespread distribution of these two neurotransmitter systems has functional implications: the modulation of glutamatergic and GABAergic neurotransmission affects many neural systems.
   b. **The second group of neurotransmitter systems comprises the cholinergic, serotonergic, noradrenergic, and dopaminergic neurons.** These four systems project to their target areas typically by long-ranging projection fibers. Since these neurotransmitter-specific projection systems reach selected neural systems, **their modulation leads to more circumscribed effects.**

III. Six Neurotransmitter Systems

A. Glutamatergic Neurotransmission

Glutamate (Glu) is the most abundant amino acid in the CNS.

1. **Anatomy. Prominent glutamatergic pathways are the corticocortical projections, the connections between thalamus and cortex, and the projections from cortex to striatum (extrapyramidal pathway) and to brainstem/spinal cord (pyramidal pathway).**

The hippocampus and the cerebellum also contain many glutamatergic neurons.

2. **Synthesis. Glutamate is synthesized in the nerve terminals from two sources: from glucose via the Krebs cycle and from glutamine by the enzyme glutaminase.** The production of glutamate in releasable pools (i.e., the neurotransmitter portion of the intracellular glutamate) is regulated by the enzyme glutaminase. **Glutamate is stored in vesicles and released by a Ca^{2+}-dependent mechanism.**
3. **Synapse. Glutamate acts at three different types of ionotropic receptors and at a family of G-protein-coupled (metabotropic) receptors.**
   a. **Binding of glutamate to the ionotropic receptor opens an ion channel** allowing the influx of Na^+ and Ca^{2+} into the cell.
   b. NMDA (*N*-methyl-D-aspartate) receptors bind glutamate and NMDA. The NMDA receptor is highly regulated at several sites.
   c. AMPA (aminomethylphenylacetic acid) receptors bind glutamate, AMPA, and quisqualic acid, while kainate receptors bind glutamate and kainic acid.
   d. The metabotropic glutamate receptor family includes at least seven different types of G-protein-coupled receptors ($mGluR_{1-7}$). They are linked to different second messenger systems and lead to the increase of intracellular Ca^{2+} or the decrease of cAMP.
   e. Glutamate is removed from the synapse by high-affinity reuptake; two transporter proteins are expressed in glial cells and one in neurons.
4. **Function. Glutamate affects many brain functions.** Some examples include:
   a. Glutamatergic neurons and NMDA receptors in the hippocampus are important in the creation of **long-term potentiation (LTP), a crucial component in the formation of memory.**
   b. **Cortical neurons use glutamate as the major excitatory neurotransmitter.** Excess stimulation of glutamatergic receptors, as seen in seizures or stroke, can lead to unregulated Ca^{2+} influx and neuronal damage.

B. GABAergic Neurotransmission

γ-Aminobutyric acid (GABA) is an amino acid with high concentrations in the brain and the spinal cord. It acts as the major inhibitory neurotransmitter in the CNS.

1. **Anatomy. GABAergic neurons can be divided into two groups: short-ranging neurons (interneurons, local circuit neurons)** in the cortex, thalamus, striatum, cerebellum, and spinal cord; **medium/long-ranging neurons** with the following projections:
   a. Caudate/putamen→globus pallidus→thalamus, substantia nigra
   b. Septum→hippocampus
   c. Substantia nigra→thalamus, superior colliculus
2. **Synthesis. GABA is synthesized via decarboxylation of glutamate by the enzyme glutamic acid decarboxylase (GAD).**
3. **Synapse. GABA acts at two types of receptors:**
   a. **The $GABA_A$ receptor is a receptor-channel complex comprising five subunits. Activation leads to the opening of the channel, allowing Cl^- to enter the cell, resulting in decreased excitability.** Five distinct classes of subunits (six variants of α, four variants of β, three variants of γ, one δ, and two variants of ρ) are known. The receptor can be modulated by various compounds that bind to several different sites:
      i. Benzodiazepines bind to the α subunit and open the channel if a γ subunit is present and if GABA is bound to the GABA site on the β subunit.
      ii. Barbiturates and ethanol bind near the Cl^- channel and increase channel open time even without GABA present.
   b. **The $GABA_B$ receptor is a G-protein-coupled receptor with similarity to the metabotropic glutamate receptor.** The $GABA_B$ receptor is linked to G_i (decreasing cAMP and opening of K^+ channels) and G_o (closing Ca^{2+} channels). The net effect is prolonged inhibition of the cell.
      i. GABA is removed from the synapse by a sodium-dependent GABA uptake transporter.
4. **Function. GABA is the major inhibitory neurotransmitter in the CNS.** Examples of normal and perturbed function include:
   a. **Cortical and thalamic GABAergic neurons are crucial for the inhibition of excitatory neurons.** Benzodiazepines or barbiturates are efficacious in the treatment and prevention of seizures.
   b. **Modulation of $GABA_B$ receptors is beneficial in the treatment of anxiety disorders, insomnia, and agitation,** most likely due to a general inhibition of neuronal activity.
   c. **Benzodiazepines and ethanol use the same mechanism to influence $GABA_A$ receptors.** This property is the basis for ethanol detoxification utilizing benzodiazepines.

C. Cholinergic Neurotransmission

Acetylcholine (ACh) has been known as a neurotransmitter since the mid-1920s. In the peripheral nervous system, ACh is found as the neurotransmitter in the autonomic ganglia, the parasympathetic post-ganglionic synapse, and the neuromuscular endplate.

1. **Anatomy. Cholinergic neurons in the CNS are either wide-ranging projection neurons or short-ranging interneurons:**
   a. Cholinergic projection neurons in the basal forebrain (septum, diagonal band, nucleus basalis of Meynert) project to the entire cortex, the hippocampus, and the amygdala.
   b. Cholinergic projection neurons located in the brainstem project predominantly to the thalamus.
   c. Cholinergic interneurons in the striatum modulate the activity of GABAergic striatal neurons.

2. **Synthesis. ACh is synthesized by the enzyme choline acetyltransferase (ChAT) from the precursors acetyl-coenzyme A (acetyl-CoA) and choline.** High-affinity and low-affinity transporters pump choline, the rate-limiting factor in the synthesis of ACh, into the cell.
3. **Synapse. ACh acts at two different types of cholinergic receptors:**
   a. **Muscarinic receptors bind ACh as well as other agonists** (muscarine, pilocarpine, bethanechol) **and antagonists** (atropine, scopolamine). There are at least five different types of **muscarinic receptors** (M_1–M_5). All **have slow response times.** They are coupled to G-proteins and a variety of second messenger systems. When activated, the final effect can be to open or close channels for K^+, Ca^{2+}, or Cl^-.
   b. **Nicotinic receptors are less abundant** than the muscarinic type in the CNS. **They bind ACh as well as agonists** (e.g., nicotine) or antagonists (e.g., d-tubocurarine). The fast-acting ionotropic nicotinic receptor allows influx of $Na^+ > K^+ > Ca^{2+}$ into the cell.
   c. **ACh is removed from the synapse through hydrolysis into acetyl-CoA and choline by the enzyme acetylcholinesterase (AChE).** Removing ACh from the synapse can be blocked irreversibly by organophosphorous compounds and in a reversible fashion by drugs such as physostigmine.
4. **Function. ACh modulates attention, novelty seeking, and memory via the basal forebrain projections to the cortex and limbic structures.**
   a. Alzheimer's disease (AD) and anticholinergic delirium are examples for a deficit state. Blocking the metabolism of ACh by AChE strengthens cognitive functioning in AD patients.
   b. Brainstem cholinergic neurons are essential for the regulation of sleep-wake cycles via projections to the thalamus.
   c. **Cholinergic interneurons modulate striatal neurons by opposing the effects of dopamine.** Increased cholinergic tone in Parkinson's disease and decreased cholinergic tone in patients treated with neuroleptics are examples for an imbalance of these two systems in the striatum.

D. Serotonergic Neurotransmission

Serotonin, or 5-hydroxytryptamine (5-HT), is a monoamine widely distributed in many cells of the body, with about 1–2% of its entire body content present in the CNS.

1. **Anatomy. Serotonergic neurons are restricted to midline structures of the brainstem.** Most serotonergic cells overlap with the distribution of the raphe nuclei in the brainstem. A rostral group (B6–8 neurons) projects to the thalamus, hypothalamus, amygdala, striatum, and cortex. The remaining two groups (B1–5 neurons) project to other brainstem neurons, the cerebellum, and the spinal cord.
2. **Synthesis. Serotonin is synthesized by the enzyme amino acid decarboxylase (AAD) from 5-hydroxytryptophan** (itself derived from tryptophan via tryptophan hydroxylase). **The rate-limiting step of the pathway is the production of 5-hydroxytryptophan by tryptophan hydroxylase.**
3. **Synapse. Serotonin acts at two different types of receptors.** With the exception of the 5-HT_3 receptor, all serotonin receptors are **G-protein-coupled receptors.**
   a. **The 5-HT_1 receptors** (5-HT_{1A-F}) **are coupled to G_i and lead to a decrease of cAMP.** The 5-HT_{1A} receptor is also directly coupled to a K^+ channel, leading to increased opening of the channel. The 5-HT_1 receptors are the predominant serotonergic autoreceptors.
   b. **5-HT_2 receptors** (5-HT_{2A-C}) **are coupled to phospholipase C and lead to a variety of intracellular effects** (mainly depolarization). Three receptors (5-$HT_{4,6,7}$) are coupled to G_s and activate adenylate cyclase. The function of the 5-HT_{5A} and 5-HT_{5B} receptors is poorly understood.
   c. **The 5-HT_3 receptor is the only monoamine receptor coupled to an ion channel, probably a Ca^{2+} channel.** It is found in the cortex, hippocampus, and area postrema. It is typically localized pre-synaptically and regulates neurotransmitter release. **Well-known antagonists are ondansetron and granisetron.**
   d. **Serotonin is removed from the synapse by a high-affinity serotonin uptake site** that is capable of transporting serotonin in either direction, depending on the concentration. **The serotonin transporter is blocked by the selective serotonin reuptake inhibitors (SSRIs), as well as by tricyclic antidepressants (TCAs).**
4. **Function. Serotonin is linked to many brain functions due to the widespread serotonergic projections and the heterogeneity of the serotonergic receptors.** Examples include:
   a. **Modulation of serotonergic receptors** and the reuptake site **is beneficial** (among others) **in the treatment of anxiety, depression, obsessive-compulsive disorder, and schizophrenia.**
   b. **Blockade of 5-HT_3 receptors** in the area postrema **decreases nausea and emesis.**
   c. **Hallucinogens** (e.g., lysergic acid diethylamide [**LSD**]) **modulate serotonergic neurons** via serotonergic autoreceptors.

E. Noradrenergic Neurotransmission

Norepinephrine (NE), a catecholamine, was first identified as a neurotransmitter in 1946. **In the peripheral nervous system it is found as the neurotransmitter in the sympathetic post-ganglionic synapse.**

1. **Anatomy. About half of all noradrenergic neurons** (i.e., 12,000 on each side of the brainstem) **are located in the locus coeruleus** (LC). They provide the extensive noradrenergic innervation of cortex, hippocampus, thalamus, cerebellum, and spinal cord. The remaining neurons are distributed in the tegmental region. They innervate predominantly the hypothalamus, basal forebrain, and spinal cord.

2. **Synthesis. NE is synthesized by the enzyme dopamine-β-hydroxylase (DβH) from the precursor dopamine** (itself derived from tyrosine via dihydroxyphenylalanine [dopa]). **The pathway's rate-limiting step is the production of dopa by tyrosine hydroxylase,** which can be activated through phosphorylation.
3. **Synapse. NE is released into the synapse from vesicles; amphetamine facilitates this release.** NE acts in the CNS at two different types of noradrenergic receptors (alpha and beta):
   a. **Adrenergic alpha-receptors can be subdivided into alpha-1-receptors** (coupled to phospholipase and located post-synaptically; prazosin is a typical antagonist) **and alpha-2-receptors** (coupled to G_i and located primarily pre-synaptically; clonidine and guanfacine are potent agonists, and yohimbine an antagonist).
   b. **Adrenergic beta-receptors in the CNS are predominantly of the beta-1-subtype.** Beta-1-receptors are coupled to G_s and lead to an increase of cAMP. cAMP triggers a variety of events mediated by protein kinases, including phosphorylation of the beta-receptor itself, and regulation of gene expression via phosphorylation of transcription factors.
   c. **NE is removed from the synapse by two mechanisms:**
      i. **Catechol-*O*-methyltransferase (COMT)** degrades intrasynaptic NE.
      ii. **The norepinephrine transporter (NET),** a Na^+/Cl^--dependent neurotransmitter transporter, is the primary way of removing NE from the synapse. The NET is blocked selectively by desipramine and nortriptyline. Once internalized, NE can be degraded by the intracellular enzyme monoamine oxidase (MAO).
4. **Function. Noradrenergic projections modulate sleep cycles, appetite, mood, and cognition by targeting the thalamus, limbic structures, and cortex.** These functions are targets of antidepressant drugs.
   a. The locus coeruleus (LC) receives afferents from the sensory systems that monitor the internal and external environments. The widespread LC efferents lead to an inhibition of spontaneous discharge in the target neurons. Therefore, the LC is thought to be crucial for fine tuning the attentional matrix of the cortex. Anxiety disorders may be due to perturbations of this system.
   b. The neurons of the LC express a variety of autoreceptors: LC firing can be decreased by clonidine and increased by yohimbine; morphine decreases LC firing and withdrawal leads to increased firing (this is the rationale for clonidine use in the treatment of opiate withdrawal).

F. Dopaminergic Neurotransmission

Dopamine (DA) was initially considered as merely an intermediate monoamine in the synthesis of norepinephrine and epinephrine. However, in the late 1950s DA was discovered to be a neurotransmitter in its own right.

1. **Anatomy. Dopaminergic neurons can be divided into three major groups based on the length of their efferent fibers:**
   a. **Ultra-short systems** in the retina and olfactory bulb
   b. **Intermediate-length systems** originating in the hypothalamus and projecting, among other areas, to the pituitary gland
   c. **Wide-ranging systems** originating from two areas:
      i. Substantia nigra (SN) neurons (= A9), projecting primarily to caudate and putamen
      ii. Ventral tegmental area (VTA) neurons (= A10) projecting to limbic areas (nucleus accumbens, amygdala)—mesolimbic projections, and cortex (frontal, cingulate, entorhinal)—mesocortical projections
2. **Synthesis. DA is synthesized by the enzyme L-aromatic amino acid decarboxylase from dopa** (which is produced from tyrosine via tyrosine hydroxylase [TH]). The turnover rate of dopa is extremely high and DA levels can be elevated if extra dopa is supplied to the brain.
3. **Synapse. DA is released into the synapse from vesicles; this process is facilitated by amphetamine and methylphenidate.**
   a. **DA acts at two different classes of DA receptors in the CNS: the D_1 receptor family and the D_2 receptor family.** The D_1 receptor family includes the D_1 and D_5 receptors. Both are coupled to G_s and lead to an increase of cAMP. The D_2 receptor family includes the D_2, D_3, and D_4 receptors. All are coupled to G_i and lead to a decrease of cAMP. There is a predilection of the different DA receptors for expression in specific brain areas:
      i. D_1: striatum, cortex, SN, olfactory tubercle
      ii. D_2: striatum, SN, pituitary gland, retina, olfactory tubercle
      iii. D_3: nucleus accumbens
      iv. D_4: GABAergic neurons in the cortex, thalamus, hippocampus, SN
      v. D_5: hippocampus, hypothalamus
   b. **Pre-synaptic dopaminergic receptors are typically of the D_2 type and are found on most portions of the dopaminergic neuron (as autoreceptors). They regulate DA synthesis and release, as well as the firing rate of DA neurons.** Autoreceptors are 5–10 times more sensitive to DA agonists than post-synaptic receptors.
   c. **DA is removed from the synapse by two mechanisms. First, COMT degrades intrasynaptic DA. Second, the dopamine transporter (DAT),** a Na^+/Cl^--dependent neurotransmitter transporter, transports DA in either direction, depending on the concentration gradient. The DAT is blocked selectively by drugs such as cocaine, amphetamine, bupropion, benztropine, and nomifensine.
4. **Function. DA affects several brain functions, primarily by modulation of other neurotransmitter systems:**
   a. **Dopaminergic neurons of the SN project to the striatum and modulate the function of striatal GABAergic neurons.** Parkinson's disease and extrapyramidal side effects due to treatment with neuroleptics are examples of decreased dopaminergic function.

b. **Dopaminergic projections of the VTA to limbic structures,** such as the nucleus accumbens, **are known to be involved in reward behavior** and in the development of addiction to drugs, such as ethanol, cocaine, nicotine, and opiates.

c. Dopaminergic projections from the VTA to the cortex play a role in the fine tuning of cortical neurons (i.e., better signal-to-noise ratio). Dopaminergic projections from the hypothalamus to the pituitary gland tonically inhibit the production and release of prolactin via D_2 receptors; blockade of these receptors leads to hyperprolactinemia.

IV. Conclusion

Psychopharmacology uses molecules to modulate human brain function. Three basic principles of neurotransmission may help to understand the current practice of clinical psychopharmacology. **First, the anatomic organization of neurotransmitter systems determines their behavioral affiliation. Second, neurotransmitter receptors modulate the electrical properties (via ion channels) or the chemical properties (via second messenger systems) of neurons. Third, the intracellular integration of receptor-mediated responses leads to immediate and/or delayed effects on neuronal function.**

Suggested Readings

Cooper, J.R., Bloom, F.E., & Roth, R.H. (1996). *The biochemical basis of neuropharmacology* (7th ed.). New York: Oxford University Press.

Hyman, S.E., & Nestler, E.J. (1993). *The molecular foundations of psychiatry*. Washington, DC: American Psychiatric Press.

Kandel, E.R., Schwartz, J., & Jessel, T. (1996). *Principles of neural science* (4th ed.). New York: Elsevier.

Nieuwenhuys, R. (1985). *Chemoarchitecture of the brain*. Berlin: Springer-Verlag.

Siegel, G.J., Agranoff, B.W., Albers, R.W., & Molinoff, P.B. (1994). *Basic neurochemistry* (5th ed.). New York: Raven Press.

Chapter 44

Treatment of Anxiety Disorders

DAN V. IOSIFESCU AND MARK H. POLLACK

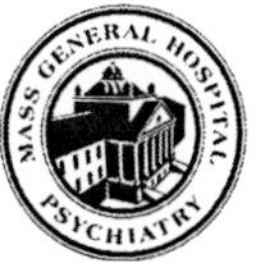

I. Introduction

Anxiety disorders tend to be chronic and to fluctuate. They are associated with considerable morbidity and impairment, yet **they respond well to pharmacological and cognitive-behavioral treatments.**

II. Panic Disorder

Panic disorder is characterized by fear of recurrent unexpected panic attacks and by a persistent concern related to the autonomic arousal which accompanies such attacks. Traditionally, **treatment of panic disorder has focused on blocking panic attacks, diminishing anticipatory or generalized anxiety and reversing phobic avoidance.** At the same time, co-morbid conditions, among which depression and alcohol abuse are particularly relevant, need to be treated.

A. Pharmacotherapy

The pharmacotherapy of panic disorder aims to prevent panic attacks and to treat co-morbid conditions, such as depression. The goal of treatment is to reduce the patient's distress and impairment to the point of remission, or to the point where the patient is capable of participating in other forms of therapy (e.g., cognitive-behavioral therapy [CBT]). (See Table 44-1 for recommended dosages of the most commonly prescribed medications.)

1. **Antidepressants.** The first medications shown to be effective in panic disorder were tricyclic antidepressants (TCAs), then monoamine oxidase inhibitors (**MAOIs**), then selective serotonin reuptake inhibitors (**SSRIs**) demonstrated efficacy.

   a. **Selective serotonin reuptake inhibitors (SSRIs)** are now the "first-line" treatment of panic disorder, which likely involves dysregulation of the central serotonergic system. Currently, paroxetine ([Paxil] and [Paxil CR]) and sertraline (Zoloft) are FDA-approved for the treatment of panic disorder, though others such as fluoxetine (Prozac), fluvoxamine (Luvox), and escitalopram (Lexapro) have also demonstrated antipanic efficacy, both in double-blind and open trials. However, direct comparisons among different SSRIs in the treatment of panic disorder are lacking.

      i. **Advantages of SSRIs** include a favorable side-effect profile, a broad spectrum of efficacy for co-morbid disorders, a low potential for abuse, safety in overdose, and once-a-day dosing.

      ii. **Disadvantages of SSRIs** include restlessness, "jitteriness," increased anxiety on initial dosing, sexual dysfunction, and a delayed onset of action (3–6 weeks).

   Given the fact that SSRIs have the potential to cause initial restlessness, insomnia, and increased anxiety, and that panic patients are sensitive to somatic sensations, the starting doses should be low (e.g., paroxetine 10 mg/day, paroxetine CR 12.5 mg/day, sertraline 25 mg/day, fluvoxamine 50 mg/day, fluoxetine 10 mg/day, citalopram [Celexa] 10 mg/day, and escitalopram 5mg/day). SSRI doses can then be titrated up, based on clinical response and side effects. The average effective doses of SSRIs are in the typical antidepressant range, and sometimes higher (e.g., paroxetine 20–40 mg/day, paroxetine CR 25–50 mg/day, sertraline 50–150 mg/day, fluvoxamine 150–200 mg/day, fluoxetine 20–40 mg/day, citalopram 20–40 mg/day, and escitalopram 10–20 mg/day).

   b. **Tricyclic antidepressants (TCAs).** Imipramine (Tofranil) was the first pharmacological agent shown to be efficacious in panic disorder. However, clomipramine is now considered to have superior antipanic properties when compared with other TCAs (possibly related to its selectivity for serotonergic uptake).

      i. **Advantages of TCAs** include their lower cost (when compared with SSRIs) and their efficacy in SSRI non-responders; in addition, they can be administered once a day, and have been well studied.

      ii. **Disadvantages of TCAs** include wide-ranging adverse effects (with anticholinergic effects, orthostatic hypotension, effects on the cardiac conduction system, weight gain, restlessness, and "jitteriness"), heightened anxiety on initial dosing, a delayed onset of action (3–6 weeks), cardiotoxicity in overdose, and a total cost of care that may be higher than that associated with SSRIs.

   The side-effect profile of TCAs accounts for a high drop-out rate (30–70%) in published studies. Treatment should be initiated with lower doses (e.g., 10 mg/day for imipramine) to minimize the "activation syndrome" (restlessness, jitteriness, palpitations, and increased anxiety) noted at the outset of treatment. Typical antidepressant doses (e.g., 100–300 mg/day for imipramine) may ultimately be used to control the symptoms of panic disorder. Blood levels of TCAs, especially for imipramine, nortriptyline (Pamelor), and desipramine (Norpramin), can be checked after a steady state (about 5 days after a dose change) is achieved, and may be useful in cases of poor response.

   c. **Monoamine oxidase inhibitors (MAOIs),** such as phenelzine (Nardil) and tranylcypromine (Parnate), are potent antipanic agents.

      i. **Advantages of MAOIs** include their efficacy in treatment-resistant patients.

      ii. **Disadvantages of MAOIs** include side effects, orthostatic hypotension, weight gain, and sexual dysfunction), the need for dietary restrictions (to prevent hy-

Table 44-1. Recommended Dosage of Most Commonly Prescribed Antianxiety Medications

Drug	*Daily Dose Range (mg)*	*Initial Dose (mg)*	*Dosing Schedule*
SSRIs			
Paroxetine (Paxil)	10–50	10	q.d.
Paroxetine CR (Paxil CR)	12.5–50	12.5	q.d.
Sertraline (Zoloft)	25–200	25	q.d.
Fluvoxamine (Luvox)	50–300	50	q.d.
Fluoxetine (Prozac)	10–80	10	q.d.
Citalopram (Celexa)	20–60	10–20	q.d.
Escitalopram (Lexapro)	10–30	5–10	q.d.
TCAs			
Imipramine (Tofranil)	100–300	10–25	q.d.
Clomipramine (Anafranil)	100–250	12.5–25	q.d.
Amitriptyline (Elavil)	100–300	10–25	q.d.
MAOIs			
Phenelzine (Nardil)	60–90	15	b.i.d.
Tranylcypromine (Parnate)	30–60	10–60	b.i.d.
Atypical antidepressants			
Venlafaxine (Effexor-XR)	75–300	37.5	q.d.
Nefazodone (Serzone)	300–600	50	b.i.d.
Benzodiazepines			
Alprazolam (Xanax)	2–10	0.25–0.5	q.i.d.
Clonazepam (Klonopin)	1–5	0.25	b.i.d.
Diazepam (Valium)	5–40	2.5	b.i.d.
Lorazepam (Ativan)	3–16	1.0	t.i.d.–q.i.d.
Azapirones			
Buspirone (Buspar)	15–60	5	b.i.d.–t.i.d.
Beta-blockers			
Propranolol (Inderal)	10–60	10–20	b.i.d.
Anticonvulsants			
Valproate (Depakote)	500–2000	250	b.i.d.
Gabapentin (Neurontin)	300–5400	300	b.i.d.–t.i.d.

pertensive crisis), drug interactions, and their toxicity in overdose.

Due to the danger associated with consumption of tyramine-containing foods while taking a MAOI and with toxicity in overdose, MAOIs are usually reserved for panic-disorder patients who remain symptomatic after treatment with safer and better tolerated agents. Optimal doses for phenelzine range between 60 and 90 mg/day, whereas doses of tranylcypromine generally range between 30 and 60 mg/day.

d. **Other antidepressants.** Venlafaxine (Effexor-XR), a dual serotonin and norepinephrine reuptake inhibitor, is generally efficacious in individuals with panic disorder at doses between 75 and 300 mg/day; its starting dose is 37.5 mg/day. Nefazodone (Serzone), a 5-HT_2 antagonist, has not demonstrated robust efficacy for panic disorder. It is efficacious and generally well tolerated for the treatment of depression at doses between 300 and 600 mg/day. Since cases of life-threatening hepatic failure have been reported with its use, monitoring of liver function tests has been advised during treatment with nefazodone. Bupropion (Wellbutrin-SR) has been considered ineffective for the treatment of panic disorder based on a small report; however, it did show efficacy in a more recent study. Treatment is typically initiated at low doses (i.e., 50–100 mg/day) to minimize early activation, with a usual target dose of 100–200 mg b.i.d.

2. **Benzodiazepines**

   a. **Initiation of treatment.** Benzodiazepines are frequently used in the treatment of panic disorder due to their efficacy, their rapid onset, and their favorable side-effect profile. Common side effects noted at the beginning of treatment include sedation and ataxia, which can be minimized by initiating treatment with low doses and by gradually titrating the dose upward. Treatment with benzodiazepines is associated with lower drop-out rates than with use of TCAs.

      i. **Advantages** include being highly efficacious, rapidly acting, and having a favorable side-effect profile.

      ii. **Disadvantages** include their association with withdrawal syndromes, potential for abuse, initial sedation and ataxia, increased sedation in the elderly, interactions with alcohol, and short-term memory impairment.

   b. **Pharmacokinetics.** High-potency benzodiazepines (e.g., alprazolam and clonazepam) are as effective as TCAs and often better tolerated in the treatment of panic disorder. Both clonazepam and alprazolam are FDA-approved for the treatment of panic disorder. Treatment with alprazolam should be started with 0.25–0.5 mg b.i.d.–t.i.d., and then gradually increased to maintenance doses (0.5–3 mg q.i.d.). However, alprazolam's short half-life may lead to interdose rebound anxiety and withdrawal symptoms. The need to treat interdose anxiety with extra medication may foster a cognitive dependence on the medication. Therefore, a longer-acting high-potency benzodiazepine, such as clonazepam, may be preferred. Clonazepam is also effective in treating panic-disordered patients; its antipanic benefits are sustained over time without escalation of the dose. Usually an initial bedtime dose of 0.25–0.5 mg is gradually raised to 1–3 mg/day, which may be given as b.i.d. Lower-potency benzodiazepines may also be effective for panic disorder at equivalent doses (e.g., 40 mg/day of diazepam).

   c. **Discontinuation syndromes. Benzodiazepines should be tapered gradually,** sometimes over as long as several months. The taper should be slower near its end. Rapid taper of benzodiazepines or abrupt discontinuation is frequently followed by a withdrawal syndrome, associated with rebound anxiety, weakness, and insomnia. The withdrawal syndrome, which has been seen after using benzodiazepines for as little as 4–8 weeks, can be severe enough to cause seizures, confusion, and psychotic symptoms, and is more intense following discontinuation of shorter-acting agents. One strategy to minimize withdrawal reactions is to switch from use of shorter-acting agents to longer-acting benzodiazepines (e.g., clonazepam) prior to initiating the taper. Symptoms that persist more than 2 weeks after discontinuation are more likely to be interpreted as a return of the underlying anxiety disorder.

   d. **Abuse and dependence.** Clinicians should consider the **potential for abuse and dependence** before prescribing benzodiazepines, especially in patients with a history of alcohol or substance abuse. A history of substance abuse is not an absolute contraindication to benzodiazepine treatment, but it warrants caution on the part of the clinician.

   e. **Use in the elderly. Benzodiazepines should be used cautiously in elderly patients,** who metabolize drugs less efficiently, may be more sensitive to sedation, ataxia, risk of falls, and memory impairment. The elderly also experience paradoxical agitation from use of benzodiazepines more often than do younger patients.

3. **Other agents.** Buspirone (Buspar) has antianxiety properties, but it does not appear to be effective in panic disorder. Beta-blockers are not useful as a primary treatment of panic, but they may reduce somatic symptoms of autonomic arousal and be used as adjuvants. Some anticonvulsants (valproate [Depakote], gabapentin [Neurontin]) have been used efficaciously in typical, atypical, and treatment-resistant panic disorder.

B. Cognitive-Behavioral Therapy

CBT models of panic disorder focus on the information-processing and behavioral reactions that characterize panic attacks. The initial panic typically emerges at a time of intense stress, which activates the firing of the fight-or-flight alarm system. In vulnerable individuals, the somatic sensations experienced during the initial episodes of panic become associated with intense stress and danger. Subsequently, catastrophic misinterpretations of the meaning of somatic sensations (e.g., "I'm going to have a heart attack") may trigger similar reactions, even in the absence of danger. The misinterpretations trigger intense anxiety, which further intensifies somatic sensations (a positive feedback loop), resulting in a dramatic increase of anxiety and the development of panic. Later in the course of panic disorder, the alarm reactions (panic attacks) may become the focus of fear.

CBT of panic disorder aims to eliminate catastrophic misinterpretations and the conditioned fear of somatic sensations, as well as to eliminate avoidance behavior. CBT for panic disorder typically lasts 12–15 sessions, and it includes four components:

1. **Informational interventions** (i.e., explanations about the nature of the disorder) aim to demystify the somatic sensations experienced during panic attacks and to instruct patients about self-perpetuating patterns that maintain the disorder.
2. **Cognitive restructuring** aims to de-catastrophize beliefs about the meaning and the consequences of somatic symptoms. Catastrophic misinterpretations distort the meaning of somatic sensations (e.g., "I'm going to have a heart attack"), or overestimate the probability or the severity of feared outcomes (e.g., "I'm going to lose control"). Patients with panic at-

tacks are asked to record their thoughts in diaries and to analyze these thoughts. The goal is to help patients reduce catastrophic interpretations and bring their thoughts in accordance with actual consequences.

3. **Exposure interventions** attempt to extinguish the conditioned response (fear) to certain somatic sensations or external situations associated with panic (i.e., agoraphobia). **Interoceptive exposure** is designed to induce somatic sensations usually associated with panic (e.g., running up the stairs to induce tachycardia). ***In vivo* exposure** targets the suffering of those with agoraphobic avoidance, by exposing them to the avoided situations. Exposure methods are utilized in a gradual manner.
4. **Anxiety management skills** (e.g., slow breathing techniques, muscle relaxation training) provide patients with skills for preventing anxious responses to initial sensations of anxiety. CBT is efficacious as an initial treatment for panic disorder, or as an adjunct to pharmacological treatment. CBT can be used also for patients who have failed to respond to pharmacotherapy or who wish to discontinue it. The integration of pharmacotherapy and CBT may produce a better outcome for some patients.

III. Generalized Anxiety Disorder

Generalized anxiety disorder (GAD) is characterized by unrealistic or excessive worry about life circumstances and is accompanied by chronic symptoms of autonomic arousal.

A. Pharmacotherapy

Most pharmacological agents used in panic disorder are also effective in GAD. However, there are some differences:

1. **Benzodiazepines** have been the mainstay of treatment for GAD; however, most current guidelines suggest use of an antidepressant that can treat the symptoms of both anxiety and depression. Nevertheless, benzodiazepines remain widely prescribed either as cotherapy or monotherapy for GAD because of their anxiolytic effect, rapidity of therapeutic onset, and favorable side effect profile. There is no evidence that any benzodiazepine is more effective than any other for GAD. However, longer-acting benzodiazepines (e.g., clonazepam, diazepam) are generally preferred for maintenance therapy, given the risk for rebound anxiety associated with short-acting benzodiazepines (e.g., alprazolam). The principles of treatment with benzodiazepines discussed for panic disorder also apply for GAD.
2. **Antidepressant agents (SSRIs, TCAs, MAOIs)** are also effective for GAD. SSRIs and SNRIs (e.g., venlafaxine) have become first-line treatment for GAD; paroxetine (Paxil) and venlafaxine (Effexor XR) have received FDA-approval for this condition. Considerations in the use of antidepressants for GAD are similar to those for panic.
3. **Buspirone,** a 5-HT_{1A} partial agonist, has proven useful in the treatment of GAD in several studies, although results in clinical practice have been considered less favorable by many clinicians. It has a gradual onset of action and a generally favorable side-effect profile. The starting dose is usually 5 mg b.i.d., which is then gradually increased to the average therapeutic dose of 10–30 mg b.i.d. (20–60 mg/day).
4. **Beta-blockers (propranolol, atenolol)** are useful as adjuvants though they are not indicated as monotherapy for anxiety; they may reduce some symptoms of autonomic arousal. When effective, beta-blockers may begin to work within the first week of treatment.

B. Cognitive-Behavioral Therapy

Many of the same CBT interventions discussed for panic disorder also apply to GAD.

1. **Informational interventions** identify maladaptive cognitions and the process of worrying as primary causes of anxiety.
2. **Cognitive restructuring.** Patients are asked to record their maladaptive cognitions as they occur in high-anxiety situations. Later, they analyze these thoughts. As patients get better at evaluating the content of their thoughts, specific "worry times" may be assigned to help them gain control over the constant tendency to worry.
3. **Exposure interventions.** Imaginary exposure to core worries is used to help patients decrease their worries about specific concerns.
4. **Anxiety management skills.** Relaxation training (e.g., slow breathing techniques, muscle relaxation training) is used to decrease the arousal that accompanies worry and to provide patients with tools to cope with anxiety-provoking situations.

IV. Social Phobia

Patients with social phobia are primarily concerned about humiliation, embarrassment, or a negative evaluation by others.

A. Pharmacotherapy

An increasing number of studies have examined the efficacy of pharmacological agents for the treatment of social phobia. **Medications with demonstrated efficacy in social phobia include MAOIs, benzodiazepines, SSRIs, beta-blockers, and gabapentin.**

1. **MAOIs.** In double-blind studies, phenelzine has proven effective in social phobia. Doses used are similar to those used for depression and for panic disorder.
2. **High-potency benzodiazepines,** especially alprazolam (Xanax) and clonazepam (Klonopin), are effective in social phobia.
3. **Beta-blockers** have been used with mixed results in the treatment of social phobia. Propranolol (10–40

mg) and atenolol (50–150 mg/day) have been shown to benefit patients with performance anxiety, but beta-blockers are not effective for the generalized subtype of social phobia.

4. **SSRIs.** All SSRIs as well as venlafaxine XR have been reported to help patients with social phobia at typical antidepressant doses. Paroxetine was the first agent to receive FDA-approval for this indication. Of note, TCAs are not generally effective for the treatment of social phobia.
5. **Gabapentin (neurontin)** (dose range, 300–3,600 mg/day) was effective in the treatment of social phobia in a randomized placebo-controlled trial.

B. Cognitive-Behavioral Therapy

Fear of critical evaluation by others in social interactions is the key cognitive aspect of social phobia. This fear motivates avoidance of social situations and ultimately prevents the acquisition of social confidence and skills. The CBT for social phobia includes:

1. **Informational interventions,** which are designed to clarify for the patient the anxiogenic nature of their thoughts and the role of avoidance in heightening phobic patterns.
2. **Cognitive restructuring,** is designed to modify the maladaptive cognitions that detract from competent social performance. Typical cognitive distortions include negative expectations of social performance ("I will not know what to say"), distorted evaluations of the self ("Everyone can do it but me"), and distorted anticipation of the reaction of others ("They will think I'm stupid"). Patients are taught to self-monitor their cognitive distortions and to analyze them logically.
3. **Exposure interventions,** aim to provide patients with the ability to practice in social situations and to evaluate their cognitions in that context. Patients rehearse feared interactions in group and homework assignments.
4. **Social skills training** includes instructions and programmed practice in a role-playing format.

V. Specific Phobia

Patients with specific phobia are fearful of circumscribed situations or objects. Those fears lead to significant distress and disability.

A. Exposure-based interventions, a form of CBT, are the mainstay of the treatment for specific phobias.

Adding medications to these interventions appears to bring no additional benefit. Benzodiazepines may be used to help an individual cope with an occasionally encountered feared event (e.g. flying in an airplane).

B. Treatment consists of systematic desensitization and participant modeling.

Systematic desensitization consists of relaxation training combined with gradual exposure (frequently imaginary) to the feared stimulus. In participant modeling, the therapist enacts a behavior and then encourages the patient to repeat that behavior.

VI. Obsessive-Compulsive Disorder

Obsessive-compulsive disorder (OCD) is characterized by recurrent, intrusive, unwanted thoughts (i.e., obsessions, such as fears of contamination) and compulsive behaviors or rituals intended to reduce the anxiety caused by obsessive thoughts.

A. Pharmacotherapy

1. **Antidepressants. Agents that inhibit serotonin reuptake are the pharmacological treatments of choice for OCD.** Clomipramine, a TCA with potent serotonin reuptake inhibition, has been studied for more than 20 years and has been proven efficacious in the treatment of OCD. The effective doses tend to be high, up to 250 mg/day.

   More recently, several SSRIs (e.g., fluvoxamine, fluoxetine, sertraline, paroxetine, and citalopram) have been shown to provide safe and effective treatment for OCD. Fluvoxamine, sertraline, and paroxetine have been FDA-approved for the treatment of OCD. SSRIs are generally effective in OCD at doses that are higher than antidepressant doses: fluvoxamine (up to 300 mg/day), fluoxetine (up to 80 mg/day), sertraline (up to 200 mg/day), and paroxetine (up to 60 mg/day).

   Few OCD patients become symptom-free in response to therapy with serotonergic agents alone; partial relief from obsessional thinking is more usual. Most patients who respond to SSRI therapy obtain partial relief from obsessional thinking; their subjective experience of anxiety and their use of compulsive behaviors are often reduced but not eliminated.

   Response to SSRI therapy may require 8–10 weeks of treatment. Failure to respond to SSRI therapy may reflect inadequate dosing or inadequate duration of treatment. If a patient does not respond to an SSRI at a high dose, use of an alternative SSRI may be successful.
2. **Buspirone,** a 5-HT$_{1A}$ partial agonist, has been helpful in treatment-refractory OCD, as an adjunct to SSRIs. It is started at a dose of 5 mg b.i.d., then gradually increased to a dose of 10–30 mg b.i.d. (20–60 mg/day).
3. **Benzodiazepines** (e.g., clonazepam) have been used successfully to treat co-morbid anxiety in OCD patients. However, benzodiazepines are ineffective when used alone for OCD. Some benzodiazepines (e.g., diazepam, alprazolam) are reported to have increased plasma levels when used in combination with SSRIs, such as fluvoxamine.
4. Other agents (e.g., trazodone, lithium, pindolol, [a beta-blocker with intrinsic sympathomimetic activity], and risperidone [an antipsychotic]) have sometimes

proven effective as adjuvants to SSRIs for the treatment of OCD.

B. Cognitive-Behavioral Therapy

The goal of CBT for OCD patients is to interrupt the chronic cycles of intrusive concerns and the compulsive rituals used by patients to ameliorate their obsessions. CBT is very effective in OCD, especially in combination with pharmacological treatment. CBT for OCD involves exposure and cognitive interventions.

1. **Exposure and response prevention.** The exposure consists of gradually confronting the patient with situations that are likely to trigger obsessive thoughts and compulsive rituals. For example, patients who fear contamination might be given a "dirty" hand towel and encouraged to hold the "contaminated" towel for an hour or longer. The response prevention used at the time of exposure requires patients to resist performing their compulsive rituals, such as hand washing, for a progressively longer period of time. The repeated exposure without performing the compulsive rituals gradually decreases anxiety.
2. **Cognitive interventions** provide patients with additional skills for breaking the link between intrusive thoughts and compulsive responses.

VII. Post-traumatic Stress Disorder

Patients with post-traumatic stress disorder (PTSD) have experienced an event that involved the threat of death, injury, or severe harm to themselves or others. The severe trauma disrupts the patient's sense of safety to the extent that the patient avoids situations that remind him or her of the trauma; he or she may become emotionally numb, irritable, hypervigilant, or have difficulties with sleep and concentration. Patients with PTSD frequently re-experience the traumatic event in the form of nightmares, flashbacks, or have marked arousal when exposed to situations reminiscent of the event.

A. Pharmacotherapy

The role of pharmacotherapy in PTSD has traditionally been related to relieve symptoms and to facilitate the onset of trauma-focused psychotherapy. However, SSRIs have recently been shown to reduce the symptoms of PTSD.

1. **Antidepressants.** TCAs (e.g., amitriptyline and imipramine) have reduced PTSD symptoms in double-blind studies. SSRIs (e.g., fluoxetine, sertraline, paroxetine), bupropion, nefazodone and MAOIs (e.g., phenelzine) have all been reported to have some efficacy in PTSD. Sertraline and paroxetine are the only pharmacological agents that have received FDA-approval for PSTD. The drugs are used in doses similar to those listed in Table 44-1; the doses for bupropion are 225–450 mg/day.
2. **Buspirone** has been reported to reduce anxiety and increased arousal in PTSD patients at doses of 30–60 mg/day. When used, it is typically co-administered with an antidepressant.
3. **Mood stabilizers, including lithium and anticonvulsants (such as carbamazepine, valproate, gabapentin, lamotrigine and topiramate), in typical therapeutic doses have demonstrated efficacy for the treatment of PTSD.** One hypothesis for the positive effects of these medications on PTSD symptoms relates to a reduction of kindling.
4. **Beta-blockers** (e.g., propranolol, nadolol, atenolol) may be useful in some patients with PTSD to decrease persistent symptoms of autonomic hyperarousal. **Clonidine,** at doses of 0.2–0.6 mg/day may also be beneficial.
5. **Benzodiazepines** can reduce anxiety and improve sleep in PTSD, but may have negative effects including disinhibition, irritability, and forestalling recovery.
6. **Neuroleptics** may reduce psychosis and impulsiveness in PTSD patients.

B. Individual Psychotherapy

General support, educating patients about the time-limited nature of many post-trauma symptoms (such as sleep disturbance), providing symptomatic relief, and making patients aware of the availability of mental health resources are reasonable management strategies for most individuals exposed to trauma. Accruing evidence suggests that broadly applied Critical Incidence Stress Debriefing in the aftermath of a trauma may not be beneficial for most patients and may actually increase the likelihood of developing PTSD. For the chronic PTSD patient, exposure-based therapies, such as CBT, appear to be the most successful.

C. Cognitive-Behavioral Therapy

CBT interventions aim to disrupt the link between trauma-related cues and the severe anxiety responses and hypervigilance which characterize PTSD.

1. **Informational interventions** aim to help patients understand their symptoms. Discussion of dissociation and flashbacks may normalize and decrease the fear triggered by these symptoms.
2. **Cognitive restructuring** aims to help patients identify cognitive distortions which may have been generated by trauma (e.g., "The world is an unsafe place" or "I am helpless").
3. **Exposure interventions** aim to help a patient's control of their emotional reactions associated with trauma. PTSD patients associate objects and situations which are only remotely linked to the trauma. With repeated exposure, patients learn to differentiate between the diffuse, exaggerated fears generated by trauma and the actual safety of current situations. The intensity of exposure therapy can vary. Implosive therapy, a more intense form of exposure therapy, is effective but depends on the ability of the patient to tolerate intense levels of arousal. Systematic desensitization involves a more

gradual exposure and can be beneficial in overcoming the phobic avoidance related to trauma.

4. **Relaxation training** may be used as in other anxiety disorders to provide patients with skills for preventing anxious responses to the initial stages of exposure treatment.

D. Group Therapy

Patients involved in group therapy experience the understanding and support provided by fellow victims; also, groups can generate and process more intense affects than can individual therapy. Some researchers also report a greater effect of group therapy on avoidance and the numbing symptoms present in PTSD, but no conclusive comparisons have been made yet.

VIII. Conclusions

Anxiety disorders benefit from a range of psychopharmacologic and psychotherapeutic interventions. For many patients, a combination of treatment modalities is the most effective treatment solution, although this issue requires further study. Most treatments have been studied for short periods, generally up to 6 months. However, a large number of patients (20–50%) experience a recurrence of their initial anxiety when treatment is interrupted. For many patients maintenance pharmacological treatment is warranted.

Suggested Readings

Fyer, A.J., Gabbard, G.O., Pine, D.S., et al. (2000). Anxiety disorders. In H.I. Kaplan, & B.J. Sadock (Eds.), *Comprehensive textbook of psychiatry* (7th ed.). Baltimore, MD: Williams and Wilkins.

Hyman, S.E., Arana, G.W., & Rosenbaum, J.F. (2000). *Handbook of psychiatric drug therapy* (4th ed.). Boston, MA: Little, Brown.

Otto, M.W., Reilly-Harrington, N.A., & Harrington, J.A. (1998). Cognitive-behavioral strategies for specific disorders. In T.A. Stern, J.B. Herman, & P.L. Slavin (Eds.), *The MGH guide to psychiatry in primary care.* New York: McGraw-Hill.

Pollack, M., Smoller, J., & Lee, D. (1998). Approach to the anxious patient. In T.A. Stern, J.B. Herman, & P.L. Slavin (Eds.), *The MGH guide to psychiatry in primary care.* New York: McGraw-Hill.

Taylor, C.B. (1998). Treatment of anxiety disorders. In A.F. Schatzberg & C.B. Nemeroff (Eds.), *The American Psychiatric Press textbook of psychopharmacology* (2nd ed.). Washington, DC: American Psychiatric Press.

Chapter 45

Antipsychotic Drugs

DAVID C. HENDERSON, LAURA KUNKEL, AND DONALD C. GOFF

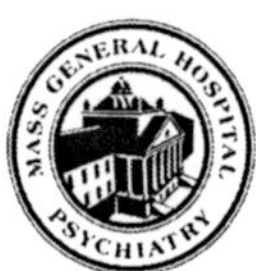

I. Introduction

Selection of antipsychotic agents has traditionally been guided by side-effect profiles, as conventional neuroleptics are all of comparable efficacy. All antipsychotic medications are more effective for acute than chronic illness and for delusions and hallucinations than for negative symptoms. In both the Written and Oral Psychiatry Boards, knowledge of different antipsychotic agents (including their generic names), mechanisms of actions, dosing schedules, side effects, drug interactions, and reasons for choosing one over another are vitally important. This chapter reviews the above areas, as well as approaches to the treatment-resistant patient.

When choosing an antipsychotic agent it is important to focus on specific target symptoms that should be monitored closely to determine efficacy for a particular agent. These target symptoms include:

A. **Psychosis** (hallucinations, delusions, and disorganization)
B. **Negative Symptoms** (apathy, flat affect, social withdrawal, and poverty of speech)
C. **Agitation** (hyperkinesis, tension, and distractibility)
D. **Cognitive Impairment** (difficulty with attention, memory, judgment, and insight)

II. Antipsychotic Agents

A. Conventional Antipsychotic Agents

Conventional (typical) antipsychotics or "neuroleptics" **are agents with dopamine D_2 antagonism** that **may produce extrapyramidal symptoms (EPS).** Conventional agents also may **elevate prolactin levels.** Finally, all conventional agents are equally effective, but they differ in their potency and their side effects. **Potency,** often described in chlorpromazine equivalents, **often determines side-effect profiles.** Table 45-1 lists common conventional agents, their dosing schedule, their potency, and their class (e.g., phenothiazine). The class of an agent is a common question on the written boards examination.

B. Atypical Antipsychotic Agents

Atypical antipsychotics (**"second generation" antipsychotics or serotonin-dopamine antagonists) are agents with dopamine D_2 and serotonin 5-HT_2 antagonism. They offer reduced or absent EPS with little or no elevation of prolactin.** They are also generally **more effective for negative symptoms** compared with conventional agents. Of note, clozapine is the only agent clearly more effective for psychotic symptoms. Finally, risperidone is more appropriately classified as a "partial atypical" as it may produce EPS at higher doses and can elevate prolactin.

III. Basic Pharmacology of Antipsychotic Agents

A. Dopamine D_2 Blockade

Conventional agents acutely block 75–90% of D_2 receptors, whereas clozapine blocks only 40–60% of D_2 receptors. Blockade of pre-synaptic D_2 autoreceptors leads to an increase in electrical activity and to release of dopamine acutely.

B. Delayed Effects

The delayed effects of conventional agents are due to an increase in the density of post-synaptic D_2 receptors (supersensitivity) and to depolarization blockade in A9 (substantia nigra) and A10 (ventral tegmental) dopamine neurons.

C. A9 and A10 Blockade

Atypical agents produce depolarization blockade only in A10 neurons. All agents increase c-fos in the nucleus accumbens, whereas conventional agents also increase c-fos in the striatum. **The A9 nigrostriatal (midbrain to neostriatum) pathway appears to be responsible for EPS. The A10 mesolimbic (midbrain to limbic structures) is possibly associated with psychosis,** and the A10 mesocortical (midbrain to frontal and temporal cerebral cortex pathway) may be responsible for negative symptoms.

D. Side Effects with Conventional Agents

1. **Dystonia, akathisia, and parkinsonism** are more commonly associated with high-potency conventional agents than with low-potency agents.
2. Low-potency agents tend to produce **sedation, hypotension, weight gain** (although molindone may produce weight loss), and **anticholinergic symptoms** (e.g., dry mouth, urinary retention, constipation, and blurred vision).
3. **Hyperprolactinemia** (associated with amenorrhea, galactorrhea, and sexual dysfunction), **tardive dyskinesia, and neuroleptic malignant syndrome** may occur with all D_2 antagonists, **unrelated to their neuroleptic potency.**
4. Other potential side effects include impaired heat regulation (i.e., **poikilothermia** with hyper- or hypothermia); **pigmentary retinopathy** (thioridazine > 800 mg/day); and **electrocardiographic (EKG) changes** (especially with pimozide, chlorpromazine, and thioridazine).

Table 45-1. Conventional and Atypical Antipsychotic Agents

Agent	*Starting Dose*	*Dose Range (mg/day)*	*Class*
Atypical			
Clozapine (Clozaril)	12.5 mg	25–900	Dibenzapine
Olanzapine (Zyprexa)	2.5–10 mg	5–20	Thienobenzodiazepine
Quetiapine (Seroquel)	25–50 mg/day	25–750	Dibenzothiazepine
Ziprasidone (Geodon)	20–40 mg b.i.d.	40–160	
Aripiprazole (Abilify)	10–15 mg/day	10–30	
Risperidone (Risperdal)	1–2 mg/day	0.5–16	Benzisoxazole
High-potency conventional			
Haloperidol (Haldol)	0.5–6 mg/day	2–100	Butyrophenone
Trifluoperazine (Stelazine)	2–10 mg/day	5–60	Phenothiazine (C)
Pimozide (Orap)	1–2	1–10	Butyrophenone
Fluphenazine (Prolixin)	2.5–10	5–60	Phenothiazine (C)
Thiothixene (Navane)	2–10 mg/day	5–60	Thioxanthenes
Mid-potency conventional			
Perphenazine (Trilafon)	8–24 mg/day	8–64	Phenothiazine (C)
Loxapine (Loxitane)	10–50 mg/day	30–250	Dibenzapine
Molindone (Moban)	50–75 mg/day	10–225	Indole
Low-potency conventional			
Chlorpromazine (Thorazine)	100–200 mg/day	100–2,000	Phenothiazine (A)
Thioridazine (Mellaril)	50–300 mg/day	100–600	Phenothiazine (B)
Mesoridazine (Serentil)	50–150 mg/day	100–400	Phenothiazine (B)

A, aliphatic phenothiazine; B, piperidine phenothiazine; C, piperazine phenothiazine.

IV. Extrapyramidal Side Effects

A. Dystonia

1. Dystonia is **an involuntary muscle contraction that may involve the tongue, neck, back, and eyes.** It is extremely uncomfortable and can jeopardize future compliance with antipsychotics. It may be life-threatening when laryngeal spasms occur. **Generally, it occurs within the first 4 days of neuroleptic treatment or following an increase in the neuroleptic dose.**
2. **Risk factors** include **youth** (age less than 40 years) and the **use of high-potency neuroleptics.** All patients under the age of 30 years started on high-potency neuroleptics should receive prophylaxis with benztropine 1–2 mg b.i.d. for 10 days, followed by a taper. Often, benztropine is initiated for prophylaxis and continued needlessly for weeks, months, or years.
3. **Treatments for acute dystonia include benztropine 1–2 mg IM or PO, diphenhydramine 25–50 mg IM or PO, or diazepam 5 mg, slow IV push.** After the initial dystonic reaction has resolved, a standing dose of benztropine or another anticholinergic agent is recommended. Dystonias are less common with atypical agents; they do not occur with clozapine. "Tardive dystonia" is a variant of tardive dyskinesia that appears to respond well to atypical agents, particularly clozapine.

B. Akathisia

1. Akathisia is **the sensation of motor restlessness which is most prominent in the lower extremities.** It is most commonly associated with high-potency agents, and it is dose-related. Akathisia is often mistaken for agitation, which may lead to a dose increase of an antipsychotic agent and worsening of akathisia.
2. **Possible treatments include** switching to an atypical agent; **lowering the neuroleptic dose;** adding a **beta-blocker** (e.g., propranolol 20 mg q.i.d.), an **anticholinergic agent** (e.g., benztropine 1 mg b.i.d.), or a **benzodiazepine** (e.g., lorazepam 0.5 mg t.i.d.).

C. Parkinsonian Symptoms

1. Antipsychotic-induced parkinsonism can be mistaken for negative symptoms or depression. Clinically, it may appear as idiopathic Parkinson's disease, with **rigidity, tremor, and bradykinesia.** It tends to be as-

sociated with use of high-potency agents and it is dose-related.

2. **Possible treatments include lowering the neuroleptic dose, switching to an atypical agent, or adding an anticholinergic agent** (benztropine 1–2 mg b.i.d.; in the elderly start with 0.25 mg) or amantadine (100–200 mg b.i.d.).
3. The elderly are most sensitive to the anticholinergic agents; therefore, long-term use of these agents should be avoided.

D. Tardive Dyskinesia

1. Tardive dyskinesia is **a late-developing involuntary choreiform movement disorder,** most commonly of the mouth, tongue, or upper extremities. Tardive dystonia is a syndrome of chronic dystonic posturing.
2. Studies suggest that **the risk for developing tardive dyskinesia is approximately 4–5% per year of exposure.**
3. **Risk factors** for tardive dyskinesia include **old age, affective disorders, being female, neuroleptic exposure of more than 6 months, a history of parkinsonian side effects, diabetes, and use of high doses of conventional agents.**
4. **Tardive dyskinesia does not appear to be associated with clozapine, olanzapine, or quetiapine,** while risperidone may also be associated with a reduced risk of tardive dyskinesia.
5. **A "withdrawal dyskinesia" may occur when a neuroleptic dose is decreased or when a switch is made to an atypical agent.** This type of dyskinesia usually resolves within 6 weeks. Anticholinergic agents may produce a reversible worsening of tardive dyskinesia. Also, tardive dyskinesia usually does not worsen with continued neuroleptic exposure.
6. **Neuroleptics should not be used if there is no clear benefit.** One should also use the lowest effective dose.
7. **The Abnormal Involuntary Movement Scale (AIMS) should be performed twice yearly** to monitor for tardive dyskinesia. Patients should also be warned and educated when taking neuroleptics for more than 6 months.
8. **Treatment for tardive dyskinesia includes discontinuation or lowering of the neuroleptic dose, addition of vitamin E** (α-tocopherol) 800–1,200 IU/day (if the duration is less than 5 years), **or switching to an atypical antipsychotic agent.**
9. Clozapine is associated with an increased rate of remission (especially with tardive dystonia). Other atypical agents are promising but their efficacy in suppressing tardive dyskinesia has not yet been established.

E. Neuroleptic Malignant Syndrome

1. Neuroleptic malignant syndrome (NMS) is **a rare, potentially lethal complication of neuroleptic treatment, characterized by hyperthermia, autonomic instability, diaphoresis, confusion, elevated creatine phosphokinase (CPK), as well as fluctuating levels of consciousness and rigidity.**
2. The symptoms may evolve over time; they usually start with mental status changes and culminate with fever and elevated CPK. **NMS represents a medical emergency** and treatment should begin, in the hospital, immediately.
3. **Treatment includes discontinuation of the neuroleptic, hydration, temperature control, and possibly bromocriptine or dantrolene** (although it is unclear if these agents improve recovery).
4. **Two weeks should elapse before restarting an antipsychotic agent.** Cases of NMS with clozapine have been reported, but the incidence appears to be lower than with conventional agents.

V. Antipsychotic Dosing

A. Dosing Schedules

In general, one should use a moderate, fixed dose (e.g., haloperidol 5–15 mg/day, risperidone 3–6 mg/day, olanzapine 10–20 mg/day) of an antipsychotic agent for an adequate period (approximately 4–6 weeks) (see Table 45-1). Benzodiazepines can also be administered for agitation (e.g., lorazepam up to 1–2 mg q.i.d.).

B. Blood Levels

Blood levels should not substitute for titration of doses based on clinical response. While some have considered there to be a "therapeutic window" (5–15 ng/mL) for haloperidol, the data are inconsistent (see Table 45-2). Blood levels may be useful in cases of non-response, non-compliance, or when drug interactions occur.

C. Metabolism

Some patients are poor metabolizers (due to low levels of P450 2D6) and may develop toxic levels even at low doses. Drug interactions range from useful, to benign, to dangerous. For example, the addition of fluoxetine may elevate haloperidol blood levels (see Table 45-3). Additionally, fluvoxamine added to clozapine has resulted in several deaths from clozapine toxicity.

VI. Patients with First-Break Psychosis

A. Response

First-break patients respond better than do chronically psychotic patients, in that 74% achieve a complete remission and 12% achieve a partial response. In general, patients with first-break psychosis respond to lower doses of antipsychotic agents.

B. Early Treatment

Early treatment is **associated with a better outcome.** When treating first-break patients, it is important to avoid side effects and to provide prophylaxis for dystonia if conventional neuroleptics are used.

Table 45-2. Potential Therapeutic Blood Levels for Antipsychotic Agents

Agent	*Therapeutic Range (ng/mL)*
Chlorpromazine	30–100
Clozapine	> 350
Fluphenazine	0.2–2.0
Haloperidol	5–15
Loxapine	30–100
Perphenazine	0.8–2.4
Thioridazine	1–1.5
Thiothixene	2–15

C. Alliance

Development of an alliance and education of the patient and family about the illness and its treatments are vital.

VII. Maintenance Treatment

A. Relapse

Relapse rates in schizophrenia range from 41% in the first year to 15% in the second year following hospital discharge. Low and conventional doses are of approximately equal efficacy against relapse in the first year, while conventional doses may be superior during the second year for the prevention of relapse. Lower doses produce significantly fewer EPS and dysphoria.

B. Depot Neuroleptics

Depot neuroleptics can be used in patients where compliance is an issue. **Fluphenazine decanoate** has a half-life of 6–9 days; its recommended injection interval is 14 days. A low dose would be 5–6.25 mg every 2 weeks, and a conventional dose would be 25 mg every 2 weeks.

Haloperidol decanoate has a half-life of 21 days; it can be given at 4-week intervals.

C. Conversion to Depot Neuroleptics

Conversion to a depot neuroleptic requires approximately four dosing intervals to achieve a steady-state blood level. In general, one should start with a loading dose and supplement with oral agents. **Tolerability with an oral preparation should be established before initiating the decanoate preparation.** The loading dose of haloperidol decanoate is approximately 20 times the oral dose that had been given, in divided doses, during the first week. The decanoate dose is then decreased by 25% for each of the next two injections. The maintenance dose (given every 4 weeks) is approximately ten times the oral dose.

VIII. Atypical Antipsychotic Agents

Atypical antipsychotic agents may be more effective than typical antipsychotic agents for the negative symptoms and cognitive impairment associated with schizophrenia.

Table 45-3. Drug Interactions with Antipsychotic Agents (Most Metabolized by Cytochrome P450 2D6)

Alcohol	Additive sedation; incoordination; haloperidol increases alcohol levels
Antacids	Impair absorption of chlorpromazine
Antiarrhythmics (class I)	Additive conduction impairment
Anticonvulsants (except valproate)	Lower antipsychotic blood levels
Antihypertensives	
Guanethidine	Reverses the antihypertensive effect
Methyldopa	Hypotension and confusion
Propranolol	Increases CPZ and thioridazine levels
Buspirone	Increases haloperidol levels
Disulfiram	Lowers chlorpromazine levels
Erythromycin	Increases clozapine levels (3A4)
Fluvoxamine	Increases clozapine levels
Ketoconazole	Increases clozapine levels (3A4)
Lithium	May increase chlorpromazine levels
SSRIs	Increase neuroleptic levels and worsen EPS
Tricyclic antidepressants	Levels increased by some neuroleptics; increase antipsychotic blood levels
Tobacco	Lowers antipsychotic blood levels

A. Clozapine

1. Clozapine (Clozaril), an atypical agent, rarely causes EPS and does not elevate serum prolactin levels. Its major benefit is that it is **more effective than conventional agents for treatment-resistant psychotic patients. A weak D_2 antagonist, with relatively greater D_1 and D_4 antagonism, clozapine does not cause D_2 receptor supersensitivity or depolarization blockade in A9 neurons.** However, it releases dopamine in the frontal cortex.

   Clozapine has significant interactions with other neurotransmitter systems; it is an alpha-adrenergic antagonist, a histaminergic (H_1) antagonist, a serotonin (5-HT_2) antagonist, and it is highly anticholinergic. Clozapine is effective in 30% of treatment-resistant patients within 6 weeks in controlled trials and in 60% at 6 months in uncontrolled trials.
2. **Clozapine appears to prevent relapse, to stabilize mood, to improve negative symptoms, to improve polydipsia and hyponatremia, and to reduce hostility and aggression, and it may reduce the risk of suicide in patients with schizophrenia. Clozapine may also reduce cigarette smoking and substance abuse in individuals with schizophrenia.**
3. **Clozapine produces many troublesome side effects,** including sedation, tachycardia, hypersalivation, dizziness, constipation, nausea, headache, hypotension, fever, dose-related seizures, weight gain, diabetes, and agranulocytosis (in approximately 1% of patients).
4. **Agranulocytosis** (granulocytes < 500/mm^3) occurs in 1.6% of patients after 1 year. The clozapine monitoring system involving weekly (for first 6 months) and biweekly (from 6 months on and for the duration of treatment) complete blood counts has reduced the incidence of agranulocytosis in the United States. Risk factors may include being an Ashkenazi Jew (with blood markers of HLA B38, DR4, DQw3) or Finnish. Usually, other cell lines (i.e. platelets and red blood cells) are preserved. The maximum risk appears to be between 4 and 18 weeks, when 77% of cases occur. Patients usually recover within 14 days if clozapine is stopped. There appears to be no cross-sensitivity with other drugs. However, carbamazepine, captopril, sulfonamides, and propylthiouracil (PTU) should be avoided in clozapine-treated patients. Guidelines for abnormal white blood count (WBC) results are presented below:
   a. WBC counts between 3,000 and 3,500, or a substantial drop in the WBCs (single drop ≥ 3,000 cells, or cumulative drop ≥ 3,000 cells within 3 weeks), or immature WBC forms and an absolute neutrophil count (ANC = [WBC] [% bands and mature neutrophils]) > 1,500/mm^3
      i. Pharmacist must confirm the plan with the physician to continue treatment.
      ii. If the WBC count is < 3,500, the physician orders twice weekly WBC counts until the WBC count is > 3,500.
      iii. If the WBC count is ≥ 3,500 when the drop is identified, the physician orders repeat the WBC.
   b. A WBC count between 2,000/mm^3 to 3,000/mm^3 or an ANC between 1,000/mm^3 to 1,500/mm^3
      i. Clozapine treatment is interrupted.
      ii. Physician orders daily WBC counts until the WBC count is > 3,000 mm^3.
   c. A WBC count < 2,000/mm^3 or an ANC < 1,000/mm^3
      i. Clozapine treatment is permanently discontinued. **The patient should never be rechallenged with the drug.**
      ii. The physician orders daily WBC counts until the WBC count is within normal limits.
      iii. The Registry should be contacted to have the patient posted immediately on the National Non-Rechallenge Masterfile.
5. Clozapine is usually started at 12.5–25 mg at bedtime. The dose is then increased by 25 mg/day as tolerated over the first week. It is best to overlap with the previous antipsychotic agent (and to watch for additive side effects) and to taper it when the clozapine dose reaches 100 mg/day. In general, clozapine should be stopped at 600 mg/day or when side effects emerge. The usual therapeutic dose is 300–600 mg/day, and the maximum dose is 900 mg/day. Clozapine is metabolized by the cytochrome P450 1A2 and 3A4 system. Agents that affect these enzymes may alter clozapine metabolism (see Table 45-3).

B. Risperidone

1. **Risperidone (Risperdal) is an atypical antipsychotic with significant 5-HT_2 and D_2 antagonism.** Risperidone antagonizes D_4, noradrenergic, and histaminergic receptors. Risperidone offers a lower incidence of EPS, which increases as doses go above 6 mg/day. Unlike other atypical antipsychotic agents, risperidone causes a sustained increase in prolactin levels in some patients. Risperidone appears to be more **effective for negative symptoms** (partly the result of fewer EPS) compared with conventional agents. It also may be more effective for psychotic symptoms in some treatment-resistant patients.
2. Side effects of risperidone include dizziness, hypotension (particularly after the first few doses), headache, nausea, vomiting, anxiety, rhinitis, coughing, hyperprolactinemia, weight gain, and QT interval prolongation (usually clinically insignificant).
3. The mean optimal dose of risperidone is 4–6 mg/day. The usual starting dose is 1–2 mg/day. Treatment-naïve patients may require only 2–4 mg/day. Elderly patients should be started at very low doses (0.5 mg/day), with a dose range of 0.5–2.0 mg/day. Risperidone is metabolized by cytochrome P450 2D6 isoenzymes, and it has a half-life of 24 hours (therefore, it can be given once daily).

C. Olanzapine

1. **Olanzapine (Zyprexa) is an atypical antipsychotic agent with a high 5-HT_2/D_2 ratio that most closely resembles clozapine.** Olanzapine possesses anticholinergic activity *in vitro* (with minimal effects *in vivo*), as well as histaminergic and alpha-adrenergic antagonism. Olanzapine exhibits antipsychotic efficacy comparable to haloperidol, yet it is more effective for negative symptoms. Olanzapine also appears to have a substantial antidepressant and antimanic effect when compared to placebo.
2. **Side effects of olanzapine** include **somnolence, dizziness** (without hypotension), **constipation, dry mouth, elevation of SGPT** (serum glutamic-pyruvic transaminase) (but without evidence of hepatotoxicity), and **weight gain. Reports of new-onset diabetes and diabetic ketoacidosis (DKA) have emerged with olanzapine, as they have with clozapine.**
3. Starting doses of olanzapine are usually 5–10 mg, and the optimal dose is 10–20 mg/day for adults. Elderly patients should be started at lower doses (2.5 mg/day), but the dose may be increased to 2.5–7.5 mg/day. Olanzapine has been associated with falls in the elderly. Olanzapine is metabolized by cytochrome P450 1A2 and 3A4 isoenzymes; it has a half-life of approximately 20 hours (therefore, it can be given once daily).

D. Quetiapine

1. **Quetiapine (Seroquel) is an atypical antipsychotic agent with a high D_2/5-HT_2 ratio** (it may be effective with < 60% D_2 blockade) and a very low incidence of EPS. Quetiapine is without significant anticholinergic effects; however, it exhibits alpha-adrenergic antagonism. It has a comparable antipsychotic efficacy to chlorpromazine and is more effective for negative symptoms.
2. Side effects include postural hypotension, somnolence, elevation of liver function tests (LFTs) (reversible), **headache, weight gain, decreased serum T_3 and T_4 levels,** and cataracts (in beagles; the risk in humans has not been established, so eye examinations are recommended every year).
3. The starting dose, in non-elderly patients, is 25 mg twice daily, after which doses are titrated upwards. Clinically effective doses range from 250 to 750-mg/day. Doses should be titrated with care to reduce the risk of postural hypotension, particularly in the elderly. Quetiapine is metabolized by the cytochrome P450 2D6 isoenzyme system; it has a half-life of approximately 6 hours (and requires multiple daily dosing).

E. Ziprasidone

1. Ziprasidone (Geodon) is an atypical antipsychotic with a high 5-HT/D_2 ratio; it may be associated with **less weight gain** than other atypical antipsychotic agents. It is associated with a **mean QTc increase of 21 milliseconds** (> 60 msec QTc increase in 21%). The incidence of QTc prolongation, i.e., > 500 milliseconds, has not differed from placebo (< 0.1%)
2. Side effects include nausea, sedation/activation, dizziness/hypotension, and prolongation of the QTc.
3. The starting dose is 20–40 mg b.i.d. Clinically effective doses range from 80–160 mg/day administered b.i.d. with meals. Ziprasidone should be used cautiously in patients with risk factors for QT prolongation (e.g., use of TCAs, low potency neuroleptics, or quinidine, cardiac disease, electrolyte disturbance [low potassium or magnesium], hypothyroidism, or substance abuse). Ziprasidone's effect on the QT interval appears to be less than what is observed with thioridazine. There have been no reported deaths associated with ziprasidone overdoses.

F. Aripiprazole

1. Aripiprazole (Abilify) is a potent (high-affinity) **partial agonist at D_2 and 5-HT_{1A}** receptors, and it is a potent **antagonist at 5-HT_{2A}** receptors. Because of its partial agonist properties, aripiprazole is hypothesized to stabilize the dopamine system (binding to D_2 receptors, increasing activation in hypodopaminergic states, and displacing dopamine in hyperdopaminergic states, thereby decreasing activation of D_2 receptors). Aripiprazole may act as a stabilizer of both dopaminergic and serotonergic neural pathways, and, therefore, function as a **dopamine-serotonin system stabilizer**.
2. Side effects include nausea, vomiting, anxiety, headache, dyspepsia, somnolence, orthostatic hypotension, tachycardia, insomnia, akathisia, EPS, and weight gain.
3. Effective doses in phase two and three clinical trials with aripiprazole have ranged from 15 mg to 30 mg/day. The recommended starting dose is 10–15 mg on a once-a-day schedule without regard to meals. Aripiprazole is metabolized by P450 2D6 and 3A4 isoenzymes.

IX. Treatment Resistance

A. Alternative Diagnoses

Patients with a poor response to treatment must have their diagnosis reassessed. Alternative diagnoses include **substance (alcohol, PCP, stimulants) abuse, neurological disorders** (e.g., partial complex seizures), **psychotic depression, drug toxicity/delirium** (e.g., steroid psychosis, anticholinergic delirium), **dissociative disorders, hysteria, and post-traumatic stress disorder.**

B. Dose Adjustment

Adjustment of the neuroleptic dose and assessment of compliance are often required. A time-limited trial at a higher dose is often indicated, if tolerated. Alternatively, if one is taking moderate to high doses, a dose reduction may provide symptomatic relief. The use of adjuvants, when symptoms persist, may help. Possible adjuvants include:

1. **Risperidone (or haloperidol/olanzapine),** added to clozapine for clozapine partial responders, may improve both positive and negative symptoms. Use of this strategy often enables the dose of clozapine to be reduced, which minimizes side effects.
2. **Lithium** (with blood levels of 0.8–1.2 mEq/L) for 3–5 weeks is necessary to determine efficacy, particularly if affective symptoms are present. Co-treatment may improve positive and negative symptoms. Drug interactions with antihypertensive agents, and non-steroidal anti-inflammatory drugs (NSAIDs) may develop.
3. **Electroconvulsive therapy** (ECT), which is helpful for catatonia and for affective symptoms, is most effective early in the course of illness. Its long-term efficacy is unclear.
4. **Antidepressants.** Tricyclic antidepressants (TCAs) may delay a positive response in acute psychosis; selective serotonin reuptake inhibitors (SSRIs) may improve depressive and negative symptoms and increase neuroleptic blood levels.
5. **Buspirone** is helpful with agitation and anxiety (15–45 mg/day).
6. **Anticonvulsants** may decrease tension, suspiciousness, manic symptoms, and electroencephalographic (EEG) abnormalities. Carbamazepine increases P450 activity, and thus may lower neuroleptic blood levels.
7. **Benzodiazepines** can decrease agitation, psychotic symptoms, and social withdrawal. Disinhibition and abuse need to be monitored.
8. **Beta-blockers,** often at high doses, may decrease agitation, violence, and impulsivity.
9. **Anticholinergics** may be used for dystonia and EPS; however, they may worsen tardive dyskinesia.

X. Alternative Medicine

A. Herbs to Treat Psychosis

Many patients self-medicate with herbal medications. Psychotic patients are no different in this regard. Herbal medications that are recommended, or are thought to have some antipsychotic properties, include:

- ***Schumanniophyton problematicum:* may potentiate the sedative effects of benzodiazepines and neuroleptics**
- ***Yangjinhua:* contains atropine and scopolamine**
- ***Rauwolfia serpentine:* High affinity for alpha-2 and D_2 receptors; reserpine (which causes depression) is derived from this plant**

B. Herbs that Cause Psychosis

Other herbal medications have been implicated or associated with psychotic symptoms, primarily during intoxication. They include:

- ***Catharanthus roseum* (periwinkle);**
- ***Cinnamomum camphora*;**
- ***Datura stramonium* (thorn apple);**
- ***Eschscholtzia California* (poppy);**
- ***Humulus lupulus* (common hop);**
- ***Hydrangea paniculata;***
- ***Mandragora officinarum* (mandrake);**
- ***Passiflora* (passion flower);**
- ***Piper methysticum* (kava, kava-kava);**
- ***Psilocybe semilanceta* (liberty cap, magic mushrooms);**
- ***Ma Huang* (Square tea, Mormon tea)**

XI. Conclusion

If treatment failure occurs, despite adequate doses of conventional agents, a switch to an atypical agent is warranted. Atypical agents differ in their patterns of efficacy; each agent is worthy of consideration. **Clozapine remains the most effective agent for treatment-resistant psychotic patients.**

Suggested Readings

Breier, A., Wolkowitz, O.M., Doran, A.R., et al. (1987). Neuroleptic responsitivity of negative and positive symptoms in schizophrenia. *American Journal of Psychiatry, 144*, 1549–1555.

Christison, G., Kirch, D., & Wyatt, R. (1991). When symptoms persist: Choosing among alternative somatic treatments for schizophrenia. *Schizophrenia Bulletin, 17*, 217–245.

Gelenberg, A.J., & Bassuk, E.L. (Eds.). (1997). *The practitioner's guide to psychoactive drugs* (4th ed.). New York: Plenum.

Goff, D.C., & Henderson, D.C. (1996). Treatment-resistant schizophrenia and psychotic disorders. In M.H. Pollack, M.W. Otto, & J.F. Rosenbaum (Eds.), *Challenges in clinical practice: Pharmacologic and psychosocial strategies*, pp. 311–328. New York: Guilford Press.

Goff, D.C., Henderson, D.C., & Manschreck, T.C. (1997). Psychotic patients. In N.H. Cassem, T.A. Stern, J.F. Rosenbaum, & M.S. Jellinek (Eds.), *Massachusetts General Hospital handbook of general hospital psychiatry* (4th ed., pp. 149–171). St. Louis: Mosby.

Kane, J.M. (1985). Antipsychotic drug side effects: Their relationship to dose. *Journal of Clinical Psychiatry, 46*, 16–21.

Meltzer, H.Y. (1987). Biological studies in schizophrenia. *Schizophrenia Bulletin, 13*, 77–110.

Chapter 46

Antidepressants and Somatic Therapies

JOSHUA ISRAEL, ANNA GEORGIOPOULOS, AND MAURIZIO FAVA

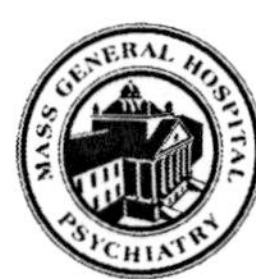

I. Overview

Antidepressants represent an effective treatment for major depression. More than 50% of depressed patients will fully recover when an adequate dose of any antidepressant is used for an adequate amount of time (at least 6 weeks); 10–15% will show some improvement, and 20–35% will not improve substantially.

After a first episode of major depression, a patient should receive at least 6 months of treatment with an antidepressant at the dosage to which they responded; any tapering of the antidepressant should be done slowly to minimize the risk of relapse.

Antidepressant medications are commonly grouped into several classes:

A. Selective Serotonin Reuptake Inhibitors (SSRIs)
B. Serotonin-Norepinephrine Reuptake Inhibitors (SNRIs)
C. Cyclic Antidepressants (most often the tricyclic antidepressants [TCAs])
D. Monoamine Oxidase Inhibitors (MAOIs)
E. Growing Category of "Others" or "Atypical Antidepressants"

II. Classes of Antidepressant Medications

A. Selective Serotonin Reuptake Inhibitors (Table 46-1)

1. **Mechanism of action. Serotonergic blockade at neuronal synaptic clefts occurs within hours of initiation of SSRI treatment.** However, the typical time to response in depression for all antidepressant medications, including the SSRIs, is 3–6 weeks; therefore, serotonin reuptake inhibition on its own cannot account for antidepressant efficacy. One postulated mechanism of action of the SSRIs involves **desensitization of serotonergic feedback receptors** in conjunction **with blockade of serotonergic neuronal reuptake;** this allows for a build-up of serotonin in the synaptic cleft with continued neuronal firing. Beta-adrenergic receptor downregulation has also been postulated, and further evidence may show that **changes in intracellular second messenger systems and gene regulation** are responsible for the therapeutic actions of these medications.
2. **Side effects.** All currently available SSRIs are equally efficacious; they differ primarily in their side effects and their half-lives. Some side effects are more common with some SSRIs than with others; however, one patient may find a particular SSRI sedating, while another might find the same SSRI activating.

   The most common side effects of all the SSRIs are nausea (which tends to be worst during early treatment), reduced appetite, weight loss, excessive sweating, headache, insomnia, jitteriness, sedation, dizziness, and sexual dysfunction (including decreased libido, impotence, and anorgasmia). Other side effects include rash, dry mouth, prolonged bleeding time, and weight gain (during long-term treatment).

   For reasons of tolerability and their benign side effect profile, the SSRIs have become the first-line treatment for depressive disorder illnesses, ranging from dysthymia to severe major depression.
3. **Half-life. Half-lives vary greatly among the SSRIs.** Although a drug's half-life does not affect its treatment efficacy or its onset of action, it is significant in terms of its side effects, its interactions with other agents, and its discontinuation-emergent symptoms. Medications with shorter half-lives may be useful when abrupt discontinuation is desired due to intolerable side effects or to medication interactions. However, medications with shorter half-lives are more likely to cause the discontinuation-emergent symptoms (e.g., tachycardia, anxiety, irritability, worsening of mood, dizziness, jitteriness, and nausea). An SSRI with a longer half-life is more likely to "self-taper" and may be beneficial for a patient who is apt to miss occasional dosages.
4. **Dosing.** Although dose-response curves have not been definitively established for the SSRIs, some patients who do not respond at a lower dose may benefit by having their dosage increased. SSRIs are hepatically

Table 46-1. Currently Available SSRIs

Available SSRIs	*Half-life (hours)*
Fluvoxamine (Luvox)	17
Paroxetine (Paxil)	21
Sertraline (Zoloft)	26 (its active metabolite has a 40-hour half-life)
Citalopram (Celexa)	36
Escitalopram (Lexapro)	27–32
Fluoxetine (Prozac; Sarafem)	84 (together with its active metabolites, *in vivo* half-life is 7 days)

metabolized and renally excreted; therefore, lower dosages may be required in hepatically-compromised patients, and this is also true to a lesser degree in patients with renal failure.

5. **Drug interactions.** SSRIs should not be co-administered with MAOIs, because of the possibility of causing a serotonin syndrome, characterized by myoclonus, tremor, hypertension, diarrhea, and confusion (see II.D below for more detail).

   Cytochrome P450 isoenzymes, including the isoenzymes 1A2, 2C, 2D6, 3A3/4, are located on microsomal membranes throughout the body. Their mechanism of metabolism is best known in the liver and bowel wall, where they oxidatively metabolize medications, as well as prostaglandins, fatty acids, and steroids. Alteration in function of these isoenzymes may cause clinically significant pharmacokinetic drug-drug interactions, via changes in drug levels. Some of the SSRIs inhibit the 2D6 and/or 3A4 isoenzymes.

B. Serotonin-Norepinephrine Reuptake Inhibitors

1. **Venlafaxine** (Effexor). **Venlafaxine inhibits both serotonin and norepinephrine uptake, though it is more selective for serotonin reuptake inhibition.** At dose ranges below 150–225 mg, it likely has the same mechanism of action as an SSRI. Its side effects are similar to those of the SSRIs: nausea, insomnia, sedation, and dizziness. **Some patients experience a sustained increase in diastolic blood pressure from baseline.** This effect is dose-dependent and may affect over 10% of patients at high doses. The half-life of venlafaxine is 5 hours, whereas that of its metabolite O-desmethylvenlafaxine is 11 hours. Venlafaxine use is contraindicated with MAOIs.
2. **Duloxetine** (Cymbalta). **Duloxetine binds selectively to both serotonin and norepinephrine transporters with high affinity, inhibiting reuptake.** Early studies of duloxetine in patients with major depression show significantly greater improvement in depressive symptoms than placebo. Adverse effects appear mild and similar to those of SSRIs, with minimal effects on blood pressure or weight. The half-life of duloxetine is 10–15 hours. Duloxetine should not be used with MAOIs.

C. Tricyclic Antidepressants

Cyclic antidepressants have been in use for nearly 50 years. **All are equally efficacious and are as effective as SSRIs. However, they have a more problematic side-effect profile and may be lethal in overdose**. The term "tricyclic" signifies a shared chemical structure with two joined benzene rings.

1. **TCA categories**
   a. **Tertiary amine TCAs**
      i. Amitriptyline (Elavil)
      ii. Clomipramine (Anafranil)
      iii. Doxepin (Sinequan)
      iv. Imipramine (Tofranil)
      v. Trimipramine (Surmontil)
   b. **Secondary amine TCAs**
      i. Desipramine (Norpramin)
      ii. Nortriptyline (Pamelor)
      iii. Amoxapine (Asendin)
      iv. Protriptyline (Vivactil)
   c. **Tetracyclic antidepressants**
      i. Maprotiline (Ludiomil) **is a tetracyclic compound composed of four benzene rings.**
2. **Categorization of side effects**
   a. **Anticholinergic effects. Anticholinergic side effects result from the affinity of TCAs for muscarinic cholinergic receptors. Anticholinergic symptoms include dry mouth, blurred vision, constipation, urinary hesitancy, and tachycardia.** Bethanechol (Urecholine), a cholinergic smooth muscle stimulant, may relieve such peripheral anticholinergic signs and symptoms. Ejaculatory difficulties and other sexual dysfunction symptoms can also occur with TCAs, possibly due to anticholinergic effects. Secondary amine TCAs tend to cause fewer anticholinergic effects than tertiary amine TCAs.
   b. **Antihistaminergic effects.** Antihistaminergic side effects result from **histaminergic H_1 receptor blockade. Common side effects include** sedation, carbohydrate craving, and weight gain. Secondary amine TCAs tend to cause less sedation than tertiary amine TCAs.
   c. **Alpha-1-adrenergic receptor blockade.** Orthostatic hypotension results from alpha-1-adrenergic receptor antagonism.
   d. **Serotonin 5-HT_2 receptor blockade.** Sedation may be related to this pharmacological action.
   e. **Cardiac effects.** Cardiac toxicity may occur in susceptible individuals and following TCA overdose; the TCAs should be avoided in patients with bifascicular heart block, left bundle branch block, or a prolonged QT interval, because they **may slow conduction through the AV (atrioventricular) node.** TCAs are **classified as class I antiarrhythmics** and must be used with great caution with other drugs from this class, including quinidine, procainamide, and disopyramide. TCAs may block the antihypertensive effects of clonidine, methyldopa, guanabenz, guanethadine, reserpine, and guanadrel and can potentiate the effect of prazosine. TCAs can cause severe orthostatic hypotension in patients with congestive heart failure due to alpha-1 receptor blockade.

   TCAs have a low threshold for toxicity; **an overdose of even a 1-week supply may be lethal.** Due to the lethality after overdose, it may be safer to treat acutely suicidal depressed patients with non-TCA antidepressants or to prescribe limited quantities of TCAs.
3. **Toxicity. Manifestations of anticholinergic toxicity** may include dilated pupils, blurred vision, dry skin, hyperpyrexia, ileus, urinary retention, confusion, delirium, and seizures. Additionally, arrhythmias, hypoten-

sion, and coma may develop. Although TCAs are highly plasma-bound and are not removed by hemodialysis, they are metabolized by hepatic microsomal enzymes. Patients who have overdosed on TCAs may require alkalinization of their serum, as well as pressors or ventilatory support to maintain survival.

TCAs should be avoided in patients with narrow angle glaucoma or prostatic hypertrophy, as symptoms related to these conditions may worsen because of anticholinergic effects. TCAs are also contraindicated with MAOIs (see below).

4. **Blood levels.** In general, **TCAs have a linear relationship between increasing levels and effectiveness. Some researchers have suggested that with nortriptyline there may be a U-shaped curve,** with decreasing efficacy at blood levels above therapeutic range, **although the evidence for this view is unconvincing due to methodological issues present in such studies.** Blood levels can guide treatment with amitriptyline, imipramine, nortriptyline, or desipramine.

D. Monoamine Oxidase Inhibitors

Monoamine oxidase (MAO) is found on the outer membrane of cellular mitochondria, where it catabolizes intracellular monoamines, including the monoamines of the central nervous system (CNS): dopamine, norepinephrine, serotonin, and tyramine. In the gastrointestinal tract and the liver, MAO catabolizes dietary monoamines, such as dopamine, tyramine, tryptamine, and phenylethylamine. The MAO inhibitors (MAOIs) are active on both MAO-A and MAO-B. The MAOIs **phenelzine** (Nardil) and **tranylcypromine** (Parnate) increase synaptic monoamine concentrations. **Both phenelzine and tranylcypromine are relatively irreversible blockers of MAO activity (A and B).**

MAOIs have a proven efficacy for unipolar major depression. **In "atypical" depression** (characterized by mood reactivity plus hypersomnia, hyperphagia, extreme fatigue when depressed, and/or rejection sensitivity), **MAOIs are more effective than are the TCAs.** The MAOIs are primarily hepatically metabolized.

1. **Side effects.** The most common side effects include postural hypotension, insomnia, agitation, sedation, impotence, delayed ejaculation, or anorgasmia. Others include weight change, dry mouth, constipation, and urinary hesitancy. Peripheral neuropathies occur and may be avoided by concomitant therapy with vitamin B_6.
2. **Toxic interactions.** When patients on MAOIs ingest dietary amines, rather than being catabolized in the intestines and the liver they are taken up in sympathetic nerve terminals and may cause the release of endogenous catecholamines with a resulting **adrenergic crisis. This is characterized by hypertension, hyperpyrexia, and other adrenergic symptoms** (e.g., tachycardia, tremulousness and cardiac arrhythmias). The amine most commonly associated with these symptoms is tyramine, but others (e.g., phenylethylalamine and dopamine) may be involved.
3. **Dietary interactions. Dietary amines can be avoided by adherence to dietary restrictions and avoiding tyramine-containing foods.** The diet must be strictly followed, but need not be as restrictive as was once thought. **Patients must be instructed to avoid:** all matured or aged cheese, fermented or dried meats (e.g., pepperoni and salami), fava and broad bean *pods* (not the beans themselves), tap beers, marmite yeast extract, sauerkraut, soy sauce and other soy products (e.g., tofu and tempe). All meats and cheese must be fresh and must have been stored and refrigerated or frozen properly. Up to *two* glasses of beer may be consumed safely; this restriction includes non-alcoholic beers.

   Since endogenous MAO activity does not return to baseline immediately upon MAOI discontinuation, 2 weeks should transpire before discontinuing the MAOI diet after MAOI discontinuation, or before beginning a contraindicated medication.
4. **Drug-drug interactions.** Avoidance of toxic drug-drug interactions with MAOIs is critical. **Medications with affinity for serotonergic receptors** (serotonergic TCAs [e.g., clomipramine], SSRIs, SNRIs, nefazodone and buspirone [Buspar]) **may result in the serotonin syndrome,** with myoclonic jerks, tremor, hypertension, diarrhea, confusion, tachycardia, fever, and ocular oscillations; in its severe form it may include hyperthermia, coma, convulsions, and death. MAOIs must be used with caution in patients with diabetes (due to possible potentiation of oral hypoglycemics and worsened hypoglycemia). Low-dose MAOIs may increase *sensitivity* to insulin, and high-dose MAOIs may increase insulin *resistance*.

   Sympathomimetics, both prescribed and over-the-counter, and relatively potent norepinephrine reuptake inhibitors, such as TCAs, may precipitate hypertensive crises. Sympathomimetics are most commonly found in nasal decongestants (e.g., pseudoephedrine, ephedrine, and oxymetazoline [Afrin nasal spray]), and also include amphetamines and cocaine. The cough-suppressant dextromethorphan can have similar toxic effects. **The hypertensive crisis is characterized by headache, stroke, pulmonary edema, and cardiac arrhythmias.** Co-administration of meperidine (Demerol) is contraindicated since it is known to cause a syndrome of fever, vascular instability, delirium, neuromuscular irritability, and death.

   The antiparkinsonian agent selegeline (Eldepryl) is an MAO-B inhibitor that becomes an MAO-A inhibitor as well at higher doses. It is not primarily used for psychiatric disorders. SSRIs and TCAs should not be given to patients on this medication due to the risk of developing a serotonin syndrome, though co-administration of bupropion is not contraindicated, at least at lower doses.

Prior to beginning an MAOI after discontinuation of a contraindicated antidepressant, the necessary drug-free time varies depending on the half-life of the previous antidepressant. At least five half-lives of the contraindicated medication are required, with two weeks required after paroxetine and five weeks required after use of fluoxetine.

5. **Medical interactions.** MAOIs are contraindicated in patients with pheochromocytoma, congestive heart failure, and hepatic disease.

E. Other Agents (Atypical Antidepressants)

1. **Bupropion** (Wellbutrin). **Bupropion increases dopamine and norepinephrine turnover in the CNS.** It is hepatically metabolized. Common side effects include agitation, insomnia, weight loss, dry mouth, headache, constipation, and tremor. It has been noted to **cause seizures, at a rate of 4/1,000 in its immediate release form. Its sustained release (SR) form is associated with a seizure risk comparable to that of the SSRIs. However, the risk of seizure markedly increases at doses > 450 mg/day in divided doses** and may be more likely to induce seizures in **patients with bulimia nervosa.** It is generally safe in overdose, though fatalities have been reported. **Bupropion is one of the safest, if not the safest, antidepressant in patients with cardiac disease.** It rarely induces sexual dysfunction, is less likely to induce it than the SSRIs, and can even be **beneficial as an adjunct in SSRI-induced sexual dysfunction.** Its use is contraindicated with the MAOIs.
2. **Mirtazapine** (Remeron). **Mirtazapine is an antagonist at inhibitory alpha-2-adrenergic auto- and heteroreceptors,** leading to increased release of both serotonin and norepinephrine at the synaptic level. It is also **a relatively potent histaminergic H_1 receptor antagonist and a serotonin 5-HT_2** and **5-HT_3 receptor antagonist.** Common side effects include somnolence, weight gain, dizziness, dry mouth, constipation, and orthostatic hypotension.
3. **Trazodone** (Desyrel). **Trazodone inhibits serotonin uptake, blocks serotonin 5-HT_2 receptors** and may act as a serotonin agonist through an active metabolite. It is also an antagonist of **alpha-1-adrenergic receptors.** Metabolism is hepatic. Trazodone is less lethal in overdose than the TCAs, though slightly more lethal than the SSRIs. **The most common side effects are sedation, orthostatic hypotension, and headache.** Priapism is a rare but serious side effect that requires immediate medical attention. Trazodone may induce arrhythmias in those with pre-existing heart disease and may increase levels of digoxin and phenytoin (Dilantin). Trazodone is **most commonly used** as an adjunctive medication **for insomnia** due to its sedating properties.
4. **Nefazodone** (Serzone). Nefazodone is **chemically related to trazodone,** with serotonin blockade but with less alpha-1 blockade. It is less likely to cause sexual dysfunction than SSRIs, and is less anticholinergic and histaminergic than the TCAs. Metabolism is hepatic. Common side effects include somnolence, dizziness, dry mouth, nausea, constipation, headache, amblyopia, and blurred vision. Nefazodone has been implicated in cases of catastrophic hepatic failure. It should be used with caution in patients with liver dysfunction, and monitoring of serum transaminases in patients taking nefazodone may be prudent. **Nefazodone is a potent inhibitor of cytochrome P450 3A4 isoenzymes,** and by interacting with cisapride (Propulsid), terfenadine (Seldane), or astemizole (Hismanal) may lead to QT prolongation and torsades de pointes. It is contraindicated with MAOIs.
5. **Psychostimulants.** Although the psychostimulants **dextroamphetamine** (Dexedrine), **methylphenidate** (Ritalin), and **pemoline** (Cylert) have not shown clear benefit in the long-term treatment of depression, they are frequently beneficial in apathetic geriatric patients, and as adjunctive medication in the treatment of refractory depression. Side effects include insomnia, tremors, appetite change, palpitations, blurred vision, dry mouth, constipation, and dizziness. Arrhythmias and tachycardia have also been reported. Pemoline has been associated with hepatic toxicity and requires monitoring of serum transaminases.
6. **Antipsychotic agents.** There is no evidence supporting the use of antipsychotic agents alone in non-psychotic, unipolar depression, though these agents are often beneficial in major depression with psychotic features and mixed episodes of bipolar disorder.

III. Special Populations

A. The Elderly

Depression in the elderly should be treated as thoroughly as it would in any patient. Since renal clearance and hepatic metabolism are frequently reduced in the elderly, lower dosages are often called for. Although TCAs are more likely to cause orthostatic hypotension than the SSRIs, they do not appear to cause a greater risk of falls.

B. Pregnancy

No clear link has been established between antidepressant treatment in pregnant women and birth defects, though the risks have not been definitively disproved either. As with all medications, it is prudent to avoid fetal exposure to psychotropics as much as possible. However, the high morbidity and mortality of depression often make this unwise. **Data regarding the TCAs, particularly imipramine, do not indicate a clear increased**

risk of fetal malformation; fluoxetine, the best studied of the SSRIs, also appears to carry no increased risk of congenital malformation. Electroconvulsive therapy (ECT) is safe to perform during pregnancy.

C. Patients with Bipolar Disorder

The risk of bipolar patients cycling into mania is 30–50% when they are treated with antidepressant medications while not on a mood-stabilizing agent. Antidepressants may even initiate and maintain rapid-cycling. The risk is improved, but not eliminated, by mood-stabilizing agents. Bupropion may have the lowest rate of "switch" into mania of the antidepressants.

D. Patients with Major Depression with Psychotic Features

Major depression with psychotic features is treated with full dosages of antidepressants. Treatment usually requires the addition of an antipsychotic as well. However, atypical antipsychotic agents, which may be associated with intrinsic antidepressant effects, may be used alone in this condition.

E. Patients with Dysthymia

Dysthymia is a chronic, mild form of depression that is associated with a high risk of superimposed major depressive episodes (double depression). There is evidence that all antidepressant classes may be useful in the treatment of this condition, although full recovery from double depression may be less likely to occur than major depression when seen alone.

F. Patients with Treatment Refractory Depression

Medical conditions, such as hypothyroidism, anemia, occult malignancy, or confounding substance abuse, must be ruled out. Often depression is labeled "refractory" before adequate medication trials have been conducted. If a patient does not respond to antidepressant treatment of adequate duration and dose, it is reasonable to increase the dosage until benefits are seen or until side effects become problematic. Duration of medication use is equally important, with at least 6 weeks of a medication trial necessary before treatment failure can be declared. A patient who has not responded to a medication in one class may still respond to a different medication of the same class, to a switch to an antidepressant of another class, or to the addition of an antidepressant which acts on different receptors, such as the addition of bupropion, mirtazapine, or a psychostimulant to an SSRI. Other options include the addition of triidothyronine (T_3), lithium augmentation, use of buspirone, or ECT.

IV. Other Indications for Antidepressants

A. Chronic Pain

TCAs are useful in many pain conditions. These include diabetic neuropathy, fibromyalgia, chronic fatigue, post-herpetic neuralgia, trigeminal neuralgia, migraine, and tension headache (for prophylaxis). Frequently TCAs have been useful for these conditions at blood levels lower than those required to achieve antidepressant response.

B. Potentiation of Pain Medications

Both the TCAs and psychostimulants potentiate narcotic analgesia.

C. Bulimia

High doses of SSRIs are effective in reducing bingeing/purging behaviors. MAOIs and TCAs may also be helpful, but the dietary restrictions associated with MAOI treatment may not be feasible among patients with eating-related impulsivity.

D. Obsessive-Compulsive Disorder

Obsessive-compulsive disorder (OCD) responds to medications with serotonergic effects, specifically SSRIs and clomipramine. Obsessions respond better than do compulsions. Typically, these medications are used in dosages higher than those needed for antidepressant response and need to be used for longer periods of time. Trichotillomania and body dysmorphic disorder may similarly respond to SSRIs.

E. Panic Disorder

SSRIs have become the first-line treatment for panic disorder. Dosing should begin at low doses, due to the jitteriness and anxiety frequently experienced at the beginning of treatment. MAOIs and TCAs are also effective, though their side effects, particularly at higher dosages, are less tolerable. It is not clear whether the atypical antidepressants are as effective as the other classes of antidepressants in this condition. Anticipatory anxiety and phobic avoidance may respond less well to antidepressant treatment and may benefit from the addition of cognitive-behavioral therapy (CBT).

F. Post-traumatic Stress Disorder

Higher dosages of SSRIs and MAOIs do not remove, but may reduce, symptomatology of post-traumatic stress disorder (PTSD). SSRIs are clearly superior to placebo.

G. Smoking Cessation

Bupropion has been shown to be effective in smoking cessation when used as part of an overall treatment program.

Suggested Readings

Alpert, J.E. (1998). Drug-drug interactions: The interface between psychotropics and other agents. In T.A. Stern, J.B. Herman, & P.L. Slavin (Eds.), *The MGH guide to primary care in psychiatry*, pp. 519–534. New York: McGraw-Hill.

Arana, G.W., Hyman, S.E., & Rosenbaum, J.F. (2000). *Handbook of psychiatric drug therapy* (4th ed.). Boston, MA: Little, Brown.

Burt, V.K., Suri, R., Altshuler, L., et al. (2001). The use of psychotropic medications during breastfeeding. *American Journal of Psychiatry, 158*(7), 1001–1009.

Fava, M., & Kendler, K.S. (2000). Major depressive disorder. *Neuron, 28*(2), 335–341.

Fava, M., & Rosenbaum, J.F. (1995). Pharmacotherapy and somatic therapies. In E.E. Beckham, & W.R. Leber (Eds.), *Handbook of depression*, pp. 280–301. New York: Guilford Publications.

Fava, M., & Rosenbaum, J.F. (1998). Approach to the patient with depression. In T.A. Stern, J.B. Herman, & P.L. Slavin (Eds.), *The MGH guide to primary care in psychiatry*, pp. 1–14. New York: McGraw-Hill.

Gardner, D.M., Shulman, K.I., Walker, S.E., & Tailor, S.A.N. (1993). The making of a user-friendly MAOI diet. *Journal of Clinical Psychiatry, 57*, 99–104.

Pearson, K.H., Nonacs, R., & Cohen, L.S. (2002). Practical guidelines for the treatment of psychiatric disorders during pregnancy. In K.H. Pearson, S.B. Sonawalla, & J.F. Rosenbaum (Eds.), *Women's health and psychiatry*, pp. 115–125. Philadelphia, PA: Lippincott Williams & Wilkins.

Preskorn, S. (1996). *Clinical pharmacology of selective serotonin reuptake inhibitors*. Caddo, OK: Professional Communications.

Rapaport, M.H., Judd, L.L., Schettler, P.J., et al. (2002). A descriptive analysis of minor depression. *American Journal of Psychiatry, 159*(4), 637–643.

Chapter 47

Electroconvulsive Therapy

LAWRENCE T. PARK, ANTHONY P. WEISS, AND CHARLES A. WELCH

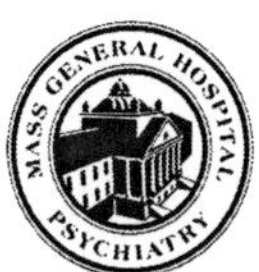

I. The Importance of Education about Electroconvulsive Therapy

A. The Expanded Role of ECT as a Psychiatric Treatment

Despite the development of several new antidepressant medications with more favorable safety and tolerability profiles, the past decade has seen a resurgence in the use of electroconvulsive therapy (ECT) in the treatment of affective illness. The reasons for this increase in the use of ECT include:

1. **Its excellent safety profile.**
2. **Its superior efficacy,** particularly in the 15–20% of depressed patients for whom adequate drug treatment is unattainable due to treatment resistance, inability to tolerate medication side effects, or an inability to take an oral medication.
3. **Its economic benefits** (due to shorter episodes of illness).
4. **The decreased societal stigmatization of ECT.**

B. Importance of Knowledge about ECT for the Practicing Psychiatrist

Since ECT remains an important part of the psychiatrist's armamentarium against severe affective illness, thorough knowledge of the indications, risks, techniques, and benefits of ECT remains an integral part of a complete psychiatric curriculum. While only a small minority of psychiatrists are involved in the actual administration of ECT, knowledge of ECT is essential for the practicing psychiatrist in order to:

1. **Know when to make appropriate referrals for convulsive therapy.**
2. **Educate the patient about the risks and benefits of this treatment.**
3. **Participate in the post-ECT management of the patient.**

II. Historical Overview

A. Early Theories

The notion that convulsions might have a beneficial effect on mental illness dates back to Hippocrates, who documented the cure of insane patients following malaria-induced seizures. The first deliberate use of convulsions as a therapeutic agent did not occur until the 1500s, when the Swiss physician Paracelsus induced seizures with oral camphor to treat mania and psychosis.

B. Meduna's Theory of "Biological Antagonism"

The use of chemically-induced seizures did not gain widespread acceptance until 1934, when a Hungarian physician, Ladislaus von Meduna, reported the beneficial effects of seizures induced by intramuscular injections of camphor in oil on a catatonic patient. Apparently unaware of previous work in this area, Meduna based his work on the idea that there was an inherent "biological antagonism" between schizophrenia and epilepsy. According to this theory, an antagonism exists between these two conditions that precluded their co-existence in an individual. While the theory was later disproved, camphor-induced seizures were nevertheless somewhat successful in treating schizophrenia.

C. Insulin Shock Therapy

Commonly known as insulin shock therapy, hypoglycemic insulin therapy for schizophrenia was **championed by Manfred Sakel, a Viennese physician, in the 1920s.** Sakel's hypoglycemic insulin therapy is often confused with convulsive therapy. In the treatment, insulin is administered to patients to induce a hypoglycemic state. This state may (or may not) be associated with seizures. Sakel distinguished between hypoglycemia with seizures (dry shock) and hypoglycemia without seizures (wet shock), and in fact thought wet shock led to more efficacious, permanent recovery.

D. Electrically-Induced Seizures

In 1937, the Italian team of Ugo Cerletti and Lucio Bini became the first clinicians to apply electricity to the head to induce a therapeutic seizure. **Like Meduna's patient, their first patient had catatonia, which quickly responded to the use of this new technique. More reliable and generally safer than the use of chemically-induced seizures, ECT rapidly gained widespread acceptance throughout Europe and the United States.**

E. Improvements in Anesthesiology

While subtle alterations in the delivery of electricity have been made since its first application (from constant-voltage sine wave stimulation to constant-current brief-pulse stimulation), the major change has come in the realm of anesthesia. Early attempts at ECT were riddled with problems, most notably bone fractures (due to the violent muscular contractions associated with the seizure), and patient discomfort (physical and mental) during the procedure. Two major breakthroughs have largely alleviated these difficulties:

1. **The use of curare as a muscle relaxant (by the psychiatrist A. E. Bennett in 1940)** allowed complete paralysis of the patient during the seizure, eliminating physical injury.
2. **The development of short-acting intravenous (IV) barbiturates in the 1950s allowed for both rapid**

induction of sedation and for amnesia surrounding the procedure.

III. Proposed Mechanisms of Action

A. Overview

Despite decades of experience with ECT, the specific mechanism of the antidepressant effect of ECT remains unknown. As noted by Sackeim (1994), more than 100 theories have been proposed to explain the therapeutic action of ECT. The most commonly cited ideas are briefly mentioned here.

B. Psychodynamic Theories

Early psychodynamic theories ascribed the beneficial effect of ECT to its fulfillment of the need for punishment in the self-loathing, depressed patient. The fact that ECT retained its effectiveness despite the use of anesthetic agents which eliminated the pain associated with ECT argues against this theory.

C. The Placebo Effect

Many writers have remarked on the dramatic and ritualized nature of ECT, believing that its beneficial effects were due to wishful thinking on the part of the staff and the patient. Several studies have demonstrated that ECT works better than "sham" ECT, largely eliminating the possibility that the beneficial effects are due solely to the placebo effect.

D. ECT as a "Memory Eraser"

Some authors have linked the beneficial effects of ECT to its ability to disturb recent memory, thereby "erasing" the recall of recent traumas that led to the depressive episode. Studies that confirmed that the efficacy of ECT were not correlated with the resultant degree of cognitive impairment debunked this theory.

E. The Seizure as Curative Agent

Since ECT is ineffective when the seizure is either pharmacologically blocked or is sub-threshold, it is clear that having a generalized seizure is crucial to the antidepressant effect of ECT. **Given the lack of efficacy when a unilateral stimulus is only marginally supra-threshold, it appears that just having a seizure alone may not be adequate.**

F. ECT as the Agent of Neurochemical Changes

ECT is associated with a myriad of biochemical changes in the brain. These changes involve the same neuroamines that are implicated in the therapeutic effect of antidepressant medication (i.e., serotonin and norepinephrine). Alteration in the concentration of these neuroamines, and upregulation of their receptors, may be at the heart of ECT's efficacy.

G. Therapeutic Effects of the Rise in Seizure Threshold

Alternatively, some believe that the chemical changes responsible for *terminating* the generalized seizure may play the largest role in ECT's effect. These chemical changes lead to a gradual rise in the seizure threshold over a course of ECT, a change that is correlated with ECT efficacy.

H. Hippocampal Neurogenesis

Some recent neuroimaging studies have demonstrated reduced hippocampal volume in depressed patients. In rat models, depression successfully treated with ECT and antidepressant medications has been associated with increased brain derived neurotrophic factor (BDNF) levels in the hippocampus and neocortex. Moreover, ECT treatment has also been associated with increased mossy fiber sprouting and neurogenesis in the hippocampus. This exciting line of research promises to augment our understanding of ECT's mechanism of action, and may shed light on the biological substrate of depression.

IV. Indications for ECT

A. Well-Established Indications for ECT

Although the exact mechanism by which ECT leads to improvement remains unclear, several neuropsychiatric illnesses are well-established indications for ECT:

1. **Major depression** (particularly with psychotic symptoms)
2. **Bipolar illness** (depressed, manic, and mixed states)
3. **Schizophrenia** (generally acute exacerbations rather than chronic illness)
4. **Catatonia** (of either organic or affective etiology)

B. Other Indications for ECT

Other illnesses for which ECT may be beneficial (but where less evidence exists) include:

1. **Parkinson's disease**
2. **Status epilepticus**
3. **Neuroleptic malignant syndrome** (in conjunction with dantrolene, bromocriptine, and intensive medical support)

C. First-Line Indications for ECT

While ECT is generally used only after medication failure, it may be regarded as a first-line therapy among patients with major depression who are:

1. **Severely malnourished or dehydrated**
2. **Medically ill and where the use of appropriate antidepressant medication is precluded (e.g., ventricular arrhythmia), and when it is not possible to take oral antidepressant medication**
3. **Delusionally depressed**
4. **Previous ECT responders**
5. **Requesting ECT**

V. Contraindications to the Use of ECT

A. Absolute Contraindications

There are no absolute contraindications to the use of ECT. **In fact, with careful anesthesia management,**

ECT has been safely applied to patients with a variety of conditions once thought to prohibit the use of ECT.

B. Relative Contraindications

Several situations do pose relative contraindications to ECT. In these cases, the risks and benefits of ECT must be carefully weighed. By reviewing the expected physiologic effects of ECT, two areas of concern become clear:

1. **Cardiovascular conditions.** Autonomic hyperactivity associated with ECT leads to significant cardiovascular effects. Initially, parasympathetic discharge predominates; it may cause bradycardia, premature ventricular contractions, or several seconds of asystole. Other signs of increased vagal tone (e.g., hypotension and salivation) may also occur. Sympathetic stimulation, an effect prolonged by circulating catecholamines, occurs later. This leads to hypertension and tachycardia. Clearly, standard ECT can place a significant strain on the cardiovascular system, and mimic the response to an exercise tolerance test. **Patients with coronary artery disease, hypertension, vascular aneurysms, and cardiac arrhythmia merit special observation and attention.**
2. **Cerebrovascular effects.** Changes in cerebrovascular dynamics can be equally dramatic, with a four-fold increase in cerebral blood flow. As a result, large rises in intracranial pressure can be seen. **Patients with space-occupying intracerebral lesions, cerebral aneurysms, or recent strokes warrant close attention.**
3. **Other conditions.** Other patients who require close anesthetic monitoring include **those who are pregnant and those who are deemed to be of high anesthetic risk** due to underlying medical or surgical conditions.

VI. Evidence for the Efficacy of ECT

A. Overview

Despite being developed for the treatment of schizophrenia, ECT has been studied predominantly in the treatment of affective disorders. While ECT remains useful and effective for a wide variety of neuropsychiatric illnesses (see IV), **the most rigorous clinical evidence exists for its use in treating major depression.**

B. Acute Treatment

ECT has been shown to be more effective than either placebo or simulated ("sham") ECT for the treatment of major depression. More important, ECT has compared favorably to several active antidepressant treatments, including tricyclic antidepressants (TCAs) and monoamine oxidase inhibitors (MAOIs). While some studies have shown no difference in the efficacy between medication and ECT, others have shown an advantage for ECT (see Janicak et al., 1997). The overall response rate for ECT is approximately 75–90%. The ongoing multi-center CORE (Consortium for Research in ECT) initiative also reports a response rate of 70–90% for major depression. Recent reports from this study have demonstrated that ECT may be particularly efficacious for elderly depressed patients. Also, for psychotic depression, response rates approach 95%.

C. Maintenance Treatment

Given the nature of major depression as a relapsing and remitting illness, treatment of the acute episode is often followed by a recurrence of depression. This may be even more of a concern after successful treatment with ECT. For this reason, the use of ECT as a maintenance treatment has been explored. At the present time, there is little prospective, randomized data to support this practice. **Existing reports, albeit largely retrospective and uncontrolled, strongly indicate the efficacy of ECT in preventing depressive relapse.**

VII. Practical Management of the ECT Patient

A. Pre-treatment Evaluation

A thorough pre-ECT evaluation is essential to the safety and efficacy of ECT. This is routinely conducted in association with an anesthesiologist and includes a complete medical and psychiatric history, full physical examination, complete blood count, determination of electrolytes, an electrocardiogram, and a chest X-ray. Depending on the patient's underlying medical condition and current medications, other tests may be indicated. The goal is to stabilize the patient's medical condition prior to ECT.

B. Informed Consent

As with any procedure, full informed consent must be obtained from the competent patient (or from a designated surrogate in the case of an incompetent patient) prior to the initiation of ECT. More than just a medico-legal formality, the process of informed consent is an opportunity for the psychiatrist to fully explain the risks and benefits of the procedure and for the patient to ask questions. Both aspects of this process help to allay patient anxiety, to improve the patient-doctor rapport, and to increase satisfaction with the treatment. Videotapes and information sheets augment, but they do not supplant, the process of informed consent.

C. Patient Care

ECT is generally administered in the early morning hours. As with any procedure that requires general anesthesia, a patient should be kept NPO for 6–8 hours prior to ECT.

D. Use of Concurrent Medications

Typically, psychotropic medications are discontinued during a course of ECT to avoid interactions. Medications often used in conjunction with ECT include:

1. **Antidepressants.** TCAs and MAOIs are discontinued routinely, largely to minimize possible cardiovascular complications. The use of newer generation selective serotonin reuptake inhibitors (SSRIs) is probably safe during ECT.
2. **Lithium.** Lithium has been known to cause delirium when co-administered with ECT; therefore, it is usually withheld during the course of ECT.
3. **Anticonvulsants.** Anticonvulsants are not contraindicated in a patient undergoing ECT, although they will raise the electrical stimulus necessary to induce a therapeutic seizure. For those patients with a pre-existing seizure disorder, it is probably safest to continue anticonvulsants and simply use a higher-intensity stimulus.
4. **Benzodiazepines. Benzodiazepines raise the seizure threshold, and may increase the degree of post-ictal confusion, particularly in the elderly patient.** Therefore, benzodiazepines are usually withheld during ECT. Pre-ECT anxiety or insomnia is often managed by prescribing a small dose of a neuroleptic or a non-benzodiazepine hypnotic, such as diphenhydramine.

E. Use of Anesthesia during ECT

The anesthetic goals for ECT are three-fold:

1. **Rapid induction with amnesia.** Over the past 20 years, **methohexital has become the agent of choice for induction of anesthesia for ECT.** As a result of its rapid onset and a short duration of action, its use is ideal for ECT. Moreover, methohexital has little impact on the seizure threshold. The usual IV dose of methohexital is between 0.5 and 1.0 mg/kg. Another widely used induction agent is propofol. The usual IV dose of propofol is between 0.5 and 2.0 mg/kg. One disadvantage of using propofol is that it raises the seizure threshold, though in most cases this does not have a significant effect on the treatment.
2. **Prevention of injury from tonic-clonic seizure activity.** While curare was the first muscle relaxant used in the modification of ECT, **succinylcholine is the most commonly used agent today.** Its popularity is based on its rapid onset, its lack of effect on seizure threshold, and its relatively low cost. In situations where succinylcholine is contraindicated (e.g., pseudocholinesterase deficiency), other agents have been used with good results.
3. **Attenuation of the sympathetic response to ECT. In patients with pre-existing cardiovascular pathology, for whom tachycardia or hypertension may be life-threatening, pre-treatment with beta-blockers may be indicated.** Labetolol (10–20 mg IV) or esmolol (100–200 mg IV) prior to induction of anesthesia have both been used to attenuate the sympathetic response to ECT.

F. Seizure Induction

1. **Electrode placement. Two standard electrode placements are currently employed for the delivery of electricity to the brain. In unilateral placement (the d'Elia placement), both electrodes are placed over the same hemisphere, typically the non-dominant right hemisphere. In bilateral placement, the electrodes are positioned symmetrically over the frontotemporal areas.**
2. **Stimulus intensity. Newer ECT devices deliver a constant-current, brief-pulse stimulus of electricity.** This technical advance has helped minimize the degree of cognitive dysfunction associated with ECT. The ability to elicit a seizure is necessary, but not always sufficient, for an antidepressant effect. Particularly with unilateral ECT, supplying a stimulus at least 50% above the seizure threshold appears to be most efficacious. This observation is complicated by the natural elevation in seizure threshold noted over the course of ECT.
3. **Seizure properties. For ECT to be effective, the induced seizure must generalize. The optimal duration of the generalized seizure is thought to be greater than 25 seconds.** Since the use of muscle relaxants started, the psychiatrist can no longer simply observe the convulsing patient to assess the quality and duration of seizure activity. In some cases, electroencephalographic (EEG) monitoring is used to determine the nature of the induced seizure. In other cases, an inflated blood pressure cuff is placed on a single extremity during the administration of succinylcholine. In this fashion, the isolated limb remains unaffected by the muscle relaxant and can be observed to convulse during the seizure.

VIII. Complications of ECT

A. Mortality

The current mortality rate of ECT is estimated at 0.01–0.03% per patient (i.e., 1–3 per 10,000). The majority of ECT-associated deaths are due to cardiovascular complications.

B. Cardiovascular Complications

The cardiovascular complications of ECT were discussed previously (see V).

C. Cognitive Complications

The cognitive side effects of ECT have been both overdramatized by detractors and under-researched by clinicians. Careful explanation of the major types of cognitive disturbance can help alleviate a patient's concern about this feared complication.

1. **Post-treatment confusion. A brief (15–30 minute) period of confusion immediately following treatment is seen in up to 10% of patients.** This is gener-

ally time-limited; it may be related to the seizure, to the effects of general anesthesia, or both factors.

2. **Delirium. Confusion associated with slowing of the EEG is common;** such confusion often delays treatment or leads to its discontinuation. The cause of post-ECT confusion is unclear, but it appears more commonly in the elderly, in patients with pre-existing dementia or neurological impairment and in those treated with bilaterally applied ECT. With cessation of ECT, delirium typically clears within days to weeks.
3. **Memory loss. ECT is associated with both anterograde and retrograde amnesia.** As with ECT-related delirium, memory impairment is more severe in association with bilateral ECT.
   a. **Anterograde amnesia.** During the course of ECT, the ability to learn new information is impaired, leading to anterograde-type amnesia. This difficulty persists briefly after ECT, and returns to baseline 2–6 months post-ECT.
   b. **Retrograde amnesia.** Loss of memory for events prior to ECT may also occur. In general, this is more severe for events closest to the time of treatment (i.e., for events leading up to hospitalization) than it is for remote events. Usually, recall is impaired for events during the previous 6 months, though memory disturbance for events occurring up to 2 years prior to ECT is not infrequently reported. For many patients, retrograde amnesia is the most significant side effect of ECT.

IX. Conclusion

ECT is the oldest biological treatment still used by psychiatrists. Although other treatments with better side effect profiles have been developed, ECT retains an important role in the treatment of affective illness.

Suggested Readings

Bremner, J.D., Narayan, M., Anderson, E.R., et al. (2000). Hippocampal volume reduction in major depression. *American Journal of Psychiatry, 157*(1), 115–117.

Dubovsky, S.L. (1995). Electroconvulsive therapy. In H.I. Kaplan & B.J. Sadock (Eds.), *Comprehensive textbook of psychiatry* (6th ed.). Baltimore, MD: Williams and Wilkins.

Hellsten, J., Wennstrom, M., Mohapel, P., et al. (2002). Electroconvulsive seizures increase hippocampal neurogenesis after chronic corticosterone treatment. *European Journal of Neuroscience, 16*(2), 283–290.

Janicak, P.G., Davis, J.M., Gibbons, R.D., et al. (1985). Efficacy of ECT: A meta-analysis. *American Journal of Psychiatry, 142*, 297–302.

Janicak, P.G., Davis, J.M., Preskom, S.H., & Ayd, F.J. (1997). *Principles and practice of psychopharmacotherapy* (2nd ed.). Baltimore, MD: Williams and Wilkins.

Miller, A.L., Faber, R.A., Hatch, J.P., & Alexander, H.E. (1985). Factors affecting amnesia, seizure duration and efficacy in ECT. *American Journal of Psychiatry, 142*, 692–696.

Nibuya, M., Morinobu, S., & Duman, R.S. (1995). Regulation of BDNF and trkB mRNA in rat brain by chronic electroconvulsive seizure and antidepressant drug treatments. *Journal of Neuroscience, 15*, 7539–7547.

O'Connor, M.K., Knapp, R., Husain, M., et al. (2001). The influence of age on the response of major depression to electroconvulsive therapy: A C.O.R.E. report. *American Journal of Geriatric Psychiatry, 9*(4), 382–390.

Petrides, G., Fink, M., Husain, M.M., et al. (2001). ECT remission rates in psychotic versus nonpsychotic depressed patients: A report from CORE. *Journal of ECT, 17*(4), 244–253.

The practice of electroconvulsive therapy: recommendations for treatment, training, and privileging (2nd ed.). (2001). A Task Force report of the American Psychiatric Association. Washington, DC: American Psychiatric Association.

Sackeim, H.A. (1994). Central issues regarding the mechanisms of action of electroconvulsive therapy: Directions for future research. *Psychopharmacology Bulletin, 30*, 281–308.

Sackeim, H.A., Devanand, D.P., & Prudic, J. (1991). Stimulus intensity, seizure threshold, and seizure duration: Impact on the efficacy and safety of electroconvulsive therapy. *Psychiatric Clinics of North America, 14*, 803–843.

Sakel, M. (1958). *Schizophrenia*. New York: Philosophical Library.

Vaidya, V.A., Siuciak, J.A., Du, F., et al. (1999). Hippocampal mossy fiber sprouting induced by chronic electroconvulsive seizures. *Neuroscience, 89*, 157–166

Welch, C.A. (1997). Electroconvulsive therapy in the general hospital. In N.H. Cassem, T.A. Stern, J.F. Rosenbaum, & M.S. Jellinek (Eds.), *The Massachusetts General Hospital handbook of general hospital psychiatry* (4th ed.). St. Louis, MO: Mosby.

Chapter 48

Lithium

DANIEL G. PRICE AND S. NASSIR GHAEMI

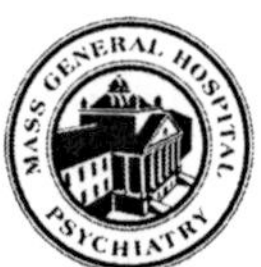

I. Overview

Lithium was the first medication to be found effective in the treatment of manic-depressive illness. It remains one of only two FDA-approved agents for mania (the other being divalproex). It is most effective in pure mania and in classical bipolar disorder (i.e., with euphoria and grandiosity). Lithium is less effective in mixed episodes, rapid-cycling disorders, or in patients with co-morbid substance abuse. Evidence exists for its prophylaxis of bipolar disorder, although naturalistic outcome studies suggest lower real-world effectiveness. Use of lithium clearly decreases the risk of death by suicide and decreases the overall mortality associated with bipolar disorder. **Unfortunately, lithium has a narrow therapeutic index, is associated with potentially life-threatening toxicity, and has numerous non-lethal side effects.** Thus, non-compliance with lithium is a major clinical problem.

II. History

In the 1940s, lithium was first reported by John Cade, an Australian physician, to be effective in mania. Double-blind studies in the 1960s led to FDA approval in 1970. Lithium was the only standard treatment for bipolar disorder until the anticonvulsant carbamazepine was found to be effective for mania in the 1980s, after which time the efficacy of valproic acid efficacy was noted in the early 1990s. **Divalproex, a formulation of valproic acid, is now the only other FDA-approved agent for use in mania.**

III. Indications

Lithium is FDA-approved for the treatment of **acute mania** and for the **maintenance and prophylaxis of bipolar disorder.** Controlled data also exist for its use in **acute depression occurring in bipolar disorder,** and to **augment antidepressants given for unipolar depression.** In addition, lithium is probably effective in the treatment of **schizoaffective disorder, bipolar type.** It has not been shown to be effective, alone or as an adjunct to other agents, in the treatment of schizophrenia, obsessive-compulsive disorder, anxiety disorders, post-traumatic stress disorder, or personality disorders.

IV. Pharmacology

Lithium is a naturally occurring cation. The standard lithium formulation is lithium carbonate. Other lithium formulations are lithium citrate, which may be better tolerated than the carbonate compound in the setting of severe nausea, and Eskalith CR, a controlled release type of lithium. Eskalith leads to lower serum peaks of lithium and may be associated with fewer cognitive side effects, such as poor concentration or sedation; however, it may be associated with more renal side effects.

The usual dosage of lithium is 900–1,200 mg/day (range 600–1,500 mg/day). It often is given 2 or 3 times daily, but it can be given as a one-time dose since its mean half-life is about 24 hours. It is dosed to a serum therapeutic range of 0.6–1.2 mEq/L (drawn 10–12 hours after the last dose), and a somewhat lower level in the elderly (0.4–0.8 mEq/L). A standard level for acute and maintenance treatment is 0.8 mEq/L (0.4 mEq/L in the elderly). **Lithium is not metabolized in the liver; it is excreted unchanged by the kidney.** Thus, its only drug interactions involve other medications that affect its renal excretion (see Table 48-1).

V. Mechanisms of Action

For many years, the mechanism of action of lithium was unknown. **Lithium has mildly pro-serotonergic effects,** but it does not significantly affect other major neurotransmitters (e.g., dopamine or norepinephrine). **Recent data strongly indicate that lithium's main effects do not occur at the synapse with neurotransmitters, but post-synaptically, at the level of G-proteins and other second messengers (e.g., phosphatidylinositol phosphate [PIP]).** It is these cellular effects that probably mediate lithium's clinical utility. **Specifically, lithium inhibits the alpha unit of G-proteins, especially those connected to beta-adrenergic receptors via cyclic adenosine monophosphate (cAMP).** By blocking the G-protein transmission of messages from these noradrenergic receptors, lithium may interfere with the neuronal activity that occurs with mania. **Similar effects on G-proteins linked to other neurotransmitters may produce lithium's antidepressant effects.** Further, lithium may inhibit PIP function when PIP is excessively active, but lithium has no effect when PIP is normally active. Thus, by its complex second messenger functions, lithium may essentially be re-establishing intracellular homeostases that underlie larger neural circuits subserving mood, accounting for its mood-stabilizing effects.

VI. Side Effects and Toxicity

Lithium has four groups of side effects: nuisance, medically serious, toxic, and teratogenic.

A. **Nuisance side effects** occur at therapeutic levels and lower, are often related to non-compliance, and are experienced as troublesome. These **include sedation,**

Table 48-1. Lithium Drug Interactions: Drugs That Increase Lithium Levels

- NSAIDs (non-steroidal antiinflammatory drugs)
- Thiazide diuretics
- ACE (angiotensin-converting enzyme) inhibitors
- Calcium channel blockers

Table 48-2. Rank Order of Reasons for Non-compliance with Lithium

- Side effects
- Indefinite intake/chronicity of illness
- Felt less creative
- Felt well, saw no need to take lithium
- Felt less productive
- Missed highs
- Less interesting to spouse
- Disliked idea of moods being controlled by medication
- Hassle to remember
- Felt depressed, thought mood would improve off medication

NOTE: Non-compliance was based on self-report by patients that they did not comply with lithium (from Jamison et al., 1979).

cognitive difficulties (e.g., poor concentration and memory), a sense of decreased creativity, dry mouth, hand tremor, increased appetite, weight gain, increased fluid intake (polydipsia), increased urination (polyuria), nausea, diarrhea, psoriasis, and acne. Polydipsia and polyuria persist in about 25% of patients during maintenance treatment with lithium. When severe, this increased urination may represent nephrogenic diabetes insipidus, a condition due to lithium's inhibition of the kidney's sensitivity to the pituitary's antidiuretic hormone (ADH, or vasopressin). Some of these side effects are treatable: sedation and cognitive effects may improve with the controlled-release formulation; dry mouth can be minimized by use of sugar-free candy; increased appetite and weight gain can be responsive to carbohydrate restriction (since lithium has a mild insulin-like effect) and exercise; nausea and diarrhea may respond to the citrate formulation; hand tremor may improve with the use of propranolol; and polydipsia and polyuria can improve with the use of thiazide diuretics (e.g., the hydrochlorothiazide/triamterene combination). **Since thiazide diuretics increase lithium levels, lithium doses should be decreased by about 50% when co-administered and lithium levels followed.** It should be noted that, because of lithium's mild insulin-like effect, the insulin regimen of diabetic patients receiving lithium may also need to be altered. Frequently, despite these measures, individuals are unable to tolerate lithium solely due to these nuisance side effects, which are the main source of lithium non-compliance (Table 48-2).

B. Medically serious side effects (excluding toxicity) fall into three categories: thyroid abnormalities, chronic renal insufficiency, and cardiac effects.

1. **Lithium's thyroid effects can occur early in treatment,** but often appear after years of use as well. Lithium has a direct reversible antithyroid effect, and thus it can lead to hypothyroidism (usually in about 5% of patients). It inhibits the thyroid gland's sensitivity to thyroid-stimulating hormone (TSH). High TSH levels on laboratory tests indicate a need to either discontinue lithium or supplement it with thyroid hormone replacement. Either T_4 or T_3 formulations can be used, alone or in combination; the most common practice is to use T_4 (L-thyroxine), since it is metabolized in the body to T_3 naturally.
2. **Lithium's effect on the kidney is more long-term,** usually seen after 10–20 years of chronic therapy. Unlike the acute direct inhibition of renal concentrating ability (including diabetes insipidus), this long-term effect of lithium is often irreversible and may involve a decrease in renal glomerular function, resulting in a mild azotemia (mildly elevated creatinine levels) in most cases. Lithium appears to reduce the glomerular filtration rate slightly. In rare instances, it can lead to severe chronic renal insufficiency and nephrotic syndrome, with glomerular pathologies of varying types. In the setting of new azotemia, the clinician needs to consider switching from lithium to another agent, although sometimes lithium can safely be continued, as long as future kidney function tests do not worsen beyond mild abnormalities.
3. **Lithium's cardiac effects** mainly consist of some decrease in cardiac conduction efficiency, which can result in **sick sinus syndrome.** Lithium can produce **blockade of the sinoatrial node,** premature ventricular beats, and atrioventricular blockade. If lithium use is essential in a patient with these effects, a cardiac pacemaker may be necessary. Otherwise, the use of a different mood stabilizer may be indicated.
4. It is noteworthy that lithium **mildly increases free calcium levels,** possibly by stimulating direct release of parathyroid hormone from the pituitary gland, but this effect has little clinical significance, and hypercalcemia is not a serious problem.
5. Lithium can also produce a **mild leukocytosis,** although this also is without clinical sequelae.

C. Toxicity

Lithium toxicity occurs in non-elderly adults, usually beginning at a level of 1.2 mEq/L (Table 48-3), with minimal side effects of tremor, nausea, diarrhea, and ataxia. Levels of 1.5–2.0 mEq/L are associated with a higher **risk of seizures.** Above 2.0 mEq/L, acute renal failure can occur and dialysis may be warranted. Above 2.5 mEq/L, coma and death can occur and dialysis is indicated. In the elderly, these signs of toxicity can occur at half the levels. **A special warning is appropriate for the elderly depressed patient who experiences diminished appetite: decreased fluid intake will quickly raise lithium levels into the toxic range.** If renal failure is produced, lithium levels rise exponentially, greatly increasing the risk of death. Dialysis is essential in such cases.

D. Teratogenicity

Early reports based on retrospective data found that lithium was associated with increased levels of congenital cardiac malformations in children of mothers treated during pregnancy. Specifically, **Ebstein's anomaly, a malformation of the tricuspid valve, was associated with lithium use in the first trimester of pregnancy.** Recent prospective studies report lower risks than in the past. However, cardiac malformations, specifically Ebstein's anomaly, are still generally thought to be a risk with lithium use during pregnancy. **These risks are probably lower than the risks of neural tube defects associated with the use of anticonvulsant mood stabilizers (e.g., divalproex and carbamazepine)** in pregnancy. Thus, in the severely ill manic patient who requires treatment, lithium use, with or without high-potency conventional antipsychotics, may at times be necessary, ideally after the first trimester of pregnancy. However, if possible, lithium use is still generally avoided during pregnancy.

VII. Clinical Effectiveness

A. Acute Mania

Lithium is quite effective in pure mania (i.e., euphoric mood), as are anticonvulsants (e.g., valproate or carbamazepine). Lithium is less effective than the anticonvulsants in mixed (depressive, dysphoric) mania.

B. Prophylaxis

Lithium has been shown in double-blind studies to **be effective in the prevention of manic and depressive episodes.** Anticonvulsants have not yet been proven in double-blind controlled studies to have this preventive effect, although clinical experience suggests that they do.

C. Acute Depression

Most studies suggest that **lithium is about as effective as tricyclic antidepressants in the treatment of bipolar depression. Lithium is safer in the treatment of bipolar depression than standard antidepressants, since those agents have a serious risk of causing mania, unlike lithium.** Lithium is also effective as an add-on treatment for unipolar depression, when given with standard antidepressants, for treatment-resistant cases.

D. Rapid-Cycling

Lithium is probably not as effective as anticonvulsants in the treatment of rapid-cycling bipolar disorder (manifest by four or more mood episodes of any kind in a year).

E. Co-morbid Substance Abuse

Co-morbid substance abuse is **a predictor of poor response to lithium.**

F. Reduction in Mortality from Suicide

Randomized prospective studies have established that lithium exerts a preventive effect on suicide, **whereas carbamazepine failed to demonstrate that effect. Lithium reduces mortality in bipolar disorder by reducing the suicide risk.** One meta-analysis of 22 studies

Table 48-3. Lithium Toxicity: Blood Levels for Non-elderly Adults (Divide Levels in Half for the Elderly)

Lithium Level (mEq/L)	*Side Effects*
Below 1.2	**Generally non-toxic**: sedation, nausea, diarrhea, cognitive effects, polyuria, polydipsia, weight gain, psoriasis, tremor
1.2–1.5	**Borderline toxicity**: moderate nausea and diarrhea, more polyuria/polydipsia, increasing tremor, mild ataxia, more severe cognitive difficulties, fine hand tremor
1.5–2.0	**Mild to moderate toxicity**: coarse hand tremor, dizziness, vomiting, severe diarrhea, ataxia, confusion
2.0–2.5	**Moderate to severe toxicity**: delirium, abnormal EEG, abnormal renal function, cardiac arrhythmias, risk of coma
Above 2.5 (dialysis indicated)	**Severe toxicity**: acute renal failure, seizures, death

SOURCE: Adapted from Maxmen, J.S. (1991). *Psychotropic drugs: Fast facts*. New York: Norton.

found a seven-fold lower suicide rate in affective disorder patients receiving long-term lithium compared to similar patients who did not receive lithium.

G. Neuroprotective Effects of Lithium

There is a growing body of literature demonstrating that **chronic lithium treatment may have neuroprotective effects.** Lithium increases levels of the protein bcl-2 (B-cell lymphoma) in frontal, hippocampal, and striatal regions. Bcl-2 is known to inhibit apoptosis and necrosis of neurons. In addition, lithium inhibits GSK-3β (glycogen synthetase kinase). GSK-3β plays a role in tau phosphorylation, an event important in the early pathophysiology of Alzheimer's disease. Magnetic resonance spectroscopy studies of the brain have shown an increase in the neuronal density marker, NAA (N-Acetyl-Aspartate), in humans treated with lithium

H. Clinical Factors Impacting Response

Chronic use of antidepressants, which often have mood-destabilizing effects, can interfere with lithium response in bipolar disorder. Psychotic features may predict sub-optimal response to lithium. Undetected or sub-clinical hypothyroidism may lead to rapid-cycling, and a poor response to lithium.

For instance, some evidence indicates that subtle thyroid dysfunction (such as a normal TSH but a low or low-normal free T_4 level) may be associated with an impaired response to, and cognitive impairment from, mood stabilizers, such as lithium. Thus, in summary, lithium response may be enhanced by minimizing antidepressant use, targeting non-psychotic patients, and optimizing thyroid function.

Suggested Readings

Bowden, C., Brugger, A., Swann, A., et al. (1994). Efficacy of divalproex vs lithium and placebo in the treatment of mania. *Journal of the American Medical Association, 271*, 918–924.

El-Mallakh, R.S. (1996). *Lithium: Actions and mechanisms*. Washington, DC: American Psychiatric Press.

Gelenberg, A.J., Kane, J.M., Keller, M.B., et al. (1989). Comparison of standard and low serum levels of lithium for maintenance treatment of bipolar depression. *New England Journal of Medicine, 321*(22), 1489–1493.

Goodwin, F.K., & Jamison, K.R. (1990). *Manic depressive illness*. New York: Oxford University Press.

Goodwin, F.K., Murphy, D.L., Dunner, D.L., et al. (1972). Lithium response in unipolar versus bipolar depression. *American Journal of Psychiatry, 129*(1), 44–47.

Harrow, M., Goldberg, J.F., Grossman, L.S., et al. (1990). Outcome in manic disorders. *Archives of General Psychiatry, 47*, 665–671.

Hetmar, O., Brun, C., Ladefoged, J., et al. (1989). Long-term effects of lithium on the kidney: Functional-morphological correlations. *Journal of Psychiatric Research, 23*(3/4), 285–297.

Jamison, K., Gerner, R., & Goodwin, F. (1979). Patient and physician attitudes toward lithium: Relationship to compliance. *Archives of General Psychiatry, 36*, 866–869.

Manji, H.K., Hsiao, J.K., Risby, E.D., et al. (1991). The mechanisms of action of lithium I: Effects on serotoninergic and noradrenergic systems in normal subjects. *Archives of General Psychiatry, 48*, 505–512.

Manji, K.H., Moore, G.J., & Chen, G. (2000). Lithium up-regulates the cytoprotective protein Bcl-2 in the CNS in vivo: A role for neurotrophic and neuroprotective effects in manic depressive illness. *Journal of Clinical Psychiatry, 61*(suppl 9), 82–96.

Manji, H.K., Potter, W.Z., & Lenox, R.H. (1995). Signal transduction pathways: Molecular targets for lithium's actions. *Archives of General Psychiatry, 52*, 531–543.

Maxmen, J.S. (1991). *Psychotropic drugs: Fast facts*. New York: Norton.

Sachs, G.S., Lafer, B., Truman, C.J., et al. (1994). Lithium monotherapy: Miracle, myth and misunderstanding. *Psychiatric Annals, 24*, 299–306.

Schou, M. (1988). Lithium treatment of manic-depressive illness. *Journal of the American Medical Association, 259*(12), 1834–1836.

Tondo, L., & Baldessarini, R. (2000). Reduced suicide risk during lithium maintenance treatment. *Journal of Clinical Psychiatry, 61*(suppl 9), 97–104.

Chapter 49

Anticonvulsants

MASON S. TURNER-TREE, ADAM SAVITZ, AND GARY SACHS

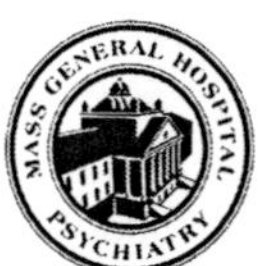

I. Introduction

Over the last 10 years, anticonvulsants have increasingly been used to treat psychiatric illness. Initially this was confined mostly to the use of carbamazepine and valproate for the treatment of bipolar disorder. More recently, with the approval of newer anticonvulsants, the use of these drugs for treatment of other disorders has expanded. This chapter focuses on both the properties and uses of different anticonvulsants. Because of the preponderance of controlled, blinded trials using carbamazepine and valproate, these agents are extensively discussed. Of the newer anticonvulsants, gabapentin and lamotrigine have been used most often and are covered in depth. Additionally, oxcarbazepine, tiagabine, and topiramate have been used for psychiatric conditions and are mentioned briefly. Clonazepam, a high-potency benzodiazepine, is also discussed because of its mood-stablizing and anxiolytic properties. **Of the drugs in this class, valproate is the only drug approved by the Food and Drug Administration (FDA) for a psychiatric illness (acute mania). All the newer anticonvulsants are FDA-approved as adjunctive medications and not as stand-alone anticonvulsants.**

We discuss each medication and compare it with the ideal anticonvulsant. The ideal anticonvulsant would have highly consistent oral bioavailability, little protein binding, a long half-life (to allow once or twice a day dosing), linear kinetics, no active metabolites, renal elimination, no hepatic enzyme induction or inhibition, and no drug interactions. The older anticonvulsants have only a few of these properties, which makes their use problematic when polypharmacy is applied in severe mental illness. Even though their efficacy in mental illness has not been demonstrated in controlled trials, the newer anticonvulsants are popular because of their ease of use.

II. Carbamazepine

A. Overview

Carbamazepine (Tegretol) is an iminostilbene anticonvulsant that is structurally similar to tricyclic antidepressants (TCAs). **It is used to treat partial seizures, with and without complex symptomatology, as well as generalized tonic-clonic seizures. Carbamazepine acts by inhibiting voltage-dependent sodium channels** (thereby decreasing the repetitive firing of neurons) **and pre-synaptic sodium channels** (preventing the depolarization of the axon terminal and the release of neurotransmitters).

B. Pharmacology

Carbamazepine is absorbed erratically and unpredictably; peak blood levels are achieved within 4–8 hours **Approximately 65–80% of the drug is protein-bound.** It is **metabolized by the liver,** resulting in an active metabolite with levels of up to 20% of the parent compound. **The initial elimination half-life is 18–55 hours;** this decreases to 5–20 hours after hepatic enzymes are induced. **Carbamazepine induces its own metabolism,** which results in the need to increase the dose after 2–3 weeks to maintain the same blood level. This enzyme induction also leads to the lower levels of many other drugs, including antipsychotics, antidepressants, benzodiazepines, oral contraceptives, other anticonvulsants, and warfarin. Co-administration of phenytoin, phenobarbital, and primidone can cause decreased levels of carbamazepine, while some selective serotonin reuptake inhibitors (SSRIs), cimetidine, erythromycin, and isoniazid lead to higher carbamazepine levels. Blood levels can be monitored to assure adequate dosing and to prevent toxicity; carbamazepine has a low therapeutic index. **When used to treat patients with epilepsy, carbamazepine's therapeutic level is 4–12 μg/mL;** although the evidence regarding treatment of bipolar disorder is less clear, the accepted carbamazepine blood level is 8–12 μg/ml. Carbamazepine is typically started at 200 mg at night and gradually increased until therapeutic levels are reached or side effects are encountered. Carbamazepine is usually given in divided dosages 2 to 3 times a day.

C. Toxicity

Carbamazepine can cause agranulocytosis and liver failure. However, these adverse effects are very rare and are thought to be prevented by routine monitoring. **Aplastic anemia and agranulocytosis occur at a rate of less than 1 in approximately 20,000 people treated. Rarer still is non-dose-related idiosyncratic hepatitis,** which can be fatal; when it occurs, it develops during the first month of treatment. To prevent a lethal outcome, a complete blood count (CBC) and liver function tests (LFTs) should be checked before starting treatment and approximately every 2 weeks after the onset of treatment for the first 2 months; thereafter, laboratory tests can be checked approximately every 3 months. **Most clinicians believe that carbamazepine should be stopped if the white blood cell count (WBC) drops below 3,000/μL, if the neutrophil count falls below 1,500/μL, or if the LFTs triple.** Common side effects include neurological (dizziness, ataxia, clumsiness, sedation, and dysarthria), gastrointestinal (nausea and gastrointestinal upset), rash (or exfoliation), metabolic (hyponatremia), and cardiovascular (intraventricular slowing of conduction, especially in overdose) problems. Side effects are usually managed by slow titration and by maintenance of the dose within the therapeutic range. Carbamazepine should be used with caution in pregnancy because it can lead to spinal malformations and possibly to liver damage.

D. Uses

Multiple studies have shown that **carbamazepine is effective for the treatment of acute mania.** Several placebo-controlled trials have demonstrated that carbamazepine works as quickly as neuroleptics in mania and may be better tolerated. Response rates are typically in the range of 55–70%. The efficacy of carbamazepine for the prophylaxis of mood swings in bipolar disorder is less clear; however, numerous studies have shown maintenance rates similar to that of lithium. Furthermore, lithium and carbamazepine have often been used in combination for the treatment of refractory bipolar illness. Some evidence shows that **carbamazepine may be better than lithium for treatment of rapid-cycling bipolar and mixed episodes.** The evidence for carbamazepine's efficacy in depression (bipolar or unipolar) is less convincing because only a minority of patients (20–50%) respond to monotherapy. Carbamazepine has also been used for the treatment of mood liability in patients with schizophrenia and schizoaffective disorder. Even with its efficacy established, carbamazepine has fallen out of favor because of its drug interactions (related to enzyme induction) and low tolerability.

However, carbamazepine may be the drug of choice for the treatment of psychiatric symptoms associated with complex partial seizures (temporal lobe epilepsy). It is better for treatment of symptoms associated with ictal events than it is for the treatment of residual inter-ictal psychotic or mood symptoms. It remains unclear if the suppression of ictal events with carbamazepine reduces or prevents the development of the inter-ictal syndrome.

Carbamazepine is also effective for treatment of pain syndromes; it was originally used to treat paroxysmal pain syndromes, such as trigeminal neuralgia (for which it is more effective than phenytoin); currently, it is used for the treatment of diabetic neuropathy, post-herpetic neuralgia, phantom limb pain, and multiple sclerosis. **Carbamazepine has also been used in the treatment of behavioral outbursts and violent behavior;** this therapeutic effect seems to be most potent in cases associated with seizures or mania. In addition, multiple uncontrolled reports have documented carbamazepine's efficacy in the treatment of behavioral outbursts in patients with head injuries, other organic syndromes, and mental retardation. Carbamazepine has also been **studied in the treatment of withdrawal syndromes,** especially those associated with high-potency benzodiazepines. One study showed that carbamazepine was as effective as oxazepam for severe alcohol withdrawal and that it produced fewer symptoms of psychological distress. Carbamazepine may also treat symptoms of protracted withdrawal.

III. Valproate

A. Overview

Valproate (valproic acid [Depakene] and divalproex sodium [Depakote]) is **an anticonvulsant used for generalized seizures (both petit mal and grand mal) and to a lesser extent for partial seizures. Its mode of action is to increase brain levels of γ-aminobutyric acid (GABA),** the principle inhibitory neurotransmitter. **It is FDA-approved for use in seizure disorders, acute mania, and migraine headache.**

B. Pharmacology

Valproate is **rapidly absorbed after oral ingestion;** peak plasma levels are achieved 1–2 hours after taking valproate on an empty stomach, and longer (3–8 hours) with food in the stomach or when the divalproex formulation is employed. **It is metabolized by the liver and has no active metabolites. Valproate is highly protein-bound,** a property that can lead to interactions with other protein-bound medications (e.g., Coumadin, digitalis, and other anticonvulsants). It has a short biological half-life (8 hours); for epilepsy, the typical dosing pattern is 3 times a day. **When used as an anticonvulsant, blood levels should typically be 50–100 μg/mL,** though they may be higher; blood levels for treatment of mania are not well established. Co-administration of enzyme inducers (e.g., carbamazepine and phenytoin) can lead to lower serum levels of valproate. Co-administration with lamotrigine leads to higher serum levels and to increased toxicity of lamotrigine. Although valproate is often started at low doses (250 mg/day) and gradually increased, valproate can be started with a loading dose of 20 mg/kg/ day for the acute treatment of mania.

C. Toxicity

The most worrisome effects of valproate are on the liver. A sizeable proportion (15–30%) of patients will develop mild and transient elevations of transaminases, which usually occur only in the first 3 months; patients generally remain asymptomatic. Cases of fatal hepatotoxicity have been reported with the use of valproate in children under the age of 10 years, usually when valproate is used along with another anticonvulsant for a neurological problem. Very rarely, major toxicities, such as hemorrhagic pancreatitis and aplastic anemia, may develop.

Side effects of valproate are most often gastrointestinal, such as nausea, vomiting, heartburn, and diarrhea (which occur less often with the divalproex formulation or when valproate is taken with food), or related to sedation, which usually improves over time. Other side effects include dizziness, ataxia, tremor, and thrombocytopenia (which rarely leads to a bleeding problem).

Long-term problems that can affect compliance are alopecia and significant weight gain (especially when used in combination with lithium). Routine monitoring with LFTs and CBCs should be done, especially during initiation of therapy.

Valproate should be avoided in pregnancy since there is a high incidence (about 4%) of neural tube defects and neonatal liver disease. Valproate may also lead to polycystic ovarian disease and to menstrual irregularities, especially in women who start the drug in their teenage years.

D. Uses

Valproate has been shown in double-blind, controlled studies to **be effective in the treatment of acute mania** at response rates similar to that seen with lithium and carbamazepine. **Valproate may be more effective than lithium in the treatment of mixed bipolar states and rapid-cycling bipolar disorder.** A few controlled studies have shown that valproate is as effective as lithium in the maintenance treatment of bipolar disorder and may be more effective in the prevention of bipolar depression. Little evidence exists for valproate's efficacy as an antidepressant.

Although not extensively studied, valproate is an adjuvant treatment for schizophrenia and schizoaffective disorder (i.e., to control mood swings and aggression). **In patients treated with more than 500 mg/d of clozapine, valproate is often added to prevent seizures.**

Valproate is also useful in the treatment of some pain syndromes. In controlled studies, prophylaxis with valproate was effective in 65% of migraine sufferers. Valproate may also be effective in the treatment of trigeminal and post-herpetic neuralgias. Two open trials have shown valproate to be efficacious for panic disorder. Case reports and a small study have shown that valproate may also be used in the treatment of benzodiazepine withdrawal. In cases of alcohol withdrawal, valproate improved symptoms more rapidly and decreased the need for benzodiazepines. Like carbamazepine, **valproate is effective in preventing complex partial seizures** and reducing the psychiatric symptoms associated with them. In addition, case reports indicate that valproate may reduce behavioral outbursts in patients, especially those with head injuries or other organic brain syndromes.

IV. Clonazepam

A. Overview

Clonazepam (Klonopin) is a high-potency benzodiazepine that is FDA-approved for the treatment of childhood epilepsy, absence seizures (petit mal), infantile spasms, myoclonic epilepsy, and complex partial seizures. Its use in epilepsy requires high doses which may lead to significant side effects. **Clonazepam acts as an agonist at the benzodiazepine-binding site of the $GABA_A$ receptor.**

B. Pharmacology

Compared with other benzodiazepines, clonazepam has an **intermediate rate of onset,** achieving peak levels within 1–3 hours. Its **biological half-life varies from 15 to 50 hours.** Clonazepam has no significant active metabolites; it is metabolized by the liver and its levels can be increased by 3A3 inhibitors (e.g., selective serotonin reuptake inhibitors [SSRIs], cimetidine, and erythromycin). Clonazepam levels can be lowered by enzyme inducers (including carbamazepine, phenytoin, and barbiturates). Clonazepam can interact with other central nervous system (CNS) depressants to cause confusion and stupor.

C. Toxicity

The most common side effects of clonazepam are **sedation and ataxia,** which occur more frequently when high doses are used. In addition, some patients become disinhibited with use of benzodiazepines. Like other high-potency benzodiazepines, clonazepam has the potential to create physiological tolerance and dependency, as well as severe withdrawal symptoms if it is discontinued suddenly. Although not well studied in pregnancy, there is some suspicion that it may be associated with cleft palates and lips.

D. Uses

Several studies have shown that clonazepam **is effective as an adjunctive agent in acutely manic patients.** Its use is associated with a reduced need for neuroleptics in manic individuals. It is unclear if clonazepam can function alone as a mood stabilizer to prevent mania or depression. A recent study in unipolar depressed patients demonstrated that addition of clonazepam to an SSRI may lead to remission of depressive symptoms sooner and prevent some SSRI side effects.

Clonazepam is **very effective in the treatment of panic and other anxiety disorders** (see chapter 44). Unlike other benzodiazepines, clonazepam seems particularly effective in treating certain neuralgias and peripheral neuropathic pain syndromes; its use is complicated by its addictive potential and by its propensity to induce sedation. It is sometimes used to facilitate withdrawal from shorter-acting high-potency benzodiazepines. Clonazepam is also used to treat neuroleptic-induced akathisia, restless leg syndrome, and some forms of agitation.

V. Lamotrigine

A. Overview

Lamotrigine (Lamictal) is a relatively new drug approved **as adjunctive treatment for refractory partial seizures. Its mechanism of action is thought to be the**

inhibition of glutamate (an excitatory neurotransmitter) release and the inhibition of voltage-gated sodium channels.

B. Pharmacology

Lamotrigine is rapidly (1–3 hours) and completely (nearly 100%) absorbed orally. It is moderately protein-bound (50–60%) and is unaffected by use of other anticonvulsants. **Its biological half-life is 25 hours,** though it is shorter (15 hours) when used with enzyme-inducing drugs. Valproate inhibits the metabolism of lamotrigine and can cause toxicity and side effects when co-administered. Lamotrigine does not affect the metabolism of other medications. It is conjugated by the liver and may cause some autoinduction at higher doses. To prevent side effects, the initial daily dose is typically 25 mg/day and increased by 25–50 mg/day every 1–2 weeks, or until a maintenance dose of 75–250 mg/day is achieved. The titration needs to be slower when used with valproate and faster when used in conjunction with an enzyme inducer. Lamotrigine can be given once or twice a day (especially with the co-administration of an enzyme inducer).

C. Toxicity

The most serious side effect of lamotrigine is rash, which may lead to Stevens-Johnson syndrome. Rash occurs in up to 40% of patients in some studies, especially when initial doses are high. A slower titration seems to reduce the incidence of rashes. Severe rashes usually appear during the first 8 weeks of treatment and require hospitalization in 3 out of 1,000 adults and in 1 out of every 100 children. Common dose-related side effects include headaches, blurred vision, ataxia, dizziness, nausea, and fatigue. Its safety in pregnancy is unknown.

D. Uses

Multiple case reports and open trials point to **lamotrigine's effectiveness in treating bipolar disorder.** These effects were initially investigated because use of lamotrigine seemed to improve energy and alertness in patients with epilepsy and may have improved some cases of depression. A recent placebo-controlled blinded trial showed that lamotrigine (200 mg/day) was effective in treating half of the patients with bipolar (type I) depression. Lamotrigine may also be beneficial in the maintenance treatment of bipolar disorder, especially among those who are rapid-cyclers. In addition, lamotrigine has been investigated in the treatment of **various pain disorders;** it seems to be effective in treating neuralgia, central pain, and neuropathic pain syndromes. In some cases, lamotrigine worked when carbamazepine and valproate failed.

VI. Gabapentin

A. Overview

Gabapentin (Neurontin) is a novel anticonvulsant indicated for **the adjunctive treatment of partial and generalized seizures.** It was synthesized as a GABA analog, but it does not modulate $GABA_A$ receptor activity. Most likely, **it interacts with the GABA transporter and increases levels of GABA.** Pregabalin is an investigational drug that is structurally similar to gabapentin and may be longer lasting and more potent.

B. Pharmacology

Gabapentin's unique properties have made it a very popular drug. The drug **is well absorbed orally** (approximately 60%). However, its absorption is non-linear because it is primarily absorbed by intestinal amino acid transporters which are saturable at higher dosages. Gabapentin is not metabolized by humans; **it is excreted unchanged by the kidneys. It does not bind to plasma proteins. Gabapentin's serum half-life is 6–7 hours,** though its CNS half-life appears to be longer. The serum level of gabapentin is increased in renal failure and is effectively cleared by hemodialysis. Its use is associated with few drug interactions. Cimetidine may decrease renal clearance, and aluminum/magnesium antacids may decrease absorption. Typically, dosing begins at 300 mg/day and is increased, as tolerated, to 900–3,000 mg/day in two to three divided dosages. Some patients cannot tolerate an initial dose of 300 mg and may need to be started at 100 mg/day.

C. Toxicity

Significant side effects are not common with gabapentin. The most common adverse effects are somnolence, ataxia, dizziness, dry mouth, and fatigue. Often these are minimized by slow titration of the dose. Systematic data have not been accumulated on gabapentin's use in pregnancy.

D. Uses

Because of gabapentin's low side-effect profile and lack of drug-drug interactions, it has been used for a wide variety of psychiatric disorders; at the present time, **there are no placebo-controlled, blinded trials of its efficacy in mental illness.** Initially, epilepsy patients treated with gabapentin showed an improved mood and quality of life. Open and retrospective trials of gabapentin in bipolar disorder have shown it to be beneficial as both adjunctive therapy and monotherapy. It seems that it may be particularly beneficial in decreasing the frequency of cycling, irritability, and anxiety. As a sole treatment of mania, it has not been effective in a large percentage of patients. In addition, case reports indicate that gabapentin can cause mood elevation and mania.

Gabapentin has been used extensively in the treatment of anxiety disorders. It has the advantage of having a high degree of safety and a lack of abusability. Although case reports and open trials of the efficacy of gabapentin exist, double-blind studies are in progress to evaluate its effects on panic disorder. One controlled study of gabapentin in social phobia showed that after 14 weeks there was a moderate response in 39% of the gabapentin group, compared with 19% in the placebo group.

Gabapentin has become the first-line anticonvulsant selected by many pain specialists. Placebo-controlled, blinded trials have shown its efficacy in treating neuropathies (diabetic and mixed) and neuralgias. Case studies of the open use of gabapentin for treatment of sedative-hypnotic withdrawal have appeared. A controlled study showed that gabapentin is effective in reducing symptoms in Parkinson's disease.

VII. Other New Anticonvulsants

A. Topiramate

Topiramate is a drug approved for the **adjunctive treatment of partial epilepsy in adults. It inhibits the rapid firing of sodium channels, enhances the GABA effect at $GABA_A$ receptors, and antagonizes kainate at AMPA (aminomethylphenylacetic acid) receptors.** It is well absorbed orally and has a half-life of 20 hours. **It has low protein-binding; 80% is excreted by the kidney unchanged, and 20% is metabolized by hepatic oxidation.** In the presence of enzyme-inducing drugs, more topiramate is metabolized by the liver, and its half-life is decreased. Although it does not induce the metabolism of other drugs, it seems to decrease the efficacy of oral contraceptives. Its main adverse effects are somnolence, dizziness, ataxia, weight loss, kidney stones, and cognitive difficulties. Cognitive difficulties affecting speech and language are insidious and affect up to 25% of patients. The typical starting dose is 25–50 mg/day, increasing slowly to 200–400 mg/day. Open studies of treatment-resistant mood disorders and mania have shown that topiramate may be effective in some patients, though the prevalence of adverse events is high.

B. Tiagabine

Tiagabine is a new adjunctive anticonvulsant whose **mechanism involves the blockade of the reuptake of GABA and elevation of extracellular levels of GABA. It is well absorbed orally with peak levels achieved in 1 hour. It is highly protein-bound (95%) and extensively metabolized by the liver.** It has **a half-life of 8 hours,** which is reduced by enzyme inducers. There are no known drug-drug interactions. The most common side effects are dizziness, somnolence, tremor, poor concentration, and confusion. One report of three patients with bipolar spectrum disorders noted improvement on low dosages.

C. Vigabatrin

Vigabatrin is an **investigational anticonvulsant available in Europe.** It works **by increasing GABA levels through the inhibition of GABA transaminase.** Like gabapentin, **vigabatrin is renally excreted, it has a half-life of 5–8 hours, and it is not protein-bound.** Side effects are common, and include weight gain, sedation, fatigue, behavioral disturbances, depression, and psychosis. Although it was withdrawn from trials in the United States because of toxicity, recent studies have shown that it may be a very effective drug for addiction; it has been studied in animal models of cocaine and nicotine addiction.

D. Oxcarbazepine

Oxcarbazepine is a **10-keto analogue of carbamazepine** that has a spectrum of action similar to that of carbamazepine but with fewer drug interactions and adverse effects. **Its only known drug interactions are an increase in plasma levels of phenytoin, phenobarbital, and valproate, and possibly decreased efficacy of oral contraceptives.** Flexibility in dosing is one advantage of oxcarbazepine, with a starting dosage of 300 mg twice daily, increasing to a maximum dose of 2,400 mg per day in twice daily divided doses. Most patients will respond to 600 mg twice daily. Oxcarbazepine does not require routine measurement of plasma levels or assessment of electrolytes, LFTs, or blood count. Rarely, hyponatremia can result with use of the drug; in high-risk populations (the elderly and those on other sodium-altering medications), routine measurement of serum sodium may be indicated. Generally, carbamazepine converts in a 1:1 ratio with oxcarbazepine and can be titrated slowly over a period of 2–3 weeks.

Suggested Readings

Deray, M., Resnick, T., Alvarez, L. (Eds.). (2001). *Complete pocket reference for the treatment of epilepsy,* pp. 92–93. Miami, FL: C. P. R. Educational Services.

Goetz, C.G., & Pappert, E.J. (Eds.). (1999). *Textbook of clinical neurology,* p. 1084. Philadelphia, PA: W.B. Saunders.

Hyman, S.E., Arana, G.W., & Rosenbaum, J.F. (1995). *Handbook of psychiatric drug therapy* (3rd ed., pp. 124–144). Boston, MA: Little Brown.

Morris, H.H. (1998). Pharmacokinetics of new anticonvulsants in psychiatry. *Cleveland Clinic Journal of Medicine, 65,* S8–15.

Perucca, E. (1996). The new generation of antiepileptic drugs: Advantages and disadvantages. *British Journal of Clinical Pharmacology, 42,* 531–543.

Sussman, N. (1998). Background and rationale for use of anticonvulsants in psychiatry. *Cleveland Clinic Journal of Medicine, 65,* S1–S7.

Chapter 50

Stimulants, Atomoxetine, Beta-Adrenergic Blocking Agents, and Alpha-Adrenergic Blocking Agents

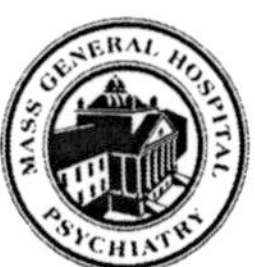

JEFFERSON B. PRINCE

I. Stimulants

A. Indications

Stimulant medication is currently FDA-approved for use in **attention deficit hyperactivity disorder (ADHD) and narcolepsy.** However, stimulants may also have efficacy **as adjunctive agents in the treatment of depression and apathy,** and they **can potentiate the effects of narcotic analgesics.** Stimulants most commonly used are **methylphenidate (short-acting forms include Ritalin and Focalin whereas extended-delivery forms include Concerta, Ritalin-LA, and Metadate-CD), dextroamphetamine (Dexedrine), a mixture of amphetamine salts (Adderall and Adderall-XR), and pemoline (Cylert)** (see Table 50-1).

B. General Properties

1. **Actions.** Stimulants have been shown to **increase intra-synaptic concentrations of dopamine (DA) and norepinephrine (NE).** Methylphenidate (MPH) primarily acts by blocking the re-uptake of DA by binding to the dopamine transporter protein on the pre-synaptic membrane. Amphetamines also diminish pre-synaptic re-uptake of DA, but they also travel into the DA neuron and cause release of DA from vesicles into the cytoplasm, prevent re-uptake from the cytoplasm into the vesicles, and cause release of more DA from pre-synaptic neurons. In addition, stimulants (amphetamine > MPH) increase levels of NE and 5-HT in the interneuronal space; compared with their effects on DA, these effects are relatively minor.
2. **Pharmacodynamics and pharmacokinetics. After oral administration, stimulants are rapidly absorbed** and preferentially taken up into the central nervous system (CNS). Food has little impact on their absorption, but lowering the pH of the gastrointestinal (GI) tract may delay the C_{max} and T_{max} of the amphetamines. Stimulants bind poorly to plasma proteins. MPH is primarily metabolized by plasma-based esterases to ritalinic acid and is excreted in the urine. Amphetamines are 80% excreted in the urine (unchanged) while 20% undergo hepatic metabolism. Acidification of the urine may enhance excretion of the amphetamines. Although the amphetamines are detected on routine urine drug screening, MPH is not usually detected.
   a. **Methylphenidate.** As it was originally formulated in 1954, methylphenidate (MPH) was produced as an equal mixture of d,l-threo-MPH and d,l-erythro-MPH. Shortly thereafter, it was realized that the erythro form of MPH produced cardiovascular side effects; thus, MPH is now manufactured as an equal mixture of d,l-threo-MPH. Studies have indicated that the primarily active form of MPH is the d-threo isomer. Therefore, the makers of Ritalin now produce Focalin (d-threo-MPH or dexmethylphenidate) as a purer form of Ritalin. Clinicians should note that in terms of potency, 10 mg of Ritalin is biologically equivalent to 5 mg of Focalin. Oral administration of immediate-release d,l-threo-MPH (available in genric MPH, Ritalin, Metadate ER, and Methylin) results in a variable peak plasma concentration within 1–2 hours, with a half-life of 2–3 hours. Behavioral effects of immediate-release MPH peak 1–2 hours after administration and tend to dissipate within 3–5 hours. Although generic MPH has a similar pharmacokinetic profile to Ritalin, it is more rapidly absorbed and peaks sooner. **Plasma levels of the sustained-release preparation of MPH (Ritalin-SR) peak in 1–4 hours, with a half-life of 2–6 hours.** Clinicians observe variability in the absorption of the SR preparation and are using it less now that several alternative extended-delivery systems are available. Peak behavioral effects of this preparation occur 2 hours after ingestion, and last up to 8 hours. Due to the wax-matrix preparation, absorption is clinically observed to be variable. Recently, several novel methods of delivering MPH and amphetamine have become available, all intended to extend the clinical effectiveness of stimulants. Even though these medications are all stimulants, their pharmacokinetic profiles differ. Concerta (Oros-MPH), the first of these novel delivery systems, has been available since August 2000. Concerta uses the OROS technology, employed by other extended delivery medications, such as Procardia-XL, Glucophage-XL, and Ditropan, to deliver a 50:50 racemic mixture of d,l-threo-MPH. An 18 mg caplet of Concerta delivers the equivalent of 15 mg of MPH (5 mg of MPH t.i.d.) providing 12-hour coverage. Initially the 18 mg caplet provides 4 mg of MPH and delivers the additional MPH in an ascending profile over 12 hours. The recommended dose of concerta is between 18 and 54 mg each day, although a recent trial in adolescents studied doses up to 72 mg each day. If Concerta is cut or crushed, its delivery system is compromised. Metadate-CD, available as a 20 mg capsule, which may be sprinkled, contains two types of beads containing d,l-threo-MPH. Metadate-CD delivers 30% or 6 mg of d,l-threo-MPH initially and is designed for 8 hours coverage. Ritalin-LA, available in

Table 50-1. Stimulants

Brand Name	*Generic Name*	*Daily Dose (mg/kg)*	*Dosing Schedule*	*Preparations Available*
Ritalin	Methylphenidate	0.3–2.0	q.d.–q.i.d.	5, 10, 20 mg regular-release tablets 20 mg sustained-release tablets
Dexedrine	Dextroamphetamine	0.3–1.0	q.d.–t.i.d.	5, 10 mg regular tablets 5, 10, 15 mg spansules
Adderall	Mixture of amphetamine salts	0.3–1.0	q.d.–b.i.d.	5, 10, 20, 30 mg scored tablets
Cylert	Magnesium pemoline	1.0–3.0	q.d.–b.i.d.	18.75, 37.5, 75 mg tablets

Generic Name (Brand Name)	*Formulation & Mechanism*	*Duration of Activity*	*How Supplied*	*Usual Absolute and (weight based) Dosing Range*
MPH (Ritalin)	Tablet of 50:50 racemic mixture d,l-threo-MPH	3–4 hours	5, 10 & 20 mg tablets	(0.3–2.0 mg/kg/d)
Dex-MPH (Focalin)	Tablet of d-threo-MPH	3–5 hours	2.5, 5, 10 mg tablets (2.5 mg Focalin equivalent to 5 mg Ritalin)	(0.15–1.0 mg/kg/d)
MPH (Methylin)	Tablet of 50:50 racemic mixture d,l-threo-MPH	3–4 hours	5, 10 & 20 mg tablets	(0.3–2.0 mg/kg/d)
MPH-SR (Ritalin-SR)	Wax-based matrix tablet of 50:50 racemic mixture d,l-threo-MPH	3–8 hours Variable	20 mg tablets (amount absorbed appears to vary)	(0.3–2.0 mg/kg/d)
MPH (Metadate ER)	Wax-based matrix tablet of 50:50 racemic mixture d,l-threo-MPH	3–8 hours Variable	10 & 20 mg tablets (amount absorbed appears to vary)	(0.3–2.0 mg/kg/d)
MPH (Methylin ER)	Hydroxypropyl methylcellulose base tablet of 50:50 racemic mixture d,l-threo-MPH; no preservatives	8 hours	10 & 20 mg tablets	(0.3–2.0 mg/kg/d)
MPH (Ritalin LA)	Two types of beads give bimodal delivery (50% immediate release and 50% delayed release) of 50:50 racemic mixture d,l-threo-MPH	8 hours	20, 30, 40 mg capsules; can be sprinkled	(0.3–2.0 mg/kg/d)
MPH (Metadate CD)	Two types of beads give bimodal delivery (30% immediate release and 70% delayed release) of 50:50 racemic mixture d,l-threo-MPH	8 hours	20 mg capsule; can be sprinkled	(0.3–2.0 mg/kg/d)
MPH (Concerta)	Osmotic pressure system delivers 50:50 racemic mixture d,l-threo-MPH	12 hours	18, 27, 36 & 54 mg caplets	(0.3–2.0 mg/kg/d)

Table 50-1. (*Continued*)

Generic Name (Brand Name)	*Formulation & Mechanism*	*Duration of Activity*	*How Supplied*	*Usual Absolute and (weight based) Dosing Range*
AMPH (Dexedrine Tablets)	d-AMPH tablet	4–5 hours	5 mg tablets	(0.15–1.0 mg/kg/d)
AMPH (Dextrostat)	d-AMPH tablet	4–5 hours	5 & 10 mg tablets	(0.15–1.0 mg/kg/d)
AMPH (Dexedrine Spansules)	Two types of beads in a 50:50 mixture short and delayed absorption of d-AMPH	8 hours	5, 10 & 15 mg capsules	(0.15–1.0 mg/kg/d)
Mixed Salts of AMPH (Adderall)	Tablet of d, l-AMPH isomers (75% d-AMPH and 25% l-AMPH)	4–6 hours	5, 7.5, 10, 12.5, 15, 20 & 30 mg tablets	(0.15–1.0 mg/kg/d)
Mixed Salts of AMPH (Adderall-XR)	Two types of beads give bimodal delivery (50% immediate release and 50% delayed release) of 75:25 racemic mixture d,l-AMPH	At least 8 hours (but appears to last much longer in certain patients)	5, 10, 15, 20, 25 & 30 mg capsules can be sprinkled	(0.15–1.0 mg/kg/d)
Magnesium pemoline (Cylert)	Tablets of magnesium pemoline	12 hours	18.75, 37.5, 75 mg tablets	Up to 3 mg/kg/d FDA recommends checking liver panel every two weeks
Atomoxetine (Strattera)	Capsule of atomoxetine	5 hour plasma half-life but CNS effects appear to last much longer	10, 18, 25, 40, 60 & 80 mg capsules	1.2 mg/kg/d

capsules of 20, 30, and 40 mg, which may be sprinkled, delivers 50% of its d,l-threo-MPH initially and another bolus approximately 3–4 hours later, thus providing approximately 8 hours of coverage. Recently, a MPH patch has shown encouraging results and may be available soon.

b. **Dextroamphetamine achieves peak plasma levels 2–3 hours after oral administration, and has a half-life of 4–6 hours.** Behavioral effects of dextroamphetamine peak 1–2 hours after administration and last 4–5 hours. For dextroamphetamine spansules, these values are somewhat longer.

c. **Adderall** is a racemic mixture of d- and l-amphetamine. The two isomers have different pharmacodynamic properties, and some children with ADHD may have a preferential response to one isomer over the other. Recent data in children with ADHD suggest that, **when compared with immediate-release Ritalin, peak behavioral effects of Adderall occur later and are more sustained.**

d. **Pemoline.** Pemoline is a CNS stimulant that is structurally different from both MPH and amphetamine and that seems to enhance central dopaminergic transmission. **Pemoline reaches peak plasma levels 1–4 hours after ingestion, and has a half-life of 7–8 hours in children and 11–13 hours in adults. A number of patients taking pemoline have developed significant hepatitis, resulting in liver failure, and in some cases death or need for liver transplant have resulted.** Given concerns regarding potential hepatic toxicity, the FDA now recommends that patients taking pemoline have liver function tests checked every 2 weeks. Although compliance with these recommendations has been scanty, pemoline has clinically become a third-line agent due to the availability of other long-acting stimulants and atomoxetine.

Tolerance to the effects of short-acting stimulants on ADHD symptoms does not appear to develop. However, this issue remains understudied, especially with the longer-acting preparations.

C. Using Stimulants

1. Attention Deficit Hyperactivity Disorder (ADHD)

a. **Short-acting stimulants are generally used for ADHD** and are typically initiated at low doses (2.5–5 mg/day for children and adolescents, 5–10 mg/day in adults), given in the morning with food. Current treatment guidelines recommend starting with longer-acting preparations in most cases. Clinicians can initiate therapy at 18 mg of Concerta or 20 mg of Metadate-CD or Ritalin-LA for MPH products or 5-10 mg of Adderall-XR or Dexedrine spansules. Every few days the dose may be increased to optimize response. While the Physicians' Desk Reference (PDR) lists maximum dosages for amphetamine products at 40 mg/d and 60 mg/d for MPH, patients often benefit form suggested daily doses of 0.3–1.5 mg/kg/day for amphetamine products and 0.5–2.0 mg/kg/day for MPH products. Frequently, patients benefit from adding immediate-release amphetamine or MPH in combination with longer-acting preparations in order to sculpt the dose to the patient's individual needs; unfortunately, the efficacy of this practice has not been well studied.

b. Numerous short-term (less than 12 weeks) clinical trials show that **approximately 70% of patients with ADHD respond to stimulant treatment;** a positive dose-response relationship is present for both the behavioral and cognitive effects of stimulants when used in children, adolescents, and adults with ADHD. Recently longer term trials have demonstrated the tolerability and continued efficacy of stimulants in patients treated continuously over the course of two years. Clinicians face a number of challenges when prescribing stimulants. Since stimulants may decrease appetite in this patient population, it is often useful to administer stimulants during or after meals. Food may even enhance their bioavailability. Stimulant-induced sleep disturbances are common and may diminish their effectiveness. Such disturbances may require alteration of the timing or amount of medication given, or require the administration of a sleep aid. Irritability or dysphoria may occur 1–2 hours after administration of stimulants, which suggests an absorption peak phenomenon which may respond to lower, more frequent doses.

2. **Co-morbidity. Usually ADHD is co-morbid with other disorders which may alter a stimulant's effectiveness.** For instance, patients with ADHD and co-morbid mood or anxiety disorders may respond differently to a stimulant, depending on the clinical state of their co-occurring disorders. In addition, **stimulants may exacerbate tics, obsessions, or compulsions**, although they are frequently used in patients with these conditions.

3. **Tolerance and abuse.** Clinicians are often concerned about growth delays, tolerance, and abuse among stimulant-treated patients. While short-term decreases in weight are often seen in children treated with stimulants, follow-up studies into adulthood have not demonstrated decreases in height ultimately attained. Although tolerance to the effects of stimulants on ADHD symptoms has been debated, **data from the NIMH Multimodal Treatment of ADHD demonstrated the persistence of the effects of stimulants.** Dextroamphetamine, Adderall, and Ritalin are schedule II medications that have the potential for abuse. While the rates of substance abuse in patients with ADHD are increased, **the use of stimulants does not appear to increase the risk of substance abuse; recent data suggest that successful stimulant treatment of children with ADHD may delay or decrease their risk of substance abuse during adolescence.** Pemoline, a schedule IV medication, has a low potential for abuse. Concerns remain regarding the addictive potential of stimulants. The design of the recently made available extended-delivery preparations make misuse of stimulants more difficult. When administered orally in their intended dosages, stimulants neither appear to cause euphoria nor appear to be addictive. The addictive potential with available preparations is thus Amphetamine > MPH > pemoline. Recent meta-analytic data show that in patients with ADHD treated for years with stimulants, the risk of substance abuse is half that of patients with ADHD who are not treated with stimulants.

4. **Narcolepsy and depression in the medically ill.** In the treatment of narcolepsy, both MPH and dextroamphetamine are used in doses of 20–200 mg/day. **Stimulants appear most effective in treating the daytime somnolence and sleep attacks associated with narcolepsy and less beneficial for cataplexy.** Recently, modafanil has become an alternative medication used in the treatment of narcolepsy. Stimulants **also have a role in the treatment of depressed, apathetic states in the medically ill or elderly, and may rapidly improve mood, interest, medical compliance, and even appetite.** Stimulants may also be **useful in reducing the narcotic requirement of terminally ill patients and diminishing the sedation associated with high doses of narcotics.**

D. Side Effects

Stimulants can cause clinically significant anorexia, nausea, difficulty falling asleep, rebound phenomena, anxiety, nightmares, dizziness, irritability, dysphoria, and weight loss. They also are associated with small increases in heart rate and blood pressure which are usually not clinically significant. Occasionally, they may elicit a depressive reaction or psychosis. Stimulant use may exacerbate tics or Tourette's syndrome. Concerns over stimulant-induced growth impairment remain, but have not been borne out. **While a physical withdrawal is not associated with stimulants, patients who have used high doses for a prolonged time may experience fatigue, hypersomnia, hyperphagia, dysphoria, and depression upon discontinuation.** Given the abuse potential of these medications, it is important to inquire about concomitant use of drugs and alcohol.

Long-term use of pemoline in children has been associated with hepatotoxicity, although reports of this are rare. Patients and parents should be educated regarding the early signs of hepatitis (e.g., change in urine and stool, abdominal discomfort, jaundice) when pemoline is being prescribed. While the usefulness of routine liver function tests remains unclear, it is prudent to obtain baseline values of serum glutamic-oxaloacetic transaminase (SGOT) and serum glutamic-pyruvic transaminase (SGPT); the FDA recommends a liver panel every two weeks.

E. Drug Interactions

The interactions of stimulants with other prescription and non-prescription medications are generally mild and not a major source of concern. Concomitant use of sympathomimetic agents (e.g., pseudoephedrine) may potentiate the effects of both medications. Concurrent use of antihistamines may diminish the effects of stimulants. Although data on the co-administration of stimulants with tricyclic antidepressants (TCAs) suggest little interaction between these compounds, careful monitoring is warranted when prescribing stimulants with either TCAs or anticonvulsants. Small cohorts taking MPH with atomoxetine demonstrated good tolerability. **Co-administration of monoamine oxidase inhibitors (MAOIs) with stimulants may result in a potentially life-threatening hypertensive crisis.** In fact, co-administration of stimulants with MAOIs is the only true contraindication to use of stimulants.

II. Atomoxetine

A. Indications

Atomoxetine (ATMX) is indicated for the treatment of ADHD (see Table 50-1). Unlike stimulants, ATMX is not a class-II medication; therefore, clinicians can provide samples and prescribe refills. Initially, ATMX was studied as an antidepressant in approximately 1,200 adults. In that trial neither ATMX nor desipramine separated from placebo, and ATMX was not pursued as an antidepressant. ATMX has also been studied, in small trials, as a treatment for enuresis.

B. General Effects

Atomoxetine acts as a selective NE reuptake inhibitor. ATMX has little affinity for other monoamine transporters or neurotransmitter receptors. It acts by blocking the NE re-uptake pump on the presynaptic membrane, thus increasing the availability of intrasynaptic NE. Data from studies in rats indicate that in addition to increasing NE in the brain, administration of ATMX leads to increased intrasynaptic DA in the pre-frontal cortex, but not in the striatum or the nucleus accumbens. This property may account for its ability to reduce ADHD symptomtology while not appearing to exacerbate tics or be addictive. ATMX is rapidly absorbed following oral administration and food does not appear to effect absorbtion; its C_{max} is 1–2 hours after dosing. ATMX is primarily metabolized via the hepatic cytochrome P450 system through the 2D6 enzyme to 4-hydroxyatomoxetine. There are a number of alternative metabolic pathways, including the 2C19 enzyme. Although ATMX is metabolized by 2D6, it neither induces nor inhibits 2D6 activity. ATMX is primarily excreted in the urine.

C. Using Atomoxetine

It is recommended that ATMX be initiated at 0.5 mg/kg/d; after a few days, it should be increased to a target dose of 1.2 mg/kg/d. Although ATMX has been studied in doses up to 2 mg/kg/d, current dosing guidelines recommend a maximum dosage of 1.4 mg/kg/d. In the initial trials ATMX was dosed b.i.d. (typically after breakfast and after dinner); however, recent studies have demonstrated its efficacy and tolerability in most patients when dosed once a day (typically after breakfast). While the plasma half-life appears to be around 5 hours, the CNS effects appear to last more than 24 hours. Therefore, most patients can be effectively treated with a single daily dose. Extensive testing was undertaken to look at the ability of patient's with relatively slow metabolic activity at 2D6 (approximately 7% of the sample) to metabolize ATMX. These studies indicated that while patients with slow metabolizer status experienced increased rates of common side effects, that these patients were generally able to tolerate ATMX. In such situations or when ATMX is co-administered with medication known to inhibit 2D6 (e.g., fluoxetine or paroxetine), clinicians should consider reducing the ATMX dose.

D. Side Effects

Compared with placebo, ATMX is associated with reduced appetite (14.1% vs. 5.8%), although height and weight in long-term use appear to be on target. Other common side effects include dyspepsia (4.5% vs. 1.4%) and dizziness (6.1% vs. 2.4%). Extensive laboratory testing suggests the ATMX causes no organ toxicity; clinical trials were not discontinued due to abnormal laboratory tests. At this time laboratory monitoring outside of routine medical care is not necessary. Similarly, the impact of ATMX on the cardiovascular system appears minimal. ATMX was associated with mean increases in heart rate of only 6 beats per minute, and increases in systolic and diastolic blood pressure averaged 1.5 mmHg. Extensive EKG monitoring indicates that ATMX has no apparent effect of QTc intervals, and EKG monitoring outside of routine medical care does not appear to be necessary.

E. Drug Interactions

Atomoxetine is metabolized primarily in the liver to 4-hydroxyatomoxetine by the cytochrome (CYP) P450 2D6 enzyme. The minor metabolite of ATMX is desmethylatomoxetine which is primarily formed by CYP 2C19. In patients with compromised CYP 2D6 functioning, multiple other enzymes were observed to be capable of forming 4-hydroxyatomoxetine. While ATMX is primarily metabolized by 2D6, it does not appear to inhibit 2D6. Although patients identified as "poor metabolizers" (i.e., low 2D6 activity) appear to tolerate ATMX, these patients do seem to have more side effects, and a reduction in dose may be necessary. Therefore, in patients who are taking medications that are strong 2D6 inhibitors (e.g., fluoxetine, paroxetine, and quinidine), it may be necessary to reduce the dose of ATMX. ATMX is contraindicated when using MAOIs. ATMX has been co-administered with albuterol (600 mcg IV) in patients with asthma. Mild elevations in heart rate and blood pressure with ATMX administration were observed. Similarly, in a small trial when ATMX was administered with MPH it appeared to be well tolerated, although co-administration of ATMX and the stimulants has not been fully studied.

III. Beta-Adrenergic Blockers

A. Indications

Beta-blockers have a variety of uses in psychiatry. They are frequently used in the treatment of performance anxiety, lithium-induced tremor, and neuroleptic-induced akathisia. They are also reported to be useful in the control of aggressive outbursts in patients with brain injury, autism, or mental retardation. They have also been used in combination with other agents in the treatment of panic disorder, generalized anxiety disorder (GAD), post-traumatic stress disorder (PTSD), ethanol withdrawal, ADHD, and with severe aggression or impulsivity. Recently, Pindolol, a beta-5-hydroxytrytamine-1A ($5\text{-}HT_{1A}$) antagonist, has been used to accelerate or enhance the antidepressive and antianxiety properties of the selective serotonin reuptake inhibitors (SSRIs). In total, the results of such trials have been mixed. Recently, propranolol, administered soon after a traumatic event, has been studied as a means of reducing the manifestations of PTSD. Their non-psychiatric uses include the treatment of hypertension, arrhythmia, neurally-mediated hypotension, migraine prophylaxis, glaucoma, symptoms of thyrotoxicosis, and acute myocardial infarction. The beta-blockers most commonly used in psychiatry include propranolol, nadolol, metoprolol, and atenolol (see Tables 50-2 and 50-3). Other options clinicans should consider include the long-acting beta-1-selective antagonist betaxolol. It has excellent oral bioavalability, a long serum half-life (16 hours), little first-pass metabolism, and it is highly beta-1-selective.

B. General Effects

Beta-blockers act as competitive antagonists of epinephrine and NE at post-synaptic beta-adrenergic receptors. Peripherally, epinephrine and NE modulate control of blood pressure and are released as stress hormones by the adrenal medulla. **Beta-1 receptors are located on the heart; they stimulate it chronotropically and inotropically. Beta-2 receptors are found in the lung and on blood vessels. Beta-2 receptor stimulation produces bronchodilation and vasodilation.** Centrally, the role of epinephrine is limited; however, the noradrenergic system is involved in the regulation of anxiety, mood, hormone release, sleep, pain, and vigilance. In the brain, beta-1 receptors are located on neurons throughout the noradrenergic system, while beta-2 receptors are primarily located on glial cells.

Beta-blockers differ in their selectivity of beta-1 and beta-2 receptor blockade, lipophilicity, route of elimination, and half-life (see Table 50-3). Propranolol and nadolol are non-selective beta-blockers, while metoprolol and atenolol are selective beta-1 receptor antagonists. These medications differ in their lipophilicity, which distinguishes their central and peripheral effects. **Propranolol and metoprolol are highly lipophilic and thus easily cross the blood-brain barrier, whereas atenolol and nadolol have very little central effect.** Propranolol and metoprolol are metabolized by hepatic enzymes, whereas atenolol and nadolol are eliminated by the kidneys.

C. Using Beta-Blockers

1. **General guidelines. Beta-blockers should be started at low doses, and gradually titrated up.** Patients should be educated about how to monitor blood pressure and pulse. Side effects (e.g., hypotension, dizziness, bradycardia, and bronchospasm) should be monitored. Doses should be held if blood pressure is less

Table 50-2. Beta-Adrenergic Blockers: Dosing Schedules

Brand Name	*Generic Name*	*Daily Dose (mg/day)*	*Dosing Schedule*	*Preparations Available (mg)*
Inderal	Propranolol	10–640	b.i.d.–t.i.d.	10, 20, 40, 60, 80, 90
Inderal-LA	Propranolol-LA	80–320	q.d.	60, 80, 120, 160
Lopressor	Metoprolol	50–450	b.i.d.–t.i.d.	50, 100
Toprol XL	Metoprolol-XL	50–400	q.d.	50, 100, 200
Tenormin	Atenolol	25–100	q.d.	25, 50, 100
Corgard	Nadolol	20–320	q.d.	20, 40, 80, 120, 160

Table 50-3. Beta-Adrenergic Blockers: Pharmacological Properties

Medication	*Selectivity*	*Lipophilicity*	*Half-life (hours)*	*Route of Elimination*
Inderal (propranolol)	Beta-1, beta-2	High	3–6	Liver
Lopressor (metoprolol)	Beta-1	High	3–4	Liver
Tenormin (atenolol)	Beta-1	Low	6–9	Kidney
Corgard (nadolol)	Beta-1, beta-2	Low	14–24	Kidney

than 90/60 mmHg or the pulse is less than 55 beats/minute.

In adults, propranolol should be started in dosages of 10 mg t.i.d. when using the regular-release preparation, or at 80 mg q.d. for the long-acting (LA) preparation. Propranolol may be titrated up (until the desired therapeutic effect is achieved) with a maximum dose of 640 mg/day of the regular preparation and 320 mg/day of the LA form. In children the dosage range is generally 1–5 mg/kg/day. Metoprolol is usually begun at 50 mg b.i.d., with a maximum dosage of 450 mg/day of the regular-release preparation; the extended-release form is begun at 50 mg q.d. with a maximum of 400 mg/day. Nadolol is started at 20 mg q.d. with a maximum of 320 mg/day. Atenolol is begun at 25 mg q.d. with a maximum of 100 mg/day.

2. **Use in selected conditions. When selecting a beta-blocker, consideration needs to be given to the desired therapeutic effect as well as to the patient's other conditions.**
   a. For **performance anxiety** a single dose of 10–40 mg of propranolol given 30 minutes prior to the event is often useful. A test dose in an anxiety-provoking environment, but prior to the actual event, is usually indicated to assess tolerability. Since most symptoms of performance anxiety are peripheral, less lipophilic compounds (e.g., nadolol or atenolol) may be equally useful.
   b. **Lithium-induced tremor** often responds to propranolol 20–160 mg/day. Nadolol or atenolol may be as effective, and lessen concern over worsening of depression by beta-blockers.
   c. For **neuroleptic-induced akathisia,** both propranolol (30–80 mg/day) and nadolol (40–80 mg/day) are reported useful.
   d. Atenolol (50–100 mg/day) has utility as an adjunct to benzodiazepines in treatment of **the hyperaroused state associated with ethanol withdrawal.** Beta-blockers are not adequate as a single medicine for detoxification.
   e. In the treatment of **ADHD,** propranolol (in dosages up to 640 mg/day) has been found to be useful in adults with severe temper outbursts. Several clinical reports indicate that combining beta-blockers with stimulants may be useful in improving the tolerability of the stimulants.
   f. There are reports of using high doses of propranolol (range 50–1,600 mg/day) to control **aggressive outbursts** in children and in adults with organic brain dysfunction.
   g. Several open case series describe the utility of propranolol (dosages 2.5 mg/kg/day) in the treatment of children with PTSD.

D. Side Effects

Beta-blockers may have a variety of clinically significant side effects, including hypotension, bradycardia, dizziness, bronchoconstriction (less problematic with selective agents), nausea, diarrhea, constipation, impotence, fatigue, depression, insomnia, vivid dreams, worsening of hypoglycemia in patients with diabetes, and rebound hypertension (if abruptly discontinued). Less frequent reactions include Raynaud's phenomenon, Peyronie's disease, psychosis, and allergic reactions. Beta-blockers may also suppress melatonin and may potentiate the effects of growth hormone. Beta-blockers have little adverse effect on memory, and they may enhance performance. Although conventional wisdom suggests that beta-blockers are associated with increased risk of depression, fatigue, and sexual dysfunction, a recent large meta-analysis of patients treated with beta-blockers for hypertension, heart failure, or after myocardial infaction observed no increase in the risk of depression and only small increases in the risk of fatigue and sexual dysfunction.

E. Drug Interactions

Beta-blockers that are metabolized hepatically (i.e., propranolol and metoprolol) are primarily metabolized by the cytochrome P450 2D6 enzyme. **Thus, medications that inhibit 2D6 activity (e.g., fluoxetine, sertraline, desipramine, clomipramine, haloperidol, fluphenazine, paroxetine, and thioridazine) will increase the levels of these beta-blockers, necessitating a decrease in dosage. Similarly, medications that induce 2D6 activity (e.g., carbamazepine, phenobarbital, phenytoin, and rifampin) may increase the metabolism of these beta-blockers, which results in decreased effects.** There have been reports of increased levels of theophylline, thyroxine, and imipramine after the addition of beta-blockers. Propranolol is highly protein-bound; this is an important factor when considering drug interactions.

IV. Alpha-Adrenergic Blockers

A. Indications

Clonidine (Catapres) has been used in the treatment of **hypertension** in adults since the 1960s. In psychiatry, clonidine has been used for **opioid withdrawal, nicotine withdrawal, Tourette's syndrome, ADHD, mania, neuroleptic-induced akathisia, behavioral dyscontrol in autism, anxiety disorders, PTSD, and sleep disturbances.** Recently, guanfacine (Tenex) has been used for PTSD, ADHD, Tourette's syndrome, and sleep disorders (see Table 50-4).

B. General Effects

Alpha-2-adrenergic receptors are widely distributed in the brain. Pre-synaptic alpha-2-adrenergic receptors are located on noradrenergic neurons in the locus coeruleus and the brainstem. These receptors function as inhibitory autoreceptors to suppress cell firing, inhibit release of NE, and downregulate central noradrenergic neurotransmission. Post-synaptic alpha-2-adrenergic receptors modulate neuronal excitability and regulate release of neurotransmitters (e.g., dopamine and serotonin) and hormones (e.g., growth hormone).

Clonidine is an imidazoline derivative with alpha-2-adrenergic agonist properties. Clonidine is almost completely absorbed after oral administration and achieves peak plasma concentrations in 1–3 hours. Clonidine's plasma half-life ranges from 8–12 hours in children to 12–16 hours in adults. Clonidine is highly lipophilic and easily crosses the blood-brain barrier. **While some clonidine is metabolized by the liver, most is excreted unchanged by the kidney.**

Guanfacine is a longer-acting, less sedating, and more selective alpha-2-adrenergic agonist. Guanfacine is eliminated by renal excretion; it has an excretion half-life of 17 hours in adults. **Guanfacine appears more selective than clonidine for the alpha-2_A-adrenergic receptor.** This characteristic may prove advantageous as these receptors appear to be located primarily in the prefrontal cortex. Thus, guanfacine may have a more selective beneficial effect on attention.

C. Using Clonidine and Guanfacine

When using these medications, it is critical to begin at a low dose and titrate upward slowly because of sedation and adverse cardiovascular effects. Clonidine is manufactured in tablets of 0.1, 0.2, and 0.3 mg. Depending on the age and size of the patient, clonidine is generally begun at one-half of a 0.1 mg tablet once or twice a day. Titration should proceed slowly and carefully until the desired benefit is reached. The behavioral effects of clonidine seem to last between 3 and 6 hours, and thus multiple daily doses are usually required. There is also a transdermal therapeutic system (Catapres-TTS). The patch provides more sustained coverage and eliminates the need for repeated doses. It should be placed on a clean, dry, hairless piece of skin. The patch can be irritating to the skin, and dermatitis can limit its tolerability. A recent multi-site trial demonstrated the efficacy of clonidine used alone and in combination with MPH to treat patients with ADHD and tic disorders. This trial is reassuring, both as a treatment for patients with ADHD and tics, as well as providing safety data regarding the combination of stimulants with clonidine.

Guanfacine is generally less sedating than is clonidine and is used in the treatment of ADHD, tic disorders, and to some degree in sleep disorders. Two uncontrolled studies noted improvements in hyperactivity, inattention, and immaturity with no effect on mood or aggression. **Guanfacine is one-tenth as potent as clonidine.** It is generally begun with one-half of a 1 mg tablet daily and gradually titrated upward until the desired benefit is achieved. It is important not to confuse the dosages of clonidine and guanfacine.

D. Side Effects

The alpha-adrenergic agonists may have several clinically significant side effects, including **dry mouth or eyes, sedation, postural hypotension, fatigue, vivid dreams or nightmares, nausea, and depression.** Cardiac side effects, including **dysrhythmia, bradycardia, non-conducted P waves, supraventricular premature complexes, intraventricular conduction delays, and T-wave abnormalities,** have been described. Rare idiosyncratic side effects include hallucinations, rash, pruritus, alopecia, hyperglycemia, gynecomastia, and an increased sensitivity to alcohol. If these medications are abruptly withdrawn, there is a risk (especially when used in doses greater than 0.6 mg/day) of a rebound hypertensive crisis. Symptoms usually begin 18–20 hours after the last dose. These medications should be tapered, not abruptly discontinued. Dermatitis may develop if the

Table 50-4. Alpha-Adrenergic Blockers

Brand Name	*Generic Name*	*Daily Dose (mg/day)*	*Dosing Schedule*	*Preparations Available*
Catapres-TTS	Catapres-TTS	0.1–0.9	One patch per week	0.1, 0.2, 0.3 mg patches
Catapres	Clonidine	0.05–2.4	q.d.–q.i.d.	0.1, 0.2, 0.3 mg tablets
Tenex	Guanfacine	0.5–3	q.d.–t.i.d.	1, 2 mg tablets

transdermal patch is used; this may be treated with hydrocortisone cream.

E. Drug Interactions

Clonidine should not be administered concomitantly with beta-blockers since severe adverse reactions have been reported. Recently, concerns have been raised regarding the concomitant administration of clonidine and MPH. However, it should be noted that in patients with conditions associated with high adrenergic output (i.e., nicotine or opioid withdrawal or cocaine overdose), clonidine is frequently administred. Similarly, in patients with clonidine overdose, beta-adreneric medications are often administered. Lastly, a recent large multi-center trial (using the combination of MPH and clonidine in the treatment of ADHD and tics) demonstrated that the combination had good tolerability and efficacy.

Suggested Readings

Hyman, S.E., Arana, G.W., & Rosenbaum, J.F. (1995). *Handbook of psychiatric drug therapy* (3rd ed.). Boston, MA: Little Brown.

Practice parameter for the use of stimulant medications in the treatment of children, adolescents, and adults. Supplement to the *Journal of the American Academy of Child and Adolescent Psychiatry*. (2002). Vol. 41 (2): 26S–49S.

Spencer, T., Biederman, J., & Wilens, T. (1997). Pharmacotherapy of ADHD: A life span perspective. In J. Oldham, & M. Riba (Eds.), *American Psychiatric Press review of psychiatry*, Vol. 18, pp. 87–128. Washington, DC: American Psychiatric Association.

Wilens, T.E., Biederman, J., & Spencer, T.J. (1997). Psychopharmacology for children and adolescents. In N.H. Cassem, T.A. Stern, J.F. Rosenbaum, & M.S. Jellinek (Eds.), *Massachusetts General Hospital handbook of general hospital psychiatry* (4th ed., pp. 467–486). St. Louis, MO: Mosby.

Wilens, T., Biederman, J., & Spencer, T. (2002). Attention deficit hyperactivity disorder. In Caskey (Ed.), *Annual review of medicine*, Vol. 53, 113–131.

Chapter 51

Drug-Drug Interactions in Psychopharmacology

JONATHAN E. ALPERT

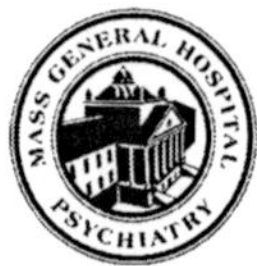

I. Introduction

Drug-drug interactions refer to alterations in drug levels and/or drug effects attributed to the administration of two or more prescribed, illicit, or over-the-counter agents in close temporal proximity. While many drug-drug interactions involve drugs administered within minutes to hours of each other, some drugs are implicated in interactions days to weeks after their discontinuation by virtue of their long half-lives and/or long-term impact on the activity of metabolic enzymes. Therefore, **recent as well as current drug use must be considered in the evaluation of potential drug-drug interactions.**

II. Relevance to Clinical Decisions

A. **Drug-drug interactions involving psychotropic medications are ubiquitous,** particularly among patients with treatment-refractory psychiatric disorders and those with co-morbid psychiatric or medical illnesses who are likely to require multiple medications.

B. Fortunately, **most drug-drug interactions between psychotropic and other medications do not contraindicate their combined use.** Rather, awareness of such interactions should prompt particularly close attention to dosing, monitoring, and patient education, and should facilitate the timely assessment and treatment of patients who present with unexpected symptomatology or blood levels.

C. The anticipated **clinical significance of drug-drug interactions must be judged in comparison with the influence of other factors** that may alter drug responses, including **age, gender, hepatic or renal disease, smoking, alcohol use, nutritional status, dietary habits, compliance with recommended dosing, and genetic polymorphisms** in the activity of metabolic enzymes. These factors often account for considerable inter-individual variability in the response to medication in the context of which the additional impact of some drug-drug interactions may be small.

D. **Consideration of potential drug-drug interactions is particularly crucial when:**

1. **Medications** (including **digoxin** [Lanoxin], **warfarin** [Coumadin], **theophylline** [Slo-bid, Theodur], **carbamazepine** [Tegretol], and **lithium** [Eskalith, Lithobid, Lithonate]) **with a low therapeutic index** (i.e., for which the margin between a toxic dose and a therapeutic dose is small) are prescribed.
2. **Medications,** such as **nortriptyline** (Pamelor), **with a narrow therapeutic margin** (i.e., drugs that are thought to be relatively ineffective at doses below and above a specified therapeutic range), are prescribed.
3. **Drugs associated with rare but catastrophic drug-drug interactions** (hypertensive crises [**monoamine oxidase inhibitors**] or cardiac arrythmias [**pimozide** (Orap), **cisapride** (Propulsid)]) are used.
4. **Medications or other substances known to be potent inducers (e.g., carbamazepine, rifampin), or inhibitors (e.g., ketoconazole) of metabolism** are used.

E. **Enhanced surveillance for drug-drug interactions is also important when:**

1. **A perplexing clinical picture** evolves, including **unexplained mental status changes, clinical deterioration** or **refractoriness to standard treatment,** or unexpectedly **extreme or erratic drug plasma levels.**
2. **Clinical states** (including liver and kidney disease, cachexia, gastrectomy, and congestive heart failure) **are present in which drug absorption, serum protein-binding, and/or elimination may be markedly altered.**
3. **Elderly or medically unstable patients** are placed at risk for adverse effects, such as hypotension or urinary retention, that pose particular hazards.
4. A **drug overdose** has occurred, in which the quantity of drug ingested may lead to significant interactions not typically observed within the usual dose range.

F. **Certain drug-drug interactions may be used to advantage** in clinical settings:

1. **Reversal of central nervous system (CNS) depression** with naloxone (Narcan) following opiate overdose or with flumazenil (Romazicon) following benzodiazepine overdose.
2. **Treatment** of anticholinergic-induced side effects (e.g., urinary retention) with bethanechol (Urecholine), or extrapyramidal symptoms associated with antipsychotic medications with benztropine (Cogentin).
3. **Enhancement of drug activity or elimination half-life,** via augmentation of conventional antidepressant medications (with agents such as lithium or buspirone), or inhibition of metabolism of cytochrome P450 isoenzyme substrates (such as cyclosporine), in the presence of specific isoenzyme inhibitors (such as ketoconazole), to reduce the need for high doses and/or to reduce the frequency of administration.

III. Classification

Drug-drug interactions may be described as idiosyncratic, pharmacodynamic, or pharmacokinetic on the basis of the presumed mechanism of interaction.

A. **Idiosyncratic interactions occur unpredictably** in a small number of patients and are **unexpected from the known pharmacokinetic and pharmacological properties** of the drugs involved.

1. **Evidence for such interactions is often inconclusive** and based upon a small number of case reports concerning complex patients on complicated medical regimens.
2. Examples include sporadically reported cases of reversible or irreversible neurotoxicity associated with the combined use of **lithium** and **verapamil** (Calan, Isoptin), or the administration of either drug with **carbamazepine** (Tegretol).

B. **Pharmacodynamic interactions involve a known, direct pharmacological effect at biologically active (receptor) sites and do not involve an alteration in drug plasma levels.** These interactions may be additive, synergistic, or antagonistic. They may occur when two or more drugs interact with the same site or when these drugs interact with interrelated sites.

1. Knowledge about pharmacodynamic interactions is often based upon prediction from basic and pre-clinical studies and subsequent confirmation in clinical case reports.
2. Examples of pharmacodynamic drug-drug interactions include:
   a. **CNS depression,** when **alcohol, benzodiazepines,** and/or **barbiturates** are used concurrently.
   b. **Cardiac conduction delays,** when **drugs with quinidine-like effects** (including **low-potency antipsychotics,** such as chlorpromazine [Thorazine], **tricyclic antidepressants** (TCAs) such as amitriptyline [Elavil], and/or **class I antiarrhythmics,** such as disopyramide [Norpace]) are co-administered.
   c. **Anticholinergic toxicity (including ileus, urinary retention, hyperthermia, and delirium)** when drugs sharing antimuscarinic properties (including **TCAs, low-potency antipsychotics, and diphenhydramine** [Benadryl]) are combined.
   d. **Hypotension,** when **drugs associated with alpha-1-adrenergic blockade** (including **atypical and heterocyclic antidepressants, such as trazodone or imipramine, low-potency antipsychotics, and atypical antipsychotics, such as clozapine** [Clozaril] **and olanzapine** [Zyprexa]) are used together.
   e. **The interference with a dopamine agonist or precursor during treatment** of Parkinson's disease or hyperprolactinemia via concurrent administration of **antipsychotic drugs.**

C. **Pharmacokinetic interactions involve a change in the plasma level and/or tissue distribution of drugs, rather than in their pharmacological activity.** Pharmacokinetic interactions are mediated by effects on drug **absorption, distribution, metabolism, or excretion.**

1. **Drug-drug interactions affecting drug absorption may reduce or enhance the bioavailability of orally administered drugs.** Examples include the effect of drugs that:
   a. **Accelerate gastric emptying (metoclopramide** [Reglan], **cisapride** [Propulsid]) or **diminish intestinal motility** (TCAs, morphine, cannabis), potentially promoting greater contact with and absorption from the mucosal surface of the small intestine.
   b. **Bind to other drugs (cholestyramine** [Questran], **charcoal, kaolin-pectin, non-absorbable fats**) forming complexes that pass unabsorbed through the intestinal lumen.
   c. **Alter gastric pH** (aluminum hydroxide, magnesium hydroxide, sodium bicarbonate), potentially altering the non-polar, unionized fraction of drug available for absorption.
   d. **Inhibit metabolic enzymes present in stomach or intestine** (e.g., monoamine oxidase and cytochrome P450 3A4), potentially retarding local degradation of certain drugs or other exogenous substances metabolized by those enzymes (e.g., tyramine), resulting in elevated concentration of these substrates that reach the portal circulation.
2. **Drug distribution from the systemic circulation to tissue depends on a variety of factors, including regional blood flow, lipophilicity, amount of drug bound to tissue and plasma proteins, and the adipose to lean body mass ratio of the individual.** Examples of drug-drug interactions that may influence distribution include:
   a. Competition for protein-binding sites by two or more drugs that may result in displacement of a previously bound drug (which, in the unbound state, becomes available for pharmacological activity). **Most psychotropic drugs are more than 80% protein-bound and many are more than 90% protein-bound ("highly protein-bound") to albumin, alpha-1-acid glycoproteins, or lipoproteins. Exceptions** include **lithium, gabapentin** (Neurontin), **topiramate** (Topamax), **oxcarbazine** (Trileptal), and **venlafaxine** (Effexor), which are minimally protein-bound, and **escitalopram** (Lexapro), **citalopram** (Celexa), **fluvoxamine** (Luvox), **bupropion** (Wellbutrin), **modafinil** (Provigil), **molindone** (Moban), **quetiapine** (Seroquel), **lamotrigine** (Lamictal), **and carbamazepine** (Tegretol), which are moderately (60–85%) protein-bound. While **potentially vital to the dosing and monitoring of drugs with a low therapeutic index** (e.g., **warfarin**), the practical significance of protein-binding interactions for clinical management is otherwise often small, since the transient rise in plasma concentrations

due to displacement of previously bound drug is offset by rapid redistribution of active drug to tissue where it is metabolized and excreted.

b. **Alterations in regional blood flow** produced by one drug may impede or enhance delivery of other drugs to relevant receptors in tissue.

c. **Competition for, or other interference with, active transport to tissue** (e.g., across the blood-brain barrier) may hinder access of some agents to relevant receptor sites. **Drug transport proteins, including P-glycoprotein, appear to play critical roles in regulating permeability of intestinal epithelia, lymphocytes, and the blood brain barrier.** Some drug interactions may involve direct effects on P-glycoprotein and related transport proteins.

3. Most drugs undergo several types of **metabolism (biotransformation),** usually enzyme-mediated, resulting in metabolites that may or may not be pharmacologically active. Many clinically important pharmacokinetic drug-drug interactions involving psychotropic drugs are based upon interference with this process.

a. **Phase I metabolic reactions (including oxidation, reduction), and hydrolysis reactions, produce intermediate metabolites which then undergo phase II metabolic reactions (including glucuronidation and acetylation), that result in highly polar, water-soluble metabolites suitable for renal excretion.** Most psychotropic drugs undergo both phase I and phase II reactions. Exceptions include the **3-hydroxy-substituted benzodiazepines (lorazepam** [Ativan], **oxazepam** [Serax], **and temazepam** [Restoril]) **and clonazepam** (Klonopin), **which undergo only phase II reactions** (glucuronidation and acetylation, respectively). **Lithium and gabapentin** (Neurontin) **are excreted by the kidneys without undergoing biotransformation in the liver.**

b. A growing understanding of metabolic enzymes, particularly the **cytochrome P450 isoenzymes,** has contributed to more rational prediction of drug-drug interactions (see IV). Other enzyme systems (including **flavin-containing mono-oxygenases** [FMOs], ***N*-acetyltransferase, glucuronyltransferases, methyltransferases, and sulfotransferases**) are also critical for the metabolism of a variety of drugs. Many drugs utilize multiple enzyme pathways for metabolism, potentially moderating the impact of drug-drug interactions that affect a single enzyme.

c. Some drugs are closely associated with metabolic induction or inhibition of other medications and are therefore frequently involved in drug-drug interactions (Tables 51-1 and 51-2). **Introduction of inducing agents results in increased synthesis of metabolic enzymes, thereby producing a slow decline over days to weeks in the blood levels of the co-administered drugs that they metabolize.** The discontinuation of inducing agents is associated with a gradual increase in those levels. **Introduction of agents that inhibit metabolic enzymes results in a typically abrupt elevation over hours to days of blood levels of co-administered drugs whose metabolism they inhibit.** The discontinuation of metabolic inhibitors is associated with a rapid fall in those blood levels.

4. **Drug-drug interactions based upon interference with renal excretion have little relevance to most**

Table 51-1. Common Inducers of Hepatic Drug Metabolism

Drugs	*Other*
Carbamazepine	Alcohol, chronic
Phenobarbital	Cigarette smoking
Phenytoin (Dilantin)	Charbroiled meats
Primidone (Myosline)	Cruciferous vegetables (e.g., broccoli)
Rifampin	St. John's wort

Table 51-2. Common Inhibitors of Drug Metabolism

- *Antifungals* (ketoconazole [Nizoral], miconazole [Monistat], itraconazole [Sporanox])
- *Macrolide antibiotics* (erythromycin, clarithromycin [Biaxin], troleandomycin [Tao])
- *Fluoroquinolones* (ciprofloxacin, norfloxacin, enoxacin)
- *Antimalarials* (chloroquine, primaquine)
- *Antituberculous drugs* (Isoniazid)
- *Protease inhibitors* (ritonavir, saquinavir, indinavir, nelfinavir)
- *Selective serotonin reuptake inhibitors* (except venlafaxine, citalopram, escitalopram)
- *Atypical* (bupropion, nefazodone, duloxetine) and *Tricyclic antidepressants*
- *Psychostimulants* (methylphenidate)
- *Phenothiazines*
- *Anticonvulsants* (divalproex sodium [Valproate])
- *Beta-blockers, lipophilic* (propranolol, pindolol, timolol, labetalol)
- *Calcium channel blockers* (diltiazem [Cardizem], verapamil [Calan])
- *Histamine blockers* (cimetidine [Tagamet])
- *Anti-arryhthmics* (quinidine, amiodarone, propafeone, mexiletine)
- Alcohol-related agents (disulfiram [Antabuse], Alcohol ingestion, acute)
- *Foods* (Grapefruit juice)

psychotropic drugs since the majority of these agents present for excretion in the form of inactive metabolites with only a small fraction of parent compound.

a. The principal **exception is lithium, for which drug-drug interactions involving renal excretion may alter lithium levels substantially** (see V.A.1).

b. Drug-drug interactions involving renal excretion are also sometimes utilized in the emergency management of drug overdose. **Acidification of urine** (with agents such as ammonium chloride) **enhances excretion of weak bases** (e.g., phencyclidine [PCP], or amphetamines), **while alkalization** (with agents such as acetazolamide) **promotes excretion of weak acids** (e.g., tricyclic antidepressants or phenobarbital).

IV. Interactions Involving Cytochrome P450 Isoenzymes

A subset of important pharmacokinetic drug-drug interactions involve the cytochrome P450 isoenzymes, a heterogeneous group of over 30 oxidative metabolic enzymes located **predominantly in the endoplasmic reticulum of hepatocytes, as well as in the gastrointestinal tract and the brain.**

A. These enzymes are involved in the **phase I metabolism** of a wide variety of drugs, as well as of endogenous substances, such as prostaglandins, fatty acids, and steroids. **The substrates, inhibitors, and inducers of P450 isoenzymes 1A2 and 2D6 and the 3A3/4 and the 2C subfamily have been particularly well characterized** (Table 51-3).

B. 2D6 and 2C19 enzymes exhibit polymorphisms, genetically-based differences in enzyme structure (isoforms) that result in altered enzyme activity and a bimodal distribution of efficient or "extensive" metabolizers and of "poor" metabolizers. Between 7% and 10% of Caucasians are "poor" metabolizers of 2D6 substrates, compared with 1–3% of African-Americans and Asian-Americans. In contrast, 15–20% of African-Americans and Asian-Americans are "poor" metabolizers of 2C19 substrates compared with 1–5% of Caucasians.

C. Extensive metabolizers will be converted, in effect, to poor metabolizers in the presence of an inhibitor of the relevant isoenzyme.

D. Poor metabolizers show higher baseline concentrations of a substrate, lower concentrations of metabolites, and little or no effect from isoenzyme inhibition or induction.

Table 51-3. Selected Cytochrome P450 Isoenzyme Substrates, Inhibitors, and Inducers

1A2	Substrates	Acetaminophen, aminophylline, caffeine, clozapine, haloperidol, olanzapine (Zyprexa), phenacetin, procarcinogens, ropinirole (Requip), tacrine (Cognex), tertiary tricyclic antidepressants, theophylline
	Inhibitors	Fluoroquinolones (ciprofloxacin), fluvoxamine (Luvox), grapefruit juice
	Inducers	Charbroiled meats, cigarette smoking, omeprazole (Prilosec)
2C	Substrates	Barbiturates, diazepam, mephenytoin, NSAIDs, propranolol, tertiary TCAs, THC, tolbutamide, warfarin
	Inhibitors	Fluoxetine, fluvoxamine, ketoconazole, omeprazole (Prilosec), oxcarbazepine, sertraline
	Inducers	Rifampin
2D6	Substrates	Atomoxetine (Strattera), beta-blockers (lipophilic), codeine, debrisoquine, donepezil (Aricept), dextromethorphan, encainide, flecainide, haloperidol, hydroxycodone, mCPP, phenothiazines, risperidone (Risperdal), aripiprazole (Abilify), SSRIs, TCAs, tramadol (Ultram)
	Inhibitors	Antimalarials, bupropion, duloxetine, fluoxetine, methadone, moclobemide, paroxetine, phenothiazines, protease inhibitors (ritonavir), quinidine, sertraline, TCAs, yohimbine
	Inducers	?
3A3/4	Substrates	Alprazolam (Xanax), amiodarone, aripiprazole (Abilify), buspirone (Buspar), calcium channel blockers, carbamazepine, cisapride (Propulsid), clozapine, cyclosporine, diazepam, disopyramide (Norpace), estradiol, HMG-CoA reductase inhibitors (lovastatin, simvastatin), lidocaine, loratadine, methadone, midazolam (Versed), progesterone, propafenone (Rhythmol), quetiapine (Seroquel), quinidine, sildenafil (Viagra), tertiary TCAs, testosterone, triazolam (Halcion), vinblastine, warfarin, zaleplon (Sonata), ziprasodone (Geodon), zolpidem (Ambien)
	Inhibitors	Antifungals (ketoconazole), calcium channel blockers (verapamil), cimetidine (Tagamet), fluvoxamine (Luvox), grapefruit juice, macrolide antibiotics (erythromycin), nefazodone (Serzone)
	Inducers	Carbamazepine, oxcarbazepine, phenobarbital, phenytoin, rifampin, St. John's wort

V. Drug-Drug Interactions According to Psychotropic Drug Class

While drug-drug interactions may be broadly classified in terms of their presumed mechanism, in clinical situations drug-drug interactions are most often discussed according to the particular classes of drugs for which they are relevant, as described below.

A. Mood Stabilizers

The principal mood stabilizers (lithium, valproate, and carbamazepine) are involved in a number of significant drug-drug interactions (Tables 51-4 through 51-6), particularly by virtue of their **distinctive pharmacokinetic properties.**

1. **Lithium is over 95% eliminated unchanged by the kidney.** It is reabsorbed in the proximal tubules and to a lesser extent in the loop of Henle; both **valproate and carbamazepine are metabolized hepatically.**
2. **Carbamazepine is a potent inducer of metabolism;** oxcarbazepine (Trileptal) may also induce metabolism via an action on P450 3A4. In addition, oxcarbazepine inhibits P450 2C19.
3. **Valproate, unlike many anticonvulsants, inhibits metabolism of other agents.**
4. **Carbamazepine is associated with an active metabolite (carbamazepine-10,11-epoxide)** which has anticonvulsant and possibly other CNS effects.
5. **Lithium, gabapentin, and topiramate are minimally protein-bound; carbamazepine and oxcarbazepine are only minimally to moderately protein-bound; and valproate is moderately to highly protein-bound.**

Table 51-4. Drug-Drug Interactions Involving Lithium

Increased lithium levels	Thiazide diuretics
	ACE inhibitors (captopril, enalapril, lisinopril)
	NSAIDs (except sulindac, aspirin)
	Metronidazole, spectinomycin, tetracycline
Decreased lithium levels	Aminophylline, theophylline
	Urinary alkalization (acetazolamide, sodium bicarbonate)
	Sodium chloride
	Osmotic diuretics (mannitol, urea)
Increased antithyroid effect	Antithyroid drugs (propylthiouracil, methimazole)
Neurotoxicity (rare)	Antipsychotics, calcium channel blockers, carbamazepine, methyldopa
Prolonged neuromuscular blockade	Neuromuscular blockers (succinylcholine, pancuronium, decamethonium)
Serotonin syndrome (rare)	SSRIs, serotonergic TCAs, tramadol (Ultram), tryptophan, venlafaxine (Effexor)

Table 51-5. Drug-Drug Interactions Involving Valproate

Increased valproate levels	Aspirin (increased unbound fraction)
	Cimetidine
	Erythromycin
	Ibuprofen
	Phenothiazines
Decreased valproate levels	Carbamazepine, phenobarbital, phenytoin
	Rifampin
Inhibited metabolism of co-administered agents	Lorazepam (Ativan), oxazepam (Serax), temazepam (Restoril), diazepam (Valium)
	Lamotrigene (Lamictal), carbamazepine (10,11-epoxide) metabolite, phenobarbital
	Tolbutamide
	Warfarin
	Zidovudine (AZT)
Absence seizures (rare)	Clonazepam (Klonopin)

Table 51-6. Drug-Drug Interactions Involving Carbamazepine

Increased carbamazepine levels	Valproate (active CBZ-E metabolite), P450 3A4 inhibitors, antifungals, macrolide antibiotics, calcium channel blockers, fluvoxamine (Luvox), grapefruit juice, isoniazid, nefazodone (Serzone), protease inhibitors
Decreased carbamazepine levels	Carbamazepine (autoinduction), phenobarbital, phenytoin (Dilantin), primidone (Mysoline)
Induced metabolism of co-administered agents	Anticonvulsants (ethosuximide [Zarontin], phenytoin, lamotrigine, valproate), antidepressants, antipsychotics, benzodiazepines, cyclosporine, glucocorticoids, methadone, oral contraceptives, warfarin

6. The putative mood-stabilizing anticonvulsant **lamotrigine** (Lamictal) **is moderately protein-bound and is metabolized by the liver, where its clearance is subject to significant inhibition by valproate** which causes lamotrigine levels to rise dramatically with increased risk of serious rash. **Lamotrigine may cause modest metabolic induction of some agents, including valproate.** In contrast, **gabapentin** (Neurontin) **is excreted largely unchanged by the kidney, and neither inhibits nor induces the metabolism of other agents. Topiramate** (Topamax) **is minimally metabolized by the liver. It also does not appear to alter the hepatic metabolism of other agents.**

B. Antidepressants

1. **The selective serotonin re-uptake inhibitors (SSRIs) have been implicated in a wide variety of pharmacokinetic interactions (mediated by the cytochrome P450 isoenzymes), as well as in the serotonin syndrome (which involves a pharmacodynamic interaction).** Selected drug-drug interactions involving the SSRIs are presented in Table 51-7.
   a. **The SSRIs, with the exception of venlafaxine** (Effexor), **citalopram** (Celexa), **and escitalopram** (Lexapro) **are moderate to potent inhibitors of P450 isoenzymes.**
   b. **The P450 isoenzyme 1A2, responsible for metabolism of theophylline and clozapine, is inhibited by fluvoxamine** (Luvox).
   c. **The 2C isoenzyme subfamily, responsible for metabolism of warfarin and diazepam, is inhibited by fluoxetine, sertraline, and fluvoxamine.**
   d. **The 2D6 isoenzyme, responsible for metabolism of TCAs, class IC antiarrhythmics, and codeine, is inhibited by fluoxetine, paroxetine, duloxetine, and, to a**

Table 51-7. Drug-Drug Interactions Involving Selective Serotonin Reuptake Inhibitors and Atypical Antidepressants That Inhibit P450 Isoenzymes

Inhibited metabolism of co-administered agents	*Antiarrhythmics* metabolized by P450 2D6 and 2C
	Antihistamines metabolized by P450 3A4 (astemizole, loratadine)
	Antipsychotics metabolized by P450 1A2 (clozapine, olanzapine, haloperidol), 2D6 (risperidone, phenothiazines), and 3A4 (quetiapine)
	Benzodiazepines metabolized by P450 2C (diazepam), 3A4 (triazolobenzodiazepines)
	Beta-blockers (lipophilic) metabolized by P450 2C, 2D6
	Calcium channel blockers metabolized by P450 3A4
	Cisapride (Propulsid) metabolized by P450 3A4
	Codeine metabolized by P450 2D6 into active (morphine) metabolite
	Methylxanthines (aminophylline, theophylline) metabolized by P450 1A2
	Secondary amine TCAs metabolized by P450 2D6
	Tertiary amine TCAs metabolized by P450, 1A2, 2C, 2D6, 3A/4
	Warfarin (variable effects)
Serotonin syndrome	*Monoamine oxidase inhibitors* (contraindicated)
	Lithium
	Serotonergic agents

lesser extent, sertraline. Citalopram (Celexa) is a weak, and probably negligible, inhibitor of 2D6 under most circumstances.

e. **The 3A3/4 isoenzymes, responsible for metabolizing pimozide** (Orap), **cisapride** (Propulsid), **carbamazepine, and alprazolam** (Xanax), **are inhibited by fluvoxamine** (Luvox), **as well as by the atypical antidepressant nefazodone** (Serzone). Other SSRIs, particularly fluoxetine and sertraline, appear to be less potent inhibitors of these isoenzymes.

f. The "serotonin syndrome" is a rare but potentially fatal pharmacodynamic complication associated with the combined use of highly serotonergic agents or the contraindicated overlapping use of MAOIs and SSRIs. **Signs and symptoms of the serotonin syndrome include myoclonus, hyperreflexia, nausea, hyperthermia, autonomic instability, agitation, delirium, and coma. In contrast to neuroleptic malignant syndrome (NMS), there are no unique laboratory findings associated with serotonin syndrome.**

2. **The TCAs are associated with a broad range of pharmacodynamic drug-drug interactions, and are also subject to drug-drug interactions involving metabolic induction or inhibition.** Significant drug-drug interactions involving TCAs and SSRIs are presented in Table 51-8.

a. **The secondary amine TCAs, including nortriptyline and desipramine, are hydroxylated by P450 2D6. Generally the more sedating tertiary amine TCAs, including amitriptyline and imipramine, are demethylated and hydroxylated by P450 1A2, 2C, 2D6, and 3A4.** In addition to serving as substrates for the P450 isoenzymes, the **TCAs are also enzyme inhibitors, particularly of P450 2D6.**

b. The potential for pharmacodynamic drug-drug interactions is higher for the TCAs than for other antidepressants by virtue of their **broad spectrum of activity on muscarinic, histaminic, and alpha-1-adrenergic receptors, and on monoamine re-uptake mechanisms and cardiac conduction.**

3. Among the psychotropics, the **MAOIs are most closely associated with potentially fatal drug-drug interactions.**

a. **Hypertensive (hyperadrenergic) crisis. Abrupt elevation of blood pressure, severe headache, nausea, vomiting, diaphoresis, cardiac arrhythmias, intracranial hemorrhage, and myocardial infarction** can occur when a variety of prescribed and over-the-counter **sympathomimetics, particularly indirect sympathomimetics,** are used concurrently with MAOIs. Sympathomimetic drugs include: **L-dopa, dopamine, cocaine, amphetamines, phenylpropanolamine, oxymetazoline** (Afrin), **phentermine, mephentermine, metaraminol, ephedrine, pseudoephedrine, phenylephrine** (Neo-Synephrine), **norepinephrine, isoproterenol, and epinephrine.** Safe over-the-counter allergy, cold and cough medications include **plain chlorpheniramine** (Chlor-Trimeton), **brompheniramine** (Dimetane), and **guaifenesin** (Robitussin). The widely available combined preparations that include decongestants or dextromethorphan must be scrupulously avoided. Although **dextromethorphan is not associated with hypertensive crises, its use with MAOIs has been linked to acute confusional states.**

b. **Serotonin syndrome may occur when highly serotonergic agents including the SSRIs and venlafaxine** (Effexor), **clomipramine** (Anafranil), **or tryptophan are combined with the MAOIs.** A minimum wash-out interval of 2 weeks is necessary following discontinuation of MAOIs before the initiation of one of these drugs. Reciprocally, **a minimum of 2 weeks must elapse after discontinuing most serotonergic drugs before starting an MAOI. In the case of fluoxetine, a minimum delay of 5 weeks is necessary because of its long half-life.** Although not associated with a "serotonin syndrome," the combination of buspirone (Buspar) with MAOIs has been associated with reported episodes of blood pressure elevation.

c. **Agitation, convulsions, blood pressure instability, hyperpyrexia, respiratory depression, peripheral vascular collapse, coma, and death may occur when meperidine** (Demerol) **is administered concurrently with the**

Table 51-8. Drug-Drug Interactions Involving Tricyclic Antidepressants (TCAs)

Increased TCA levels	Antifungals, beta-blockers (lipophilic), calcium channel blockers, cimetidine, macrolide antibiotics, methylphenidate, phenothiazines, quinidine, SSRIs
Decreased TCA levels	Carbamazepine, phenytoin, phenobarbital, primidone, rifampin
Prolonged cardiac conduction	Antiarrhythmics (type I), antipsychotics (low potency), calcium channel blockers
Hypotension	Antihypertensives, antipsychotics (low potency, atypicals), trazodone, MAOIs, vasodilators
Attenuated antihypertensive effects	Clonidine, guanethidine
Anticholinergic toxicity	Antipsychotics (low potency), benztropine (Cogentin), diphenhydramine (Benadryl), mirtazapine (Remeron)

MAOIs. Their combined use is absolutely contraindicated. Other narcotic analgesics (e.g., codeine, morphine) appear to be safer, although their analgesic and CNS depressant effects may be potentiated and dose adjustments may be necessary.

d. **Cases of adverse, though reversible events, including fever, delirium, convulsions, hypotension, and dyspnea have been reported when MAOIs and TCAs have been combined.** The concurrent use of these two classes of antidepressant is generally contraindicated. However, very cautious addition of an MAOI to an established treatment with a TCA has been carried out successfully in the treatment of exceptionally treatment-resistant depressed patients.

e. The effects of **CNS depressants, insulin, sulfonylurea hypoglycemic drugs, antihypertensive, or vasodilator medications may be potentiated,** with the exception of guanethidine (Esimil, Ismelin) whose antihypertensive effects may be blocked. There have been reported cases of hypertension and bradycardia on beta-blockers, and of hypertension and mental status changes with reserpine and methyldopa. The beta-agonistic effects (including tachycardia, palpitations, and anxiety) of methylxanthines and inhaled bronchodilators may be enhanced. Phenelzine (Nardil) may potentiate neuromuscular blockade on succinylcholine.

4. The atypical antidepressants include several agents with P450 inhibitory properties, particularly **nefazodone** (Serzone), a P450 3A4 inhibitor, **bupropion** (Wellbutrin) and **duloxetine,** both P450 2D6 inhibitors. Mirtazepine (Remeron) is a potent antagonist of the alpha-2-adrenergic receptor like yohimbine (Yocon); it also blocks the histamine, muscarinic, and alpha-1-adrenergic receptors, properties shared with many TCA antidepressants and antipsychotic agents. Thus, pharmacodynamic interactions with these agents would be expected. While relatively little is known about interactions of MAOIs with atypical antidepressant drugs, concerns about serious toxicity generally contraindicate their co-administration.

C. Antipsychotics

Drug-drug interactions involving antipsychotics are presented in Table 51-9.

1. The **lower-potency agents,** such as chlorpromazine, and the **atypical antipsychotics,** are generally more likely than are the high-potency agents, such as haloperidol, to participate in **pharmacodynamic interactions with drugs (such as TCAs) that cause anticholinergic effects, sedation, hypotension, and prolonged cardiac conduction. Nevertheless, potentially fatal cardiac arrhythmias have occurred due to drug interactions with pimozide** (Orap), a P450 3A4 substrate.
2. **Clozapine, olanzapine** (Zyprexa), **and haloperidol involve multiple pathways, including P450 1A2.** Their clearance may therefore be **inhibited by fluvoxamine** (Luvox) and **fluoroquinolone antibiotics** (e.g., ciprofloxacin [Cipro]), and may be **induced by omeprazole** (Prilosec) and by **cigarette smoking.**
3. **Phenothiazines** (e.g., perphenazine [Trilafon] and chlorpromazine [Thorazine]) **are both substrates and inhibitors of P450 2D6. Risperidone** (Risperdal) **is also a 2D6 substrate.**
4. **Quetiapine** (Seroquel) **and ziprasidone** (Geodon) **are P450 3A4 substrates,** whose serum concentrations may be increased by isoenzyme inhibitors (e.g., **erythromycin**), and decreased by inducers (e.g., **carbamazepine** and **rifampin**).
5. **Aripiprazole** (Abilify) is a substrate of both P450 3A4 and P450 2D6.

D. Anxiolytics

1. **Pharmacodynamic interactions**

a. The most common and potentially serious drug-drug interactions involving benzodiazepines are the **additive CNS depressant effects** that result when these agents are co-administered with **barbiturates, ethanol, narcotics,**

Table 51-9. Drug-Drug Interactions Involving Antipsychotic Medications

Increased antipsychotic levels	Inhibitors of P450 1A2, 2D6, 3A4 including fluoxetine, paroxetine, fluvoxamine, nefazodone, bupropion, duloxetine, fluoroquinolones and macrolide antibiotics, antifungals
Decreased antipsychotic levels	Beta-blockers (lipophilic), carbamazepine, phenobarbital, phenytoin, rifampin
Interference with antipsychotic drug absorption	Antacids (aluminum, magnesium)
Prolonged cardiac conduction	Calcium channel blockers, TCAs, inhibitors of P450 isoenzyme activity (cf. above)
Hypotension	Antihypertensives, MAOIs, TCAs, trazodone, vasodilators
Anticholinergic toxicity	TCAs, benztropine, diphenydramine, mirtazapine
Interference with dopaminergic effects	Bromocriptine, L-dopa, pramipexole, ropinirole
Additive risk of myelosuppression (clozapine)	Carbamazepine, AZT

antihistamines, TCAs, and zolpidem (Ambien). These effects commonly include sedation and psychomotor impairment. At high doses or in severely compromised patients, fatal respiratory depression may occur.

b. **Flumazenil** (Romazicon) is a **competitive inhibitor of the benzodiazepine receptor;** therefore, it antagonizes benzodiazepine effects. The anticholinesterase **physostigmine also blocks benzodiazepine binding in brain** and can also reverse CNS depression caused by benzodiazepines.

2. **Pharmacokinetic interactions.** While rarely life-threatening, alterations in blood levels of the benzodiazepines may account for the emergence of side effects, such as unsteadiness or slurred speech, or for loss of antianxiety or hypnotic efficacy when a new drug is co-administered.
   a. **Antacid suspensions** (aluminum and magnesium hydroxide) **may delay the rate, but less likely the extent, of absorption** of orally administered benzodiazepines, a property **more important for single, as-needed (p.r.n.) dosing rather than for maintenance dosing** of benzodiazepines.
   b. **Inducers of phase I metabolic processes (including carbamazepine, phenobarbital, and rifampin) may reduce the levels of the majority of benzodiazepines, which are subject to oxidative metabolism,** while leaving levels of lorazepam, oxazepam, and temazepam unchanged.
   c. Inhibitors of metabolism account for a variety of drug-drug interactions with benzodiazepines.
      i. **Specific inhibitors of the cytochrome P450 3A3/4 subclass** (Table 51-3) (including the **macrolide antibiotics, antifungals, nefazodone** [Serzone], **fluvoxamine** [Luvox], **and grapefruit juice) may increase plasma levels of the triazalobenzodiazepines (alprazolam** [Xanax], **triazolam** [Halcion], **and midazolam** [Versed]) by interfering with hydroxylation.
      ii. **Specific inhibitors of the cytochrome P450 2C class** (Table 51-1) (including **omeprazole** [Prilosec], as well as **ketoconazole** and certain SSRIs, including **fluoxetine, fluvoxamine** [Luvox], and **sertraline**) may increase plasma levels of **diazepam** (Valium) by interfering with the *N*-demethylation.
      iii. **Inhibitors of glucuronide conjugation** (phase II metabolism), including **valproate** and **probenecid,** may increase plasma levels of the **3-hydroxy-substituted benzodiazepines (lorazepam, oxazepam, and temazepam)** which are not altered by inhibitors of phase I metabolism.
3. **Idiosyncratic interactions. Absence seizures** have been described in some patients receiving both **valproate** and **clonazepam** (Klonopin), although this drug combination is widely and safely used in many patients with bipolar disorder or seizure disorders.

E. Miscellaneous

1. St. John's wort has been implicated in serious drug interactions that appear to be related to P450 3A4 induction of metabolism of other agents as well as a direct effect on the drug transport protein, P-glycoprotein. **Diminished levels and/or effectiveness of the following agents have been reported in individuals taking St. John's wort: cyclosporine, antiretrovirals, anticoagulants, theophylline, digoxin, and oral contraceptives.**
2. **Zolpidem** (Ambien) and **zaleplon** (Sonata). Additive CNS-depressant effects are likely to occur when other sedating agents (including **alcohol, barbiturates,** and **benzodiazepines**) are co-administered with zolpidem or zaleplon, which interact with the $GABA_A$-benzodiazepine complex. Their sedative-hypnotic effects are reversed by the benzodiazepine receptor antagonist **flumazenil** (Romazicon). Like the triazalobenzodiazepines, **zolpidem and zaleplon levels are potentially affected by drug-drug interactions involving cytochrome P450 3A4.**
3. **The psychostimulants, particularly methylphenidate** (Ritalin, Concerta), **appear to inhibit metabolism of a large number of substances including SSRIs, TCAs, anticoagulants, and anticonvulsants,** thereby elevating the levels of these co-administered agents.
4. **Modafinil** (Provigil) **may induce the activity of P450 3A4 with long-term use** and therefore may reduce levels and effectiveness of important substrates, including oral contraceptives.
5. **Atomoxetine (Strattera) is a substrate of P450 2D6** whose levels may rise in the setting of inhibition by fluoxetine, paroxetine, bupropion, and other 2D6 inhibitors. It may also potentiate the effects of $beta_2$-agonists and of pressors. Co-administration of atomoxetine with MAOIs is contraindicated.
6. **Rivastigmine** (Exelon) **is not a substrate, inhibitor, or inducer of the P450 isoenzymes. Tacrine** (Cognex) is a **substrate for cytochrome P450 1A2** and may compete with other drugs for this hepatic microsomal isoenzyme. Elevated levels of **theophylline** have been reported in this context. Both **galantamine** (Reminyl) and **donepezil** (Aricept) are **substrates for 2D6 and 3A4;** their clearance is therefore susceptible to inhibition by such agents as **fluoxetine** and **ketoconazole.** Neither galantamine nor donepezil appear to inhibit or induce the metabolism of other agents. **Cholinergic toxicity is possible when cholinesterase inhibitors are combined with other cholinomimetic agents** (e.g., **bethanechol** [Urecholine]). **Conversely, drugs with anticholinergic properties may interfere with the activity with these medications.**
7. **Codeine is a substrate for P450 2D6 which converts it into its active form (morphine). Hence the analgesic effect of codeine may be substantially diminished when co-administered with P450 2D6 inhibitors. Methadone is a substrate for cytochrome P450 isoenzyme 3A4 and, to a lesser extent, 2D6.** It is **also a 2D6 inhibitor** which can potentially interfere with the clearance of other 2D6 substrates (e.g., desipramine).

8. **Disulfiram** (Antabuse). **In addition to inhibiting aldehyde dehydrogenase,** thereby resulting in the accumulation of acetaldehyde following ethanol ingestion, **disulfiram inhibits other hepatic microsomal enzymes that interfere with the metabolism of a variety of drugs** (including **warfarin, phenytoin, benzodiazepines, antipsychotics,** and **antidepressants**). The severity of the **disulfiram-alcohol reaction is increased by a variety of agents (including MAOIs, vasodilators, alpha- or beta-adrenergic antagonists, and paraldehyde).** Severe **confusional states may occur when metronidazole has been administered within 2 weeks of disulfiram; therefore, its concurrent use is contraindicated.**
9. **Sildenafil (Viagra) is a P450 3A4 substrate** whose levels may be increased by inhibitors including erythromycin or nefazodone. **As it potentiates the hypotensive effects of nitrates, their combined use is absolutely contraindicated.**

Suggested Readings

Alpert, J.E., Bernstein, J.G., & Rosenbaum, J.F. (1997). Psychopharmacological issues in the medical setting. In N.H. Cassem, T.A. Stern, J.F. Rosenbaum, & M.S. Jellinek (Eds.), *Massachusetts General Hospital handbook of general hospital psychiatry* (4th ed.), pp. 249–303. St. Louis, MO: Mosby.

Callahan, A.M., Marangell, L.B., & Ketter, T.A. (1996). Evaluating the clinical significance of drug interactions: A systematic approach. *Harvard Review of Psychiatry, 4,* 153–158.

Ciraulo, D.A., Shader, R.I., Greenblatt, D.J., et al. (Eds.). (1995). *Drug interactions in psychiatry* (2nd ed.). Baltimore, MD: Williams and Wilkins.

Cozza, K.L., & Armstrong, S.C. (2001). *The cytochrome P450 system: Drug interaction principles for medical practice.* Washington, DC: American Psychiatric Press.

DeVane, C.L., & Nemeroff C.B. (2000). 2000 guide to psychotropic drug interactions. *Primary Psychiatry, 7*(10).

Ereshefsky, L. (1996). Drug interactions of antidepressants. *Psychiatric Annals, 26,* 342–350.

Gardner, D.M., Shulman, K.I., Walker, S.E., & Tailor, S.A. (1996). The making of a user-friendly MAOI diet. *Journal of Clinical Psychiatry, 57,* 99–104.

Jefferson, J.W. (1998). Drug interactions—Friend or foe? *Journal of Clinical Psychiatry, 59*(suppl 4), 37–47.

Keck, P.E., & Arnold, L.M. (2000). The serotonin syndrome. *Psychiatric Annals,* 333–343.

Livingston, M.G., & Livingston, H.M. (1997). Monoamine oxidase inhibitors. An update on drug interactions. *Drug Safety, 14,* 219–227.

Markowitz, J.S., & DeVane, C.L. (2001). The emerging recognition of herb-drug interactions with a focus on St. John's wort (hypericum perforatum). *Psychopharmacology Bulletin, 35,* 53–64.

Markowitz, J.S., & Patrick, K.S. (2001). Pharmacokinetic and pharmacodynamic drug interactions in the treatment of attention deficit hyperactivity disorder. *Clinical Pharmacokinetics, 40,* 753–772.

Meyer, M.C., Baldessarini, R.J., Goff, D.C., & Centorrino, F. (1996). Clinically significant interactions of psychotropic agents with antipsychotic drugs. *Drug Safety, 15,* 333–346.

Richelson, E. (2001). Pharmacology of antidepressants. *Mayo Clinic Proceedings, 76,* 511–527.

Robinson, M.J., & Qaqish, R.B. (2002). Practical psychopharmacology in HIV-1 and acquired immunodeficiency syndrome. *Psychiatric Clinics of North America, 25,* 149–175.

Spina, E., & Perucca, E. (2002). Clinical significance of pharmacokinetic drug interactions between antiepileptic and psychotropic drugs. *Epilepsia, 43*(suppl 2), 37–44.

Von Moltke, L.L., & Greenblatt, D.J. (2000). Drug transporters in psychopharmacology—Are they important? *Journal of Clinical Psychopharmacology, 20,* 291–294.

Wang, P.W., & Ketter, T.A. (2002). Pharmacokinetics of mood stabilizers and new anticonvulsants. *Psychopharmacology Bulletin, 36,* 44–66.

Chapter 52

Cardiovascular and Other Side Effects of Psychotropic Medications

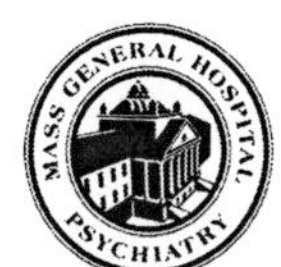

Edward R. Norris, Ned H. Cassem, Jeff C. Huffman, and Theodore A. Stern

I. Introduction

Psychiatric illness is regularly complicated by medical symptoms and disorders. The more severe the medical illness, the more frequent is the impact on psychiatric disorders. In a fashion similar to primary psychiatric disorders, proper management of many combined medical and psychiatric disorders requires use of medications. Physicians have long feared the effects of psychotropics in medically ill patients; they continue to be wary of them in severely medically compromised patients. Historically, many psychotropics have been recognized for their potential adverse effects on the cardiovascular (CV) system and on other organ systems. Knowledge of side effects and their prevalence is a requirement for safe and effective treatment of all patients.

II. Management of Side Effects

Safe administration of psychotropics involves management of potential side effects. **Attention to several general principles will enhance safety and compliance.**

A. **Anticipate, and inform the patient about probable side effects;** include a review of the most common side effects. Reassure the patient that there are strategies to minimize the adverse effects of medications.

B. **Select drugs that have the smallest chance of exacerbating current medical problems.**

C. **Use the lowest effective dose and gradually titrate the dose.** This may minimize side effects because side effects are often dose-related. **"Start low, go slow,"** especially in the elderly, the neurologically impaired, and the medically ill.

D. **Manage side effects with adjunctive agents** rather than switching to another agent that may delay the therapeutic response.

E. **Reassure the patient.** Although this is a temporary strategy for management of side effects, it may allow time for treatment and for side effects to abate.

F. **Instruct the patient regularly that psychiatric symptoms often mirror common medication side effects.** Clearly written patient instructions will increase medication compliance. **Symptoms that begin after medication initiation or worsen with dose escalation are likely to be medication-related.**

III. Effects on the Cardiovascular System

A. Hemodynamic Effects

1. **Orthostatic hypotension (OH) is correlated with alpha blockade and to alpha-noradrenergic receptor affinity.** OH is of greatest concern for the elderly, for those on antihypertensive medications, and for patients with cardiovascular disease. Many antidepressants, especially tricyclic antidepressants (TCAs) and monoamine oxidase inhibitors (MAOIs), cause OH.
   a. **TCAs.** Imipramine, desipramine, and amitriptyline are equally likely to produce OH. For TCAs, the incidence of OH in patients with a normal electrocardiogram (ECG) is 7%; with a bundle branch block (BBB), it is 32%, and with congestive heart failure (CHF), it is 50%. Doxepin and trazodone are also apt to cause OH. **Among the TCAs, nortriptyline is the least likely to induce OH.**
      i. A pre-drug orthostatic fall in blood pressure (BP) increases the risk of OH in patients and predicts response to TCAs.
      ii. Unrelated to age or gender, OH occurs before the therapeutic effect of TCAs.
      iii. Over time, the objective fall in BP will persist, but subjective complaints will diminish.
   b. **MAOI**-induced OH is common, but is not predicted by a pre-drug orthostatic fall in BP. Mild OH occurs in 47% of patients, and severe OH occurs in 5–10% of MAOI-treated patients. The maximum effect appears after 3–4 weeks, and OH can subside after 6 weeks.
   c. **Other antidepressants.** Among other antidepressants, nefazodone and mirtazapine are associated with a low incidence of OH, while fluoxetine, sertraline, paroxetine, citalopram, escitalopram, bupropion, fluvoxamine, and venlafaxine are not associated with OH. However, data indicate that SSRI-treated patients may have as many falls as TCA-treated patients. The mechanism is unknown and the topic is still under debate.
   d. **Antipsychotics.** Low-potency neuroleptics can cause significant OH, especially in patients who are dehydrated or who are taking other BP-lowering agents. While high-potency agents are much less likely to lower BP, clozapine causes significant OH. Therefore, it is recommended that the starting dose be low and that it be titrated slowly.
      i. The atypical antipsychotics risperidone, ziprasidone, and quetiapine can cause OH to a lesser extent; olanzapine is uncommonly associated with OH.
   e. **Benzodiazepines and stimulants** rarely cause OH.

2. **Essential hypertension** may arise with use of some medications.
   a. Venlafaxine produces a dose-related elevation of supine diastolic BP in 7% of patients taking doses of 200–300 mg/day. It occurs in up to 13% in those with daily doses greater than 300 mg/day.
   b. Buspirone in combination with a MAOI or another serotoninergic drug can cause hypertension.
   c. Psychostimulants can aggravate hypertension; however, the stimulant pemoline appears to have minimal effects on BP or other cardiovascular parameters.
3. **Hypertensive crisis, a potentially fatal interaction, is characterized by an elevation of BP, severe headache, nausea, vomiting, and diaphoresis.** It occurs when patients on MAOIs ingest large amounts of tyramine-containing foods. Hypertensive crisis requires immediate medical attention to reduce BP with the alpha-1-adrenergic antagonist phentolamine.
4. Another potentially fatal interaction, **serotonin syndrome,** produces hypertension, tachycardia, hyperpyrexia, delirium, agitation, myoclonus, and hyperreflexia. In severe cases, seizures may result. Serotonin syndrome most often occurs when MAOIs and other serotonergic agents (such as SSRIs, TCAs, or buspirone), are co-administered. However, serotonin syndrome may occur when any two or more serotonergic agents are taken concurrently, and, rarely, there have been cases of serotonin syndrome with MAOI or SSRI monotherapy.

B. Cardiac Conduction System

MAOIs, bupropion, venlafaxine, fluoxetine, sertraline, citalopram, escitalopram, paroxetine, and fluvoxamine appear to have very few or no cardiac conduction system effects. Clinically, the low-potency neuroleptics produce more cardiovascular effects than do high-potency neuroleptics. Benzodiazepines have no adverse effects on the heart. Buspirone and naltrexone have no direct effects on the heart.

1. **Heart rate** can be affected by neuroleptics and anticholinergic medications.
   a. Tachycardia, arising from anticholinergic vagolytic effects, can pose additional risk to the cardiac patient. While **low-potency neuroleptics and TCAs produce a statistically significant increase in heart rate,** several atypical antipsychotics increase the heart rate as well. Clozapine causes sustained tachycardia of 10–15 beats/minute in 25% of patients, and olanzapine can cause a small amount of tachycardia. **Tachycardia** has also occurred in patients using psychostimulants.
   b. Bradycardia has occurred rarely with SSRI administration, usually in elderly patients or with significant overdose.
2. Although major depression is associated with a higher prevalence of **ventricular arrhythmias,** including ventricular tachycardia and reduced heart rate variability, psychotropic medications also interfere with cardiac conduction. All TCAs appear to prolong both atrial and ventricular depolarization by sodium and potassium channel inhibition.
   a. The main effect of TCAs is the prolongation of the conduction in the His-ventricular portion of the His bundle, as occurs with the group IA antiarrhythmic drugs. The hydroxy metabolites of TCAs also prolong conduction. **Although nortriptyline is the least cardiotoxic TCA, all TCAs should be avoided in patients with ventricular arrhythmias.** Trazodone, given after myocardial infarction, has been reported to aggravate pre-existing premature ventricular contractions (PVCs).
   b. All low-potency neuroleptics slow cardiac conduction to the same degree as do the TCAs, and high-potency neuroleptics are preferred for patients with conduction disturbances. However, pimozide, risperidone, and clozapine can slow cardiac conduction; clozapine has caused reversible electrocardiographic (ECG) changes. Carbamazepine can produce conduction abnormalities at toxic doses. In patients with pre-existing abnormalities, even therapeutic levels of carbamazepine can result in conduction abnormalities. Prolonged cardiac conduction, caused by TCAs, low-potency neuroleptics, pimozide, clozapine, risperidone, and ziprasidone, increases the risk of death from re-entrant ventricular arrhythmias by 3%.
3. The **prolongation of the QT_c interval** can lead to torsades de pointes and sudden death. Patients are at higher risk if their QT_c is greater than 440 milliseconds. Patients with liver dysfunction, those on cisapride, patients on cardioactive drugs, and those who are female are at higher risk for QT_c prolongation.
   a. **All TCAs cause prolongation of the QT interval,** especially in combination with neuroleptics.
   b. **Antipsychotics can prolong the QT interval,** and low-potency antipsychotics (especially thioridazine) convey a higher risk.
   c. Atypical antipsychotics also appear to have a higher risk of QT interval prolongation. In healthy volunteers, ziprasidone has caused the greatest mean QT_c prolongation, followed by quetiapine, risperidone, and olazapine; each of these causes greater mean QT_c prolongation than orally administered haloperidol.
   d. However, intravenous (IV) haloperidol, often used in emergency situations, carries a risk of QT_c prolongation and torsades de pointes (especially at higher doses).
   e. With lengthening of the QT interval, potassium and magnesium levels need to be checked and repleted prior to treatment.
4. Less severe atrial arrhythmias occur with psychotropics.
   a. Lithium can cause sinus node dysfunction and first-degree atrioventricular block. The elderly are especially prone to the inhibitory effects of lithium on impulse generation within the atrium.
   b. Valproic acid in overdose has been associated with heart block.

c. Amoxapine has been the subject of case reports of atrial flutter and fibrillation.

5. **Clozapine** has been associated with a number of adverse cardiovascular effects. In addition to causing OH, tachycardia, and QT_c prolongation, **clozapine has been associated with the development of myocarditis** in otherwise healthy patients. Therefore, the diagnosis of myocarditis should be considered in patients with unexplained fatigue, dyspnea, fever, chest pain, or other symptoms of heart failure while taking clozapine. Clozapine has also been associated with cardiomyopathy, pericarditis, and pericardial effusion.

C. Cardiovascular Disease

All psychotropics should be used with caution for 4–6 weeks after myocardial infarction.

1. **TCAs should be used with extreme caution in patients with coronary artery disease (CAD).**
   a. TCAs and low-potency antipsychotics increase the risk of angina or myocardial infarction (MI) because of tachycardia induced by anticholinergic vagolytic effects.
   b. **Selective serotonin reuptake inhibitors (SSRIs) appear to be safe in patients with CAD** and may have favorable effects on platelet aggregation. A recent large trial found sertraline to be safe and effective in patients who began treatment four weeks post-MI.
   c. Disulfiram (Antabuse) is contraindicated in patients with significant CAD.
   d. Psychostimulants should also be used with caution in this population because of their effects on heart rate and blood pressure.
2. **Congestive heart failure.** TCAs may exacerbate congestive heart failure (CHF), as can low-potency antipsychotics and clozapine, by virtue of their anticholinergic potency and the tachycardia associated with this effect.
3. **Left ventricular dysfunction.** Even in patients with left ventricular (LV) dysfunction, ejection fraction does not change during imipramine treatment; however, imipramine-treated patients are susceptible to severe OH.

IV. Central Nervous System Effects

A. A high-frequency tremor can occur as a side effect of TCAs, SSRIs, MAOIs, bupropion, lithium, valproic acid, carbamazepine, lamotrigine, and antipsychotics. Tremor can also be exacerbated by caffeine or by anxiety. The use of low-dose beta-blockers (e.g., propranolol 10 mg t.i.d.) or low-dose benzodiazepines can minimize the tremor.

B. Increased anxiety and jitteriness may be seen during the initiation of TCAs, SSRIs, venlafaxine, bupropion, risperidone, and ziprasidone. These symptoms often remit within a few weeks, and they can be minimized by starting at low doses or by co-administering benzodiazepines.

C. Parkinsonism, acute dystonia, and akathisia are common movement disorders caused by use of neuroleptics, especially high-potency typical neuroleptics.

1. When parkinsonism appears, the dose of neuroleptic medication should be reduced, anticholinergic medication should be added, or a switch to another agent should be considered.
2. Acute dystonia is an emergency; treatment involves the use of anticholinergic and antihistaminergic medications.
3. Akathisia is characterized by the subjective feelings of restlessness or the appearance of restlessness. Besides dose reduction or a change of medication, use of beta-adrenergic blocking drugs and benzodiazepines is often helpful. These extrapyramidal symptoms are somewhat less common with risperidone (especially at daily doses of 6 mg or less) and ziprasidone, and are quite rare with olanzapine, quetiapine, and clozapine. Some patients on SSRIs experience an akathisia-like motor restlessness that may respond to low-dose propranolol or to benzodiazepines.

D. Neuroleptic-induced tardive dyskinesia (TD) is a late-appearing disorder of involuntary movements. The most common movements involve the face, fingers, and toes. TD is most common with typical antipsychotics; the risk of developing TD on these agents appears to be 4–5% per year for at least the first four years. Atypical neuroleptics appear to have lower rates of TD, with risperidone having approximately one-sixth the risk of TD compared with typical agents, and olanzapine and quetiapine having approximately one-twelfth the risk. Clozapine has not been associated with TD. Other risk factors for TD include greater duration of treatment with neuroleptics, female gender, increasing age, and the presence of mood or cognitive disorders.

E. Neuroleptic malignant syndrome (NMS) is a life-threatening complication of antipsychotic medications. The symptoms include muscular rigidity with increased creatine phosphokinase (CPK), dystonia, agitation, delirium, and autonomic dysfunction. In addition, fever and alteration of the WBC may be present; supportive medical treatment, discontinuation of the neuroleptic, and dantrolene or bromocriptine should be employed.

F. Fatigue and sedation can be manifestations of psychiatric symptoms or medication side effects. TCAs, MAOIs, trazodone, nefazodone, mirtazapine, lithium, valproic acid, topiramate, and antipsychotics are each likely to produce sedation. The side effect of sedation can be used to induce sleep in some patients.

G. **Sleep disturbances** can be related to antidepressant treatment and these may improve if the medication is taken earlier in the day. Insomnia can also occur with SSRIs, bupropion, venlafaxine, and MAOIs. Psychostimulants and ziprasidone have been associated with insomnia and sleep disturbance. Reducing caffeine, eliminating daytime naps, and practicing good sleep hygiene (e.g., restricting activities in the bedroom to sleep or sexual relations) can be effective.

H. **Hypomania or mania** related to antidepressant use occurs in less than 1% of patients without a history of bipolar disorder. Patients with bipolar disorder who are not on a mood stabilizer are at much higher risk. Switching of mood states can occur with the use of TCAs and are least likely with bupropion and paroxetine.

I. **Reduction in the seizure threshold** can be seen in patients taking bupropion and clozapine. Doses of bupropion greater than 150 mg (and daily doses of greater than 450 mg) should be avoided to reduce the risk of seizures; similarly, doses of clozapine should not exceed 600 mg.

J. **Cognitive slowing** has been described with a variety of psychotropic medications. It may be difficult to distinguish the effects of fatigue, sedation, loss of hypomanic symptoms, and other effects of treatment from "true" cognitive dysfunction, but a number of agents have been associated with cognitive slowing.

1. **Among the mood-stabilizing agents, topiramate has been most strongly associated with cognitive impairment.**
2. Lithium, valproic acid, and carbamazepine have also been associated with poor concentration, attention, and memory.
3. Lamotrigine and gabapentin appear to have few negative cognitive affects.
4. The anticholinergic effects of TCAs may impact cognitive function, while SSRIs, bupropion, venlafaxine, and other antidepressants do not appear to adversely impact cognition.
5. Finally, conventional antipsychotics (especially those with anticholinergic effects) have been associated with cognitive impairment, whereas the atypical agents may be associated with mild improvements on neuropsychological batteries.

V. Anticholinergic Effects

Anticholinergic activity varies greatly among psychotropics. **It is greatest for the tertiary amine TCAs** (amitriptyline, imipramine, doxepin) **and typical antipsychotics,** and minimal for the newer antidepressants (SSRIs, venlafaxine, bupropion, mirtazapine, and nefazodone (see Table 52-1)). Alprazolam and stimulants have essentially no anticholinergic effects. Tolerance often develops to many of the anticholinergic side effects over time.

A. **Dry mouth** (xerostomia) can result in bad breath, stomatitis, and dental caries. Often sugarless gum or hard candy can stimulate salivation. Dry eyes can be treated with artificial tears.

B. **Blurred vision** usually lessens with time, but when persistent, it can be managed by addition of pilocarpine 1% drops or bethanechol. Patients with narrow-angle glaucoma may experience dangerous elevations of intraocular pressure when anticholinergic medications are used.

C. **Urinary hesitancy and retention** can occur in patients on anticholinergic medications. This can be complicated by urinary tract infection and even renal damage. Elderly patients and those with prostatic hypertrophy or other outflow problems are at higher risk. Severe urinary retention mandates the discontinuation of the antidepressant.

D. **CNS anticholinergic toxicity can present with confusion, memory loss, delirium, and psychosis.** Usually this is accompanied by other signs of anticholinergic excess (increased temperature, dry skin, flushing, and urinary retention). Elderly patients, children, and brain-injured patients are at increased risk.

1. Management includes reducing or discontinuing the dose and use of **physostigmine** (1–2 mg IV push over 2 minutes). This requires close careful monitoring of vital signs, hemodynamics, and mental status.

VI. Gastrointestinal Adverse Effects

These effects can occur with all psychotropics but usually they disappear within a few days or weeks.

A. **Nausea and dyspepsia are common** side effects and can be relieved by the use of divided dosing or dosing with meals. Adjuvant treatment includes use of over-the-counter antacids, bismuth salicylate, and H_2 blockers. Cisapride should be avoided in patients on fluvoxamine or nefazodone because these agents can significantly increase cisapride levels, risking cardiotoxicity.

B. **Diarrhea** is more commonly seen with use of newer serotonergic antidepressants, such as the SSRIs, that lack anticholinergic activity. Management strategies include the use of antidiarrheal agents.

1. For SSRI-induced diarrhea, *Lactobacillus acidophilus* culture and cyproheptadine (a serotonin and histamine antagonist) have been helpful.
2. Diarrhea and other gastrointestinal side effects associated with lithium may respond to a change in the preparation (e.g., from lithium carbonate to Eskalith

Table 52-1. Side Effect Profiles of Psychotropic Medications

Drug	*Sedation*	*Anticholinergic Potency*	*Hypotension*	*Hypertension*	*Tachycardia*	*Conduction Slowing*
Antidepressants (cyclics)						
Amitriptyline (Elavil)	+++	+++	+++	–	+++	Yes
Amoxapine (Asendin)	+	+	+++	–	+	Yes
Clomipramine (Anafranil)	+++	+++	+++	–	+++	Yes
Desipramine (Norpramin)	+	+	+++	++	+	Yes
Doxepin (Sinequan)	+++	+++	+++	–	+++	Yes
Imipramine (Tofranil)	++	++	+++	–	++	Yes
Maprotiline (Ludiomil)	++	+	++	–	+	Yes
Nortriptyline (Pamelor)	+	+	+	–	+++	Yes
Protriptyline (Vivactil)	+	+++	++	–	+++	Yes
Trimipramine (Surmontil)	+++	++	++	–	++	Yes
Antidepressants (SSRIs)						
Citalopram (Celexa)	+	–	–	–	–	–
Escitalopram (Escitalopram)	+	–	–	–	–	–
Fluoxetine (Prozac)	+	–	–	–	–	–
Fluvoxamine (Luvox)	+	–	–	–	–	–
Paroxetine (Paxil)	+	–	–	–	++	–
Sertraline (Zoloft)	+	–	–	–	–	–
Antidepressants (MAOIs)						
Phenelzine (Nardil)	+	+	+++	+	–	–
Tranylcypromine (Parnate)	+	+	++	+	–	–
Antidepressants (other)						
Bupropion (Wellbutrin)	+	–	–	–	–	–
Mirtazapine (Remeron)	++	+	+	–	–	–
Nefazodone (Serzone)	++	–	+	–	–	–
Trazodone (Desyrel)	+++	–	++	–	–	Yes
Venlafaxine (Effexor)	+	–	–	++	–	–
Antipsychotics (phenothiazines)						
Chlorpromazine (Thorazine)	+++	++	+++	–	+++	Yes
Mesoridazine (Serentil)	++	++	++	–	++	Yes
Perphenazine (Trilafon)	+	+	+	–	+	Yes
Thioridazine (Mellaril)	+++	+++	+++	–	+++	Yes
Antipsychotics (butyrophenone)						
Droperidol (Inapsine)	+	–	+	–	–	Yes, with IV form
Haloperidol (Haldol)	+	–	+	–	–	Yes, with IV form
Antipsychotics (thioxanthene, dibenzazepene, indolone)						
Loxapine (Loxitane)	++	++	++	–	++	Yes
Molindone (Moban)	++	++	+	–	++	Yes
Pimozide (Orap)	+	+	+	–	+	Yes
Thiothixene (Navane)	+	+	+	–	+	Yes

(continued)

Table 52-1. (*Continued*)

Drug	*Sedation*	*Anticholinergic Potency*	*Hypotension*	*Hypertension*	*Tachycardia*	*Conduction Slowing*
Antipsychotics (atypical)						
Clozapine (Clozaril)	+++	+++	+++	–	+++	Yes
Olanzapine (Zyprexa)	+	++	+	–	++	–
Quetiapine (Seroquel)	++	–	++	–	+	–
Risperidone (Risperdal)	+	–	++	–	+	Yes
Ziprasidone (Geodon)	+	–	+	–	+	Yes
Mood stabilizers						
Carbamazepine (Tegretol)	++	–	++	–	–	Yes
Lamotrigine (Lamictal)	+	–	–	–	–	–
Lithium (Eskalith)	++	–	–	–	–	Yes
Topiramate (Topamax)	+	–	–	–	–	–
Valproic acid (Depakote)	++	–	–	–	–	–
Psychostimulants						
Dextroamphetamine (Dexedrine)	–	–	–	+++	++	–
Methylphenidate (Ritalin)	–	–	–	++	++	–

KEY: +, weak; ++, moderate; +++, strong.

CR, or vice versa); similarly nausea, vomiting, and diarrhea with valproic acid may resolve with a switch to divalproex sodium (Depakote).

C. **Constipation** is common with TCAs, but it can be seen with all antidepressants. In the elderly, severe constipation and paralytic ileus can be a serious health risk. Hydration and adequate over-the-counter bulk laxatives (Metamucil) or stool softeners may be useful. Bethanechol relieves the constipation caused by anticholinergic antidepressants. Constipation can also be seen with other anticholinergic agents, such as clozapine, olanzapine, and low-potency typical antipsychotics.

D. **Hepatotoxicity**

1. **Dose-dependent rises in liver functions occur, but they rarely cause fatal hepatotoxicity.**
2. Carbamazepine causes an idiosyncratic dose-related hepatitis.
3. Antipsychotics have been associated with cholestatic jaundice, which presents with nausea, malaise, fever, pruritus, abdominal pain, and jaundice within the first two months of antipsychotic treatment.
4. **The antidepressant nefazodone is also associated with elevated rates of hepatotoxicity;** this usually occurs within the first six months of treatment.
5. Disulfiram and naltrexone have also been associated with dose-related elevation of liver enzymes and rare hepatotoxicity, though these effects usually occur at doses higher than those typically used.

VII. Hematological Effects

Agranulocytosis is a potentially life-threatening hematological side effect seen most commonly with clozapine and rarely with phenothiazines. A white blood cell (WBC) count drop of 50% or a count of less than 3,000 should lead to immediate discontinuation of the offending agent. When agranulocytosis occurs, the causative agent should be resumed only with great caution.

A. Carbamazepine is associated with benign and severe hematological toxicities and with depression of red blood cells, white blood cells, and platelets. Evaluation of a complete blood count (CBC), closer evaluation of the patient with baseline abnormalities, and regular monitoring is required.

B. Valproic acid can cause thrombocytopenia or platelet dysfunction; only rarely has it been associated with bleeding problems. Patients on valproic acid should have their platelet count and bleeding time checked before any surgery.

C. Mirtazapine has been rarely associated with agranulocytosis and with neutropenia. Such hematological effects appear to resolve when mirtazapine has been discontinuated.

D. Lithium can produce a benign, relative leukocytosis without impairing leukocyte function. The WBC rarely exceeds 15,000 as a result of lithium treatment alone.

VIII. Renal Effects

A. Although lithium commonly causes defects in urine-concentrating ability, it rarely causes renal failure in patients whose lithium levels are maintained in the therapeutic range. The amount of renal damage is higher in those patients who receive lithium in divided doses as opposed to once-daily dosing.

B. **The most common renal problem due to lithium is polyuria.** This may be due to lithium's effect on antidiuretic hormone, leading to an inability to concentrate urine. **Polyuria can occur in up to 70% of patients with long-term lithium treatment;** 10% of lithium-treated patients are diagnosed with **nephrogenic diabetes insipidus** (DI), a urine output of greater than 3 L/day. Treatment includes maintaining the lowest effective lithium level, administering the drug at a single bedtime dose, and using **diuretics (amiloride and hydrochlorothiazide) to markedly reduce urine volume caused by DI.**

C. Lithium also causes an occasional acute rise in serum creatinine, which abates with lithium discontinuation. Lithium-induced nephrotic syndrome has also been reported.

IX. Weight Gain

Weight gain is a common cause of medication noncompliance.

A. Among antidepressants, weight gain is most strongly associated with tertiary amine TCAs (e.g., amitriptyline, imipramine, and doxepin), MAOIs (phenelzine), and mirtazapine. Weight gain may be related to a drug's antihistaminic or serotonergic effects. The SSRIs, venlafaxine, nefazodone, and, especially, bupropion are less likely to cause weight gain. Among mood-stabilizing agents, both lithium and valproic acid have been associated with long-term weight gain; carbamazepine is less commonly associated with weight gain. Lamotrigine appears to be weight-neutral, and topiramate is associated with weight loss.

B. Weight gain is a serious problem with all typical antipsychotics except molindone (Moban). Of the typical antipsychotics, low-potency agents (phenothiazines) have been shown to increase appetite in a dose-related manner and have been associated with significant weight gain; high-potency agents are associated with less weight gain. The atypical antipsychotics have also been linked to significant weight gain. Of the atypical agents, clozapine appears to have the greatest propensity to cause increased weight. Over 75% of patients on clozapine gain weight, with an average increase of 9–25 pounds. Olanzapine is also strongly associated with weight gain, with an average weight gain of approximately 8 pounds in the first 10 weeks of treatment, and more than half of patients gain more than 7% of their body weight (at least 12 pounds for the average subject) with maintenance treatment. Quetiapine and risperidone are also associated with significant weight gain, though less than with clozapine and olanzapine. Ziprasidone appears to be weight-neutral.

C. If weight gain occurs, dietary modification and increased exercise are effective countermeasures. There is little experience with the combination of weight loss agents and antidepressants. Topiramate has been used with some success in the treatment of psychotropic-associated weight gain. Package labeling contraindicates the use of D-fenfluramine with SSRIs because of the risk of serotonin syndrome.

X. Dermatological Effects

A. **Up to 10% of patients experience cutaneous reactions to psychotropic medications.** The usual reaction is an erythematous maculopapular rash that tends to occur early in treatment and usually it is self-limited with most medications. The decision to continue depends on the agent used, the level of discomfort, evidence of systemic involvement, and the patient's history. Rashes that are associated with mood-stabilizing agents most often require discontinuation of the offending agent.

B. **Systemic involvement (fever, leukocytosis, and elevated liver function) usually indicates a generalized immune response** and discontinuation of the offending medication is necessary. Severe reactions, including generalized urticaria, erythema multiforme, and toxic epidermal necrolysis, may occur.

C. **Lamotrigine has been associated with the development of serious dermatological reactions, including Stevens-Johnson syndrome and toxic epidermal necrolysis.** Furthermore, approximately 10% of patients taking lamotrigine may have a maculopapular rash or erythema. Such dermatological reactions usually occur in the first eight weeks of treatment; they are approximately three times more common in children than in adults. The risk of rash can be minimized with slow upward titration of the dose. Carbamazepine has also been associated with the development of dangerous dermatological reactions, such as Stevens-Johnson syndrome, though it occurs less commonly than with lamotrigine.

D. **Cutaneous erythematous plaques with atypical and lymphoid infiltrates and pseudolymphomas have been reported** in some patients on SSRIs and benzodiazepines. The development of severe atypical dermatologic reactions requires discontinuation of the offending agent and dermatologic consultation. Development and exacerbation of acne has occurred in patients taking lithium.

XI. Endocrinological Side Effects

A. **Antipsychotics have been associated with the development of type 2 diabetes mellitus (DM).** Many of the atypical antipsychotics have been associated with the development of new-onset DM, with **clozapine and olanzapine being the most commonly implicated agents.** Quetiapine, risperidone, and typical neuroleptics have also been associated with the development of type 2 DM. The manifestations of this antipsychotic-associated DM have ranged from borderline abnormalities of glucose regulation to full-blown diabetic ketoacidosis (DKA). The mechanism(s) for the development of DM in association with antipsychotics is unclear, but may be related to overutilization of insulin (as a result of weight gain) or the development of insulin resistance. Treatment usually involves standard dietary and pharmacologic interventions and, where possible, switch from the offending agent.

B. **Hyperprolactinemia can result from the use of dopamine-blocking agents. Typical neuroleptics and risperidone** have been associated with the development of prolonged elevation of prolactin levels. This effect appears to be greatest with risperidone. The mechanism of this effect is related to the action of dopamine in the tuberoinfundibular tract. Dopamine typically inhibits the release of prolactin in this tract; however, when dopamine-blocking agents are administered, prolactin release into the bloodstream is increased. Clinical consequences of hyperprolactinemia can include galactorrhea, amenorrhea, gynecomastia, and impotence. Other atypical antipsychotics—quetiapine, ziprasidone, clozapine, and olanzapine—have not been associated with hyperprolactinemia.

XII. Sexual Side Effects

Sexual dysfunction occurs in roughly one-third of patients treated with antidepressants. Sexual side effects have been noted with SSRIs, TCAs, MAOIs, and venlafaxine. Nefazodone, mirtazapine, and bupropion are not associated with decreased sexual desire or function. Sexual dysfunction can occur in up to 60% of all patients on antipsychotic medications. Sexual dysfunction is under-reported unless it is specifically asked about. Sexual dysfunction can lead to medication non-compliance if not addressed by the physician.

A. **Decreased libido** can be a symptom of depression or medication. If it persists after improvement of mood symptoms, a medication effect should be suspected.

B. **Erectile dysfunction** may result from the anticholinergic or anti-alpha-adrenergic effects of medications.
   1. **Priapism** can occur with antidepressants or antipsychotics. It is most frequently reported with trazodone use (1 in 1,000 men). All men who receive trazodone should be warned that priapism is a medical emergency which requires evaluation by a urologist.

C. **Delayed orgasm and anorgasmia** may be serotonergically mediated. It is associated with TCAs, MAOIs, SSRIs, and atypical antidepressants.

D. **Treatment of sexual side effects involves use of adjunctive agents or the discontinuation of the offending medication.** A variety of adjunctive agents have been used in the treatment of antidepressant-induced sexual dysfunction.
   1. Agents with dopamine or noradrenergic agonism (e.g., bupropion, psychostimulants, and amantadine), serotonergic agents (e.g., cyproheptadine and buspirone), and agents acting on nitric oxide (e.g., sildenafil) have proved useful.
   2. Yohimbine, an alpha-2-adrenergic antagonist, can improve erectile and orgasmic dysfunction at doses of 5.4 mg t.i.d. Yohimbine is contraindicated in patients taking MAOIs.
   3. Cholinergic agonists (e.g., bethanechol, 10–80 mg/day) can enhance libido and improve erectile function and ejaculatory problems.

XIII. Conclusions

A. Knowledge of the risk of side effects is a requirement to the safe and effective treatment of all patients.

B. **One should anticipate the side effects likely to develop and select drugs that have the smallest chance of exacerbating medical problems.**

C. **The lowest effective dose should be used and gradually titrated to an effective dose.**

D. Many psychotropics interfere with the CV system, and patients at higher risk for falls or heart disease should be monitored closely. Psychotropic medications with minimal CV effects should be administered.

Suggested Readings

Allison, D.B., Mentore, J.L., Heo, M., et al. (1999). Antipsychotic-induced weight gain: A comprehensive research synthesis. *American Journal of Psychiatry, 156,* 1686–1696.

Alpert, J.E., Bernstein, J.G., & Rosenbaum, J.F. (1997). Psychopharmacologic issues in the medical setting. In N.H. Cassem, T.A. Stern, J.F. Rosenbaum, & M.S. Jellinek (Eds.), *The Massachusetts General Hospital handbook of general hospital psychiatry* (4th ed., pp. 249–303). St. Louis, MO: Mosby.

Caroff, S.N., Mann, S.C., Campbell, E.C., et al. (2002). Atypical antipsychotics and movement disorders. *Journal of Clinical Psychiatry, 63*(suppl 4), 12–19.

Grebb, J.A. (2000). General principles of psychopharmacology. In H.I. Kaplan, & B.J. Sadock (Eds.), *Comprehensive textbook of psychiatry* (7th ed., pp. 2235–2250). Philadelphia, PA: Lippincott, Williams and Wilkins.

Hyman, S.E., Arana, G.W., & Rosenbaum, J.F. (1995). *Handbook of psychiatric drug therapy* (3rd ed.). Boston, MA: Little, Brown.

Lindenmayer, J.P., Nathan, A.M., & Smith, R.C. (2002). Hyperglycemia associated with the use of atypical antipsychotics. *Journal of Clinical Psychiatry, 62*(suppl 23), 30–38.

Perlis, R.H., Fava, M., Nierenberg, A.A., et al. (2002). Strategies for treatment of SSRI-associated sexual dysfunction: A survey of an academic psychopharmacology practice. *Harvard Review of Psychiatry, 10,* 109–114.

Tesar, G.E. (1998). Cardiovascular side effects of psychotropic agents. In T.A. Stern, J.B. Herman, & P.S. Slavin (Eds.), *The MGH guide to psychiatry in primary care,* pp. 497–517. New York: McGraw-Hill.

Chapter 53

Natural Medications in Psychiatry

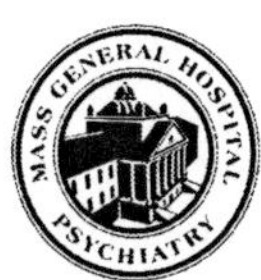

DAVID MISCHOULON AND ANDREW A. NIERENBERG

I. Introduction

A. Definition

The term **"natural medication,"** as used here, **refers to medications derived from natural products, but not approved by the Food and Drug Administration (FDA)** for their purported indication. **These medications include plants and herbs, hormones and vitamins, fatty acids, amino acid derivatives, homeopathic preparations, as well as other products.**

B. The Popularity of Natural Remedies

Natural medications, in use for thousands of years, are still quite popular in Europe, Asia, and South America. Recently, their use has increased dramatically in the United States. Widely featured on television, in newspapers, books, and Internet sites, these agents are now used by the majority of the world's population. The National Institutes of Health (NIH) recently recognized that one-fourth of the people in the United States seek and obtain non-traditional treatments (including natural medications), and **more than 70% of the population worldwide uses non-traditional treatments. In 1990, more visits were made to alternative practitioners nationwide than to primary care physicians (PCPs).** Unfortunately, traditional medical education has largely neglected the topic of natural remedies in didactic curricula. As psychiatric practitioners, we need to inform ourselves about the topic from medical, scientific, and cultural standpoints.

C. Features That Contribute to Widespread Use of These Agents

1. **A growing dissatisfaction with the medical profession** and with orthodox medicine, which in recent years has been perceived as being more preoccupied with managed care and with profits than with healing.
2. **A recent trend to have patients be more proactive in their treatment,** rather than to assume the traditional "passive" stance when working with a physician.
3. **The ready availability of natural medications without a prescription,** and the heightened sense of independence associated with the ease of access and the ability of patients to "prescribe" for themselves if they wish to bypass the medical establishment.
4. **An increasing number of non-physician practitioners who recommend these medications** without the need to consult with a medical doctor.
5. **Ease of treatment, often at a lower cost.**

II. Problems Associated with Use of Natural Medications

A. Efficacy

Several problems arise when attempting to determine the efficacy of natural medications.

1. **The benefits of natural remedies are not clear.**
2. Manufacturers, suppliers, and the federal government have typically avoided sponsoring clinical research on the benefits of natural remedies.
3. Few systematic studies have addressed whether they are efficacious or whether they are superior to placebo.
4. Most of the data on natural medications are derived from reports and uncontrolled trials (often with small samples), and not from double-blinded, placebo-controlled studies.

B. Safety

1. **Most people mistakenly believe that "natural" means "safe."**
2. Although relatively few reports of serious adverse effects from these medications exist, some individuals who have taken more than the recommended dosage, or even the recommended dosage, have become toxic.
3. Limited data regarding the safety and efficacy of combining natural medications with conventional medications are available.
4. Natural medications are not regulated by the FDA (although homeopathy is regulated).
5. Systematic study to determine optimal doses, contraindications to use, drug-drug interactions, and potential toxicities is lacking.
6. **A variety of preparations are available; they vary in potency, quality, and purity, and hence in their efficacy.**

C. Cost

1. **Some treatments can be quite expensive; they may even cost more than conventional medications.**
2. Insurance companies generally do not reimburse subscribers for these treatments, so **out-of-pocket payments are required.**
3. Natural remedies may prove less cost-effective in the long run, particularly if they are unhelpful to patients.

III. What Are the Indications for Natural Medications?

Although natural medications are said to help almost any medical problem, **there are relatively few psychiatric disorders for which natural medications are useful.** Psychiatric conditions for which these agents are used include dementia and disorders of mood, anxiety, and sleep, and possibly psychoses. Natural treatments have not been well explored for obsessive-compulsive disorder (OCD).

IV. Natural Antidepressants

A. St. John's wort (extract of *Hypericum perforatum L.*)

1. **Efficacy**
   a. Based on results of more than ten placebo-controlled trials from Europe, St. John's wort (SJW) has been **shown to be effective for mild-to-moderate depression,** and to be more effective than placebo; roughly two-thirds of patients responded to SJW.
   b. Shown to be as effective as low-dose tricyclics (imipramine 75 mg, maprotiline 75 mg, or amitriptyline 75 mg) in five active control studies; response rates were about 64% (for hypericum) vs. 59% (for tricyclics). Results against amitriptyline were not as encouraging.
   c. Recent head-to-head, large-scale clinical trials comparing SJW against the selective serotonin reuptake inhibitors (SSRIs) (fluoxetine and sertraline) and placebo have yielded mixed results. In two studies, SJW yielded a comparable response rate to fluoxetine and sertraline. However, a recent study comparing SJW with sertraline and placebo suggested no advantage for either medication when compared with placebo in moderately severe major depressive disorder (MDD). In two recent studies comparing SJW to placebo, SJW failed to separate from placebo in one study, but demonstrated a statistically significant advantage over placebo in another study. Some of these studies included individuals with more severe depression, and this may have influenced the results. The data overall appear to suggest a similar trend to that of the early European studies. Additional studies are underway.
2. **Presumed active components**
   a. The presumed active components of SJW are **polycyclic phenols, hypericin, pseudohypericin, and hyperforin.**
   b. Hypericin is generally believed to be the main active component.
   c. However, recent studies of hyperforin suggest this is a key antidepressant component (better results have been obtained with preparations containing 5% vs. 0.5% hyperforin).
3. **Possible mechanisms of action include:**
   a. The inhibition of cytokines (which changes levels of interleukins IL-6, IL-1β, and decreases cortisol).
   b. A decrease in serotonin (5-HT) receptor density.
   c. A decrease in re-uptake of neurotransmitters.
   d. A result of these components having minimal monoamine oxidase inhibitor (MAOI) activity. (Note: As a result, SJW should not be combined with a SSRI, because of the possibility of development of serotonin syndrome.)
   e. Although the metabolism of SJW is not well understood, it is presumed to be hepatic, because none has been found in urine.
4. **Suggested dose**
   a. Suggested doses of SJW range from **900 mg/day** (about 900 μg of hypericin), **to 1,800 mg/day, divided on a b.i.d. or t.i.d. basis.** However, preparations of SJW differ in the amount of active components.
5. **Adverse effects**
   a. The adverse effects of SJW may include **dry mouth, dizziness, constipation, and phototoxicity.**
   b. No data are yet available on overdose.
   c. A switch to mania in bipolar patients may be induced by SJW.
   d. A number of cases of adverse **drug-drug interactions** with SJW have emerged. Hyperforin induces CYP-3A4 expression, and may reduce the therapeutic activity of a number of medications, including warfarin, cyclosporine, oral contraceptives, theophylline, fenprocoumon, digoxin, indinavir, and camptosar. There are cases of transplant rejection resulting from SJW-cyclosporine interactions. Transplant recipients and HIV-positive individuals receiving protease inhibitors should not use SJW.
6. **Summary**
   a. SJW **appears better than placebo, and equivalent to low-dose tricyclics (and probably SSRIs) for the treatment of depression.** It may be most effective for milder forms of depression. **It is apparently safe to use, but care must be taken with drug-drug interactions.** More controlled studies are needed.

B. S-Adenosyl Methionine (SAMe)

1. **Efficacy**
   a. SAMe has demonstrated a **mood-elevating effect** in depressed patients. A small number of clinical studies suggest that **doses up to 1,600 mg/day** of parenteral (intravenous [IV] or intramuscular [IM]) and oral SAMe preparations are superior to placebo and as effective as tricyclic antidepressants (TCAs).
   b. However, some early studies are problematic, due to **instability of oral SAMe preparations.**
   c. SAMe may have a relatively **faster onset of action** than conventional agents; some patients have shown improvement in as little as one to two weeks. The combination of SAMe and low dose TCAs may result in earlier onset of action than with a TCA alone.
   d. **Other indications** for SAMe may include treatment of cognitive deficits in dementia, relief of distress during the purpuerium, reduction of psychological distress during opioid detoxification, antidepressant benefit for the alcoholic, use in medically ill depressed patients for whom conventional antidepressants may be contraindicated, and relief from arthritis or other disease of the joints.
2. **Mechanism of action**
   a. SAMe is a major **methyl donor** in the brain. It donates methyl groups to hormones, neurotransmitters, nucleic

acids, proteins, and phospholipids. SAMe levels depend on levels of the **vitamins folate and B_{12}.** Deficiencies in folate and B_{12} are also associated with development of depression and/or refractoriness to treatment (see section C).

b. SAMe may exert its antidepressant effect by donating methyl groups in the reactions that result in the **synthesis of norepinephrine, serotonin, and dopamine,** deficiencies of which have been associated with mood disorders.

3. **Suggested doses**

a. Recommended doses of SAMe, based on clinical studies, **range from 400–1,600 mg/day.** Clinical experience suggests that **some patients may need even higher doses.** SAMe is relatively expensive ($0.50–1.25 for a 200 mg tablet), and the cost may be prohibitive to many patients, particularly those requiring higher doses.

4. **Side effects and toxicity (rare)**

a. SAMe is **relatively free of adverse effects,** and has no apparent hepatotoxicity. Side effects include mild insomnia, lack of appetite, constipation, nausea, dry mouth, sweating, dizziness, and nervousness. There are some reports of increased **anxiety, mania, or hypomania** in patients with bipolar depression.

b. So far, there **are no reports of adverse drug-drug interactions** with SAMe.

5. **Summary**

a. SAMe appears to be safe and effective for depression, but larger studies are needed to establish this with certainty.

C. Folate and Vitamin B_{12}

1. **Folic acid**

a. Folic acid is required for the synthesis of SAMe, which is needed for synthesis of norepinephrine (NE), dopamine (DA), and serotonin (5-HT).

b. **Between 10% and 30% of depressed patients may have low levels of serum folate.**

c. **Patients with low folate levels respond less well to antidepressants than those with normal folate levels.**

d. The recommended dose of folate is **400 μg/day.**

e. Folate may potentiate the effect of conventional antidepressants in non-folate-deficient individuals.

2. **Vitamin B_{12}**

a. Vitamin B_{12} is converted to methylcobalamin, a substance that is involved in the synthesis of central nervous system (CNS) neurotransmitters.

b. Vitamin B_{12} deficiency may result in an earlier age of onset of depression.

c. The recommended dose of Vitamin B_{12} is **6 μg/day.**

3. **Summary**

a. Physicians should check levels of vitamin B_{12} and folate in patients with treatment-resistant depression, particularly if they have concurrent medical illness.

b. **Correction of folate and Vitamin B_{12} deficiency may improve depressive symptoms and one's response to antidepressant therapy.**

D. Dehydroepiandrosterone (DHEA)

1. **Characterization of DHEA**

a. DHEA is **an adrenal steroid,** which is converted to testosterone and estrogen.

2. **Efficacy**

a. An open treatment study of six middle-aged and elderly depressed patients with 30–90 mg/day of DHEA for 4 weeks resulted in improvement in depressive symptoms and memory.

3. **Mechanism of action**

a. Mechanisms of DHEA may include GABA (γ-aminobutyric acid) antagonism, NMDA (*N*-methyl-D-aspartate) potentiation, increase in brain serotonin and dopamine activity.

4. **Suggested doses**

a. Suggested doses of DHEA are **5–100 mg/day.**

b. Over-the-counter strength and purity are not regulated.

5. **Adverse effects**

a. Side effects **include acne, irritability, insomnia, headaches, menstrual irregularities, increased ocular pressure, and palpitations.**

6. **Summary**

a. Early data on DHEA are promising, but larger studies are needed. Its role for the treatment of women is unclear.

E. Phenylethylamine (PEA)

1. **Mechanism of action**

a. PEA is **a neurohormone** believed to maintain energy, attention, affect, and courage.

b. PEA's action is probably related to catecholamine release from sympathetic nerves, in a fashion similar to that of amphetamine; it has no tolerance or reinforcement patterns.

c. Deficiency of PEA may have a role in development of depression.

2. **Efficacy**

a. Open studies show that **administration of oral PEA in combination with low-dose MAOI is effective in 60% of depressed patients.** (Note: PEA is metabolized by MAO; it is therefore necessary to either give high doses of PEA or concomitant doses of a MAOI.)

b. Mood elevation associated with use of PEA may occur in 1–2 days; full remission requires 2 weeks.

3. **Suggested doses**

a. The suggested dose of PEA is **10–60 mg/day,** given along with 5–10 mg of selegiline.

4. **Adverse effects**

a. **Mild anorexia** is the only reported adverse event.

5. **Interactions with other psychotropics**

a. Co-administration of MAOIs, and TCAs can increase PEA levels.

b. Co-administration of lithium may decrease PEA levels.

c. Use of alcohol or marijuana may increase PEA levels.

6. **Manufacturing/distribution issues**

a. PEA is generally not distributed to drug stores.

b. The physician must order powder in bulk from a manufacturer, and enlist a pharmacist to prepare PEA in tablet form; then the patient must buy the medication at that pharmacy.

7. **Summary**
   a. While data on the use of PEA are promising, anecdotes about its use are not as encouraging.
   b. Logistics of PEA administration and distribution are a limitation to its use.

F. Essential Fatty Acids (EFAs)

1. **Classification**
   a. EFAs (primarily omega-3 and omega-6) are **polyunsaturated lipids derived from fish oil.**
   b. **Eicosapentanoic acid (EPA)** and **docosahexanoic acid (DHA)** are thought to be psychotropically active omega-3 fatty acids.
2. **Efficacy**
   a. Omega-3 fatty acids **may have a protective role against depression and bipolar disorder,** based on lower rates of depression in countries where large amounts of fish are consumed.
   b. Recent double-blind placebo controlled trials of **eicosapentanoic acid (EPA)** suggest efficacy in **major depression and schizophrenia.**
   c. Omega-3 fatty acids may also have a role in the treatment of **bipolar disorder.** One small double-blind, placebo-controlled trial with 30 bipolar-disordered patients revealed that, of those who received the omega-3 mix, only one had a recurrence; subjects in this group also had a longer period of remission.
   d. Omega-3 and omega-6 mixtures may help alleviate psychotic symptoms. Case reports with EFAs show variable results when used alone or as an adjunct to antipsychotics.
3. **Mechanisms of action**
   a. **EFAs may function in a fashion similar to mood stabilizers. They seem to inhibit G-protein signal transduction via reduced hydrolysis of phosphatidylinositol and other membrane phospholipids,** which are precursors to second messengers.
4. **Suggested dosing**
   a. Commercially available preparations of omega-3 may have **up to 1,000 mg (1 g) of omega-3, with varying ratios of EPA:DHA. Individual preparations of EPA and DHA are becoming available.**
   b. Recent evidence suggests that psychotropically active doses of omega-3 may be in the range of **1–2 g/day.**
5. **Adverse effects**
   a. Mild dose-related **gastrointestinal distress** appears to be the only side effect associated with use of EFAs.
6. **Summary**
   a. Overall, the use of EFAs is promising, particularly in view of the wide variety of illnesses potentially treatable with these substances. However, larger studies are needed.

G. Inositol

1. **Classification**
   a. Inositol is **a polyol precursor of second messenger systems** in the brain.
2. **Mechanism of action**
   a. Levels of inositol in the cerebrospinal fluid (CSF) may be decreased in the presence of depression.
   b. Administration of inositol may reverse the desensitization of serotonin receptors.
3. **Efficacy**
   a. Inositol has been studied in a variety of conditions.
      i. Depression. In a double-blind, controlled trial of 12 g/day for 4 weeks, inositol was shown to be superior to placebo (28 patients).
      ii. Panic disorder. In a double-blind, controlled trial of 12 g/day for 4 weeks, inositol administration resulted in a decrease in frequency and severity of panic attacks and agoraphobia (21 patients).
      iii. Obsessive-compulsive disorder (OCD). In a double-blind, controlled trial of 18 mg/day for 6 weeks, inositol resulted in alleviation of symptoms associated with OCD (13 patients).
      iv. No effect was apparent in schizophrenia, attention deficit hyperactivity disorder (ADHD), Alzheimer's disease, autism, or electroconvulsive therapy (ECT)–induced cognitive impairment.
4. **Side effects and toxicity**
   a. **No apparent toxicity** has been associated with use of inositol; it has a mild side-effect profile.
5. **Summary**
   a. **Overall, inositol is a promising treatment with multiple possible indications.** However, trials so far have been small; larger patient samples are required for a better understanding of this drug's efficacy.

V. Natural Anxiolytics

A. Valerian *(Valeriana officinalis)*

1. **Efficacy**
   a. Valerian is **sedating** and a mild hypnotic.
   b. It is not ideal for acute treatment of insomnia, but it does promote natural sleep after several weeks of use.
   c. Valerian is very popular among Hispanics.
   d. There are only a few (about ten) small, controlled, clinical trials regarding use of valerian. It decreases sleep latency and improves sleep quality; apparently there is no dependence or daytime drowsiness.
   e. When compared with flunitrazepam in one study, it was found to have the same efficacy but with fewer side effects.
2. **Mechanism of action**
   a. Valerian's efficacy is attributed to valepotriates, and sesquiterpenes, but it may function in a fashion similar to benzodiazepines.
   b. It decreases GABA breakdown, and causes changes in the electroencephalogram (EEG) during sleep.
   c. Its metabolism is not well understood.
3. **Suggested doses**
   a. The suggested dose for valerian is **450–600 mg, taken 2 hours before bedtime.**

Table 53-1. Natural Medications and Their Indications and Usage

Medication	*Active Components*	*Putative Indications*	*Possible Mechanisms of Action*	*Suggested Doses*	*Adverse Events*
Black cohosh (*Cimicifuga racemosa*)	Triterpenoids, isoflavones, aglycones	Menopausal symptoms	Suppression of luteinizing hormone	40 mg/day	Gastrointestinal upset, dizziness, headache, weight gain
Chaste tree berry (*Vitex agnus castus*)	Unknown	Premenstrual symptoms	Prolactin inhibition, interaction with dopaminergic receptors	200–400 mg/day	None
Dehydro-epiandrosterone (DHEA)	Adrenal gland steroid hormone	Depression and dementia	GABA antagonism, NMDA potentiation, increase in brain serotonin and dopamine activity	5–100 mg/day in b.i.d.–t.i.d. dosing	Acne, irritability, insomnia, headaches, menstrual irregularities, increased ocular pressure, palpitations
Fatty acids	Essential fatty acids (primarily omega-6 and omega-3)	Depression (docosahexanoic acid–omega-3) Mania (omega-3 fatty acid mix) Psychosis (omega-3 and omega-6)	Inhibition of membrane signal transduction	1,000–2,000 mg/day	Gastrointestinal upset
Folic acid	Vitamin	Depression	Neurotransmitter synthesis	400 μg/day	None
Ginkgo biloba	Flavonoids, terpene lactones	Dementia	Nerve cell stimulation and protection, membrane/receptor stabilization, free-radical scavenging, PAF inhibition	120–240 mg/day in b.i.d.–t.i.d. dose	Mild gastrointestinal upset, headache, irritability, dizziness
Homeopathy	Various herbs and minerals	Various disorders	Unknown	Varies with preparation	Mild transient worsening of target symptoms
Inositol	Second messenger precursor	Depression, panic, OCD	Second messenger synthesis, sensitization of serotonin receptors	12–18 g/day	Mild
Kava (*Piper methysticum*)	Kavapyrones	Anxiety	Central muscle relaxant, anticonvulsant, GABA receptor binding	60–120 mg/day	Gastrointestinal upset, allergic skin reactions, headaches, dizziness, ataxia, hair loss, visual problems, respiratory problems, dermopathy, severe liver toxicity
Melatonin	Pineal gland hormone	Insomnia	Circadian rhythm regulation in suprachiasmatic nucleus	0.25–0.3 mg/day	Sedation, confusion, inhibition of fertility, decreased sex drive, hypothermia, retinal damage

(continued)

Table 53-1. *(Continued)*

Medication	*Active Components*	*Putative Indications*	*Possible Mechanisms of Action*	*Suggested Doses*	*Adverse Events*
Phenylethylamine (PEA)	Neurohormone, amino acid derivative	Depression	Catecholamine release	10–60 mg/day, with 5–10 mg/day of selegiline	Mild anorexia
St. John's wort (*Hypericum perforatum* L.)	Hypericin, hyperforin, polycyclic phenols, pseudohypericin	Depression	Cytokine production, decreased serotonin receptor density, decreased neurotransmitter reuptake, MAOI activity	900–1,800 mg/day in b.i.d.–t.i.d. dosing	Dry mouth, dizziness, constipation, phototoxicity, serotonin syndrome when combined with SSRIs, adverse interactions with other drugs
Valerian (*Valeriana officinalis*)	Valepotriates, sesquiterpenes	Insomnia	Decrease GABA breakdown	450–600 mg/day	Blurry vision, dystonias, hepatotoxicity, mutagenicity?
Vitamin B_{12}	Vitamin	Depression	Neurotransmitter synthesis	6 µg/day	None

4. **Side effects and toxicity (rare)**
   a. Side effects include **blurry vision, dystonias, and hepatotoxicity.**
   b. Since Mexican or Indian valerian may pose a mutagenic risk, these preparations should not be used.
5. **Summary**
   a. Overall, data on valerian are promising; double-blind trials and trials comparing valerian to more conventional anxiolytic/hypnotics are needed.
   b. Unfortunately, the logistics of creating a double-blind trial are complicated by valerian's distinctive and powerful smell (due to isovaleric acid). A placebo with a similar smell will need to be created.

B. Kava *(Piper methysticum)*

1. **Kava originated in the Polynesian Islands.** It was originally prepared by virgins of the tribe, who chewed kava roots, placed the mash in a fermenting pot, and then prepared a tealike drink that was consumed by all tribe members (kava is not prepared this way in the United States!).
2. **Efficacy**
   a. Kava is **believed to have a calming and relaxing effect** ("With kava in you, you can't hate"), without altering consciousness.
   b. Controlled, double-blind studies (about six trials) suggest it may be helpful for mild anxiety states, including agoraphobia, specific phobias, generalized anxiety disorder (GAD), and adjustment disorder.
3. **Mechanism of action**
   a. Kava's mechanism of action is thought to be a result of **kavapyrones.**
   b. These agents are central muscle relaxants and anticonvulsants.
   c. They are involved with GABA receptor binding, and norepinephrine uptake inhibition.
   d. They reduce the excitability of the limbic system, perhaps as well as benzodiazepines do, but they are not associated with either dependence or withdrawal.
   e. The half-life of kava varies from 90 minutes to several hours.
   f. Bioavailability can vary up to ten-fold, depending on the preparation.
4. **Suggested doses**
   a. The suggested dose of kava is **60–120 mg/day.**
5. **Side effects (mild)**
   a. Mild side effects are possible, and **include gastrointestinal upset, allergic skin reactions, headaches, and dizziness.**
6. **Toxic reactions**
   a. Toxic reactions may occur with high doses or prolonged use, and **include ataxia, hair loss, visual problems, respiratory problems, and a kava dermopathy** (transient yellowing of the skin, perhaps related to cholesterol metabolism).
   b. These toxic effects are reversible if the use of kava is discontinued.
   c. Recently, there have emerged at least two dozen cases of **severe hepatotoxicity** related to kava; in some cases **liver transplant** has been required. A direct relationship between kava and liver disease was not uniformly clear, and some individuals may have been taking excessive doses. Several countries have since removed kava from the market, and the U.S. FDA is investigating its safety.
   d. The sudden emergence of kava-related liver toxicity may reflect increasing use of kava in the absence of physician

supervision. Physicians should proceed with caution regarding prescription of kava. **It is recommended that duration of use of kava not exceed three months.** Individuals with a history of liver disease or alcohol use, or those who are taking concurrent medications with potential liver toxicity, should avoid kava.

7. **Summary**
   a. Kava appears to be **more effective than placebo for mild anxiety states;** studies are needed to compare it with other anxiolytics.
   b. The **safety** of kava for over-the-counter use is currently under scrutiny.

C. Melatonin

1. **Definition**
   a. Melatonin is **a hormone derived from serotonin;** it is made in the pineal gland.
2. **Efficacy**
   a. Melatonin is involved in the organization of circadian rhythms.
   b. It is commonly used by travelers to reset their biological clocks when traveling across time zones; this is the main source of melatonin's popularity.
   c. It is **believed to be an effective hypnotic;** it works within 1 hour of administration, regardless of the time of day it is taken.
   d. It may be **more effective for people with insomnia caused by circadian rhythm disturbances.**
3. **Mechanism of action**
   a. The effects of melatonin may involve interaction with the suprachiasmatic nucleus.
   b. It seems to reset the circadian pacemaker and attenuates an alerting process.
   c. There may also be a direct soporific effect.
4. **Recommended doses**
   a. The recommended dose of melatonin for decreasing sleep latency is **0.25–0.30 mg/day.**
   b. Many melatonin preparations have as much as 5 mg of melatonin.
5. **Side effects and toxicity**
   a. Side effects and toxicity are rare. However, they may **include daytime sleepiness or confusion with high doses, inhibition of fertility, decreased sex drive, hypothermia, and retinal damage.**
6. **Contraindications**
   a. Contraindications to use of melatonin **include pregnancy and an immunocompromised status** (e.g., human immunodeficiency virus [HIV]-positive individuals, or people who take steroids or other immunosuppressant drugs).
7. **Summary**
   a. Melatonin is an agent that is promising, and is generally **accepted as safe and effective.**
   b. It may also have a potential use in children with sleep disorders.

VI. Medications for Pre-menstrual/ Menopausal Symptoms

A. Black Cohosh (*Cimicifuga racemosa*)

1. **Efficacy**
   a. Black cohosh comes from an herbaceous plant that is used for alleviation of menopausal symptoms (physical and psychological).
   b. Five placebo-controlled studies show black cohosh to be **efficacious,** as measured by changes in various psychometric scales, **in doses of 40 mg/day.**
2. **Active ingredients**
   a. Its active ingredients are **triterpenoids, isoflavones, and aglycones.**
3. **Mechanism**
   a. Its mechanism of action may involve suppression of luteinizing hormone (in the pituitary gland); speculation has been raised that it may also have an antibreast cancer effect.
4. **Suggested dose**
   a. Its suggested dose is **40 mg/day.**
5. **Side effects (mild)**
   a. Side effects are mild and **include gastrointestinal upset, headache, dizziness, and weight gain.**
6. **Toxicity**
   a. No specific toxicity has been associated with black cohosh, but data are limited.
7. **Contraindications**
   a. Contraindications to use **include pregnancy, the presence of heart disease, and hypertension.**
8. **Summary**
   a. So far, the use of black cohosh is promising, but further study is needed.
   b. Because of limited data on safety, duration of use is not recommended to exceed three months.

B. Chaste Tree Berry (*Vitex agnus castus*)

1. **Classification**
   a. The dried fruit of the chaste tree was reported to help medieval monks keep the vow of chastity (via decreasing their sex drive).
2. **Efficacy**
   a. **Used for the alleviation of pre-menstrual syndrome (PMS),** based on PTMS scale. One controlled double-blind study (175 mg/day chaste berry vs. pyridoxine) has revealed a decrease in symptoms of PMS.
3. **Mechanism**
   a. Although its clinically active ingredient is not known, its effect may be due to prolactin inhibition (one study of women); its relation to D_2 dopaminergic receptors is under investigation.
4. **Dosing**
   a. Suggested dosing is **200–400 mg/day.**
5. **Adverse effects**
   a. **No adverse events** have been reported.
6. **Summary**
   a. More systematic trials of chaste tree berry are needed.

VII. Cognition-Enhancing Remedies

A. Ginkgo Biloba (Seed from *Ginkgo biloba* Tree)

1. **Efficacy**
   a. Ginkgo biloba has been used in Chinese medicine for over 2,000 years, for treatment of cognitive deficits and affective symptoms in organic brain diseases (e.g., Alzheimer's disease and vascular dementias).
      i. **Target symptoms include memory, abstract thinking, and affective symptoms.**
      ii. Ginkgo may also improve learning capacity.
   b. Ginkgo's potential role in the treatment of antidepressant-induced sexual dysfunction is under study.
      i. In males and females on several antidepressants, low-dose ginkgo has resulted in improvement in all aspects of sexual dysfunction (desire, arousal, orgasm, and resolution).
2. **Active components**
   a. The active components of ginkgo **include flavonoids and terpene lactones.**
3. **Mechanisms of action**
   a. Ginkgo **stimulates still functional nerve cells.**
   b. **It protects them from pathologic effects, such as hypoxia, ischemia, seizures, and peripheral damage.**
   c. As membrane/receptor stabilizer, it appears to be a **free-radical scavenger.**
   d. Ginkgolide B **inhibits platelet activating factor;** ginkgo should therefore be avoided in individuals with a bleeding disorder.
4. **Efficacy**
   a. Many double-blind trials have suggested that **symptoms of dementia improve with use of ginkgo** (more than 30 trials).
   b. However, standards for testing the response to treatment have changed over time.
   c. The German Federal Health Agency Mandates of 1991 reported that improvement in dementia *symptoms* (e.g., memory, abstract thinking) is not enough. We also need to see improvement in activities of daily living (ADLs) and a reduced need for care.
   d. Many older studies have therefore been uninformative as they have not met new methodological criteria.
5. **Recent studies**
   a. A year-long randomized, double-blind study of 309 patients suggests that ginkgo may stabilize and improve cognitive performance and social functioning in demented patients. Changes were modest but significant, and were noticeable by caretakers.
   b. Some studies have compared ginkgo against other nootropics (e.g., ergot alkaloids, nicergoline, and nimodipine).
      i. Studies showed comparable efficacy; ginkgo seems to have had fewer side effects.
      ii. For these reasons, 24–28% of physicians recommend ginkgo.
      iii. Family physicians in particular tend to favor ginkgo over other nootropics.
6. **Suggested dose**
   a. Suggested doses of ginkgo are **120–240 mg/day** (on a b.i.d.-t.i.d. basis).
   b. At least an 8-week course is recommended. The patient should be re-evaluated after three months of use; full assessment of effect may require up to one year of use.
7. **Side effects include mild gastrointestinal upset, headache, irritability, and dizziness.**
8. **Summary**
   a. Overall, ginkgo **appears to be effective, with a very low rate of toxicity.** No interactions with other drugs have been detected.
   b. A potential role in the amelioration of antidepressant-induced sexual dysfunction has been studied.
   c. Its full role remains to be clarified.

VIII. Homeopathy

A. History

1. Developed in Germany 200 years ago by Samuel Hahnemann, **homeopathy is the second most utilized health care system worldwide.**
2. It is **derived from plants and minerals.**
3. It is regulated by the FDA, and sold over-the-counter.

B. Principles and Paradoxes of Homeopathy

1. **Potency is believed to be proportional to the degree of dilution.**
2. Preparation, therefore, involves dilution to minute quantities.
3. **Principle of similars**
   a. **Symptoms represent the body's attempt to heal itself.**
   b. **Therefore, the medication must paradoxically cause the symptoms it intends to alleviate.**
4. The homeopath obtains a careful history, with the goal of finding the one medication or combination of medications that will help the body heal its symptoms.
   a. Personality, diet, sleep pattern, reaction to temperature, and weather are considered (use of milk products is often an issue).
   b. Homeopathic remedies are administered orally, and allowed to dissolve on, or under, the tongue.
   c. **Improvement tends to be gradual, on the order of weeks to months.**
   d. **A transient aggravation of symptoms may occur early in treatment.**

C. Mechanism of Action

1. Its mechanism of action is controversial and **not well understood.** It has drawn on various disciplines to explain it, but none is entirely convincing.
   a. Quantum theory
   b. Water clathrate formation (small amounts of crystals can cause lattice change in water, therefore, small amounts of medication may cause major changes in disease)
   c. Thalamic neuron theory

D. Efficacy

1. Most research has focused on physical health rather than on mental health.
2. One study examined 12 patients with various psychiatric disorders, including social phobia, panic, major depressive disorder (MDD), attention deficit disorder (ADD), and chronic fatigue.
3. There is also a meta-analysis of 107 trials.
4. These data suggest that homeopathy may be useful, but most studies are not rigorously designed.

E. Adverse Effects

1. Apparently, **side effects are benign, except for the initial worsening of symptoms,** which can often result in discontinuation of treatment.
2. No known drug interactions or overdose risk have been reported.

F. Summary

1. Homeopathy reveals promising results in some cases, but further studies are needed.
2. For long-term use of these remedies, many seek assistance from a homeopathic practitioner in view of the frequent need for combination treatments.

IX. Recommendations for Practitioners

A. Routinely inquire about patients' use of natural medications, as many patients will not volunteer information about their use of these remedies.

B. Monitor patients who are on multiple medications. Be alert for potential adverse drug-drug interactions.

C. Emphasize to patients that these alternative medications are relatively untested.

D. State that it is unclear whether natural medications are appropriate or even preferable to conventional psychotropics.

X. Candidates for Alternative Treatments

A. Mildly symptomatic patients with a strong interest in natural remedies.

B. Patients who have failed multiple trials of conventional remedies, or who are highly intolerant of side effects.

1. Keep in mind that these patients are often the most difficult to treat, and alternative agents seem best suited to the mildly ill.

XI. Conclusions

A. Natural medications are a growing field in psychopharmacology, and, in time, they may prove a valuable addition to the pharmacological armamentarium.

B. Early research data and anecdotal reports are promising, particularly with mild-to-moderate illness.

C. To recommend them as effective and safe, we need more systematic, controlled studies on adequate patient samples.

D. The NIH and NIMH have begun to support large-scale studies, and these will hopefully result in more useful guidelines and recommendations for clinicians.

Suggested Readings

Alpert, J.E., & Fava, M. (1997). Nutrition and depression: The role of folate. *Nutrition Review, 55,* 145–149.

Alpert, J.E., Mischoulon, D., Rubenstein, G.E.F., et al. (2002). Folinic acid (Leucovorin) as an adjunctive treatment for SSRI-refractory depression. *Annals of Clinical Psychiatry, 14,* 33–38.

Benjamin, J., Agam, G., Levine, J., et al. (1995). Inositol treatment in psychiatry. *Psychopharmacology Bulletin, 31,* 167–175.

Chatterjee, S.S., Bhattacharya, S.K., Wonnermann, M., et al. (1998). Hyperforin as a possible antidepressant component of hypericum extracts. *Life Science, 63,* 499–510.

Cohen, A. (1996). Treatment of antidepressant-induced sexual dysfunction: A new scientific study shows benefits of ginkgo biloba. *Healthwatch, 5*(1).

Comas-Diaz, L. (1989). Culturally relevant issues and treatment implications for Hispanics. In D.R. Koslow, & E.P. Salett (Eds.), *Crossing cultures in mental health,* pp. 31–48. Washington, DC: SIETAR International.

Crone, C.C., & Wise, T.N. (1998). Use of herbal medicines among consultation-liaison populations. *Psychosomatics, 39,* 3–13.

Davidson, J.R., Morrison, R.M., Shore, J., et al. (1997). Homeopathic treatment of depression and anxiety. *Alternative Therapy Health Medicine, 3,* 46–49.

Eisenberg, D.M. (1997). Advising patients who seek alternative medical therapies. *Annals of Internal Medicine, 127,* 61–69.

Eisenberg, D.M., Kessler, R.C., Foster, C., et al. (1993). Unconventional medicine in the United States: Prevalence, costs, and patterns of use. *New England Journal of Medicine, 328,* 246–252.

Ernst, E. (1998). Harmless herbs? A review of the recent literature. *American Journal of Medicine, 104,* 170–178.

Farrel, R.J., & Lamb, J. (1990). Herbal remedies. *British Journal of Medicine, 300,* 47–48.

Fava, M., Borus, J.S., Alpert, J.E., et al. (1997). Folate, B_{12}, and homocysteine in major depressive disorder. *American Journal of Psychiatry, 154,* 426–428.

Furnham, A., & Bhagrath, R. (1993). A comparison of health beliefs and behaviours of clients of orthodox and complementary medicine. *British Journal of Clinical Psychology, 32,* 237–246.

Furnham, A., & Smith, C. (1988). Choosing alternative medicine: A comparison of the beliefs of patients visiting a general practitioner and a homeopath. *Social Science Medicine, 26,* 685–689.

Itil, T., & Martorano, D. (1995). Natural substances in psychiatry (Ginkgo biloba in dementia). *Psychopharmacology Bulletin, 31,* 147–158.

Jenike, M.A. (1994). Hypericum: A novel antidepressant. *Journal of Geriatric Psychiatry Neurology, 7,* S1–S68.

Jonas, W., & Jacobs, J. (1996). *Healing with homeopathy.* New York: Warner.

Kleijnen, J., Knipschild, P., & ter Riet, G. (1991). Clinical trials of homeopathy. *British Medical Journal, 302,* 316–323.

Krippner, S. (1995). A cross cultural comparison of four healing models. *Alternative Therapy Health Medication, 1,* 21–29.

Laakmann, G., Schule, C., Baghai, T., et al. (1998). St. John's wort in mild to moderate depression: The relevance of hyperforin for the clinical efficacy. *Pharmacopsychiatry, 31*(suppl 1), 54–59.

Leathwood, P.D., & Chauffard, F. (1985). Aqueous extract of valerian reduces latency to fall asleep in man. *Planta Medicine, 2,* 144–148.

LeBars, P.L., Katz, M.M., Berman, N., et al. (1997). A placebo-controlled, double-blind, randomized trial of an extract of Ginkgo biloba for dementia. North American EGb Study Group. *Journal of the American Medical Association, 278,* 1327–1332.

Lecrubier, Y., Clerc, G., Didi, R., & Kieser, M. (2002). Efficacy of St. John's wort extract WS 5570 in major depression: A double-blind, placebo-controlled trial. *American Journal of Psychiatry, 159*(8), 1361–1366.

Linde, K., Ramirez, G., Mulrow, C.D., et al. (1996). St. John's wort for depression—An overview and meta-analysis of randomized clinical trials. *British Medical Journal, 313,* 253–258.

MacGregor, F.B., Abernethy V.E., Dahabra, S., et al. (1989). Hepatotoxicity of herbal medicines. *British Medical Journal, 299,* 1156–1157.

Mathews, J.D., Riley, M.D., Fejo, L., et al. (1988). Effects of the heavy usage of kava on physical health: Summary of a pilot survey in an aboriginal community. *Medical Journal of Australia, 148,* 548–555.

Matsumoto, J. (1995). Molecular mechanism of biological responses to homeopathic medicines. *Medical Hypotheses, 45,* 292–296.

Maurer, K., Ihl, R., Dierks, T., & Frolich, L. (1997). Clinical efficacy of Ginkgo biloba special extract EGb 761 in dementia of the Alzheimer type. *Journal of Psychiatry Research, 31,* 645–655.

National Institutes of Health Office of Alternative Medicine. (1997). Clinical practice guidelines in complementary and alternative medicine. An analysis of opportunities and obstacles. Practice and Policy Guidelines Panel. *Archives of Family Medicine, 6,* 149–154.

Nierenberg, A.A. (1998). St. John's wort: A putative over-the-counter herbal antidepressant. *Journal of Depressive Disorders: Index Review, 3*(3), 16–17.

Norton, S.A., & Ruze, P. (1994). Kava dermopathy. *Journal of the American Academy of Dermatology, 31,* 89–97.

Packer-Tursman, J. (2002, January 22). Anxiety over kava. *Washington Post,* p. HE01.

Peet, M., Brind J., Ramchand, C.N., et al. (2001). Two double-blind placebo-controlled pilot studies of eicosapentaenoic acid in the treatment of schizophrenia. *Schizophrenia Research, 49*(3), 243–251.

Peet, M., Horrobin, D.F. (2002). A dose-ranging study of the effects of ethyl-eicosapentaenoate in patients with ongoing depression despite apparently adequate treatment with standard drugs. *Archives of General Psychiatry, 59*(10), 913–919.

Peet, M., Laugharne, J.D., Mellor, J., & Ramchand, C.N. (1996). Essential fatty acid deficiency in erythrocyte membranes from chronic schizophrenic patients, and the clinical effects of dietary supplementation. *Prostaglandins Leukotrienes Essential Fatty Acids, 55,* 71–75.

Sabelli, H., Fink, P., Fawcett, J., & Tom, C. (1996). Sustained antidepressant effect of PEA replacement. *Journal of Neuropsychiatry Clinical Neuroscience, 8,* 168–171.

Sack, R.L., Hughes, R.J., Edgar, D.M., & Lewy, A.J. (1997). Sleep-promoting effects of melatonin: At what dose, in whom, under what conditions, and by what mechanisms? *Sleep, 20,* 908–915.

Schulz, V., Hänsel, R., & Tyler, V.E. (1998). *Rational phytotherapy: A physicians' guide to herbal medicine* (3rd ed.). Berlin: Springer.

Schwartz, G.E., & Russek L.G. (1997). Dynamical energy systems and modern physics: Fostering the science and spirit of complementary and alternative medicine. *Alternative Therapy Health Medicine, 3,* 46–56.

Singh, Y.N. (1992). Kava: An overview. *Journal of Ethnopharmacology, 37,* 13–45.

Stoppe, G., Sandholzer, H., Staedt, J., et al. (1996). Prescribing practice with cognition enhancers in outpatient care: Are there differences regarding type of dementia? Results of a representative survey in lower Saxony, Germany. *Pharmacopsychiatry, 29,* 150–155.

Volz, H.P. (1997). Controlled clinical trials of hypericum extracts in depressed patients—An overview. *Pharmacopsychiatry, 30*(suppl 2), 72–76.

Wetzel, M.S., Eisenberg, D.M., & Kaptchuk, T.J. (1998). Courses involving complementary and alternative medicine at US medical schools. *Journal of the American Medical Association, 280,* 784–787.

Whitmore, S.M., & Leake, N.B. (1996). Complementary therapies: An adjunct to traditional therapies [letter]. *Nurse Practictioner, 21,* 12–13.

Williams, L.L., Kiecolt-Glaser, J.K., Horrocks, L.A., et al. (1992). Quantitative association between altered plasma esterified omega-6 fatty acid proportions and psychological stress. *Prostaglandins Leukotrienes Essential Fatty Acids, 47,* 165–70.

Wolkowitz, O.M., Reus, V.I., Roberts, E., et al. (1997). Dehydroepiandro-sterone (DHEA) treatment of depression. *Biologic Psychiatry, 41,* 311–318.

Wooltorton, E. (2002). Herbal kava: Reports of liver toxicity. *CMA Journal, 166,* 777.

Chapter 54

Suicide

Roy H. Perlis and Theodore A. Stern

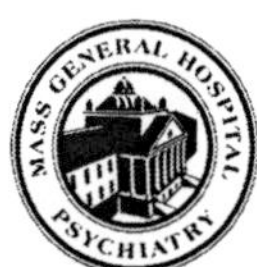

I. Overview

As the **eleventh leading cause of death** in the United States, suicide represents a significant public health problem. **Each year, some 29,000 people commit suicide; for every attempt that is successful, between 10 and 25 will fail.**

Up to two-thirds of those who commit suicide visit a physician in the month prior to making an attempt, though this visit is often not associated with psychiatric complaints. Screening for suicidal ideas and assessing for risk factors provides an opportunity to intervene before an attempt occurs. Such screening is essential in psychiatric populations, as **up to 90% of patients who commit suicide carry at least one major psychiatric diagnosis.**

II. Epidemiology (see Table 54-1)

Population-based studies demonstrate that suicide rates vary widely among different demographic groups.

A. Gender

Although females *attempt* suicide at a rate three times that of males, males are four times more likely to succeed. This difference has been attributed to the more lethal means often chosen by men.

B. Age

In general, suicide rates increase with age, with the greatest rates seen in those over the age of 60 years. Those age 15–24 years represent an important exception to this trend, as suicide has become the third leading cause of death in this group. Moreover, for every completed attempt among adolescents, there are 100–200 unsuccessful attempts. Among depressed patients, however, one major study showed a mean age of 36 years in men and 45 years in women.

C. Ethnicity

In the United States, suicide rates are highest among Caucasian and Native American populations. Outside of the United States, reported suicide rates show wide variation. Reasons for variation among ethnic and cultural groups are unknown.

D. Individual Factors

According to population studies, individuals who are divorced or widowed, who are unemployed or in financial difficulty, or who live alone, also have higher suicide rates. For example, suicide rates are four times greater in those who are divorced, compared with those who are married.

III. Evaluation (see Table 54-2)

Unfortunately, the demographic factors mentioned earlier are of limited utility in identifying particular patients at risk for suicide. Moreover, people who are contemplating suicide are often reluctant to reveal suicidal thoughts, particularly to clinicians with whom they do not have a long-standing relationship. Thus, suicide risk must be assessed even in those who do not express suicidal ideas.

A. Survivors of a Suicide Attempt

Those patients who have already attempted suicide or inflicted self-harm should be assessed as soon as possible.

B. Individuals who Express Thoughts of Suicide or Hopelessness

Those who openly express suicidal thoughts or hopelessness should be asked specifically about suicidal intention and plans.

Table 54-1. Selected Epidemiologic Risk Factors for Suicide

Demographic
Male gender
Age > 60 years
White or Native American
Personal
Widowed or divorced
Living alone
Unemployed or having current financial difficulties
Recent loss (e.g., of job or close relationship)

Table 54-2. Key Elements of the Suicide Evaluation

- Assess the degree of suicidal ideas
- Inquire about the details of the plan, the access to means, and the possibility of rescue
- Identify the precipitants for suicidal thinking
- Screen for the presence of major psychiatric illness
- Inquire about past suicide attempts
- Screen for risk factors (see Tables 54-1 and 54-3)
- Identify the extent of social supports
- Perform a complete mental status examination

C. Individuals who Exhibit Excessive Risk-Taking

Patients who exhibit excessive risk-taking or who appear accident-prone may be motivated by thoughts of suicide. Frequent automobile accidents or increasing substance use, for example, may presage a suicide attempt.

D. Patients with Psychiatric Illness

Patients with any type of psychiatric illness should be asked directly about suicidal thoughts at initial evaluation as well as follow-up visits.

IV. Approach to the Suicidal Patient

A. General Strategies

1. **Establish rapport first.** A calm, non-judgmental, empathic approach is usually helpful in this regard. However, it is important to note that **suicidal patients commonly elicit strong feelings** (e.g., anger or anxiety) **in clinicians.** An awareness of these feelings can help to minimize their interference with the evaluation.
2. **Begin with general questions.** When conducting the interview, it is often useful to **proceed from asking general questions about suicidal thoughts to asking specific questions about plans and circumstances.** A question such as, "Have you had thoughts that life is not worth living?" can be a useful starting point. Sometimes it will be necessary to rephrase questions or to inquire multiple times, as some patients who initially deny being suicidal may reveal these thoughts once they feel more comfortable during the interview. Inquiring about suicide does not prompt patients to consider the idea for the first time. In fact, some patients are relieved by the opportunity to discuss these feelings.
3. **Gather information from collateral sources.** Since some patients in acute care settings deny being suicidal, **collateral informants** (e.g., family members, friends, or outpatient treaters) **can be essential to the assessment of risk.** Most patients who suicide have communicated their intent to others within six months of an attempt.

B. Goals of the Assessment

The goals of assessment include identification of the degree of acute, short-, and long-term risk for suicide, and determination of ways in which each may be diminished. The stress-diathesis model is commonly applied to understand suicide risk. This model considers acute precipitants (the stress) in the context of underlying risks or vulnerabilities for suicide (the diathesis).

C. Specific Elements of History

1. **Determine the nature of suicidal thoughts or attempts.** The intensity, frequency, and duration of suicidal thoughts may reveal acuity and patterns of risk. A simple notation such as "suicidal ideation is present" is insufficient.
2. **Learn the details of the plan,** including when, where, and how a patient intends to commit suicide, as they can suggest the potential lethality of a plan and the possibility of its success. This concept is sometimes quantified as a **risk/rescue ratio,** in which the highest risk is associated with more lethal means and with a small chance for rescue. For example, a patient who plans to drive his truck to a remote country road and shoot himself in the head would have a high risk/rescue ratio. If, instead, he planned to take a few extra capsules of a multivitamin while sitting in his therapist's office, his risk/rescue ratio would be low.
3. **Determine the methods used in attempted suicide.**
   a. **Firearms are used most commonly** as the agent of suicide by both genders; they account for nearly 60% of completed suicides in the United States. Adolescents with a gun in the household have suicide rates between 4 and 10 times greater than other adolescents.
   b. **Poisoning is the second most common means of suicide for women, compared with hanging for men.**
   c. **Among attempts that do not succeed, drug ingestion is the most common means, used in 70% of failed attempts.** The medications used most commonly include antidepressants, non-narcotic analgesics, and benzodiazepines; typically these agents are used in combination.
4. **Clarify the expectations of the suicide attempter.** In assessing risk, it is essential to consider a patient's beliefs about a suicide plan, not merely the objective risk that the plan would pose. A patient who genuinely believes that the ten tablets of vitamin C he ingested should have been fatal will still be at significant risk for suicide, even though the objective risk posed by such an "overdose" might be minimal.
5. **Uncover the motivation for actions;** knowledge of these motivations may suggest possible interventions.
   a. **The wish to escape from suffering,** or the wish to be reunited with loved ones, are examples often cited by suicidal patients.
   b. **Hopelessness, or a negative view of the future, is an even stronger predictor of risk than is depression itself.** A patient should be asked about future plans; when one sets affairs in order or says "good-bye," it is often in anticipation of an imminent suicide attempt.
   c. **Recent loss of a relationship** (e.g., through death or divorce) is a risk factor, particularly among substance-abusing patients.
   d. **Manipulative suicide attempts** are common, particularly among patients with personality disorders. **Deliberate self-harm, without clear intent to die, is sometimes referred to as parasuicide.** However, such attempts must still be addressed seriously, as even chronically suicidal patients may commit suicide.
6. **Perform a careful psychiatric review of systems, which may suggest the presence of major psychiatric illness. Psychiatric illness represents the most**

powerful risk factor for suicide attempts and for completed suicide. Among patients who commit suicide the prevalence of psychiatric illness is greater than 90%; the greatest risk is associated with major depression, substance abuse, anxiety and panic, and psychotic disorders.

7. **Evaluate psychosocial supports** and the patient's ability and willingness to take advantage of them; these factors may help to prevent suicide.
8. **Identify individual risk factors** based upon a detailed history and mental status examination.

D. Additional Measures

In an effort to standardize and to refine the assessment of suicide risk, a number of rating scales have been studied, including the Beck hopelessness and depression scales and the Linehan Reasons for Living scale. These measures augment, but do not replace, thorough history-taking. Generally more severe depression and hopelessness and fewer reasons for living correlate with suicide risk.

V. Risk Factors for Suicide (see Table 54-3)

Overall, a clinician's ability to predict suicide remains poor. One 5-year study of risk factors found a false-positive rate of 30% (suicide was predicted but did not occur) and a false-negative rate of 44% (suicide was not predicted but occurred). **However, a careful assessment of risk factors remains crucial in estimating risk and planning interventions. Not surprisingly, past suicide attempts and current suicidal ideas are the best predictors of suicidal behavior.**

A. Psychiatric Disorders

1. **Around 60% of completed suicides occur in patients with a mood disorder, who have a lifetime risk of suicide as high as 15%. Co-morbid anhedonia, anxiety or panic attacks, and alcohol abuse** may significantly increase the likelihood of suicide attempts within one year after an attempt. The presence of psychotic symptoms also increases risk.
   a. Of note, **suicide rates during depressive episodes are roughly equivalent in major depressive disorder and bipolar depression.**
   b. **Manic states are very rarely associated with suicide;** the risk in mixed states is related to the magnitude of depressive symptoms.
2. **Substance abuse, particularly of alcohol or multiple drugs, is a factor in at least 25% of cases; alcohol abusers have a lifetime risk of suicide as high as 18%.** An important associated risk factor is recent personal loss or onset of medical complications; suicide among substance abusers often occurs later in the disease course. Even among patients without a longstanding pattern of substance abuse or dependence, substance use greatly increases the risk of suicide. The impaired judgment and impulsivity associated with **acute intoxication play a role in 20% (and possibly up to 50%) of completed suicides.**
3. **Anxiety disorders may play a role in 15–20% of suicides.** The risk posed remains significant even after controlling for co-morbid depression and substance abuse; when anxiety is combined with depression, the risk of suicide may be additive.
4. **Psychosis contributes to 10% or more of suicides, with a lifetime risk among schizophrenics of 15%.**
   a. In contrast to patterns seen in the general population, the schizophrenic patient who commits suicide is most likely to be a young male with high pre-morbid functioning.
   b. **Akathisia and abrupt neuroleptic discontinuation significantly increase the risk of suicide,** as does onset of depression following the resolution of an acute psychotic episode.
   c. **Command hallucinations for self-harm may signal imminent risk.**
   d. Recently, use of clozapine has been associated with a decreased lifetime risk of suicide.
5. **Having a personality disorder, particularly borderline personality disorder or antisocial personality disorder, contributes to 5–10% of suicides.** Chronic suicidal ideas, as well as impulsive and often life-threatening manipulative acts, are particularly common in this patient group. Such attempts may "accidentally" succeed and cannot be ignored.

Table 54-3. Psychiatric Diagnoses Associated with Suicide

- Major depression or bipolar disorder
- Schizophrenia
- Alcohol or other substance abuse
- Anxiety disorder
- Personality disorder (borderline or antisocial)

B. Prior Suicide Attempts

Prior suicide attempts predispose to suicide; 50% of suicides occur in patients who have made at least one prior attempt. In the year following an attempt, the risk may be up to 100 times that of the general population.

C. Past and Current Medical History

Medical disorders can be identified in up to 40% of patients who make suicide attempts; typically, the medical disorder is chronic in nature. In patients over the age of 60 years, up to 70% of suicides are associated with medical illness. Associations have been demonstrated with many illnesses, including chronic renal failure, acquired immunodeficiency syndrome (HIV infection/AIDS), epilepsy, cancer, lupus, multiple sclerosis, Huntington's disease, and chronic pain.

D. Family History

Whether through dynamic or genetic mechanisms, several aspects of family history influence suicidality. **A family history of suicide itself increases risk, as does a history of any psychiatric illness, independent of particular diagnosis.** Twin and adoption studies suggest some genetic basis for this risk. An additional risk is conferred by a chaotic early family environment, which includes abuse of any kind.

E. Social History

Epidemiologic data show an association between suicide and marital status; **the greatest risk of suicide occurs in widowed, divorced, or separated individuals. Both social isolation and living alone similarly increase the risk of suicide. Unemployment** and **financial or legal difficulties** are also associated with increased suicide risk. On the other hand, suicide rates are lower for parents of children under age 18 years. Statistics aside, the presence or absence of supports plays a powerful role in modifying suicide risk. The involvement of family, friends, or outpatient care providers with whom a patient has an alliance may increase the degree of safety.

F. Abnormal Elements of the Mental Status Examination

1. **Gross alterations in attention,** awareness, and arousal, such as seen in delirium or acute intoxication, can impair judgment and precipitate a suicide attempt; they require prompt evaluation and intervention.
2. **Evidence of psychiatric illness** (e.g., **mood, anxiety, or psychotic symptoms**) can compound suicide risk.
3. **Motor restlessness** may suggest an anxious or agitated depression, or indicate underlying akathisia. Any of these states presents significant risk.
4. **Impulsivity,** poor judgment, and lack of insight may contribute to lethal acts.

VI. Management of the Suicidal Patient

A. Stabilize Medical Conditions

A patient who is treated for a suicide attempt may require concurrent medical evaluation and treatment. At times, a patient who has expressed suicidal ideas will have already taken some action; the examiner needs to maintain a high index of suspicion for unsuspected or unreported drug ingestions.

B. Ensure Safety

1. **Before an evaluation can proceed, both the patient and the examiner must be protected from harm.** A patient may be incredibly resourceful in this regard; almost any setting can be lethal in the right circumstances. Sharp objects may be used to cut; pills or other small objects can be ingested. Falls and hanging are also commonly attempted in hospital settings.
2. **The least restrictive means necessary to ensure safety should be employed.**
   a. **Frequent supervision** may be adequate for reliable patients who do not appear to be at acute risk.
   b. While **one-to-one supervision** allows for greater patient freedom, it may be inadequate for large or impulsive patients.
3. **Use of medications** may be extremely helpful for treating anxiety or agitation in suicidal patients.
4. **Physical restraints** may be required if a patient continues to resist attempts at containment. However, they cannot substitute for supervision, particularly when intoxication is suspected.

C. Rule Out Intoxication or Withdrawal

A patient should be monitored closely for physiological signs of intoxication or for withdrawal reactions; serial mental status exams should be performed. **When sober, many patients retract suicidal statements. However, a complete evaluation for safety is still required.**

VII. Disposition and Treatment

A. Make Thoughtful Clinical Decisions

The assessment and treatment of suicidal thinking and behavior is fundamentally a question of clinical judgment, guided by an understanding of known risk factors and tailored to the individual patient. By themselves, risk factors alone or in combination have extremely high false positive and false negative rates. Because of the importance of clinical judgment, the **thought process behind clinical decisions should be carefully documented.**

B. Review Treatment Options

1. **Location of treatment.** A number of treatment locales are available for suicidal patients. A general hospital admission may be necessary for a patient who has made an attempt and who requires medical treatment. A patient who is acutely at risk generally requires **hospitalization on a locked psychiatric unit.** An individual who refuses treatment typically requires involuntary commitment. Of note, **the risk of suicide does not subside following admission: 5% of suicides occur among psychiatrically ill inpatients.**

   At times, a patient who requires less containment but is unable to return home may be managed in a partial hospital or in a day-treatment program. Finally, if increased supports may be arranged, a patient may be managed at home.
2. **Psychosocial treatment.** Psychosocial interventions can be extremely useful while maintaining the safety of a suicidal patient. Involving family and close friends, as well as outpatient treaters, can be particularly helpful.

3. **Pharmacological and other somatic interventions**
   a. **Pharmacological interventions depend on the underlying psychiatric illness.** Antidepressants are commonly used, sometimes in combination with anxiolytics. Choice of medications should be guided by a consideration of their lethality in overdose. Thus, selective serotonin reuptake inhibitors (SSRIs) are usually considered as first-line therapy for the depressed patient. **Most patients who suicide have not had any recent antidepressant treatment.**
   b. **The impact of medications on the long-term risk of suicide** has recently become a focus of investigation. Among patients with bipolar disorder, **lithium maintenance** has been shown to decrease the risk of suicide. Among schizophrenic patients, **clozapine** may similarly decrease risk. Whether other medications share these benefits, and whether lithium and clozapine have a direct anti-suicide effect rather than simply efficacy in the underlying mood disorder, remain unknown.
   c. **Electroconvulsive therapy (ECT)** is sometimes utilized in acutely suicidal individuals, because the onset of antidepressant effect is much more rapid than with pharmacotherapies.

C. Complete a Checklist Prior to Discharge

Whatever the disposition, the key factors in decision-making and the plans for maintaining safety should be documented in the medical record. Both the patient and outpatient treaters should participate as much as possible in planning.

While some clinicians utilize **"contracts for safety,"** which represent a verbal or written contract with a suicidal patient, there is **no evidence of their efficacy** in reducing suicide attempts. Moreover, they may be **falsely reassuring** to clinicians, as they cannot substitute for a true alliance.

When planning for hospital discharge clinicians should:

Make the potential means of suicide inaccessible.
Address the precipitants for suicidal ideas and behavior, if possible.
Treat the underlying psychiatric illness, including substance abuse.
Develop or enhance outpatient supports.
Arrange for close follow-up, including a plan for management of recurrent suicidal ideas.

VIII. Neurobiology of Suicide

A. Abnormalities in serotonin neurotransmission. Early investigations found that patients who committed suicide, particularly using violent means, had lower levels of a serotonin metabolite (5-hydroxyindoleacetic acid, or 5-HIAA) in cerebrospinal fluid than did control patients. Subsequent studies have suggested other abnormalities in serotonin neurotransmission (e.g., decreased expression of serotonin transporter in the brain). Abnormalities in noradrenergic neurotransmission, and in the hypothalamic-pituitary-adrenal axis have also been described.

B. Genetic contributions to suicide risk. A portion of suicide risk may be familial: individuals who commit or attempt suicide are more likely than are those of the general population to have family members who have committed suicide. Twin and adoption studies likewise suggest some heritable risk for suicide. Efforts to identify the specific genes that confer this risk are ongoing.

Suggested Readings

Hirschfeld, R.M.A., & Russell, J.M. (1997). Assessment and treatment of suicidal patients. *New England Journal of Medicine, 337*, 910–915.

Hyman, S.E. (1994). The suicidal patient. In S.E. Hyman, & G.E. Tesar (Eds.), *Manual of psychiatric emergencies* (3rd ed., pp. 21–27). Boston, MA: Little, Brown.

Lagomasino, I.T., & Stern, T.A. (1998). Approach to the suicidal patient. In T.A. Stern, J.B. Herman, & P.L. Slavin (Eds.), *The MGH guide to psychiatry in primary care*, pp. 15–22. New York: McGraw-Hill.

Mann, J.J. (2002). A current perspective of suicide and attempted suicide. *Annals of Internal Medicine, 136*, 302–311.

Maris, R.W. (2000). Suicide. *Lancet, 360*, 319–326.

Roy, A. (1995). Suicide. In H.I. Kaplan, & B.J. Sadock (Eds.), *Comprehensive textbook of psychiatry* (6th ed., pp. 1739–1752). Baltimore, MD: Williams and Wilkins.

Stern, T.A., Lagomasino, I.T., & Hackett, T.P. (1997). Suicidal patients. In N.H. Cassem, T.A. Stern, J.F. Rosenbaum, & M.S. Jellinek (Eds.), *Massachusetts General Hospital handbook of general hospital psychiatry* (4th ed., pp. 69–88). St. Louis, MO: Mosby.

Chapter 55

Psychiatry and the Law I: Informed Consent, Competency, Treatment Refusal, and Civil Commitment

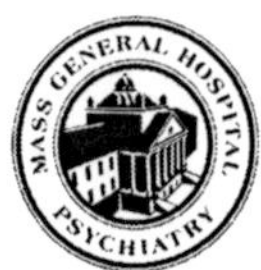

RONALD SCHOUTEN

I. Overview

Psychiatrists interact with the legal system on a regular basis. **Issues related to informed consent, competency to consent to treatment, treatment refusal, and civil commitment are important aspects of daily clinical practice.** These four topics are reviewed in this chapter. Forensic psychiatry, the subspecialty of psychiatry devoted to the application of clinical principles and practice to the legal system, includes these topics, along with **criminal competencies and criminal responsibility.**

II. Informed Consent

A. Relevance

1. **Case law, also known as common law, prohibits the touching of another person unless consent has been obtained or there is some justification.** In the absence of consent or justification, **the unpermitted touching is a battery and gives rise to a right to sue for damages.**

   Consent can be expressed (the patient explicitly consenting to treatment) **or implied** (e.g., a patient standing in a clearly marked line to get an inoculation). Justification occurs when there is an emergency—i.e., failure to act would likely have an imminent, serious negative effect on the patient's condition.
2. **Informed consent is an ethical concept** that was made operational by American courts beginning in the 1960s when it began to be converted to a legal duty on the part of physicians. From a clinical and ethical standpoint, informed consent arises from the physician's obligation to respect the **autonomy** of the patient. **Lack of informed consent is a basis for alleging medical malpractice.**

B. Defining Informed Consent

Informed consent is a process through which the physician gets the permission of the patient or a substitute decision-maker to provide treatment to the patient. The decision-maker must be *competent* (i.e., have the capacity to make the decision), must be given enough *information* to make an informed decision, and must make the decision *voluntarily.* The legal requirements of informed consent are likewise information, competency, and voluntariness. Each of these is described in more detail.

1. **Information**
   a. **The amount and type of information that must be given to the patient in order to meet the requirements of informed consent varies among jurisdictions.** Three basic standards are used in this area:
      i. **Professional standard:** the amount of information a reasonable professional would provide under similar circumstances.
      ii. **Materiality standard:** what the average patient would require to make a decision under the same circumstances. This is also referred to as a **patient-oriented standard.** In some jurisdictions (e.g., Massachusetts), the concept is extended to require provision of the information that would be material to the particular patient's decision.
      iii. **Combined standard:** requires the information that the reasonable medical practitioner would provide but also examines whether it was "sufficient to ensure informed consent."
   b. **Providing the following information to patients will fulfill the information requirements in most jurisdictions.**
      i. **The nature of the condition to be treated and the treatment proposed.**
      ii. **The nature and probability of the risks associated with the treatment.** Minor risks or side effects that occur frequently (e.g., dry mouth) and significant risks that occur infrequently (e.g., hepatic failure secondary to sodium valproate) should be reviewed with the patient.
      iii. **The inability to predict the results of the treatment.**
      iv. **The irreversibility of the procedure, if applicable.**
      v. **The alternative treatments available,** including no treatment. This should include a discussion of the risks and benefits associated with these options.
2. **Competency.** For a patient to give adequate informed consent, **he or she must have the physical and mental capacity to make informed treatment decisions. How much capacity is required depends on the nature of the condition and the risks of the proposed treatment.** Less capacity is required for low-risk treatments with high likelihood of a good result (e.g., intravenous fluids for dehydration). A higher level of capacity is required when the treatment is of higher risk or is more invasive, and the results are less likely to be favorable (e.g., amputation in an elderly diabetic patient with renal failure).
   a. Technically, **competency is a legal term not a clinical term,** although these terms tend to be used interchange-

ably in the clinical setting. **A legal declaration of incompetence strips a person of certain rights and privileges normally accorded to adults** (e.g., making treatment decisions, making contracts, voting, or executing a will).

i. **All adults are presumed to be competent to make their own treatment decisions in the eyes of the law.**

ii. **Only a judge can declare a person legally incompetent.** However, **clinical assessments of capacity (competency evaluations) are the first step toward a legal declaration of incompetence** and often indicate the likely outcome of any legal proceedings.

- Competency/capacity evaluations are used as evidence in judicial proceedings on the question of competency.
- A competency evaluation that concludes that a patient has the capacity to make treatment decisions can allow treatment to proceed if there are doubts about the patient's mental status.
- A conclusion that the patient lacks the capacity to give informed consent requires the choice of an alternative decision-maker except in an emergency or where the patient has a valid advance directive.

b. **Competence (capacity) can be global or task specific.**

i. **Global capacity** refers to the ability to undertake and carry out all the normal responsibilities and rights of an adult. A declaration of global incapacity strips an individual of his or her rights as a **legal person.**

ii. **Specific capacities** include the following:

- **Testamentary capacity is the capacity to execute a will.** Specific legal standards for testamentary capacity apply in all jurisdictions and may vary. The usual standards require that the person executing the will know the nature of the document being executed, know the contents of the estate, and know the persons who would normally inherit from him or her (the natural objects of his or her bounty).
- **Testimonial capacity is the capacity to serve as a witness in court.**
- **Capacity to make treatment decisions.**

c. **Evaluating the capacity to make treatment decisions** (Appelbaum and Grisso, 1988)

i. Does the patient express a preference?

ii. Is the patient able to attain a factual understanding of the information provided?

iii. Is the patient able to appreciate the seriousness of the condition and the consequences of accepting or rejecting treatment?

iv. Can the patient manipulate the information provided in a rational fashion and come to a decision that follows logically from that information considered in the context of the individual's personal beliefs, experience, and circumstances?

- It is the process of reaching a decision, not the decision itself, that must be rational. Competent people have a right to make decisions for themselves that may seem irrational to the rest of the world.
- Disagreement with the treating clinician's recommendations is not a basis, in and of itself, for saying that a patient is irrational.

d. **Consequences of a finding of incapacity**

i. **Guardianship of the person**

- The person declared incompetent is the **ward.**
- The **guardian** is the party appointed by the court to make decisions on behalf of the ward.
- Depending on the jurisdiction, the guardian may make decisions based upon the perceived **best interests of the ward** or by means of a **substituted judgment** analysis (what the ward would have decided if he or she were competent to make the decision). In cases involving extraordinary or invasive treatment, the substituted judgment analysis may be carried out by a judge rather than by the guardian.

ii. Guardianship of the estate (conservatorship).

iii. Appointment of an agent to act on behalf of the incompetent pursuant to a **durable power of attorney, health care proxy, or other form of advance directive.**

3. **Voluntary**

a. Simply means free of coercion by those proposing the treatment.

b. Persuasion by family members does not void informed consent so long as the circumstances do not put the physician on notice that the treatment is being imposed against the patient's will or indicate that the patient is incompetent.

C. Exceptions to the Requirement of Informed Consent

1. **Emergency situations**

a. When failure to act would result in a serious and imminent deterioration in the patient's condition.

b. The emergency exception allows for initiation of treatment and stabilization, not for ongoing treatment without obtaining proper consent.

2. **Waivers**

a. The patient may defer to someone else's judgment.

b. Waiver may be implied (e.g., presenting oneself to the emergency room after being injured).

3. **Therapeutic privilege**

a. **Where the process of providing information and obtaining consent would result in a serious risk of deterioration in the patient's condition, that process can be deferred until the patient's condition has improved sufficiently.**

b. The possibility that providing the information might lead to treatment refusal is not sufficient to invoke therapeutic privilege.

III. Treatment Refusal

A. All competent people have a right to make their own medical treatment decisions, and all adults are presumed to be competent.

1. This applies even where the individual is suffering from serious mental illness or is civilly committed.
2. The presumption of competency persists until a court has declared a person to be incompetent, as noted above.
3. When a patient is believed to be incapacitated from making treatment decisions, an alternative decision-maker should be sought rather than relying on the presumption of competence and allowing the patient to continue making treatment decisions.

B. Individuals who are incompetent still have a right to individual autonomy, which can be honored by following their preferences for treatment expressed when they were competent or to the extent they can be determined in the absence of prior expression.

C. The law concerning treatment-refusal varies among the states.

1. States generally draw a distinction between routine and ordinary medical care (e.g., antibiotics or minor surgery) and extraordinary or invasive care (e.g., cancer chemotherapy or coronary artery bypass grafting) when determining what can be done when a patient refuses treatment.
   a. Benzodiazepines and antidepressants are generally considered to be routine, ordinary, and non-invasive.
   b. Antipsychotic medication, electroconvulsive therapy, and psychosurgery are considered to constitute extraordinary, dangerous, and invasive treatments in many states.
2. States differ in terms of what legal steps must be taken before a patient's refusal of treatment can be overridden.
   a. The basic rule in all states is that **competent individuals have a right to make their own treatment decisions, including refusal of treatment that others believe is in the patient's best interest.** Exceptions to this rule exist in matters involving criminal law and the correctional system.
   b. When a patient who appears to lack the capacity to make treatment decisions refuses routine and ordinary care, physicians can generally rely upon family members or significant others who know the patient to make a decision.
   c. When the care to be provided is extraordinary, invasive, or dangerous, many states require that a formal guardian be appointed to make the treatment decisions.
      i. Guardianship is established after a hearing at which family members, treaters, and sometimes the patient, will testify.
      ii. Not all states allow the guardian, once appointed, to make all decisions on behalf of the patient. In some states, extraordinary, invasive, or dangerous care can only be authorized by a judge after a full trial on the issue, with the guardian assigned to monitor the care (Rogers v. Commissioner [Mass., 1983]).
      iii. While some states require full adversarial proceedings and judicial involvement in these matters, others (including federal courts) believe that professional judgment and administrative review satisfy the due process requirements without going to court (Rennie v. Klein [3rd Circuit, 1981]; U.S. v. Charters [4th Circuit, 1988]).
      iv. Refusal of treatment by those awaiting trial or already convicted of a crime has been the subject of considerable judicial attention.
         - Antipsychotic medications may be administered over the refusal of convicted prisoners, competent or incompetent, if an independent review panel agrees that the prisoner suffers from a serious mental illness, is dangerous to himself or others, or is gravely disabled, and the medication proposed is in the prisoner's best interests (Washington v. Harper [U.S., 1990]).
         - Forced administration of antipsychotic medication for the purpose of rendering the inmate competent to be executed violates the Louisiana state constitutional right to privacy and constitutes cruel, excessive, and unusual punishment (Louisiana v. Perry [La., 1992]).
         - Forced administration of antipsychotic medication in order to render a defendant competent to stand trial violated the rights of the defendant under the Sixth and Fourteenth Amendments to the U.S. Constitution absent a showing by the state that the treatment was both medically necessary and appropriate (Riggins v. Nevada [U.S., 1992]).

IV. Civil Commitment

The process of hospitalizing a person against his or her will is referred to as involuntary civil commitment. Civil commitment statutes are similar in the various jurisdictions, as commitment can only occur when the patient poses a danger to him- or herself or others.

A. Legal Restrictions on Civil Commitment

1. Confinement of an individual against his or her will is considered to be a deprivation of fundamental rights guaranteed under the Constitution of the United States and state constitutions.
   a. Civil commitment is considered to be an act of the state government because it occurs under the authority of the state.
   b. Before a state can deprive someone of their fundamental rights, proper procedural protections (e.g., a court or administrative hearing before a neutral fact finder) must be granted. Such procedures collectively constitute **due**

process, which is guaranteed by the Constitution (Vitek v. Jones, 445 U.S. 480 [U.S., 1980]). Commitment to a mental hospital entails a massive curtailment of liberty and requires due process protection.

2. **In non-emergencies, the patient is entitled to a full hearing before he or she can be confined.**
3. Lawsuits for deprivation of civil rights, false imprisonment, and negligence can arise from improper civil commitment.
4. **An individual can only be involuntarily committed if he or she is a danger to self or others.** The fact that a patient may demonstrate a clear-cut clinical need for treatment, in the absence of dangerousness, is not sufficient.
   a. A state cannot constitutionally confine a non-dangerous individual who is capable of surviving outside the hospital setting on his own or with the help of friends (O'Connor v. Donaldson [U.S., 1974]).
   b. **The standard of proof in civil commitment cases is "clear and convincing" evidence,** more than is required in ordinary civil cases and less than the criminal standard of beyond a reasonable doubt (Addington v. Texas [U.S., 1979]).

B. The details of the commitment process vary among the states.

1. For example, in California an emergency commitment is valid for 72 hours, during which time the patient is evaluated to determine whether further commitment is necessary and justified. In Massachusetts, the emergency commitment is for four days.
2. States also differ in how mental illness is defined. Some states, for example, do not consider substance abuse and disorders like Alzheimer's disease as mental illnesses for the purpose of civil commitment.
3. Where a patient is offered an opportunity to sign himself into a state hospital voluntarily and does so while lacking the capacity to make an informed decision, he has a constitutional right to due process of law prior to the deprivation of a liberty interest, and the state and its agents can be held liable for a violation of the patient's federal civil rights (Zinermon v. Burch [U.S. 1990]).

C. The Dangerousness Criteria

While the details differ, all states use the criteria of danger to self or others as the basis for involuntary commitment. The danger must be the result of mental illness, rather than ordinary anger or antisocial behavior. For example, a hired killer would not be an appropriate candidate for involuntary commitment to a psychiatric hospital should his murderous intentions become known, absent evidence that a mental illness other than a personality disorder contributed to his dangerousness. However, an individual convicted of a violent crime may be committed to a hospital if it is determined that he poses a danger to himself or others.

1. **Danger to self means attempts at serious self-harm or suicide or credible threats to cause such self-harm.**
2. **Danger to others generally refers to threats or attempts to cause physical harm to others, or actual harm already inflicted.** In addition, it may include situations in which others are placed in reasonable fear that they will be harmed by the patient.
3. **Individuals may also be involuntarily committed if they pose a substantial risk of harm because they are unable to provide for their own well-being in the community.** In some states, this criterion is referred to as the **gravely disabled** criterion.
   a. Generally, mere difficulty caring for oneself is not enough to meet this criterion. **The risk of harm** (e.g., believing that one is invincible and therefore can walk into traffic) **must be substantial and imminent.** A likelihood of harm in the distant future is not sufficient.
   b. Civil commitment under this criterion, as well as the others, is **permissible only if no less restrictive alternative is available in the community** (Lake v. Cameron [D.C. Circuit, 1966]). Alternatives to civil commitment may include increased outpatient visits, voluntary hospitalization, day hospital programs, custodial care by relatives, or shelters.

D. Civil commitment of criminal defendants and convicted individuals has been the subject of important court decisions.

1. Due process clause requires that the reason for confinement and the nature of the confinement be of reasonable relevance to the purpose of confinement (Jackson v. Indiana [U.S., 1972]).
   a. Jackson was deaf, with limited ability to sign, and had limited intellectual resources. He had been found incompetent to stand trial on charges of shoplifting, and was committed to the state hospital until he was restored to competency, a state that everyone agreed was unattainable under the circumstances.
   b. If the state wanted to continue to confine Jackson to a mental institution, he must meet standard criteria for civil commitment.
2. "The Constitution permits the Government, on the basis of the insanity judgment, to confine (a defendant) to a mental institution until such time as he has regained his sanity or is no longer a danger to himself or society. This holding accords with the widely and reasonably held view that insanity acquittees should be treated differently from other candidates for civil commitment" (Jones v. United States, 463 U.S. 354 [1983]).
   a. Insanity acquittee may be held as long as he is mentally ill and dangerous, but no longer.
   b. This is a post-Hinckley case arising in DC; many scholars attribute the reasoning to the climate created by the successful insanity plea of attempted presidential assassin John Hinckley.

3. Louisiana statute violated the Due Process Clause of the U.S. Constitution where it allowed a criminal defendant found not guilty by reason of insanity to be returned to the hospital, even if a hospital review committee found him no longer mentally ill and/or if he was determined at a court hearing to be dangerous (Foucha v. Louisiana [U.S., 1992]).
   a. A hospital psychiatrist testified that Foucha had recovered from the drug-induced psychosis that had formed the basis for his insanity defense, but also testified that Foucha had been in altercations at the hospital, had an antisocial personality disorder that was not a mental disease and was untreatable, and the psychiatrist would not "feel comfortable in certifying that he would not be a danger to himself or to other people."
   b. Continued confinement in a mental institution is improper without a determination in civil commitment proceedings of current mental illness and dangerousness.
   c. The state's legitimate interest in imprisoning convicted criminals for retribution and deterrence does not exist in the case of an insanity acquittee, who has not been found guilty and cannot be punished.
   d. The state may legitimately detain people who are unable to control their behavior and thereby pose a danger to public safety, provided the confinement takes place pursuant to proper procedures and evidentiary standards.
4. Kansas's Sexually Dangerous Predator Act is not unconstitutional where it establishes procedures for the civil commitment of persons who, due to a "mental abnormality" or "personality disorder," are likely to engage in "predatory acts of sexual violence" (Kansas v. Hendricks [U.S., 1997]; Kansas v. Crane [U.S., 2002]).
   a. Involuntary civil confinement, which follows conclusion of criminal sentence if the individual is found to be a sexually dangerous person, did not constitute additional punishment for criminal behavior as it does not have the goals of retribution or deterrence.
   b. Procedures provided by the state, including the right to immediate release when the detainee proves he is no longer sexually dangerous, are adequate.
   c. It is a sufficient basis for commitment that the convicted defendant has a mental illness or personality disorder that makes it difficult to control his predatory behavior.

Suggested Readings

Appelbaum, P.S., & Grisso, T. (1988). Assessing patients' capacities to consent to treatment. *New England Journal of Medicine, 319,* 1635–1638.

Appelbaum, P.S., Lidz, C.W., & Meisel, A. (1987). *Informed consent: Legal theory and clinical practice.* New York: Oxford University Press.

Grisso, T., & Appelbaum, P.S. (1998). *Assessing competence to consent to treatment.* New York: Oxford University Press.

Gutheil, T.G., & Appelbaum, P.A. (2002). *Clinical handbook of psychiatry and the law* (3rd ed.). Baltimore, MD: Lippincott, Williams and Wilkins.

Spring, R.L., Lacoursiere, R.B., & Weissenberger, G. (1997). *Patients, psychiatrists, and lawyers: Law and the mental health system* (2nd ed.). Cincinnati, OH: Anderson Publishing.

Winick, B.J. (1997). *The right to refuse mental health treatment.* Washington, DC: American Psychological Association.

Chapter 56

Psychiatry and the Law II: Criminal Issues and the Role of Psychiatrists in the Legal System

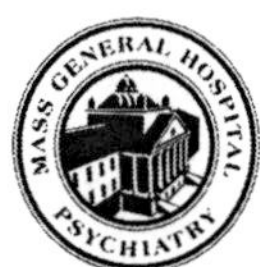

RONALD SCHOUTEN

I. Overview

Psychiatrists play a prominent role in the courts as expert witnesses in both civil and criminal litigation. **This chapter focuses on the subjects of criminal competencies, criminal responsibility, the psychotherapist-patient privilege, and the role of the psychiatrist in court.**

II. Competency in the Criminal System

A. Competency to Stand Trial

1. The basic standard
   a. **Whether the defendant "has sufficient present ability to consult with his lawyer with a reasonable degree of rational understanding, and whether he has a rational as well as a factual understanding of the proceedings against him"** (Dusky v. United States [U.S., 1960]).
   b. **This standard applies in all states, the District of Columbia, and federal courts.** States may use their own criteria, so long as those criteria provide as much, or more, protection of the defendant's rights than the federal standard.
   c. **Minimal capacity is required.** In practice, the threshold for competency is low. But see Cooper v. Oklahoma (U.S., 1996) described below, holding that the standard of proof for incompetence is "preponderance of the evidence" and not some higher standard.
2. **The rationale for requiring that the defendant meet basic standards of mental capacity** before he or she can be put on trial (Drope v. Missouri [U.S., 1975]).
   a. The fact-finding portion of the proceedings can only be accurate if the defendant can work with his or her attorney with an understanding of the proceedings.
   b. Only a competent defendant can exercise the constitutional rights to a fair trial and to confront his or her accuser in a meaningful way.
   c. The integrity and dignity of the legal process are preserved by ensuring that the defendant is competent to stand trial.
   d. The purposes of retribution and individual deterrence are served only if the convicted defendant was competent to stand trial.
3. **The competency decision**
   a. **The defendant may be ordered by the judge to undergo an evaluation.** This can be done on an outpatient basis, but is more commonly conducted on an inpatient unit with special capabilities to conduct forensic evaluations.
   b. The defendant's consent is not necessary for a competency evaluation; the court can order it over the defendant's objection (United States v. Hugenin [1st Circuit, 1991]).
   c. The defendant has a right to consult with counsel before the competency evaluation pursuant to the Sixth Amendment, but no right to have counsel present at the evaluation in federal courts. States may provide this right if they choose (Buchanan v. Kentucky [U.S., 1987]).
   d. **The focus of the competency evaluation is the defendant's mental state at the time of the proceedings, not at the time of the alleged criminal act.**
   e. **The decision whether or not the defendant is competent to stand trial is made by the trial judge.**
   f. If the defendant is found to be incompetent to stand trial, he or she is committed to a state or federal hospital to be treated and restored to competency.
   g. If the defendant cannot be restored to competency, he or she cannot be convicted and must be released from the hospital. However, the defendant can be held in the facility if he or she meets the usual criteria for civil commitment.
4. **Key cases on competency to stand trial**
   a. **The trial judge must raise the issue of competency if either the court's own evidence or that presented by the defense or prosecution raises a *bona fide* doubt of the defendant's competency** (Pate v. Robinson [U.S., 1966]).
      i. The question of competency can be raised at any point in the trial process.
      ii. The prosecution may raise the question of competency.
   b. **A defendant found incompetent to stand trial and committed to a state facility cannot be held indefinitely if there is no hope of restoration of competency, unless he is committed under the usual civil commitment standards in a regular civil proceeding** (Jackson v. Indiana [U.S., 1972]).
      i. Jackson was deaf, with limited ability to sign, and had limited intellectual resources. He had been found incompetent to stand trial on charges of shoplifting, and was committed to the state hospital until he was restored to competency, a state which everyone agreed was unattainable under the circumstances.
      ii. If the state wanted to continue to confine Jackson to a mental institution, he had to meet the standard criteria for civil commitment. Otherwise, the continued confinement would be in violation of the due process clause of the federal constitution.

c. **The defendant's statements made during a competency to stand trial evaluation cannot be used against the defendant in the guilt or sentencing stages of the proceeding** (Estelle v. Smith [U.S., 1981]).
   i. Using the information in that way would violate the Fifth Amendment protection against self-incrimination.
   ii. Limitations on this protection:
      - Fifth Amendment rights are not violated if the psychiatrist's testimony is limited to the question of competency to stand trial.
      - If the defendant requested the psychiatric evaluation and presents the evidence at trial, the prosecution may use the report of the evaluation to rebut the evidence offered by the defendant [Buchanan v. Kentucky (U.S. 1987)].

d. **If an indigent defendant cannot afford to hire a psychiatric expert to assist in the case, the state must provide "at a minimum . . . access to a competent psychiatrist who will conduct appropriate examination and assist in evaluation, preparation, presentation of the defense"** (Ake v. Oklahoma [U.S., 1985]).
   i. This rule applies whenever a mental health issue may be relevant (e.g., competency, criminal responsibility, aid in sentencing).
   ii. The court may appoint the psychiatrist. The defendant is not constitutionally entitled to select a psychiatrist of his own choosing or to receive funds to hire one of his own.

e. **The standard of proof for competency to stand trial is the preponderance of the evidence,** not the higher standards of clear and convincing evidence or proof beyond a reasonable doubt (Cooper v. Oklahoma [U.S., 1996]).
   i. The defendant exhibited bizarre behavior before and during his trial, including refusing to talk to his attorney, responding to hallucinations, eating his feces, and expressing his belief that his defense counsel had tried to murder him.
   ii. At an initial competency hearing, Cooper was found incompetent and sent to the state hospital for treatment. He was found competent to stand trial at four subsequent hearings where he failed to meet the Oklahoma statutory requirement that the defendant establish lack of competency by "clear and convincing evidence."
   iii. The due process clause of the Fourteenth Amendment was violated by the application of a clear and convincing standard of proof because it created the risk that an individual would be forced to stand trial who was more likely than not incompetent.

B. Competency to Plead Guilty or Serve as One's Own Attorney (Godinez v. Moran [U.S., 1993])

1. The defendant, who was taking a number of psychotropic medications, asked to discharge his attorney, to represent himself, and to plead guilty after he was assessed to be competent to stand trial by two psychiatrists.
2. The Supreme Court held that **the mental capacity involved in competency for pleading guilty or waiving the right to counsel is the same as for competency to stand trial. No higher standard applies.**

C. Competency to Be Sentenced/Executed

1. **The standard and rationale**
   a. **The standard: whether the convicted individual has an understanding of the nature of the proceedings and an ability to participate in the process.**
   b. The rationale for requiring that the convicted individual be competent for the sentencing and punishment phases:
      i. To preserve the integrity of the sentencing and punishment process.
      ii. To ensure that the convicted individual will have the ability to contest the decision through all stages of appeal prior to imposition of punishment.
      iii. The deterrent function of punishment is served by only punishing those who have the requisite mental capacity to be sentenced or punished.
2. **The APA position on ethical issues in death penalty cases.** The Ethics Committee's opinion (1990) was as follows:
   a. **It is unethical for a psychiatrist to participate in executions.**
   b. **It is not unethical for a psychiatrist to conduct a competency evaluation in which the prisoner is told of the interview's purpose and the limitations on confidentiality.**
3. **Key cases on competency to be sentenced/executed:**
   a. **Estelle v. Smith (U.S., 1982).** Smith's Fifth Amendment right to be free from self-incrimination and Sixth Amendment right to assistance of counsel were denied when the state's psychiatrist, who had examined him solely for the purpose of assessing competency to stand trial, was allowed to testify as to Smith's dangerousness at the penalty phase and **defendant was not informed of the purpose of the evaluation or right to the presence of counsel.**
   b. **Barefoot v. Estelle (U.S., 1983). Even though the state cannot compel a defendant to undergo a psychiatric evaluation, there is no constitutional barrier to allowing psychiatric experts to testify to the defendant's future dangerousness** at the penalty phase based on hypothetical questions.
      i. The APA filed an *amicus curiae* (friend of the court) brief pointing out the unreliability of dangerousness predictions.
      ii. The court rejected the arguments in that brief, holding that such assessments are not so inherently unreliable that they should be excluded totally and that the lack of reliability can be addressed as a credibility issue on cross-examination.
   c. **Ford v. Wainwright** (U.S. 1986)

i. Execution of a prisoner who is insane constitutes cruel and unusual punishment in violation of the Eighth Amendment.

ii. A prisoner is entitled to a full and fair hearing on the issue of competency to be executed.

d. **Satterwhite v. Texas (U.S., 1988). Admission of testimony based on a psychiatric evaluation conducted without the knowledge of the defendant's attorney constituted a basis for reversal of the conviction,** where it could not be assured that this inadmissible evidence had not influenced the jury.

e. **Atkins v. Virginia** (U.S., 2002)

i. Imposition of the death penalty upon a mentally retarded individual constitutes "cruel and unusual punishment" in violation of the Eighth Amendment to the U.S. Constitution.

ii. This decision, which marked a reversal of the Court's prior decisions on this issue, was based upon (a) changes in attitudes and approaches by society and legislatures, (b) the likelihood that the permissible deterrent and retribution effects did not apply with this population, (c) this population was at increased risk of receiving a death sentence because of a diminished ability to establish mitigating factors.

f. **Forced administration of antipsychotic medication for the purpose of rendering an inmate competent to be executed violates the Louisiana state constitutional right to privacy and constitutes cruel, excessive, and unusual punishment (Louisiana v. Perry [Louisiana, 1992]).**

g. **Forced administration of antipsychotic medication in order to render a defendant competent to stand trial violated the rights of the defendant under the Sixth and Fourteenth Amendments to the U.S. Constitution,** absent a showing by the state that the treatment was both medically necessary and appropriate (Riggins v. Nevada [U.S., 1992]).

III. Criminal Responsibility

A. In order for an act to be criminal, there must be both a guilty act and guilty intent.

1. ***Actus reus:*** the harmful act itself
2. ***Mens rea:*** a guilty mind, guilty or wrongful intent

a. *Mens rea,* in the narrow sense, is the mental state required as an element of a specific crime (e.g., larceny—knowingly taking possession of property that is not yours, for your own use, and with the intent of depriving the true owner of its use).

b. **In the general sense, *mens rea* refers to blame-worthiness or legal liability.** An individual who takes someone else's car for his own use when directed to do so by auditory hallucinations is unlikely to be found blame-worthy.

B. The defense of lack of criminal responsibility/not guilty by reason of insanity is based on the concept that some individuals who commit criminal acts should not be held morally blame-worthy because they cannot be considered moral agents due to their mental state (Moore, 1984).

C. Voluntary intoxication is not a basis for an insanity defense, although it may provide a basis for a diminished capacity defense. Mental illness caused by substance abuse, exacerbation of an existing mental illness due to intoxication, and pathologic intoxication can all provide a basis for an insanity defense.

D. Evolution of the Standards

1. **The M'Naghten test** (England, 1843). "To establish a defense on the ground of insanity, it must be clearly proved that, at the time of the committing of the act the party accused was laboring under such a defect of reason, from disease of the mind, as not to know the nature and quality of the act he was doing, or, if he did know it, that he did not know he was doing what was wrong."

a. It is a cognitive test, focusing only on whether the defendant knew what he was doing or that what he was doing was wrong.

b. It was adopted after the insanity acquittal of the would-be assassin of Prime Minister Robert Peel, who instead assassinated Peel's secretary.

2. **Irresistible impulse/loss of control test.** A defendant with a mental disease or defect would be held not responsible for criminal acts, even if he could tell right from wrong, if such disease or defect deprived him of power to choose right from wrong and the alleged crime was so connected with the mental disease as to have been the product of it solely.

a. The focus is on the existence of a mental illness and on a resulting loss of control over behavior.

b. The volitional test: a lack of knowledge of wrongfulness is not required.

3. **The New Hampshire and Durham tests** (Durham v. United States [D.C. Circuit, 1954])

a. **An accused is not criminally responsible if his unlawful conduct was the product of a mental disease or defect.**

b. This test is still used in New Hampshire.

4. **The Model Penal Code** (American Law Institute) combines two older tests: cognitive and volitional.

a. **A person is not responsible for criminal conduct if at the time of such conduct as a result of mental disease or defect he lacks substantial capacity either to appreciate the criminality (wrongfulness) of his conduct or to conform his conduct to the requirements of the law.**

As used in this Article, the terms "mental disease or mental defect" do not include an abnormality manifested only by repeated criminal or otherwise antisocial behavior.

b. Basic elements involve:

i. A mental disorder (but not antisocial personality disorder).

ii. An impairment in functioning as a result of the disorder, but the impairment need not be complete.

iii. A clear and direct causal connection or relationship between the behavioral impairment and the act.

5. **APA/Federal Court test.** It is an affirmative defense to a prosecution under any federal statute that, **at the time of the commission of the acts constituting the offense, the defendant, as a result of a severe mental disease or defect, was unable to appreciate the nature and quality or the wrongfulness of his acts.**
   a. This was passed by Congress in response to the insanity acquittal of John Hinckley after his failed assassination attempt on President Reagan.
   b. **It requires an <u>inability</u> to appreciate the nature and quality or wrongfulness, not merely a lack of substantial capacity.**
   c. **The mental disease or defect must be severe.**

E. Consequences of a Finding of Insanity

1. **An insanity acquittee is remanded to a correctional facility, often a forensic hospital, where there is assessment of dangerousness and the level of security needed.**
2. See chapter 55 (IV.D) for key cases on continued commitment of insanity acquittees.

F. Guilty but Mentally Ill (GBMI)

1. This category was developed as an alternative to the insanity defense, but it may be offered by a state as an additional option for the trier of fact (judge or jury).
2. **An individual found GBMI is not legally insane and is held responsible for the act, but is acknowledged to have been mentally ill at the time of the act.**
3. It has been adopted in a limited number of states.

G. Diminished Capacity

1. **Diminished capacity can be raised where an individual suffers from a mental illness or cognitive deficit that does not meet the requirements of the insanity defense, but nevertheless provides a basis for not holding the person fully responsible for the behavior.**
2. **The result is usually to reduce the level of the conviction** (e.g., reduction of the finding of guilt from first- to second-degree murder).

H. Demographics of the Insanity Defense

1. **One-tenth of 1% of felony trials; two insanity pleas per 1,000 felony arrests.**
2. Success rate varies by state.
3. Juries hand down only 5%, 40–50% by judges; the rest of the pleas are bargained.
4. Not a "rich man's defense": acquittees tend to be young (20–30 years), white, with on average an eighth-grade education, and to be employed as unskilled laborers.

IV. The Role of Psychiatrists in the Legal System

A. The Psychotherapist-Patient Privilege

1. **Definition**
   a. **Psychiatrists have an obligation to keep matters revealed by patients in the course of treatment confidential.** A corollary to confidentiality is the concept of **privilege.** Whereas confidentiality is an ongoing obligation on the part of the physician, **privilege is a right that belongs to the patient that must be raised by the patient before it comes into play. Privilege is the right to have matters revealed to a physician or therapist held in confidence and not revealed against the patient's will, except under certain circumstances.**
   b. **Testimonial privilege:** the right of a patient to prevent his or her therapist from testifying in an administrative or judicial proceeding about information revealed during the course of therapy. The privilege belongs to and can only be raised or waived by the patient. If the patient does not raise the privilege, the physician may be compelled to testify.
2. **Exceptions to the privilege**
   a. **Expressed waiver by the patient.**
   b. Where the patient has put his or her mental status at issue in the course of litigation (e.g., claiming emotional damages in a personal injury suit).
   c. Mandated reporting, as in cases of child abuse.
   d. Statutory exceptions (e.g., when the patient is involved in billing disputes or malpractice litigation against the physician).
3. Exists in all 50 states, the District of Columbia, and all federal courts (<u>Jaffee</u> v. <u>Redmond</u> [U.S., 1996]).
4. Rationale for the psychotherapist privilege
   a. From a societal standpoint, in instances where preservation of the psychotherapist-patient relationship is more important than the information that will be excluded from the trial.
   b. The privilege protects the privacy of a special relationship.

B. The Psychiatrist as Forensic Evaluator/Expert Witness

1. **Forensic evaluations: any psychiatric evaluation connected with litigation or for the purpose of providing an expert clinical opinion to assist a deliberative body.**
   a. **Not a doctor-patient relationship as there is no clinical care involved.**
   b. The Double Agent problem. A treating clinician has a fiduciary obligation to act only in the best interests of the patient; **the forensic evaluator's obligation is to the party requesting the evaluation.**
      i. **The client is the attorney, court, agency, etc., that has retained the psychiatrist.**
      ii. **Confidentiality is absent in the forensic evaluation. As a result, the forensic evaluator has an ethical**

obligation and, in some states, a legal obligation to obtain informed consent from the evaluee before conducting the examination. This includes warning the evaluee about the limitations on confidentiality.

iii. **No criminal evaluations should be conducted until the defendant has had an opportunity to meet with his or her attorney.**

2. **The expert witness**
   a. **An expert witness is a witness who has knowledge related to the subject matter of the litigation beyond that of the average juror or judge, who can offer information that will be useful to the judge or jury in reaching a decision in the matter.**
   b. Anyone with such additional knowledge can technically be accepted as an expert, although the credibility of the expert may be attacked. For example, a medical student might be accepted as an expert in medicine based on his or her studies, but the credibility of that expert will be attacked based on the lack of experience.
   c. Experts may use any information they would normally use in the course of an evaluation as a basis for testimony, including hearsay (information that they did not obtain first-hand, but rather obtained through the reports of a third party).
3. **The role of the expert witness**
   a. **Provide scientifically and clinically accurate testimony.**
   b. **Provide testimony in an ethically responsible manner.**
   c. **Provide answers to the legal questions raised in the proceeding, to the extent possible.**
   d. **The psychiatrist, once designated as an expert witness, can provide the court with an expert opinion on an issue before the court—e.g., whether the care of a patient was below the standard of care (malpractice), whether the defendant has a mental illness that rendered him unable to conform his behavior to the requirements of the law (criminal responsibility). The fact witness (see below) is not allowed to offer such opinions.**

C. The Psychiatrist as Fact Witness

1. **A fact witness is an individual who has information related to the matter being litigated.**
   a. **There are no special requirements to be a fact witness, other than first-hand knowledge relevant to the case.** Anyone, including a child, can be a fact witness.
   b. A fact witness cannot offer an expert opinion or use hearsay.
2. The treating psychiatrist may be called to testify about the mental condition of a patient in a wide variety of settings (e.g., personal injury litigation, workmen's compensation claims, administrative hearings, criminal cases).
3. The rules of the psychotherapist-patient privilege apply *if* the patient raises it. The court may decide that the privilege does not apply and order the psychiatrist to testify. **Refusal to testify can lead to a finding of contempt of court, justifying a fine or jail time.**
4. **The rules and exceptions regarding privilege apply.**
   a. If a patient is in litigation related to a motor vehicle claim, but does not raise emotional damages as a claim, the records of the treating physician generally cannot be obtained.
   b. If, in connection with the litigation, the patient claims emotional damages, the other side may obtain the records and testimony of the treating physician.

Suggested Readings

Almanzor, M.C. (1997). The effect of intoxication as a "mitigating factor" for murder and manslaughter. *New England Law Review, 31,* 1079.

American Medical Association Council on Ethical and Judicial Affairs. (1997). *Code of medical ethics* (Annotation 2.06). Chicago: AMA.

Levine, A.M. (1998). Denying the settled insanity defense: Another necessary step in dealing with drug and alcohol abuse. *Boston University Law Review, 78,* 75.

Moore, M.S. (1984). *Law and psychiatry: Rethinking the relationship.* Cambridge: Cambridge University Press.

Perlin, M.L. (1997). "The borderline which separated you from me": The insanity defense, the authoritarian spirit, the fear of faking, and the culture of punishment. *Iowa Law Review, 82,* 1375.

Reider, L. (1998). Toward a new test for the insanity defense: Incorporating the discoveries of neuroscience into moral and legal theories. *UCLA Law Review, 46,* 289.

Schouten, R. (1998). The psychotherapist-patient privilege. *Harvard Review of Psychiatry, 6,* 44–48.

Thomason, S.C. (1998). Criminal procedure—crazy as I need to be: The United States Supreme Court's latest addition to the incompetency doctrine. *University of Arkansas Little Rock Law Journal, 20,* 349.

Chapter 57

Patient Compliance

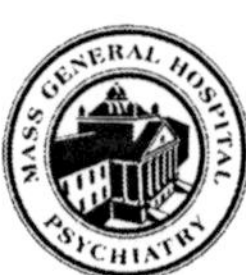

CRISTINA GALARDY, DOMINIC J. MAXWELL, AND JOHN B. HERMAN

I. Overview

Compliance (and its more recent synonym, "adherence") refers to the extent to which a patient's behavior coincides with medical advice. An often under-appreciated aspect of medical care, compliance has significant effects on diagnostic and therapeutic interventions. The patient's trust and confidence in the treating clinician is the single most positive predictor of compliance.

Although often thought of as applying only to medication regimens, **compliance refers to any recommendation** (be it to avoid caffeine, to take daily exercise, or to limit exposure to sunlight) **delivered by the physician.** Compliance with medical instructions begins with clear communication between doctor and patient. **The patient must understand not only the recommendation, but also the illness,** as well as the options and choices and the risks and benefits of the recommendation. **The patient then needs to have the ability and desire to remember and follow through with the recommendation.**

The physician's role is to recognize disease and to advise the patient to accept a treatment recommendation.

Non-compliance is common in all branches of clinical medicine (most studies cite non-compliance rates of between 25% and 75%), **and costly,** leading to increased morbidity, additional diagnostic tests, and increased rates of hospitalization. Among psychiatric patients, non-compliance results in suboptimal treatment of mental illness, increased risks of suicidal and violent behaviors, and more frequent hospitalizations. **Non-compliance** is manifest by failure to arrive for appointments, by not filling prescriptions, and by over-dosing, under-dosing, or prematurely discontinuing medications.

II. Why Do Patients Fail to Adhere to Treatment Recommendations?

Reasons for non-compliance are varied. There are no significant differences in compliance rates between psychiatric and non-psychiatric populations. Moreover, there are no demographic variables (e.g., income, socioeconomic class, occupation, level of education, or type of illness) that affect rates of non-compliance to any significant degree. The etiology of the non-compliance may be intentional or unintentional, and, it may be conscious or unconscious. **Causes of non-compliance may be subdivided into three categories:**

A. **Miscommunication or distrust between doctor and patient.** Clear communication minimizes misunderstanding between the two parties, with regard to both illness and treatment, and is fundamental to compliance. A positive doctor/patient relationship is also essential.
B. **Pychosocial and cultural factors.** Economics (the cost of a medication), a patient's cultural beliefs about illness, family pressures, and stigma all play large roles. Other factors include a desire to avoid acknowledgment of an illness requiring treatment, a need to assert control over the doctor-patient relationship, or a need to retain symptoms for secondary gain.
C. **Medical/psychiatric factors.** Unpleasant effects or side effects of prescribed treatments, cognitive deficits due to illness and psychiatric symptoms (e.g., hopelessness, psychosis, or memory impairment) may make compliance difficult, if not impossible.

Exploring the underpinnings of a patient's unwillingness or inability to comply is crucial to improving compliance. Non-compliance always conveys important information to the physician, be it about the state of the doctor-patient relationship, the cultural background and belief system of the patient, or the patient's pathology. Recognizing non-compliance and considering its genesis is an essential step toward correcting it.

III. What Can You Do about Non-compliance?

The physician's first step when addressing non-compliance is to recognize it. Non-compliance should always be considered when a patient's condition unexpectedly worsens or when things just "don't add up." **Fostering good compliance is an art, reflecting the dynamic equilibrium between doctor and patient and between science and interpersonal relationships.** Fewer patients are willing to take their doctor's word unquestioned; most have a greater access to medical information and a greater need for maintaining or asserting control. With such patients it is important that the caregiver be flexible and open-minded and that he or she demonstrate a willingness to elicit and address the patient's concerns. By uncritically acknowledging the potential for non-compliance, improvement of the behavior can be facilitated (e.g., "A lot of patients often miss medication doses from time to time, Do you?"). It is important to encourage a healthy curiosity about decision-making, and, to whatever extent is possible, it is also helpful to share your reasoning with your patient. Including the patient in the decision-making process can be empowering, and can facilitate a subjective feeling of independence and control that is commonly threatened by the presence of the illness itself.

In the case of medication prescribing, **non-compliance has been called the first barrier to bioavailability. Chronic non-compliance may reflect as much about a patient's pathology as the state of the doctor-patient relationship.** While there is no guarantee to patient compliance, **the following recommendations can help to maximize compliance:**

A. **Give clear, simple, written instructions.** Ask the patient to repeat the instructions to confirm a clear understanding.
B. **Avoid complicated dosing schedules;** be realistic! Instruct the patient and encourage the use of pill boxes and other reminders ("with meals" as opposed to "three times a day," or "when you take the dog out" instead of "in the morning").
C. **Explain your rationale for treatment** recommendations. Pictures and diagrams are often useful.
D. **Inform the patient of common side effects.**
E. **Inquire about financial burdens or resources that impact affordability of treatment.**
F. **Actively solicit a patient's fears, anxieties, and concerns about the treatment plan.**
G. **Offer easy availability,** frequent follow-up visits, availability by phone, prompt return of pages regarding concerns about treatment and illness. Surprise and (generally) delight your patient by initiating a phone call or an e-mail to inquire about their condition.
H. **Ask** whether a patient is deviating from treatment recommendations, e.g., ***"How is it going with the [medicine]"?***

In all circumstances, non-compliance provides the clinician with vital data about the patient that need to be recognized and acted upon. When non-compliance is addressed, communication, care, and trust between the doctor and the patient will be improved.

Suggested Readings

Conrad, P. (1985). The meaning of medications: Another look at compliance. *Journal of Science and Medicine, 20,* 29–37.

Cramer, J.A. & Spilker, B. (Eds.). (1991). *Patient compliance in medical practice and clinical trials.* New York: Raven Press.

Eisenthal, S., Emery, R., Lazare, A., et al. (1979). "Adherence" and the negotiated approach to patienthood. *Archives of General Psychiatry, 36,* 393–398.

Meichenbaum, D., & Turk, D.C. (1987). *Facilitating treatment adherence: A practitioner's guidebook.* New York: Plenum Press.

Chapter 58

An Overview of the Psychotherapies

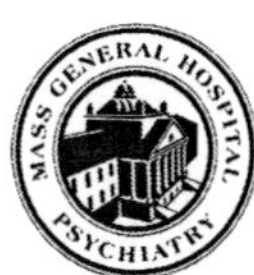

ROBERT S. ABERNETHY III AND STEVEN C. SCHLOZMAN

I. Overview

Psychotherapies are most often categorized by their fundamental theoretical elements. These classifications include treatments (e.g., psychoanalytic psychotherapy, behavioral and cognitive-behavioral therapy [CBT], and interpersonal therapy). Other classifications reflect **their duration of treatment** (e.g., brief or short-term psychotherapy) **or the patients in attendance** (e.g., group, couples, or family therapy).

This chapter describes the nine common forms of psychotherapy: **psychoanalytic or psychodynamic psychotherapy, behavior therapy, cognitive and CBT, interpersonal therapy, dialectical behavior therapy (DBT), psychoeducational psychotherapy, supportive psychotherapy, multisystemic treatment, and integrative psychotherapy.** Discussion includes which patients are referred for which therapy, and, when possible, to what extent each form of therapy has been studied in terms of efficacy and cost-effectiveness.

II. Psychoanalytical Psychotherapy (Expressive or Psychodynamic Psychotherapy)

A. Overview

1. Psychoanalytic psychotherapy is probably the **most commonly practiced type of psychotherapy in the United States. It is based on the Freudian tradition of uncovering unconscious aspects of a patient's mental life. Unconscious conflicts, repressed feelings, family issues from early in a patient's life, and difficulty with current relationships are the themes commonly addressed in this therapy.** Typically, the therapist takes a **non-directive posture,** paying close attention to **transference, countertransference, resistance, free association, and dreams** as a means of understanding and delineating unconscious conflicts.
   a. **Transference:** the unconscious redirection of feelings and desires retained from the past that are redirected toward the therapist.
   b. **Countertransference:** the unconscious association of feelings or desires from the past that the therapist develops for the patient.
   c. **Resistance:** those forces within the patient, conscious and unconscious, that oppose the purpose of the patient's evaluation and the goals of treatment.
   d. **Free association:** the undirected expression of conscious thoughts and feelings as a means of gaining access to unconscious processes.
2. **Severe and chronic personality disorders, as well as persistent problems in coping with life events, may be approached with psychoanalytic psychotherapy.** Anorexia nervosa also can be managed with long-term psychoanalytic psychotherapy.
3. The length of therapy varies from a **few months to a few years.**
4. Although some **research has supported the efficacy of this form of treatment,** it is important to remember that the nature of psychodynamic psychotherapy makes controlled studies difficult to conduct. Lack of research does not necessarily correlate with lack of efficacy. Based on existing data, cognitive and behavioral therapies (see below) may be more efficient in terms of symptom reduction and length of therapy, and have more rigorous research evidence of effectiveness. Although mood and anxiety disorders may respond to psychoanalytic psychotherapy, combinations of medication and cognitive or behavioral therapy may be more effective and efficient and cost less. Although few insurance programs pay for this type of treatment, many patients pursue and pay out-of-pocket for psychoanalytic psychotherapy because they find it emotionally and intellectually compelling.
5. There are **four principal subtypes of psychoanalytic or dynamic psychotherapy** associated with the following theoreticians:
   a. **Classical psychotherapy: Sigmund Freud**
   b. **Ego psychology: Anna Freud**
   c. **Object relations psychotherapy: Melanie Klein and Donald Winnicott**
      i. Melanie Klein is commonly associated with concepts such as the **depressive, paranoid, and schizoid positions.**
      ii. Donald Winnicott is commonly associated with concepts such as the **transitional object** and the **good-enough mother.**
   d. **Self-psychology: Heinz Kohut**
      i. Kohut is commonly associated with the concept of **mirroring.**

III. Behavior Therapy

A. Behavior therapy is based on **reducing symptoms by learning relaxation techniques, changing factors that reinforce symptoms, and giving the patient graduated exposure to distressing stimuli. Joseph Wolpe** published the first book on behavior therapy, and **Isaac Mark** demonstrated the effectiveness of behavior therapy on simple phobias.

B. Behavior **therapists usually are directive and encourage homework experimentation. Homework** may involve exposure to a feared situation (e.g., speaking out during a committee meeting). The purpose of this suggestion is to reduce the reinforcing expectation that catastrophe would occur if one speaks out. **Mental imaging** allows the patient to learn how to relax while imagining the feared situation. Behavior therapy equips the patient with concrete strategies that can be used after the termination of therapy.

C. Behavior therapy is **generally brief,** requiring **six to twenty sessions.**

D. Research evidence has repeatedly demonstrated **efficacy for behavior therapy** for a variety of **anxiety disorders, depression, and some psychosomatic symptoms (e.g., pain).** Behavior therapy is manual driven; each session has a documented direction and goal. **Manual-driven therapies more easily lend themselves to systematic study and research.**

IV. Cognitive Therapy and Cognitive-Behavioral Therapy

A. Cognitive therapy is **based on the assumption that negative thoughts promote depression or anxiety.** Ideally, these negative thoughts are documented by the patient during depressing or anxious experiences that occur between visits, and, during therapy sessions, patients are encouraged to challenge these negative ideas. **Aaron Beck** first described cognitive therapy and demonstrated its effectiveness with controlled research.

B. **Research evidence has demonstrated that cognitive therapy is an effective treatment for depression.** Cognitive therapy is also indicated for **anxiety states** and problems related to **substance abuse. Cognitive-behavioral therapy (CBT)** is the term used to describe the combination of cognitive and behavioral therapies. CBT is **effective for anxiety disorders, such as obsessive-compulsive disorder (OCD) and depression.**

C. Cognitive therapy generally requires ten to twenty sessions.

D. Cognitive therapy is a manual-driven psychotherapy.

V. Interpersonal Psychotherapy

A. Interpersonal psychotherapy **addresses relationships in the "here and now"** that may contribute to depression. Four common interpersonal issues are reviewed to discover the best focus of therapy: **grief, role transition, role dispute, and interpersonal deficits. Gerald Klerman** is credited with the early description and research on interpersonal psychotherapy.

B. Interpersonal psychotherapy has been **used primarily in the treatment of depression.**

C. This is a **brief therapy** with an active focus. The usual duration is twelve sessions.

D. There is good research evidence that this manual-driven psychotherapy is effective.

VI. Dialectical Behavior Therapy

A. **Dialectical behavior therapy (DBT) is an individual and group program for borderline personality disorder. The main goals of DBT are the reduction of self-injurious behavior and of hospitalizations.** This is a **manual-driven therapy with a psychoeducational focus** on mindfulness, interpersonal effectiveness, emotion regulation, and distress tolerance. **Marsha Linehan** originally described DBT and has demonstrated its effectiveness with borderlines in a controlled research protocol.

B. **DBT was designed especially for borderline personality disorder.**

C. DBT is typically longer than other manual-driven therapies, with a **duration of at least 1 year.**

D. **Controlled research designs** have demonstrated that DBT is **effective with borderline personality disorder at reducing self-injurious behavior and hospitalizations.**

VII. Psychoeducational Therapy

A. This form of **therapy is used to support and educate patients and families** about ways to manage and understand emotional or physical problems.

B. **Psychoeducational therapy has been used with schizophrenic patients and their families to teach *low-expressed emotion* strategies.**

C. Research has demonstrated the effectiveness of low-expressed emotions with schizophrenics.

D. This is usually **a long-term therapy** used for chronic psychiatric problems.

VIII. Supportive Psychotherapy

A. Supportive psychotherapy is **usually brief,** with an **active focus on helping the patient deal with a life crisis.** The therapist offers **advice, sympathy, and support while reinforcing the patient's strengths.**

B. Supportive psychotherapy is anecdotally extremely helpful, but **formal research to demonstrate its effectiveness is lacking.** Supportive psychotherapy appears **especially effective for acute grief reactions.**

IX. Multi-systemic Treatment

Multi-systemic treatment involves multiple and active interventions for young people who commit violence. **It has attracted increasing attention during the past decade. Unlike traditional models, where social service organizations and clinicians meet with young people in separate settings, multi-systemic treatment** involves direct intervention in the settings in which the child has encountered the most problems. Interventions encourage a more structured parenting style **and communication and affection within the family, foster positive peer relations, and establish lines of communication between parents and teachers by using such programs as after-school activities to promote academic growth. Recent studies suggest that multi-systemic treatment** reduces violent behavior, decreases the costs of caring for potentially violent youth, and improves academic performance.

X. Integrative Psychotherapy

A. Integrative psychotherapy represents **a combination of some or all of the therapies** described above and offers a multi-modal approach to the patient's problem. Integrative psychotherapy is widely practiced but has not been formally researched to demonstrate its effectiveness. **Virtually any psychiatric problem can be treated** with a combination of integrated psychotherapies and appropriate pharmacotherapy. **Arnold Lazarus and Paul Wachtel** were early writers on integrative or multi-modal psychotherapy.

B. Integrative psychotherapy varies in length from brief to long-term.

XI. Brief Psychodynamic Psychotherapies

A number of theorists have developed a variety of brief psychodynamic psychotherapies.

A. Peter Sifneos: short-term **anxiety-provoking psychotherapy** that focuses on **unconscious oedipal issues.**

B. David Malan: time-limited psychotherapy that focuses on **triangles of conflict** (wish, threat, defense) and on **triangles of insight** (therapist, current, and past relationships).

C. Habib Davanloo: intensive short-term dynamic psychotherapy **that focuses on breaking through defenses** to unlock the unconscious.

D. Lester Luborsky: supportive expressive psychotherapy that focuses on the core conflictual relationship **theme.**

E. James Mann: time-limited psychotherapy that focuses on **time and loss.**

F. Hans Strupp: time-limited dynamic psychotherapy that focuses on **cyclical maladaptive patterns.**

XII. Group Therapies

Group therapy has been used for a **variety of Axis I conditions, such as mood disorders, anxiety disorders, and schizophrenia.** Groups have also been useful in the **long-term management of personality disorders and in grief work.** Some groups are comprised of patients with different diagnoses, some with the same diagnoses. Groups have been **useful for support and education for patients with medical conditions such as breast cancer and acquired immunodeficiency syndrome (AIDS). David Spiegel's** research has focused on the efficacy of group therapy for women with breast cancer. **Groups can be open-ended, with new patients beginning and other patients terminating over time. Other groups are time-limited, with all patients beginning at the same time and the group terminating at a predetermined date.** Group therapists may address the group as a whole or may focus on individual patients in the group. Finally, groups may embrace any of the theoretical orientations outlined above.

Suggested Readings

Abernethy, R.S. (1992). The integration of therapies. In S. Rutan (Ed.), *Current trends in psychotherapy*. New York: Guilford Press.

Alonso, A., & Swiller, H.I. (1993). *Group therapy in clinical practice*. Washington, DC: American Psychiatric Press.

Basch, M.F. (1988). *Understanding psychotherapy: The science behind the art*. New York: Basic Books.

Beck, A.T. (1976). *Cognitive therapy and the emotional disorders*. New York: Meridian.

Borduin, C. (1999). Multisystemic treatment of criminality and violence in adolescents. *Journal of the American Academy of Child and Adolescent Psychiatry, 39*(a3), 242–249.

Gabbard, G.O., Gunderson, J.G., & Fonagy, P. (2002). The place of psychoanalytic treatments within psychiatry. *Archives of General Psychiatry, 59*(6), 505–510.

Hellerstein, D., Pinsker, H., Rosenthal, R., & Kee, S. (1994). Supportive therapy as the treatment model of choice. *Journal of Psychotherapy Practice Research, 3*, 300–306.

Klerman, G., Weissman, M., Rounsaville, B., & Chevron, E. (1984). *Interpersonal psychotherapy of depression*. New York: Basic Books.

Linehan, M.M. (1993). *Cognitive-behavioral treatment of borderline personality disorder.* New York: Guilford Press.

Mann, J. (1992). *Time-limited psychotherapy*. Cambridge, MA: Harvard University Press.

Rutan, J.S. (1992). *Psychotherapy for the 1990s*. New York: Guilford Press.

Sperling, M.B., & Sack, A. (2002). Psychodynamics and managed care: The art of the impossible? *American Journal of Psychotherapy, 56*(3), 362–377.

Wachtel, P.L. (1977). *Psychoanalysis and behavior therapy: Toward an integration.* New York: Basic Books.

Chapter 59

Planned Brief Psychotherapy: An Overview

MARK A. BLAIS AND JAMES E. GROVES

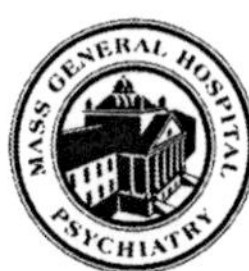

I. Overview

Interest in planned brief psychotherapy has grown enormously in the last few decades. Unfortunately, this interest has been fueled more by changing patterns of health care reimbursement than by an appreciation of the clinical value inherent in brief psychotherapy. This chapter provides an overview of an eclectic approach to planned brief psychotherapy. By presenting the important features of brief therapy in a general manner (rather than as a specific school of brief therapy), the essential features of this form of psychotherapy can more easily be assimilated into one's ongoing psychotherapy practice. Still, **to understand even an eclectic version of short-term therapy, one must have an historical context within which to place it.**

II. A Brief History of Brief Psychotherapy

Toward the end of the nineteenth century, **when Breuer and Freud were busy inventing psychoanalysis, hysterical symptoms defined the focus of the work.** These early treatments were brief and symptom-focused, the therapist was active, and, basically, desperate patients selected themselves for the fledgling venture. **In time, free association, exploration of the transference, and dream analysis replaced hypnosis and direct suggestion** as the method of treatment, and the duration of treatment was greatly increased and therapist activity decreased. **Franz Alexander's manipulation of the interval and spacing of sessions was one of the major events in the development of modern short-term therapy. Decreased frequency, irregular spacing, therapeutic holidays, and therapist-dictated scheduling (rather than patient- or symptom-dictated scheduling) all enhanced the reality orientation of therapy.** World War II saw a glut of patients needing treatment for "shell shock" and "battle fatigue." New concepts and theories emerged from treating so many patients so rapidly. **Grinker and Spiegel's treatment of soldiers and Lindemann's work with survivors of the Coconut Grove fire** highlight this period in the development of brief treatment. Finally, **in the early 1960s, Sifneos and Malan independently developed the first theoretically coherent short-term psychotherapies.**

III. The Modern Brief Psychotherapies

Although this chapter focuses on an eclectic approach to brief therapy, it is important to have some sense of the **current brief psychotherapy schools.** There are basically four schools of brief psychotherapy: psychodynamic, cognitive-behavioral, interpersonal, and eclectic. **All four of these orientations share the essential features of brief therapy: brevity, patient selection, treatment focus, and high levels of therapist activity.**

A. **The psychodynamic short-term therapies** (see Sifneos, 1992; Malan, 1976; Davanloo, 1980) **feature psychoanalytic interpretation of defenses and unconscious conflicts** as their main "curative" agent. **Sifneos's anxiety-provoking therapy** is an ideal example of a brief psychodynamic psychotherapy. This treatment runs for 12–20 sessions and focuses narrowly on issues such as the failure to grieve, fear of success, or triangular, futile love relationships. The therapist serves as a detached, didactic figure who holds to the focus and challenges the patient to relinquish both dependency and intellectualization, while confronting anxiety-producing conflicts. One can think of this method as a classical oedipal level defense analysis with all the lull periods removed. One limiting feature is that it serves only 2–10% of the population, the subgroup able to tolerate its unremitting anxiety.

B. **The cognitive-behavioral brief therapies** (see Beck and Greenberg, 1979) **aim at bringing the patient's "automatic" (pre-conscious) thoughts into awareness and demonstrating how these thoughts impact behavior and feelings.** This style of therapy is much more broadly applicable in terms of both patients and problems. The basic thrust of cognitive therapy, according to Beck and Greenberg, is to get the automatic thoughts more completely into consciousness, to challenge them consciously, and to practice new behaviors that change the picture of the world and the self in it. The patient is actively helped to challenge these automatic thoughts.

C. **Brief interpersonal therapy was developed by Klerman (1984) and is a highly formalized (manualized) treatment. Interpersonal psychotherapy (IPT) focuses not on mental content but on the process of the patient's interaction with others.** In IPT, behavior and communications are taken at face value. IPT was developed primarily to treat patients with depressive episodes related to either grief or loss, interpersonal disputes, or interpersonal skill deficits.

D. **The "eclectic" brief therapies are characterized by combinations and integrations of multiple theories and techniques. Budman and Gurman**

(1988) present one very popular version of eclectic brief therapy which focuses on three dimensions of mental life: the interpersonal, the developmental, and the existential. The model of Budman and Gurman pursues a systematic approach, beginning with the individual's reason for seeking therapy at this time. Major changes in the patient's social support are reviewed. A major feature here is the belief that maximal benefit from therapy occurs early, and the optimal time for change is early in treatment.

IV. The Natural Course of Psychotherapy

Despite the common perception that psychotherapy is a long-term, even timeless, enterprise, most of the existing **data indicate that psychotherapy as it is practiced in the real world has a time-limited course.** For example, using national outpatient psychotherapy utilization data obtained in 1987 (before the nationwide impact of managed care), **Olfson and Pincus found that 70% of psychotherapy users received ten or fewer sessions.** In fact, only 15% of their sample received 21 or more sessions. These data are highly consistent with earlier studies showing a median number of eight sessions for outpatient psychotherapy. Clearly then, in the real world, the majority of patients have a time-limited or brief psychotherapy experience. The material presented in this chapter will help you deliver psychotherapy in a planned and thoughtful manner, which is better matched to psychotherapy's natural course.

V. The Brief Therapy Mind-set

A certain mind-set needs to be adopted by a therapist hoping to successfully learn and practice brief treatment.

A. **From the start there must be a willing suspension of disbelief and cynicism about brief therapy.** An example of this would be a willingness to consider a quick positive response as something other than a temporary "flight into health."
B. **Therapy must be conceptualized as a time-limited enterprise,** as something that will end at a known planned date. This appears deceptively simple, but in practice it is actually a difficult cognitive change to make and one that has ramifications for all your treatment decisions, particularly your activity level as the therapist. To illustrate, briefly consider how you might approach a new patient if from the start you knew that the therapy would last 14 sessions.
C. **The therapist must expect and accept that patients will return to therapy periodically across their lifespan** (sometimes called intermittent brief therapy across the life-cycle). This relates to the notion of cure and what is an acceptable outcome for treatment. This is often the easiest of the three components to accept.

VI. The Essential Features of Brief Therapy

A. Patient Evaluation and Selection

1. **Initial evaluation. Patient selection is the art of finding the right patient with the right problem for brief psychotherapy** and it starts with the initial evaluation. A **two-session evaluation** format is recommended for determining if a patient is appropriate for brief therapy. This format allows the clinician to conduct a complete psychiatric evaluation and assess the appropriateness of the patient for brief psychotherapy without feeling too much time pressure. To guide you in the selection of patients, we present a number of inclusion and exclusion criteria (see Table 59-1). These criteria are fairly general, covering most forms of brief therapy, and restrictive—many patients will be screened out. However, for the new or novice brief therapist the use of these criteria will provide nearly ideal brief therapy patients.
2. **Exclusion criteria.** Here is a short list of exclusion criteria. **The brief therapy patient should not be actively psychotic, abusing substances, or at significant risk for self-harm.** The actively psychotic patient will not be able to make adequate use of the reality-oriented/logical aspects of the brief treatment. Substance-abusing patients should be directed to substance-abuse treatment prior to undertaking any form of psychotherapy. Patients at significant risk for self-harm are not appropriate for brief therapy due to possible complications with the ending of their treatment at a planned time. These factors should be considered categorical in nature; the presence of any one of them

Table 59-1. Patient Selection Criteria for Brief Therapy

Exclusion criteria
Active psychosis
Substance abuse
A significant risk of self-harm
Inclusion criteria
Moderate emotional distress
A desire for relief
A specific or circumscribed problem
History of positive relationship
Function in one area of life
Ability to commit to treatment

should rule out a patient for brief psychotherapy. This is especially true for a therapist just beginning to learn brief treatment.

3. **Inclusion criteria.** These criteria can be thought of as dimensions, with each patient being rated on how much of each dimension they have. The potential candidate for brief therapy should:
   a. Be in moderate emotional distress, as this provides the motivation for treatment.
   b. Personally want relief from his or her emotional pain; they should not have been sent to therapy reluctantly by a boss or spouse.
   c. Be able to articulate a fairly specific cause of their pain or a circumscribed life problem (or be willing to accept your specific formulation of their difficulty); this helps provide a treatment focus.
   d. Have a history of at least one positive (mutual) interpersonal relationship.
   e. Still be functioning in at least one area of life.
   f. Have the ability to commit to a treatment contract.

   As stated earlier, patients should be rated for their standing on all of these dimensions. The more of these qualities (amount and number) that a patient has, the better the candidate for brief therapy he or she is.

B. Developing a Treatment Focus

Developing a treatment focus is probably the most misunderstood aspect of brief therapy. Many writers talk about "the focus" in a circular and mysterious manner, as if the whole success of the treatment rests on finding *the* one correct focus (Hall, Arnold, & Crosby, 1990). This can be confusing and intimidating to those just learning brief therapy. Rather, **what is needed is the establishment of a focus that both the therapist and the patient can agree upon and that fits the therapist's treatment approach.** This can be called **a functional focus.** The main technique for finding a functional focus is the "Why now?" technique developed by Budman and Gurman (1988). **This technique is applied by repeatedly asking the patient "Why did you come for treatment now?"** "Why today rather than last week, tomorrow, etc. . . . ?" (You really need to try this simple technique a few times to see how effective and powerful it can be.) The goal is to find out what the triggering event for therapy was, as this might provide an ideal treatment focus.

Budman and Gurman (1988) also describe **four common treatment foci:**

1. **Losses,** past, present, or pending. These can be interpersonal (e.g., the loss of a loved one), intrapersonal (e.g., the loss of a psychological ability, the social loss of a support network), or functional (as in the loss of specific abilities or capacities).
2. **Developmental desynchronies** (being out of step with expected developmental stages). This is often seen in the professional who required extensive periods of education prior to initiating an adult lifestyle.
3. **Interpersonal conflicts,** usually repeated interpersonal disappointments, either with loved ones or bosses.
4. **Symptomatic presentations.** Many patients present for psychotherapy simply with the desire for symptom reduction. It is helpful to memorize these four common foci and review them in your head while conducting an initial evaluation assessment of their relevance to the patient. The most important thing to remember is that you are not finding *the* focus, only *a* focus for the therapy.

C. Completing the Initial Evaluation

By the completion of the second evaluation session you need to:

1. **Decide if the patient is appropriate for brief treatment.**
2. **Select an agreed-upon focus.**
3. **Have a clearly stated treatment contract,** including the number of sessions, how missed appointments will be handled, and how post-termination contact will be handled.

The two-session evaluation format also allows you to see how the patient responds to you and to the therapy. In fact, it can be very enlightening to give the patient some kind of homework to complete between the two sessions. An initial positive response, and feeling a little better in the second session, bodes well (while a strong negative reaction conveys a worse prognosis). A more ambivalent response, such as forgetting the task, may signal problems with motivation and should be explored.

D. Being an Active Therapist (see Table 59-2)

Conducting a brief (12–16 sessions) psychotherapy requires that the therapist be very active. The therapist performing such therapy must keep the treatment focused and the process of treatment moving forward. Several techniques have been designed to structure and to direct the therapy. These include beginning each session with a summary of the important points raised during the last session, and restating the focus. Assignment and review of homework (out of session assignments designed to transfer gains from therapy to the patient's life) are tasks that characterize the activity of the therapist. Interven-

Table 59-2. Types of Therapist Activity
• Structuring sessions
• Use of homework
• Developing the working alliance
• Limiting silences
• Clarification of vague responses
• Addressing positive and negative transference quickly
• Limiting psychological regression

tions that focus on the "working alliance" are important, as are timely interventions, which limit silences and deviations from the focus.

The goal of eclectic brief therapy is to restore or improve pre-morbid adaptation and function. Efforts are made by the therapist to limit and check psychological regressions. **Asking, "What did you think about that?" rather than about feelings and affect (e.g., "How did that make you feel?") can help with the exploration of potentially regressive material.** Limited within-session regression is acceptable and often necessary in brief therapy; however, prolonged regressions accompanied by decreased function are to be avoided.

Clarification is important in brief therapy. Requests for clarification should be made whenever a patient produces vague or incomplete material. This would include asking for examples or for specifics, and empathically pointing out contradictions and inconsistencies.

Transference occurs in all treatments, including brief psychotherapy. **Despite the fact that many aspects of brief therapy are designed to discourage the development of transference, the therapist must be ready to deal with it when it develops.** Two forms of transference are particularly important to recognize quickly: negative and overly positive transferences. Negative transference can be suspected when the patient responds repeatedly with either angry or devaluing statements or when he or she experiences the therapy as humiliating. Overly positive transference is signaled by repeated and excessively positive comments (e.g., "Oh, you know me better than anyone ever has"). Both of these forms of transference should be dealt with quickly from the perspective of reality. The therapist should review the patient's feelings and reasoning and relate these to the actual interaction. For example, if the therapist was inadvertently offensive, this should be admitted to, while pointing out that the therapist's motive was to be helpful.

VII. Phases of Planned Brief Therapy

Three traditional phases of psychotherapy as they apply to brief treatment need review.

A. **The initial phase (from the evaluation to session two or three) principally includes evaluation and selection of the patient, selection of the focus, and establishment of a working alliance.** This phase is usually accompanied by some mild reduction in symptoms and a low-grade positive transference, particularly as a working relationship develops. The goal is to set the frame and the structure of the therapy, while also giving the patient hope.

B. **The middle phase** (session four to eight or nine). In the middle phase, the work gets more difficult. **The patient usually becomes concerned about the time limit, feeling that the length of treatment will not be sufficient.** Issues of separation and aloneness come to the fore and compete with the focus for attention. It is important for the therapist to reassure the patient (with words and a calm, understanding demeanor) that the treatment will work, and direct their joint attention back to the agreed-upon focus. The patient often feels worse during this phase and the therapist's faith in the treatment process is often tested.

C. **The termination phase** (session eight to twelve or sixteen). In this phase the therapy usually settles down. **The patient accepts the fact that treatment will end as planned, and his or her symptoms typically decrease.** In addition to the treatment focus, post-therapy plans and the situational loss of the therapy relationship are explored. At or around the actual termination of treatment, it is not unusual for the patient to present some new and often interesting material for discussion. While the therapist may be tempted to explore this new material and thereby extend the treatment, doing so is usually (but not always) a mistake. Interest in the new material should be shown, but, if it is not clinically important, treatment should end as planned.

D. **Post-treatment Contact**

Within the eclectic brief therapy framework, it is acceptable for patients to return to therapy at multiple points during their life. When a therapy is completed, a patient should wait about 6 months before considering further therapy. This allows the patient to practice his or her newly learned psychological insights and skills in the real world and time to assess their new level of adaptation and function. In considering post-treatment contact, you should strive to help patients with psychological troubles whenever they develop across the lifespan.

Suggested Readings

Beck, S., & Greenberg, R. (1979). Brief cognitive therapies. *Psychiatric Clinics of North America, 2,* 11–22.

Blais, M. (2000). Planned brief therapy. In J. Jacobson, & A. Jacobson (Eds.), *Psychiatric secrets* (2nd ed.). Philadelphia, PA: Hanley & Belfus.

Book, H. (1998). *How to practice brief psychodynamic psychotherapy: The core conflictual relationship theme method.* Washington, DC: American Psychological Association.

Budman, S., & Gurman, A. (1988). *Theory and practice of brief therapy.* New York: Guilford Press.

Burk, J., White, H., & Havens, L. (1979). Which short-term therapy? *Archives of General Psychiatry, 36,* 177–186.

Crits-Christoph, P. (1992). The efficacy of brief dynamic psychotherapy: A meta-analysis, *American Journal of Psychiatry, 149,* 151–158.

Davanloo, H. (1980). *Short-term dynamic psychotherapy.* New York: Jason Aronson.

Davanloo, H. (1987). Intensive short-term dynamic psychotherapy with highly-resistant depressed patients: Part I. Restructuring ego's regressive defenses. *International Journal of Short-term Psychotherapy, 2,* 99–13.

Groves, J. (1992). The short-term dynamic psychotherapies: An overview. In S. Rutan (Ed.), *Psychotherapy for the 90s.* New York: Guilford Press.

Groves, J. (1996). *Essential papers on short-term dynamic therapy.* New York: New York Universities Press.

Hall, M., Arnold, W., & Crosby, R. (1990). Back to basics: The importance of focus selection. *Psychotherapy, 27,* 578–584.

Klerman, G., Weissman, M., Rounsaville, B., & Chevron, E. (1984). *Interpersonal psychotherapy of depression.* New York: Basic Books.

Leibovich, M. (1981). Short-term psychotherapy for the borderline personality disorder. *Psychotherapy Psychosomatics, 35,* 257–264.

Malan, D. (1976). *The frontier of brief psychotherapy.* New York: Plenum Medical Book.

Malan, D., & Osimo, F. (1992). *Psychodynamics, training and outcome in brief psychotherapy.* London: Butterworth-Heinemann.

Mann, J. (1991). Time-limited psychotherapy. In P. Crits-Christoph, & J.P. Barber (Eds.), *Handbook of short-term dynamic psychotherapy,* pp. 17–44. New York: Basic Books.

Mann, J., & Goldman, K. (1982). *A case-book in time-limited psychotherapy.* New York: McGraw-Hill.

Olfson, M., Pincus, H.A. (1994). Outpatient psychotherapy in the United States, II: Patterns of utilization. *American Journal of Psychiatry, 151*(9), 1289–1294.

Sifneos, P. (1992). *Short-term anxiety provoking psychotherapy: A treatment manual.* New York: Basic Books.

Winston, A., Laikin, M., Pollack, J., et al. (1994). Short-term psychotherapy of personality disorders. *American Journal of Psychiatry, 151,* 190–194.

Chapter 60

Couples Therapy

ANNE K. FISHEL

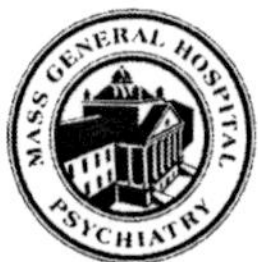

I. Introduction

Couples therapy is a clinical subspecialty that most clinicians engage in, but few do so with any formal training. **Couples therapy focuses on the pattern of interactions between two people while taking into account the individual history and contribution of each member.**

Clinical work with couples is typically part of child evaluation, ongoing child and adolescent psychotherapy, divorce mediation, crisis work, or child custody evaluation. Couples therapy is also an important component in the treatment of sexual dysfunction, alcoholism and substance abuse, the disclosure of an infidelity, depression and anxiety disorders, infertility, and serious medical illness. Couples therapy is also useful in resolving polarized relational issues, such as the decision to marry or divorce, the choice to have an abortion, or the decision to move to a distant city for one partner's career. The term "couples therapy" rather than "marital therapy" is deliberately used throughout this chapter to include therapy with homosexual couples and unmarried heterosexual couples.

A. Organizing Principles for Couples Therapists

1. **Attraction and mate choice. The couple's therapist often locates the origins of the current dilemma in the nature of the initial attraction.** Two common explanations of attraction are "opposites attract" (elaborated by the psychodynamic construct "projective identification") and "repetition compulsion."
   a. **Projective identification:** the idea that individuals unconsciously look for something in the other that is difficult for the self and then act to elicit the very behavior in the other that has been disavowed. So, for example, a shy, self-effacing man may be attracted to a self-confident, ambitious woman, but over time complains that she is too self-absorbed. She may initially find his steadiness and calm attractive, only to later criticize him for his cold remove. What is problematic for the self becomes contentious between the couple.
   b. **Repetition compulsion or re-enactment:** the idea that one falls in love with someone who resembles a loving caretaker from childhood, or who resembles an abusive caretaker with whom one wants a second chance to master the abuse. Murray Bowen, a psychodynamic therapist, observed that **individuals at a similar level of psychological functioning tend to marry.**
2. **Contribution from family of origin. Regardless of theoretical orientation, most couples' therapists posit a connection between past family experiences and current marital functioning.** Beginning with the choice of a mate, each member of the couple brings an unconscious template of lover and then proceeds to distort the other to conform with the self's needs. The process of couples therapy is, in large part, one of distinguishing between those distortions based on past familial relationships and the reality of one's actual partner.
3. **Life cycle context. A couple's relationship takes place within the context of changes in each individual and changes in the wider context of family.** Since individuals' psychological growth may take place at different rates, relationships must be able to tolerate divergent growth trajectories, as, for example, when one partner is ready for children, or for retirement, before the other.

   Life-cycle theorists have posited several predictable stages of development for intact middle-class couples with children. Life events and a particular set of psychological tasks that require change prompt these stages. It is assumed that **it is in the transition from one stage to another that couples and families are most at risk for divorce and the appearance of individual symptomatology.**
   a. The stages, with the principal concomitant emotional task required, are outlined by Carter and McGoldrick (1999):
      i. Young adults leave home: accepting emotional and financial responsibility for the self.
      ii. Families join through marriage: committing to and forming a new marital system.
      iii. Families have young children: making room for new members in the marital system.
      iv. Families have adolescents: increasing the flexibility of family boundaries to include adolescents' independence, as well as grandparents' dependence.
      v. Children get launched and move on: re-evaluating marriage and career issues, as parenting roles diminish.
      vi. Families exist later in life: accepting the shifting of generational roles to care for the older generation and face aging and loss in middle generation.
   b. As the larger social context changes, the parameters of these stages shift as well. At present, e.g., couples can expect an average of 20 years from the time their youngest child marries until retirement, as compared with only 2 years for this launching stage at the turn of the century. The lengthening of this stage is due to longer life expectancy and women ending their childbearing at a relatively young age, with fewer children.

4. **Gender.** After decades of overlooking the contribution of gender differences to couples relationships, there has been a burgeoning of writings over the last two decades (Barnett and Rivers, 1996; Carter and McGoldrick, 1999; Luepnitz, 1988; Tannen, 1990; Walters et al., 1988). The influence of gender has been documented in at least two areas:
   a. The effect of marriage and divorce on men's and women's health and well-being. Several researchers have noted that **married men experience better health and greater marital satisfaction than do their female counterparts.** Also, married men achieve greater occupational success than single men, while the opposite is true for married women. Even in dual-career marriages, women continue to do the lion's share of household and child care tasks, particularly the daily and routine tasks (e.g., cooking and laundry). **The effects of divorce on women are far more devastating than they are on men;** men experience a 42% average rise in their standard of living after divorce, and women experience an average 75% decline in financial resources (Weitzman, 1985).
   b. The effect of gender socialization on communication, roles, and violence. **Boys, in general, are encouraged to be more aggressive and independent, and discouraged from focusing on their emotional worlds. Girls, by contrast, are raised to focus more on their relationships with others and to be concerned with understanding the needs of others. These distinct paths of socialization lead to the creation of two cultures,** making most heterosexual marriages essentially cross-cultural. Tannen (1990) has observed the misunderstandings that can result from this cultural difference, with men arguing and interrupting more and women eager to compromise and capitulate. With the rapid societal changes over the last few decades bringing increasing numbers of mothers into the workplace and the demand that fathers be more emotionally available in the family than their own fathers were, many couples are experiencing additional stress and confusion about their gender roles.
   c. **The effects of gender socialization can be seen in domestic violence as well.** In domestic violence, 95% of all cases are perpetrated by men against women. Goldner and colleagues (1990) argue that such violence can best be understood in terms of gender socialization. Men who were raised to feel shamed by expressing feelings may defend against perceived feminine threats of dependency and vulnerability by asserting their masculinity through violence.
5. **What is a good relationship?** In recent years, several therapists have grappled with defining healthy marital functioning. In *The Good Marriage*, Wallerstein and Blakeslee (1995) interviewed 50 happily married couples and concluded that these **couples had dealt successfully with nine tasks:**
   a. They detached emotionally from each member's family of origin.
   b. They built intimacy while preserving a sense of autonomy.
   c. They relaxed the boundaries of the couple's relationship to allow children in while maintaining the emotional richness of marriage.
   d. They confronted the inevitable developmental changes of aging, loss, illness, and came out of crisis with renewed strength.
   e. They safely expressed difference, anger, and conflict without violence or capitulation.
   f. They established a pleasurable sexual relationship that changed in response to the stressors of aging, work, and family life.
   g. They shared laughter and humor.
   h. They provided emotional nurturance and encouragement.
   i. They allowed the marriage to be renewed by the elements of fantasy and attraction that first drew the partners to one another.
6. **Communication. Early models of couples therapy stressed the importance of developing communication skills, sometimes at the expense of other relational dimensions like gender, sex, and family of origin issues.** The emphasis on communication stressed the importance of each partner being able to speak openly and frankly while the other listened with undefensive empathy. In part, this emphasis belies a bias about intimacy: that closeness can be achieved only through the full and open disclosure of each partner's innermost feelings. **More recent interpretations of the role of communication include a wider range of issues: not only talking and listening, but also refraining from making hurtful comments and focusing on non-verbal action, including acts of affection and sexuality, the giving and receiving of generous acts, and the sharing of mutually enjoyed activities, even if they do not include self-disclosing conversation** (Weingarten, 1990).

II. Conducting an Evaluation

A couple's evaluation should contain an opportunity for the couple to discuss their relationship together and to explore their individual histories separately. The evaluation offers a balance between clinical understanding and empathy on the one hand, and prodding the couple into thinking about their relationship in new, more flexible ways, on the other. Throughout the evaluation, the clinician looks for opportunities to re-establish hope, to point out resources and strengths of the couple, and to provide a forum for each partner's position to be heard without judgment. The clinician will also look for opportunities to transform individual explanations of a problem into systemic, interactive descriptions. **A successful evaluation will determine the motivation of each partner to participate in ongoing treatment and tease out when couples therapy is con-**

traindicated and when individual, group, or no therapy should be recommended instead.

A. The First Session (both members of the couple)

1. **Providing a context of safety and comfort.** The clinician should set a time frame, ask each member to introduce him- or herself separate from the problems that bring them in, and offer certain rules of discourse:
   a. **The "I pass" rule can be introduced.** If anyone is asked a question that feels too intrusive, he or she is encouraged to "pass."
   b. **Setting the expectation that whatever is said in the individual meetings will be shared in the wrap-up meeting.** This guideline prevents the therapist from getting in the untenable position of sharing a secret with one member of the couple about the other.
   c. **Summarizing any contact the therapist has already had with one member of the couple** to demonstrate the therapist's commitment to openness and equity.
2. **Getting each couple member's definition of the problem.** It is essential that the clinician convey that both partners' perspectives will be respected and contained, and that the therapist will not play the role of a judge, arbitrating two adversaries. Each individual should have an opportunity to tell his or her version without interruptions and qualifications by the other.
   a. As an opening question, the clinician might ask: "Often in couples, each member has a different view of the problem and different hopes for change. I'd like to hear from each of you how you see your difficulties."
   b. **It is important to determine whether both parties are engaged in the evaluation process** or whether one member has been dragged, coerced, or threatened by the other. The clinician might ask: "I'd like to hear how you made the decision to give me a call and whose idea it was."
   c. **The therapist will want to know about the larger context** in which the couple lives in order to understand other resources and other stressors. The therapist might ask: "Who else has been concerned and given advice or offered help?" And, "Have there been any other changes in the family in the last year?" (e.g., illnesses, job loss, deaths, moves, infertility, births). Often, a request for couples therapy will coincide with an accumulation of other stressors.
3. **Expanding the couple's view of the problem.** An evaluation should offer the couple ample opportunity to share their working, rehearsed definitions of the problem as well as a chance to have their ideas challenged and stretched in order to create new strategies for change. Several questions help make the shift from the couple's current view to a more flexible, often interactional definition that paves the way for each member of the couple to change in order to alter the pattern between them rather than the pathology within one. Here are some examples:
   a. **"If you were to be in couples therapy for 6 months and at that point you declared that the therapy had been a wild success, what would I notice that would let me know that your relationship had changed in important ways?** What, for example, would you be talking about or doing with each other or noticing about the other that is not happening now?" (see De Shayzer, 1994). With these questions, the couple is asked to envision a solution and a way of knowing when the therapy would be over.
   b. Since a majority of couples will experience sexual difficulties at some point in their relationship, it is worth asking every couple during an evaluation, even if it is not part of the stated problem: **"Is there anything you would like to change about your sexual relationship?"**
   c. **Since one can often detect the seeds of the current dilemma in the story of the couple's initial attraction to one another, it is useful to ask: "What first attracted you to one another?"** Furthermore, most couples, no matter how upset or angry, will brighten and soften toward one another in answering this question. When there is not a palpable shift toward more positive affect, the therapist may be concerned that there is an absence of affection and friendship to draw on.
   d. Mark Karpel, in *Evaluating Couples,* suggests that the therapist ask each member of the couple: "What is it like being married to you?" **When each member's version of the self matches the partner's view, the therapy is far more straightforward.** When these versions do not match, the therapist will have to attend to the fact that there is no agreement on the relational problem.
   e. **Where is the couple developmentally?** Attending to normative responses to life-cycle changes will alert the therapist to inquire about commonly occurring reactions to these events. For example, if a couple has small children, one will want to ask how their sexual relationship has changed, and do they have fights about the equity of child care and housework.
   f. **"What can you tell me about the family you grew up in that will help me understand your current dilemma?"** This question probes for the themes and issues that each individual brings to the relationship and sets the groundwork for later exploration of projective identification.
   g. **"Tell me about an instance when the problem did not occur."** "What did you notice that each of you was doing differently?" These questions, derived from narrative therapy (White and Epston, 1990), ask the couple to stand apart from their problem and notice the positive examples of their interactions. In addition, such an inquiry guides members to reflect on his or her contribution to the pattern between them.
   h. **Over the course of a marriage, 50% of couples will be unfaithful, so there is a strong possibility that any couple seeking therapy may have an infidelity going on.** It is unlikely, however, that if you ask about a secret affair in the presence of the couple, that you will be told the truth. If you ask in an individual meeting about infidelity, you will more likely hear the truth, but you will be stuck with

having a secret that will make you collude with one member and likely enrage the other if the secret comes out. An alternative to asking directly about infidelity is to test the waters by inquiring, "Has fidelity been a challenge for either of you to maintain?" "What has been your understanding about what constitutes infidelity?" **When there is an ongoing affair or, when one member is suspicious of the other's fidelity, these questions will often elicit non-verbal cues of anxiety or anger.**

B. The Two Individual Sessions (one member at each)

These sessions offer an opportunity to get to know the individuals better and to give them a chance to bring up whatever they want without having to share the time with their partner. In addition it is useful to ask about:

1. Each individual's current level of commitment to the relationship.
2. Each member's history of, and current use of, drugs and alcohol.
3. Previous and current experiences with therapy and psychiatric hospitalizations.
4. Any history of depression, suicidality, anxiety, or other mental illness.
5. Any history of sexual abuse.
6. Any current medical problems.
7. Particularly with women: "Do you ever feel afraid of your partner? Do you feel sexually coerced by your partner? Do you feel free to make decisions? Do you have access to financial resources? Has your partner ever been violent toward you, your children, or inanimate objects?"

C. The Fourth Wrap-up, Feedback Session (both members of the couple)

When one partner has been dragged to couples therapy, the evaluation may be the end of the line and the feedback can give the couple ideas to work with even if they forgo further couples therapy.

1. **Comment on positive aspects of the relationship.** Conveying an appreciation of the couple's positive qualities diminishes defensiveness, promotes hopefulness, and places the focus on the relationship. The therapist might note, e.g., how intently the couple listened to one another, or how courageous it was for them to come to therapy or how well they use humor.
2. **Give a reading of the affective temperature of the relationship.** It is crucial that the therapist accurately interpret the couple's level of distress. Is this a couple on the verge of a break-up, in need of a tune-up in a few areas, or in conflict about the extent of the overhaul needed?
3. **Identify the stressors and place the problem in a developmental perspective.**
4. **Offer a relational description of the problem** that includes both perspectives and points to areas of change.
5. **Make recommendations for treatment.**
   a. **When to refer for couples therapy:**
      i. When the therapist and the couple can agree on an interactional definition of the problem.
      ii. When there is irreconcilable disagreement, as with a stalemate about whether to marry, to divorce, or to have children.
      iii. With particular complaints, such as sexual difficulties, chronic fighting, adjustment to serious medical illness in one partner, or the aftermath of the disclosure of an affair.
      iv. When the couple is having difficulty negotiating a life transition; e.g., when a couple fears the dissolution of their marriage as they anticipate their oldest child's leave-taking, or when a couple with a newborn feels overwhelmed by the intensity of their fights with one another.

   b. **When to refer for individual therapy:**
      i. If one partner is motivated for therapy and the other is not.
      ii. If an individual symptom requires specialized treatment, as when one member is clinically depressed, has an uncontrolled temper, or is experiencing post-traumatic stress disorder (PTSD).
      iii. If one member is maintaining a secret affair and is conflicted about whether to end it and work on the marriage.

   c. **When couples therapy is contraindicated** (Note: to recommend against couples therapy is not the same as recommending that a couple separate or divorce):
      i. When only one member can identify a wish to change or make a commitment to working on the relationship.
      ii. When there is ongoing violence and the violent partner is unwilling or unable to negotiate a convincing no-violence contract. When there is history of lethality, such as substance abuse, restraining orders, weapons, threats to kill self or other, obsession with the partner, or violence that has lead to injury (Bograd and Mederos, 1999).
      iii. When there have been repeated failed attempts at couples therapy and a chronic relational problem with a high degree of mistrust and a lack of any positive feelings between them.

III. Treatment Interventions

Each of the interventions listed below belongs to a distinct theoretical orientation. Couples therapists will offer a more thoughtful, coherent treatment if their interventions derive from theory than if they use an array of techniques in a trial and error fashion. These interventions represent only a sampling of those available.

A. Interpretation of unconscious processes that distort the ability of each member of the couple to perceive the other for who she or he really is (**psychodynamic model**). The distortions derive largely from unresolved family-of-origin issues. **Therapeutic work focuses on interpretation of projective identification and transference** (with interpretations made between the members of the couple as well as between the couple and therapist).

B. Communication Skills Training (Cognitive-Behavioral Model)

1. **Active listening.** Each partner practices, both in the session and outside, how to listen with empathy and curiosity to the other. They take turns being speaker and listener, with the latter demonstrating understanding by paraphrasing what was said and asking for confirmation from the speaker.
2. **Developing a marital *quid pro quo*.** Each individual makes a list of behaviors that are pleasing to him or her. Then, **the therapist negotiates an increase in pleasing behaviors on the part of each that is contingent on the other emitting comparable behavior.** For example, one spouse may agree to make dinner in return for the other being physically affectionate.
3. **Learning to fight constructively by following certain rules,** such as sticking to one issue at a time, eliminating name-calling or sarcasm, asking for a specific change, and asking for and giving feedback.

C. Role-Playing and Other Action-Oriented Techniques (Experiential Model)

1. **Psychodrama.** Each member of the couple may enact a present interaction that is repeatedly unsatisfactory or a situation from his or her family of origin that connects to a current marital dilemma. Each member of the couple can then enroll the other in a rewritten enactment that corrects a past injustice. Or, if the husband directs his wife to role-play him, he can show her the way he would like to be responded to.
2. **Role reversal.** Switching of roles can enhance empathy, increase the behavioral and affective repertoire of each member of the couple, and loosen polarized positions.

D. Paradoxical Interventions (Strategic Model)

These are based on the premise that couples request and shun change simultaneously. To deal with this common dual agenda, strategic therapists offer paradoxical interventions, which mirror the couple's conflicting requests to get out of their mess but without having to change. For example, **with an intervention, known as the "therapeutic double bind," the therapist may tell the symptomatic member not to change because the symptom is accomplishing an important function for the marriage.** If the individual resists the intervention, then change occurs. If he complies, change still occurs, because the symptom will be viewed differently, as being under voluntary control.

E. Narrative Approaches (Narrative Model)

1. **Externalizing the problem. The therapist and couple collaborate on a name for the problem and attribute negative intentions to it.** For example, a couple with chronic fighting might be asked, "Describe the ways that you let your habit of bickering with one another ruin the rest of your relationship."
2. **Exploring the unique outcome.** There are times when the couple has resisted the problem's pull or when the couple's life was not dominated by the problem. The couple is asked to speculate about what made it possible at those times to resist the usual pattern.
3. **Using small shifts in language to construct a different view of the problem** that is less constraining and more amenable to solutions.

Suggested Readings

Barnett, R.C., & Rivers, C. (1996). *She works/he works: How two income families are happier, healthier and better off.* San Francisco, CA: Harper.

Bograd, M., & Mederos, F. (1999). Battering and couples therapy: Universal screening and selection of treatment modality. *Journal of Marital and Family Therapy, 25*(3), 291–312.

Carter, B., & McGoldrick, M. (Eds.). (1999). *The changing family life cycle: A framework for family therapy* (3rd ed.). Boston, MA: Allyn and Bacon.

De Shayzer, S. (1994). *Words were originally magic.* New York: Norton.

Goldner, V., Penn, P., Sheinberg, M., & Walker, G. (1990). Love and violence: Gender paradoxes in volatile attachments. *Family Process, 29,* 343–364.

Gottman, J. (1994). *Why marriages succeed or fail.* New York: Simon and Schuster.

Hetherington, M.E., Kelly, J. (2002). *For better or for worse: Divorce reconsidered.* New York: W.W. Norton.

Karpel, M. (1994). *Evaluating couples: A handbook for practitioners.* New York: Norton.

LoPiccolo, J., & LoPiccolo, L. (Eds.). (1978). *Handbook of sex therapy.* New York: Plenum.

Luepnitz, D. (1988). *The family interpreted.* New York: Basic Books.

Tannen, D. (1990). *You just don't understand: Women and men in conversation.* New York: William Morrow.

Wallerstein, J., & Blakeslee, S. (1995). *The good marriage: How and why love lasts.* Boston, MA: Houghton Mifflin.

Wallerstein, J.S., Lewis, J., & Blakeslee, S. (2000). *The unexpected legacy of divorce: A 25 year landmark study.* New York: Hyperion.

Walters, M., Carter, B., Papp, P., & Silverstein, O. (1988). *The invisible web: Gender patterns in family relationships.* New York: Guilford.

Weingarten, K. (1991). The discourses of intimacy: Adding a social constructionist and feminist view. *Family Process, 30,* 285–305.

Weitzman, L. (1985). *The divorce revolution.* New York: Free Press.

White, M., & Epston, D. (1990). *Narrative means to therapeutic ends.* New York: Norton.

Chapter 61

Family Therapy

Lois S. Slovik and James L. Griffith

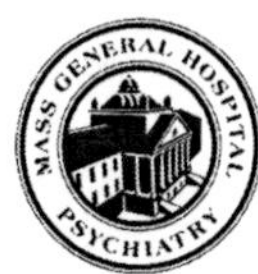

I. Introduction

Family therapy is not new. Originally done by social workers in the late 1800s, what we today call family (or systems) therapy had a resurgence in the late 1940s and evolved from the intersection of societal needs and scientific thinking. The scientific perspective included **Ludwig von Bertalanffy's general systems theory and Norbert Wiener's cybernetic theory, which had as its focus communication, control, patterning, and the activity of feedback cycles.** From a societal perspective, the sudden reuniting of families at the conclusion of World War II created problems for which the public turned to mental health professionals, and for which individual therapy was insufficient. The focus of the request was interpersonal, and included help with marital discord, divorce, delinquency, and emotional breakdowns in family members. Thus, modern-day family therapy was reborn.

This chapter is written from the idea of "drawing distinctions." Human beings punctuate or draw boundaries around particular actions, bring them to the foreground, and give them meanings. **Therapists from each of the "schools" of family therapy have particular distinctions** (like the imprint of a cookie-cutter on rolled-out dough) in mind when they assess or treat a family. **Their theory** (what they think about) **controls what they look for. Once a pattern is "seen," strategies and techniques are used to create change. This chapter is organized as to what therapists from each of the listed schools of family therapy "think about," "look for," and "do."**

II. Psychodynamic Family Therapy

A. What They Think About

1. Strategies and techniques are based upon **object relations and Freudian theory.**
2. **The family is viewed as a system that is composed of individuals embedded within a social context.** They consider an **individual's purposes, feelings, and meanings** as critical factors in the formulation of a family's situation, **with culture as a critical constraint.**
3. The health of the family is considered in the context of its life-cycle, within and across generations.
4. Problems are thought to occur through **multi-generational family failure.**
5. **Interpersonal functioning is tied to attachments to past figures** (incorporation/introjection) from which the family member(s) need to be freed.
6. **Internal processes affect a person's view of the world** and controls his behavior. These can get acted out through the process of projective identification.
7. Traumatic events, either on an individual, family, or societal level, are associated with intense anxiety and helplessness that often cannot be discussed but are represented by repetitive patterns of action that are dysfunctional (repetition compulsion).
8. **Pathology is thought to result from a combination of an individual's or a family's developmental arrest, plus stress.**
9. **Change occurs through gaining conscious insight into previously unconscious processes and by reclaiming projections.**

B. What They Look For

1. **Historical information.** It is important to take an extensive history. **Each person has an experiential map (transference) of the world,** which contains meanings for actions and sequences of behaviors, rules of how people are expected to respond, models for being (e.g., a man/woman, husband/wife, mother/father, parent/child). This map develops out of each person's history and lies embedded in relationships among introjects of important early figures.
2. **Projective identification (PI).** An activity of the ego that modifies the perception of the other (person), and, in a reflexive fashion, alters one's image of the self. This conjoined change in perception influences behavior of the self toward the other (person) (Zinner & Shapiro, 1972).
3. **Unresolved loss/grief.** When a family member(s) has not fully grieved the loss of a relationship, a current relationship can become emotionally charged at points where they too closely resemble (or fail to resemble closely enough) the lost relationship. Similar to projective identification, interactions between family members tend to enhance the personality qualities in a living member that resemble the member who has died or has been lost (e.g., a child that may have qualities of the absent parent in a divorce becomes more like that parent).
4. **Clarity of ego boundaries.** The lack of clarity of ego boundaries leads to the use of projection, to distortion of reality testing, and to the need for other methods (or defenses) in order to stabilize emotional distance.

C. What They Do

1. **Take a verbal history and/or do a genogram.**
2. **Clarify communication** process between family members.
3. **Interpret the transference** (Note: family members' transference objects are in the room), and encourage insight.

4. **Use of psychodramatic techniques,** such as the double or role reversal.

D. Representative Therapists

1. **Nathan Ackerman** (interlocking pathology)
2. **Norman Paul** (unresolved mourning)
3. **James Framo** (family of origin)
4. **Ivan Nagy** (the "family ledger" and contextual family therapy)
5. **Murray Bowen** (multi-generational transmission through fusion/differentiation and emotional triangles)
6. **J.L. Moreno** (psychodrama)

III. Symbolic-Experiential Family Therapy

A. What They Think About

1. Based on early exposure to play therapy and to children's metaphorical, non-analytical emotional processes, the focus of the therapy is on the **here-and-now. "Learning" takes place spontaneously in the therapy room through the direct effort of the therapist, who sets the context for growth experiences.**
2. Symbolic/experiential therapists consider themselves to be **"atheoretical."**

B. What They Look For

1. They set out to identify the prominent areas of distress by **experiencing the rigid, repetitive cycling of interaction among family members.**

C. What They Do

1. Use one's self.
2. Use spontaneity to:
   a. **Disorganize rigid, repetitive cycling of interaction through the use of play and experimentation.**
   b. **Highlight covert family conflicts.**
   c. **Activate and allow constructive anxiety or confusion** in family members other than the symptom-bearer. They tend to increase the focus on others instead of on the scapegoat and to avoid blame of the care-taking parent (or spouse).
3. **Re-define the symptoms as efforts for growth.**
4. **Model fantasy alternatives** to real stress, replacing key players in certain conflicts with the therapist. They also tend to encourage and support any new decisions.
5. **Create transgenerational boundaries.** They are known for encouraging extended family reunions.

D. Representative Therapists

1. **Carl Whitaker** (theater of the absurd); Whitaker along with Napier is the author of *The Family Crucible.*
2. **Walter Kempler** (Gestalt).
3. **Virginia Satir** (master communicator) clarified communication and encouraged affect. A physically active therapist, she created a therapy that was both affirming and positively focused. She is known for her book *Conjoint Family Therapy.*
4. **J.L. Moreno** (psychodrama).

IV. Behavioral Family Therapy

A. What They Think About

1. Behavior, particularly maladaptive or problematic, is learned through **reinforcement (conditioning) or modeling.** This behavior can be extinguished and replaced by new learned behavior patterns.

B. What They Look For

1. Maladaptive here-and-now behaviors that are reinforced.

C. What They Do

1. Treatment is primarily cognitive, with the use of positive and negative behavioral reinforcement.

D. Representative Therapists

1. **Robert Liberman and Richard Stuart** (behavioral marital therapy/social exchange theory)
2. **Gerald Patterson** (behavioral parent skills training)
3. **James Alexander** (functional family therapy)
4. **Ian Falloon** (expressed emotion [EE])

V. Structural Family Therapy

This therapy evolved out of work with "psychosomatic families" (e.g., those with asthma, diabetes, or anorexia) and multi-problem families, especially those with delinquent children. Structuralists have a relatively fixed image of a normal family with respect to the life-cycle and cultural norm.

A. What They Think About

The **focus for change is the family's "structure,"** which is considered to be a manifestation of the transactional patterns (actions) between the family members.

B. What They Look For

1. Structuralists set out to identify the **"rules" that regulate family relationships** through observing repetitive patterns of behavior. These include:
   a. **Boundaries:** who participates in a given activity and how. When a group of people participate in a set of repetitive transactions, they form a subsystem. Each subsystem has rules (expectations) for behavior and function; e.g., the parental system is in charge of those actions related to nurturance, guidance, and control. The spousal, parental, and child subsystems are the most important. The function of the boundary is to protect the differentiation of the subsystem from interference, allowing for contact between subsystem members and others. Clear boundaries are necessary for proper functioning. Three major types of boundaries exist along a continuum: the disengaged, the permeable, and the enmeshed.
   b. **Alignment:** the joining or opposition of a family member in relation to another. These include **alliances** (with another) and **coalitions** (against another).
   c. **Power/hierarchy:** this relates to the relative influence of each family member in relation to the others.
2. The following transactional patterns have been identified in psychosomatic and dysfunctional families:

a. **Enmeshment:** poorly differentiated, weak, and easily crossed subsystem boundaries. (Note: this type of boundary would be considered normal between mother and infant, and dysfunctional between parent and adolescent.)

b. **Overprotectiveness:** excessive "nurturance" is constantly elicited and supplied. Family members are hypersensitive to signs of distress in each other. This often occurs at the cost of autonomy and boundary differentiation.

c. **Rigidity:** retaining accustomed ways of interacting when they are no longer appropriate. Here, transactions and rules do not have the flexibility to change when changes in family structure are called for (e.g., during a shift from latency age to adolescence).

d. **Lack of conflict resolution:** problems that are left unresolved consistently reappear and reactivate the system's avoidance circuits. Three types of avoidance mechanisms have been described:

i. **Triangulation:** a person is caught in a disagreement between two others and is simultaneously asked to side with each.

ii. **Parent-child coalition:** a child is in a fixed alliance with one parent and against the other parent when needed.

iii. **Detouring:** a person (often a parent) may detour conflict through their attention to another, often a child.

C. What They Do

1. **The therapist acts as a master director who, in a problem-oriented way, helps change the family's structure (patterns of interaction) through in-session moves and out-of-session tasks.** When pathologic interactions no longer exist, the symptom (seen as a transactional pattern between persons) is no longer needed to stabilize the system.
2. Therapy is done through:

a. **Joining** (relating personally for professional purposes) in order to assess the family's structure (subsystems, boundaries, hierarchy and power).

b. Creation of an in-session **enactment** (asking or provoking family members to act out the problem in the therapy room).

c. **Tracking of sequences** (elucidating individuals' beliefs and repetitive actions that reinforce the stability of the problem).

d. **The setting of goals** including the family's overt goal and (often) the therapist's covert goal.

e. Once the above are accomplished, the therapist then sets out to restructure the family's transactions through **reframing the problem and using in-session tasks and out-of-session homework assignments.**

D. Representative Therapists

1. **Salvador Minuchin** (published works include *Families and Family Therapy, Families of the Slums, Family Therapy Techniques, Psychosomatic Families*)
2. **Stanton and Todd** (drug addiction)
3. **Aponte, Fishman, Montalvo, and Rossman** (multiproblem families, troubled adolescents)

VI. Family Psychoeducational Treatment

Psychoeducational treatment is a strategy for treating disabling, chronic illnesses (e.g., schizophrenia) with functional impairment. The focus of attention is shifted from the etiology of the illness to the determinants of the course of the illness and to the social processes (e.g., family interactions) that influence it.

A. What They Think About

1. **The central notion is that families and other natural social groups can be trained to create an intentional environment that compensates for, and may partially correct, functional disability in a member of the group.**
2. George Brown, in London, hypothesized that affective factors (**expressed emotion [EE]**) might account for relapse. Expressed emotion consists of both an attitudinal aspect (e.g., highly critical views of the patient) and a behavioral component (e.g., a tendency to be "overinvolved"—highly protective, attentive, or reactive) in relation to the patient. He found that, when expressed emotion is high, relapse occurs more frequently.

B. What They Look For

1. **Level of the family expressed emotion.**
2. **Assessment of family structure** (boundaries, alignment, power/hierarchy).
3. **Assessment of communication processes,** especially the presence of blaming, or the ability to make requests for changes in behavior, to admit vulnerability, to stay on the topic, or to get a consensus on resolution of conflict and problems.
4. **Knowledge** about the illness and the possession of **coping skills.**

C. What They Do

1. **They work both with individual families and with family groups.**
2. **There are four phases of treatment:**

a. **Engagement** with the family, usually at the time of an acute psychotic episode.

b. **Education** workshops in which clinicians present information and didactically describe key behavioral guidelines.

c. A re-entry period, with biweekly sessions focused on stabilization of the patient outside the hospital.

d. A **rehabilitation** phase that consists of sessions that emphasize the slow and careful raising of the patient's level of functioning.

3. Work is done directly to decrease the expressed emotion and to help the family resolve conflicts and clarify communication.

D. Representative Therapists

1. **William McFarlane**
2. **Ian Falloon**
3. **Carol Anderson**

VII. Milan Systemic Therapy

The Milan Systemic Therapy began with four Italian psychoanalysts (Selvini-Palazzoli, Boscolo, Cecchin, and Prata). They worked as co-therapy teams, with one team conducting the interview and the other team observing from behind a one-way mirror. In the process, the team behind the mirror noticed ("discovered") the circular pattern of interaction that exists between family members, and between family members and the therapist. They are particularly known for the idea that the therapist is an integral part of the system, and for the development of circular questioning.

A. What They Think About

1. The mental significance of any particular behavior or event that may be derived from its social context. Behavioral effects and not intentions are evaluated.
2. **Circular patterns of interaction** exist between family members and between the family and the therapist. **The observer is part of the system being observed.**
3. **Patterns co-evolve** between family members and become redundant. If the family is unable to adopt new patterns of action when change is needed, and instead continue to do more of what they are already doing, they become "stuck." This intensified redundancy of actions develops into a "symptom."
4. **Change of beliefs leads to behavioral change.**
5. Solutions, and the ability to change, reside within the family, not the therapist.
6. Spontaneous change can occur.
7. There is no one truth (taken from constructivism).
8. The **"team," "family game," and "invariant prescription"** are associated with this school.

B. What They Look For

1. **Systemic therapists focus on recursive actions, the circular relationships among the family members, and the beliefs that control the family members' actions.**

C. What They Do

1. Milan systemic therapists are **known for using a team approach, the one-way mirror, and for conducting "long-term brief"** (long sessions with a month between each meeting) **therapy.**
2. Sometime during the session the family therapist(s) stops the interview and confers with the team members behind the mirror. At the end of the interview, a message, composed by the team, is read or sent to the family. This often includes a **paradoxical or positively connoted intervention.**
3. The sessions are noted for **"hypothesizing,"** for **"circularity,"** and for **neutrality** (not allying with the reality of any particular family member).
4. Systemic therapists are particularly known for the use of **"circular questions,"** which move the listener to an observing position.
   a. Circular questions are questions about relationships. They are circular because they attempt to make explicit the implicit circular connectedness of actions and of relationships.
   b. This form of questioning allows the physician and family members to experience themselves within the context of their relationships, particularly how they recursively or reciprocally influence each other.
   c. A circular question asks one person to consider the perceptions or beliefs of another person (e.g., family member, peer, medical staff) who is in relationship with the patient or his illness; e.g., What do you think concerns your wife most about your illness? or If your illness improves, whose life would change the most? In what way?
5. Attention is paid to the family's simultaneous and paradoxical request for **change/no change.**

D. Representative Therapists

1. **Milan Team (Mara Selvini-Palazzoli, Boscolo, Cecchin, and Prata)**
2. **Peggy Papp and Peggy Penn** (the Greek Chorus)

VIII. Strategic Family Therapy

A. What They Think About

1. The focus of attention is on **problem-solving.**
2. **Life-cycle transitions, both predictable (e.g., marriage, birth of a child, adolescence) and unpredictable (e.g., loss of a job, illness, death), demand shifts in how people perceive and relate to each other. At these times, new behavioral ways of relating (solutions for problems) must come into play. If new behaviors don't occur the family becomes "stuck" and a symptom develops.**
3. Problems are perceived as misguided attempts at changing an existing difficulty. **"The solution becomes the problem"** (Watzlawick, Weakland, & Fisch, 1974) when family members persist in trying to change a current difficulty by applying a solution that had worked in other situations, but works poorly for the current problem. The family members' understanding (belief) of "common sense" supports their persistent (behavioral) efforts, even though they are not achieving success. The individual(s) within the family becomes locked into this (now pathologic) sequence or pattern of behaviors and cannot see a way to alter them (like a tire spinning in the mud).
4. **Strategic therapists believe that an individual can't be expected to change unless the system that sustains his or her symptoms changes.** They believe that problems cannot be considered apart from the context in which they occur and the functions for which they serve. Thus, **a detailed analysis of the current context of the problem is more important than a detailed history of the problem.**
5. The problem is often the result of a **double bind** (a conflict in the content and relationship levels of a message). The person(s) caught in double bind can neither solve the problem nor leave the field.

6. **Pragmatics is important, insight per se is not.**
7. Strategic therapy has been strongly influenced by hypnosis, and the work of **Milton Erikson.**

B. What They Look For

1. Strategic therapists are interested in the here-and-now: **the temporal relationships and repetitive series of actions that maintain the problem.** They are particularly sensitive to the issues of **power** and to those that involve either paradox or a double bind.
2. **Solution-focused strategic therapists** show preferential interest in discovering **"exceptions to the rule"** (when the problem would be expected to occur, but doesn't). Rather than focusing upon an analysis of the behavioral sequences maintaining the problem, they seek to identify naturally occurring behavioral sequences that take place when the problem doesn't happen, and therefore might serve as candidate solutions.

C. What They Do

1. Their **focus is on solving the problem (symptom).** The problem as the family describes it must be changed into a solvable form, one that is co-created by the therapist and the family.
2. Through **questions, enactments, and homework assignments,** the therapist tries to discover the "unseen" problem: the family's maladaptive effort to solve what is maintaining the problem. Strategic therapists are interested in who, what, when, where, and in what way people are involved.
3. Strategies are aimed at **tracking and disrupting the sequences of behavior and meanings** that maintain the problem, and interventions are aimed at **restructuring** the family's transactional sequences in a healthier way.
4. **Psychoeducation and compliance-based directives are both used.**
5. Strategic therapists are best known for their **defiance-based, paradoxical directives.** They include:
   a. **Re-framing or relabeling the symptom.** By changing the context of the sequence of actions that constitute the symptom one can change the meaning of the event; e.g., telling an adolescent who consistently comes in past her curfew that she is doing her younger brother a huge favor as her action binds her parents' attention, allowing him to do what he wants without being noticed.
   b. **Prescribing the symptom.** The therapist encourages or instructs the family member(s) to engage in the specific behavior that needs to be eliminated using a "new" rationale that is acceptable in its logic, but makes the old behavior(s) unacceptable; e.g., telling the older sister how wonderful she is to sacrifice herself for her younger brother and to continue her (negative) behavior.
   c. **Restraining the system.** The therapist attempts to discourage or even deny the possibility of change, therefore hoping the family will defy him/her and continue to change.
   d. **Positioning.** The therapist attempts to shift a problematic "position" (usually an assertion that the patient is making about himself, the problem, or another family member), by accepting and exaggerating that position. This is used when one family member's position is considered to be maintained by a complementary or opposite response in the other; e.g., telling the person who is a penny-pincher to be even more frugal because it allows the spendthrift more money to spend.
6. The new **solution-focused strategic therapists focus on identifying, amplifying, and predicting the "exceptions"** to the rule (occasions when the problem or symptom might have been expected to occur, but doesn't). This allows alternative perceptions, possibilities, and "stories" to be uncovered. The following questions are often used by these therapists:
   a. "Between now and the next time that we meet, I would like you to observe, so that you can describe to us next time, what happens when (e.g.) you would expect John to lie and he doesn't."
   b. **The miracle question:** "Suppose that one night, while you were asleep, there was a miracle and this problem was solved. How would you know? What would be different?" The therapist then negotiates with the family members what part of this new reality they would be willing to implement the next day, as if the miracle had occurred.

D. Representative Therapists

1. The Mental Research Institute (**MRI**) in California (Gregory Bateson, Don Jackson, Jay Haley, Paul Watzlawick, and John Weakland)
2. **J. Haley and Cloe Madanes** (paradox and ordeal therapy)
3. **Steve deShazer, Inso Berg, and Michelle Weiner-Davis** (solution-focused strategic therapy)

IX. Narrative Family Therapy

A. What They Think About

Narrative therapists conduct their therapy from a position of "not knowing." That is to say, the therapist does not have any set ideas about what and how change should occur. The therapy is "co-created" by the therapist and family and takes its shape according to the emergent qualities of the conversation that inspires it.

1. The **dominant narratives of an individual's life organizes his/her perceptions and behaviors.**
2. The perceptions that family members have of themselves and others are structured, and limited by the stories, the language, and the metaphors they use.
3. A problem occurs when:
   a. The **narratives available** for guiding perception, cognition, and action **preclude interactions** other than with the ones seen.
   b. Family members lack either the needed emotional vocabulary or narrative skills to make the story of their experience understandable to others.

c. Family members have become positioned in the relationship where they have stopped talking or listening.

d. **Therapy provides a context where self-narratives can be told, heard, or expanded in meaning.**

B. What They Look (or Listen) For

1. **Dominant narratives that constrain the relationship.**
2. **Alternative narratives** in unnoticed or forgotten experience.
3. **Through the use of questions that evoke curiosity and reflection, the therapist attempts to understand the way in which the family members' ideas and beliefs are patterned.**
4. Narrative therapists are particularly attentive to listen for **emotionally charged words, and for specific language or metaphors** used in describing the problem. Implicit metaphors serve as maps that are embedded in language, and language always influences the selection of life events that are noticed. The events noticed contain meaning and dictate the selection of behaviors available.

C. What They Do

1. **The therapist and family members work to co-create (jointly develop) new, more useful, life stories.**
2. **Questions are used not to seek information from the listener, but rather to change how the listener processes information.** Karl Tomm (1987) introduced the term "interventive interviewing" to describe the use of these questions.
3. **Narrative therapists consider themselves to be collaborative, respectful, and less hierarchical than the earlier family therapists.**
4. Narrative therapists have been known to make use of the **reflecting team** (Andersen, 1987). Midway through a family meeting, the team behind the one-way mirror changes places with the therapist and family. The family and therapist now observe behind the mirror as the team discusses (reflects on) them. When the reflections are completed, the family and team again change places and the therapist asks the family what they found to be useful. The idea is that family member(s) are only able to take in the new ideas that they are ready to hear.
5. **Externalize the problem.** Michael White and David Epston have created a series of questions that separate the problem from the person. These include:
   a. **Relative influence questions** that are designed to compare the influence of the problem over the life of the family member(s) and the influence of the family member(s) over the problem.
   b. **Unique outcome questions,** which ask for exceptions to the usual descriptions of failure in the struggle with the problem. These exceptions can nearly always be identified, but often go unnoticed when one has accepted a life narrative of failure.

D. Representative Therapists

1. **H. Goolishian and H. Anderson** (the problem-oriented system)
2. **Tom Andersen** and the Tromsø team (reflecting team)
3. **Michael White and David Epston** (externalizing the problem)
4. **Karl Tomm** (interventive interviewing)

X. Family Resilience Therapies

A. What They Think About

While family psychoeducation approaches have focused on roles that families can play in reducing the frequency of illness relapse or buffering its severity, **family resilience interventions extend this strategy to identify family processes that not only buffer severity of illness, but prevent its onset for those at risk. Family resilience refers to coping and adaptational processes that already exist in the family as it operates as a functional unit.**

1. **Key processes can be identified that enables couples and families facing disruptive crises or persistent stresses to strengthen their relationships, regain function, and further the growth of individual members.**
2. A **stressor affects at-risk children only to the extent that they disrupt crucial family processes** that otherwise would neutralize or buffer the stressor.
3. The **hardiness of individuals is best understood as a mutual interaction of individual, family, and environmental process.**
4. In addition to posing risks for individual dysfunction, **crisis and persistent stresses affect the entire family by causing relational conflict and family breakdown.**
5. Family processes mediate the impact of stress on all members and their relationships. **Protective processes foster resilience by buffering stress and fostering resilience.**
6. **All families have the potential for resilience.** Resilience can be maximized by encouraging the family's best efforts. In addition, the communicational and relational systems of the person's family and social networks are strengthened.

B. What They Look For

1. **Identification of risk factors and protective factors for onset of illness.** For example, factors conferring protection upon children at risk for depression were identified by Beardslee as:
   a. **Becoming activists and doers**
   b. **Becoming heavily involved in school and extracurricular activities**
   c. **Developing deep commitments to and involvement in interpersonal relationships**

d. **Seeking self-understanding as a way to deal with a parent's depression**
e. **Expressing articulate understandings of the parent's illness and the problems that are derived from it**
f. **Refusing to feel blame or guilt for the parent's illness**

C. What They Do

1. Use **family based cognitive-behavioral interventions that attempt to educate families about the illness,** either using a clinician visit or group lecture as a format to enhance understanding of the illness.
2. **Conduct an assessment of all family members,** not only the at-risk family member.
3. **Link the educational material directly to the family's unique life experiences.**
4. **Counsel family members to counter feelings of guilt and blame.**
5. **Encourage the development of relationships both within and outside the family.**

D. Representative Therapists

1. **William Beardslee** (childhood depression)
2. **Froma Walsh**
3. **S. Wolin**
4. **J.I. Griffith** (family centered approaches in international mental health)

XI. Conclusion

Family therapy, although still recognizable, is very different now than it was at its inception. The evolution and current integration of theory and clinical need have created a therapy that is more collaborative, respectful, and less hierarchical than earlier forms of family therapy. Therapeutic attention is more focused on strengths and resources and less on pathology. Although the therapist is no longer considered to be the one who holds "the truth," he or she continues to develop ideas and skills useful for healing.

Suggested Readings

Andersen, T. (1987). Dialogue and meta-dialogue in clinical work. *Family Process, 26,* 415–428.

Aponte, H., & VanDeusen, J. (1981). Structural family therapy. In A. Gurman, & D. Kniskern (Eds.), *Handbook of family therapy.* New York: Brunner/Mazel.

Beardslee, W.R. (1998). Prevention and the clinical encounter. *American Journal of Orthopsychiatry, 69*(4), 521–533.

Beardslee, W.R., Swatling, S., Hoke, L., et al. (1998). From cognitive information to shared meaning: Healing principles in prevention intervention. *Psychiatry, 61,* 112–129.

Beardslee, W.R., Versage, E.M., Salt, P., et al. (1999). The development and evaluation of two preventive intervention strategies for children of depressed parents. In D. Cicchetti, & S.L. Toth (Eds.), *Rochester symposium on developmental psychopathology: Vol. 9, Development approaches to prevention and intervention,* pp. 111–151. Rochester, NY: University of Rochester Press.

Bodin, A. (1981). The interactional view: Family therapy approaches of the Mental Research Institute. In A. Gurman, & D. Kniskern (Eds.), *Handbook of family therapy.* New York: Brunner/Mazel.

Bowen, M. (1978). *Family therapy in clinical practice.* New York: Jason Aronson.

deShazer, S. (1985). *Keys to solution in brief therapy.* New York: Norton.

deShazer, S., Berg, I., Lipchik, E., et al. (1986). Brief therapy: Focused solution development. *Family Process, 25,* 207–223.

Goldenberg, I., & Goldenberg, H. (Eds.). (1980). *Family therapy: An overview.* Monterey, CA: Brooks/Cole.

Goolishian, H., & Anderson, H. (1987). Language systems and therapy: An evolving idea [special issue: Psychotherapy with families]. *Psychotherapy, 24,* 529–537.

Griffith, J.L. (2002). Living with threat and uncertainty: What the Kosovars tell us. *Family Process, 41,* 24–27.

Griffith, J.L., Blyta, A., Ukshini, S., et al. (2002, May 21). Promoting family resistance to effects of culturecide: The Kosovar Family Professional Educational Collaborative. Paper presented at the 154th Annual Meeting of the American Psychiatric Association, Philadelphia, PA.

Griffith, J.L., & Slovik, L. (2003). Family therapy. In A. Tasman, I. Kay, & L. Lieberman (Eds.), *Psychiatry.* New York: Wiley Publishers, 2003.

Hoffman, L. (1990). Constructing realities: An art of lenses. *Family Process, 20,* 1–13.

Madanes, C. (1981). *Strategic family therapy.* San Francisco, CA: Jossey-Bass.

Minuchin, S. (1974). *Families and family therapy.* Cambridge, MA: Harvard University Press.

Penn, P. (1982). Circular questioning. *Family Process, 21,* 267–280.

Selvini-Palazzoli, M., Boscolo, L., Cecchin, G., & Prata, G. (1980). Hypothesizing-circularity-neutrality: Three guidelines for the conductor of the session. *Family Process, 19,* 3–12.

Slovik, L., & Griffith, J. (1992). The current face of family therapy. In S. Rutan (Ed.), *Psychotherapy for the 1990s.* New York: Guilford Publications.

Stanton, M.D. (1981). Strategic approaches to family therapy. In A. Gurman, & D. Kniskern (Eds.), *Handbook of family therapy.* New York: Brunner/Mazel.

Tomm, K. (1987). Interventive interviewing: Part I. Strategizing as a fourth guideline for the therapist. *Family Process, 26,* 3–14.

von Bertalanffy, L. (1968). *General systems theory: Foundation, development, applications.* New York: Brazillier.

Walsh, F. (1998). *Strengthening family resilience.* New York: Guilford Press.

Watzlawick, P., Weakland, J., & Fisch, R. (1974). *Change: Principles of problem formation and problem resolution.* New York: Norton.

Weiner, A. (1961). *Cybernetics.* Cambridge, MA: MIT Press.

Whitaker, C., & Napier, A. (1978). *The family crucible.* New York: Harper and Row.

White, M. (1988). Negative explanation, restraint, and double description: A template for family therapy. *Family Process, 125,* 169–184.

White, M. (1988). The process of questioning: A therapy of literary merit. *Dulwich Centre Newsletter* (Winter), 8–14.

White, M. (1988/89). The externalizing of the problem and the re-authoring of lives and relationships. *Dulwich Centre Newsletter* (Summer).

Wolin, S., & Wolin, S. (1993). *The resilient self: How the survivors of troubled families rise above adversity.* New York: Villiard Books.

Zinner, J., & Shapiro, R. (1972). Projective identification as a mode of perception and behavior in families and adolescents. *International Journal of Psychoanalysis, 53,* 523–530.

Chapter 62

Group Psychotherapy

Anne Alonso

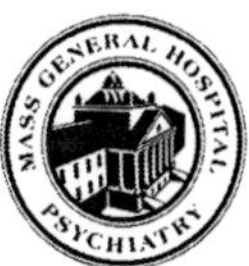

I. Introduction

A. Overview

People thrive best in a community that values their participation and protects their dignity. The stresses that impinge on individuals are defined in part by their biology, in part by their family dynamics, and also by the culture in which they live. The integration of mind, body, and social context is vulnerable to assault from problems in any one of these dimensions. **Group psychotherapy offers the opportunity for purposefully created, closely observed, and skillfully guided interpersonal interaction.** Such interactions can positively influence the countless varieties of human distress and malfunction. Distorted perceptions of others, insufficient communications, inadequately discharged affects, stereotyped behaviors, impulsive actions, and alienation can all be addressed and modified within the therapeutic group (see Table 62-1). In addition, the events of 9/11 and its aftermath have provided dramatic examples of the ways that groups for trauma patients have been of great use to "normal populations facing abnormal situations."

B. What Is a Therapy Group?

A therapy group is a collection of patients selected and brought together by the leader for a shared therapeutic goal (see Table 62-1).

C. What Are Common Therapeutic Assumptions?

Group therapy rests on some common assumptions and principles across the whole panoply of therapeutic groups:

1. **A universal and primary need for attachment. The need for attachment is seen as primary** by a whole host of group theorists; the press for belonging is that which yields a sense of cohesion that can help the individual stay with the anxious new moments in a group of strangers.
2. **Contagion. For better and for worse, people who wish to belong to a cohesive community are apt to mimic and to identify with the feelings and beliefs of other members of that community.** At its best, this process allows for new interpersonal learning; at its worst, it raises the specter of dangerous mobs.
3. **Amplification. An increasing exposure to feelings, needs, and drives increases the individual's awareness of his or her own passions,** and allows for a more direct and conscious management of those impulses.
4. **Intimate exchanges.** Of necessity **the members of a cohesive group experience their own approaches to intimacy with others and with the self, and receive immediate feedback on the impact they have on important others in their surround.**

D. How Do These Intimate Exchanges Heal?

Close interactions between the members of a group yield beneficent effects **by generating intrapsychic and interpersonal situations that:**

1. Reduce isolation.
2. Diminish shame.
3. Evoke early familial interactions and feelings.
4. Expand the individual's emotional and behavioral repertoire.
5. Provide support and empathic confrontation.
6. Help people grieve.

E. What Aspects of Groups Are Therapeutic?

Whatever the model, group therapy rests on the assumptions that there are healing factors that emerge and operate in all groups, and that some of these can be brought into play to allow the individual within the group to grow and to develop beyond the constrictions in life that brought that person into treatment. While some group theorists rely on a cluster of factors relevant to their models of the mind and of pathology, all utilize some of the whole group of therapeutic factors identified in Table 62-2.

II. Creation and Goals of Groups

A. How Does the Therapist Plan and Organize a Group?

Before approaching the concrete work of planning and organizing a psychotherapy group, **the goals of the group must be clearly understood and developed by the leader.** These goals in turn will be dependent on the setting, the population, the time available for treatment, and on the training and capacity of the leader(s).

B. What Are the Goals of Groups?

Therapists form groups for a whole range of therapeutic purposes. The main ones are to:

1. **Re-establish pre-morbid levels of functioning. People in acute and immediate distress often find support in groups that have as their main goal a re-establishment of a person's equilibrium.** Patients who have suffered a breakdown of their lives and who have needed hospitalization can utilize groups within the inpatient or partial hospital setting. These groups have as their primary focus the restructuring of the patient's sensorium, the management of acute distress, and the planning for a return to the community. These patients also need help in dealing with the shameful

Table 62-1. Comparison of Different Types of Group Psychotherapy

Parameters	*Day Hospital/Inpatient Group*	*Supportive Group Therapy*	*Psychodynamic Group*	*Cognitive-Behavioral Group*
Frequency	3–5 times/week	Once a week	1–3 times/week	Once a week
Duration	1 week to 6 months	Up to 6 months or more	1–3+ years	Up to 6 months
Indications	Acute or chronic major mental illness	Shared universal dilemmas	Neurotic disorders and borderline states	Phobias, compulsive problems, etc.
Pre-group screening	Sometimes	Usually	Always	Usually
Content focus	Extent and impact of illness; plan for return to baseline	Symptoms, loss, life management	Present and past life situations; intragroup and extragroup relationships	Cognitive distortions, specific symptoms
Transference	Positive institutional transference encouraged	Positive transference encouraged to promote improved functioning	Positive and negative to leader and members, evoked and analyzed	Positive relationship to leader fostered; no examination of transference
Therapist activity	Empathy and reality testing	Strengthen existing defenses by actively giving advice and support	Challenge defenses, reduce shame, interpret unconscious conflict	Create new options, active and directive
Interaction outside of group	Encouraged	Encouraged	Discouraged	Variable
Goals	Reconstitute defenses	Better adaptation to environment	Reconstruction of personality dynamics	Relief of specific psychiatric symptoms

consequences of hospitalization, and with the sometimes elusive process of establishing outpatient treatment that will support them upon discharge. A benevolent inpatient or partial hospital group experience will be of special value with the latter problem, since affordable treatment will be primarily offered in group therapy for the foreseeable future.

Many patients who have been hospitalized after an acute illness, or who attend partial hospitalization programs, need to regain equilibrium, deal with the shame inherent in losing the ability to live independently, and prepare to re-enter the world outside of the therapeutic environment.

2. **Support targeted patient populations.** Since the time that Dr. Pratt offered his "classes" for tubercular patients at the Massachusetts General Hospital in 1905, **people have come together to commiserate with one another around common problems,** to share information, and to learn how to deal with the impact of those problems on their lives. **Groups have been organized around medical illnesses** (such as cancer, diabetes, and acquired immunodeficiency syndrome [AIDS]), **around psychological problems** (such as bereavement), **and around psychosocial sequelae of trauma** (such as war or natural disasters). The goals of such groups are to provide support and information embedded in a socially accepting environment with people who are in a position to really understand what the others are going through. The treatment may emerge from cognitive-behavioral principles, psychodynamic principles, or psychoeducational ones. Frequently, these groups tend to be time-limited; members often join at the same time and terminate together. The problems addressed in these groups are found in a broad variety of patients, from the very healthy to the more distressed, and cut across other demographic variables, such as age and culture. Increasingly, research data have shown that involvement in

Table 62-2. Some Therapeutic Factors in Group Psychotherapy

Factor	*Definition*
Acceptance	The feeling of being accepted by other members of the group; differences of opinion are tolerated, and there is an absence of censure.
Altruism	The act of one member's being of help to another; putting another person's need before one's own and learning that there is value in giving to others. The term was originated by August Comte (1798–1957), and Freud believed it was a major factor in establishing group cohesion and community feeling.
Cohesion	The sense that the group is working together toward a common goal; also referred to as a sense of "we-ness"; believed to be the most important factor related to positive therapeutic effects.
Contagion	The process in which the expression of emotion by one member stimulates the awareness of a similar emotion in another member.
Corrective familial experience	The group re-creates the family of origin for some members who can work through original conflicts psychologically through group interaction (e.g., sibling rivalry, anger toward parents).
Empathy	A capacity of a group member to put himself or herself into the psychological frame of reference of another group member and thereby understand his or her thinking, feeling, or behavior.
Imitation	The emulation or modeling of one's behavior after that of another (also called role modeling); also known as spectator therapy, as one patient learns from another.
Insight	Conscious awareness and understanding of one's own psychodynamics and symptoms of maladaptive behavior. Most therapists distinguish two types: (1) intellectual insight—knowledge and awareness without any changes in maladaptive behavior; (2) emotional insight—awareness and understanding leading to positive changes in personality and behavior.
Inspiration	The process of imparting a sense of optimism to group members; the ability to recognize that one has the capacity to overcome problems; also known as instillation of hope.
Interpretation	The process during which the group leader formulates the meaning or significance of a patient's resistance, defenses, and symbols; the result is that the patient develops a cognitive framework within which to understand his or her behavior.
Learning	Patients acquire knowledge about new areas, such as social skills and sexual behavior; they receive advice, obtain guidance, attempt to influence, and are influenced by, other group members.
Reality testing	Ability of the person to evaluate objectively the world outside the self; includes the capacity to perceive oneself and other group members accurately.
Ventilation	The expression of suppressed feelings, ideas, or events to other group members; the sharing of personal secrets that ameliorate a sense of sin or guilt (also referred to as self-disclosure).

these groups can have remarkably positive effects on extending survival and on the quality of life for the severely ill (e.g., a woman with end-stage breast cancer).

3. **Provide relief for certain symptoms.** Group treatment may target specific symptoms. This approach to psychopathology is congruent with categorical nosological systems, such as the DSM-IV. Diagnosis here is seen as symptomatic rather than developmental; treatment goals include alleviation of symptoms. For example, patients with eating disorders or specific phobias are clustered in groups which can then promote skills for self-monitoring and for replacement of an automatic symptom with a more adaptive set of behaviors and cognitions. These groups may include members with a broad range of intrapsychic development, which is not the primary focus of the group. At the same time, some people who work successfully in these groups may want to continue the work of personality change in open-ended dynamic groups when their symptoms are relieved.
4. **Encourage and stimulate character change. Character difficulties are tenacious for all human beings,** from the healthiest neurotic to the most regressed patient. For all individuals, character problems are:
   a. Outside of the patient's awareness.
   b. Syntonic and perceived as "Who I am" when brought into awareness.
   c. Resistant to change, even when the patient wants to make such a change.
   d. Repeated compulsively until worked through; that is, they are robbed of some of their power with each experience of successful change to better alternatives.

e. Difficult to change without strong motivation to overcome psychological inertia.

The neurotic patient will find intrapsychic conflicts emerging in the interpersonal field of group, and make use of the group's curative factors to overcome the resistances to newer intimacies. Some of the earlier literature on group treatment expressed doubts about the appropriateness of this "uncovering" kind of group for sicker patients. More recently, group theorists have argued that the distributed transferences in a group mitigate an overly threatening regression for such patients. Character problems have a tenacity that is difficult to reorganize in brief treatment. Instead, the process requires frequent regressions in the service of the ego, and attempts to work through the same characterological habits again and again. At the same time, brief analytic and cognitive-behavioral group models have been used to address sectors of the personality difficulties, to good effect.

C. How Should a Therapy Group Be Conducted?

The success of a group depends on the ability of the therapist to provide a safe context and meaning for the therapy group. This is done by designing a contract around the group goal(s) and by carefully selecting members that are suitable for that group. For example, in a symptom-specific group, members should have similar symptoms and concerns; in a more psychodynamic group, members should be selected from a fairly homogeneous level of ego development, although their symptoms and character styles may differ along a wide spectrum. The latter group is focused on changing and expanding internal defenses to promote a greater capacity to love and to work.

D. What Are the Roles of the Group Leader?

Before the group begins, the leader must make several decisions that will have major implications for the whole enterprise. Beyond the obvious focus on the kind, duration, and theoretical underpinnings, **the leader must then decide on matters of:**

1. **Membership**
2. **Logistics (e.g., place, time, and fees)**
3. **Whether to work alone, or with a co-therapist.**
4. **Whether patients will be treated in group therapy alone or in some combination of group therapy, individual therapy, pharmacotherapy, or self-help group.**
5. **Managing records, and protecting confidentiality.**

In addition to the logistical decisions listed above, the leader's stance needs to be consistent with the goals of the group. A leader of a psychodynamic, open-ended group will probably be more likely to sit back and allow the group's associations to lead the way for the group's work while he or she comments, like a critic at a concert. On the other hand, such a stance makes little sense for the leader of a cognitive-behavioral group, who is engaged in conducting desensitization exercises, and in providing cognitive restructuring, including homework exercises to meet the goals of that therapeutic endeavor.

E. How Should Patients Be Prepared for a Group?

Both anecdotal and empirical evidence shows that investment of significant amounts of time in preparation of a patient for group therapy will improve the chances of a successful entry and retention into a group. In addition to the usual history-taking, it is very helpful to examine the patient's fantasies and biases about groups and to collect the history of their participation in all kinds of groups (e.g., family, school, sports, work, and friendships). This is the time to discuss the group's agreements and the rationale that underlies them, and to elicit the patient's collaboration in the enterprise by making as much information available as possible. Patients are helped by knowing how the group works, by knowing what the leader's role might be, and by knowing what they might expect for themselves.

A typical agreement includes expectations about constant attendance, the duration of the group, the content of the patient's discussions, and the commitment to confidentiality and to financial obligations. Beyond those, each specific group will have more particular expectations; e.g., a cognitive-behavioral group may expect "homework" from the members, a more psychodynamic group may encourage dream analysis.

F. How Does the Group Deal with Authority and Group Leadership?

A group leader must exercise authority over each of the above factors if the group is to be safe and containing for its members. Whether a member who is difficult in the group stays or leaves or whether a new member enters must not be left to a vote, just as such decisions are not made within a family. The privilege and burden of administrative and inclusion/exclusion matters is a serious responsibility of the group leader, as is the question of single or co-therapy leadership. It is important to remember that the leader is not a member of the group, despite the ambivalent entreaties of the members to bring the leader into the group. The clearer the leader is about the boundaries, the safer are the members to indulge their fantasies of wanting to corrupt the process, or to overcome the leader's authority.

The fiduciary responsibilities of the leader are better maintained to the extent that the leader exercises restraint and relative neutrality in the sense of non-judgmental listening and responding to the patients' struggles. By remaining warm and neutral, the leader is in a position to listen non-judgmentally to all aspects of the whole group's impulses and resistance, without taking sides or carrying the burden of somehow policing the group, and deciding which are good feelings and interactions, and which are not.

G. How Does a Group Deal with the Incorruptibility of the Leader?

In a therapy group, as in any therapeutic work, **the leader must remain as pure as Caesar's wife;** dual roles are unacceptable, no overly familiar incursions into the members' personal lives, nor those of the leader are tolerated. No special fee arrangements that are not in the awareness of the group can be tolerated without damaging the integrity of the group boundaries. In short, all group business that cannot be conducted in the group ought not to be conducted at all. This refusal to hold secret any extra-group contacts sets a fine model that says the group is a safe therapeutic agent.

H. How Does One Deal with the Question of Co-therapy?

As in many clinical decisions, **the question of leading alone or with a colleague depends in part on the model, in part on the context and setting, in part on the availability of an appropriate co-therapist, and the system's support,** administrative and otherwise, for committing two professionals to the same task at the same time.

Inpatient or partial hospitalization groups tend to meet several times a week, and, for those groups, co-therapy is a useful way to ensure continuity of leadership. On the other hand, some analytic group leaders avoid co-therapy because of the splitting of the patient-to-leader transferences. There are no rigid rules, but certain caveats must be observed.

Co-therapists work best when:

1. They are truly co-therapists, of relatively equal status and experience. In cases where a student and a supervisor work together, it is useful to acknowledge this reality.
2. They share a common theory base.
3. They are willing to dedicate an hour or so per week to working out their collaborative problems and their perceptions of the group.
4. They are comfortable in sharing the fee.

Failure to observe these agreements may leave the patients low on the priority list of therapeutic concern while the co-therapy pair compete or otherwise undercut one another. On the more positive side, when co-therapy works well, both clinicians and patients have the advantage of two professional heads and hearts working in concert for the benefit of all.

III. Who Should Be Treated in Group Therapy?

A. Indications for Group Treatment

Most people who are appropriate for individual psychotherapy are also appropriate for group therapy; the questions are what kind of group, and under which circumstances. **In a psychodynamic group where early developmental conflicts and relationships are assumed to interfere with the here-and-now of the patient's life, it will be important to organize a group that is reasonably homogeneous for the level of ego development and heterogeneous in every other regard.** Mixing people of differing gender, cultures, and/or ages can be extremely useful so long as these patients emerge from a similar developmental spectrum. The differences among them can then be addressed and exploited to the advantage of the members in the group. However, when patients diverge sharply in levels of ego development, group cohesion and universality will be compromised. For example, a group of patients who experience severe anxiety around loss consequent to serious abandonment throughout their lives will do well to work together in a group. On the other hand, to mix two or three such patients in a group of people who are conflicted around intimacy and sustained relationships may well result in two subgroups, neither of which has an easy empathic rapport with the other's internal dilemmas. The specific symptom or population designation of other groups points the way by definition to patient selection.

B. Who Should *Not* Be Treated in Group Therapy?

Some patients are unable to make good use of group therapy without prior clinical interventions. For example, the actively manic patient may be more overstimulated than helped in a group. Another category of patients frequently referred to groups includes severely schizoidal people who have really never developed sustained human relationships. To place these patients in a group overrides their capacity and sets them up for early failure. Acutely disturbed patients may need and deserve individual attention prior to entry into an ongoing therapy group. In all of these cases, prior treatment, either psychopharmacological and/or individual supportive therapy, may increase the likelihood of the patient succeeding in the therapy group further down the road.

IV. Combined Therapies

A. Group Therapy Combined with Individual Therapy

Occasionally, patients are treated in both individual and group therapy, either by the same therapist or by two different ones. This option is useful for a variety of patients:

1. **The over-intellectualized patient.** For some patients, insight becomes a way to avoid feeling. When it does, it is very useful to place these patients in a therapy group where they can see how they are in the interaction with others who will offer feedback and affective resonance.
2. **The patient who cannot tolerate the dyadic transference of individual treatment.** Dyadic treatment can threaten the fragile ego boundaries of patients who are either very needy, or who are overstimulated by the

apparent promises of the individual work. These patients often flee treatment, or regress to terrifying actions that can be life-threatening in what approaches psychotic levels of transference. Adding group therapy can distribute the transferences across the spectrum of all the members of the group and the group leader, and may enable the individual and the group treatment to proceed more safely and more productively.

B. Collaboration between the Two Therapists

It is crucial that the two therapists collaborate by frequent phone calls and by avoiding the patients' likely attempts to split them. In the case where the two therapists do not agree, or do not respect the other's work, then the patient is potentially at great risk of harm, or at least in a stalemate that is iatrogenic in origin.

C. Combined Treatment with the Same Therapist

Patients will sometimes be seen in both individual and group therapy with the same therapist. There are many advantages and, as always, some costs to this treatment plan.

It is illuminating to deal with the intrapsychic dimensions of the patient in the individual hour, and then observe the same patient express those internal dilemmas and live them out in the interactions with members of the group. For example, a mild and extremely gentle individual might startle his or her therapist by launching a very aggressive attack on one or more members of the group when the shy facade is challenged.

For some patients, however, sharing the therapist's attention can be so distressing that the work of therapy is stalled. It may be far better for that patient to be referred to another leader's group, or to defer group treatment to a more secure time.

D. Boundaries in Combined Treatment

Clinicians struggle with how much to preserve the privacy of what they know about the patient from the dyadic hour when the patient enters the group, and how much to disclose. **While there are no hard and fast rules, what matters is consistency, and the prior agreement with the patient about this matter.** Many clinicians opt to protect the information while urging the patient to bring the problems into the group. One major exception is the case where the group or one of its members is at risk; as usual, the rules of confidentiality are suspended when there is any threat to safety of any of the participants. It is very useful to agree that all treaters will be in regular contact with one another in order to work for the patient's advantage.

E. Is Group Therapy Primary or Adjunctive Treatment?

As in most treatments that adhere to the biopsychosocial model, psychosocial treatment has an impact on the biology of the patient, as well as on the psychology and the social adjustment of that person. In cases of more severe distress, a combination of group treatment, psychopharmacological treatment, and, occasionally, individual treatment, may be ideal. However, **given the cost constraints that delimit most mental health care, group therapy remains a very impressive primary treatment** for a whole host of patient situations and needs.

V. Legal and Ethical Considerations in Group Therapy

A. The Leader and Confidentiality

The group leader is bound by the usual rules of confidentiality in the group as in any other clinical encounter with the patient. With the exception of a threat to a person or persons, this confidentiality holds and is usually elaborated in the Code of Ethics of the therapist's professional organization. The same pertains to any conduct of the therapist that violates the code of ethics relative to sexual or other extra-professional contact with a patient.

B. Group Members and Confidentiality

The bigger challenge is confidentiality among members. **Aside from stressing the importance of protecting the identities of patients in the group, there is little that the leader can do to ensure compliance, nor is it against the law for members to break confidentiality.** Group therapists worry about whether the group can become a pool of witnesses in the case of a subpoena. Some states extend the same protection to the members that they do to the leader, namely, the patient-therapist privilege, but this has not been tested and may not apply with all professionals across the disciplines.

VI. Research, Outcome, and Evaluation

Research on group therapy has focused mostly on outcomes. More recently, measures have been developed that seek to relate the patient's sense of belonging and feeling valued in the group with the effectiveness of the treatment. Studies continue to support the importance of group cohesion on group effectiveness; feeling valued is seen as a statement of cohesion. Research also indicates greater confidence in the efficacy of group treatment, and shows no appreciable differences between individual, or group therapy, and pharmacotherapy. However, these studies remain problematic, given the problems that bedevil most social science research: It is difficult to control for therapist differences, and attempts to do so by providing manuals for intervention become different models than what happens in real life. Non-specific factors are elusive, but seem to indicate that **patients progress when they feel cared about, when the leader is warm and somewhat structured, when the match with colleagues in the group is appropriate, and when the goal and direction of the group are clear and consistent.**

Researchers have moved beyond the question of do groups work, to a finer look at how they work, in what circumstances, and for whom. Proper and careful screening and otherwise preparing a patient to enter a group results in a greater chance of success in entering and staying. **Members who are at about the same level of ego development do better in open-ended groups than they do in groups with a large disparity of ego levels of development.** Short-term, focused groups are more successful if leaders are structured as to agenda, and time boundaries, and if the patients are more homogeneous with regard to the problem being addressed.

Research instruments are useful for measuring patient satisfaction, and self-reports of increased well-being. The Clinical Outcome Results battery developed by the American Group Psychotherapy Association is but one example; it utilizes such measures as the Symptom Checklist 90-Revised (SCL-90R), The Social Adjustment Scale Self Report (SAS-SR), The Multiple Affect Adjective Check List-Revised (MAACL-R), and the Global Assessment Scale (GAS). More recently, measures, such as the Structured Analysis of Social Behavior and the Group Climate Questionnaire (GCQ), have been used extensively by MacKenzie (1992, 1997) and others who work with patients in structured time-limited groups.

A major shortcoming in group therapy research stems from the pragmatics of conducting research over a long time, and with more amorphous goals. Thus, most of the data emerges from research on time-limited groups, usually within the cognitive-behavioral or interpersonal model. While those findings are very important to secure, they have limited applicability for the more open-ended dynamic models of group treatment. That research remains to be enlarged upon. Of particular interest is the emerging research on recovery from severe physical illness (e.g., women with metastatic breast cancer). Women from that population were found to double their survival time, and to decrease their need for pain medication, if they also participated in group therapy along with their usual oncologic treatments.

VII. Consultation and Supervision for Group Therapy

It is often difficult for group leaders to ask for help, as it is difficult for most professional helpers, once they have gone beyond their formal training years. But failure to find help in conducting a group can increase the strain on the leader exponentially given the number of people in the consultation room and the multiplicity of countertransference vectors. **A well-running group can look deceptively autonomous of the leader's impact, but the truth is that the leader's calmness and full attention is the platform on which the group grows.** Occasional consultations and/or ongoing peer supervision is a safe, judicious practice. It is also a way for the leader to take advantage of his or her affiliative needs and to avoid using the patient group for dealing with the loneliness of the well-functioning group leader. In addition to departmental faculty with group therapy expertise, there are professional organizations that offer ongoing training and supervision for group leaders at all levels of seniority.

Suggested Readings

Alonso, A., & Swiller, H.I. (Eds.). (1993). *Group therapy in clinical practice.* Washington, DC: American Psychiatric Press.

Bion, W.R. (1961). *Experiences in groups.* London: Tavistock.

Bloch, S., & Crouch, E. (1985). *Therapeutic factors in group psychotherapy.* New York: Oxford University Press.

Brabender, V., & Fallon, A. (1993). *Models of inpatient group psychotherapy.* Washington, DC: American Psychiatric Press.

Durkin, H. (1964). *The group in depth.* New York: International Universities Press.

Ezriel, H. (1973). Psychoanalytic group therapy. In L.R. Wolberg, & E.K. Schwartz (Eds.), *Group therapy: 1973. An overview,* p. 183. New York: Intercontinental Medical Book Corp.

Foulkes, S.H. (1961). Group process and the individual in the therapeutic group. *British Journal of Medical Psychology, 34,* 23.

Freud, S. (1962). Group psychology and analysis of the ego. *Standard edition of the complete psychological works of Sigmund Freud.* London: Hogarth.

Gans, J.S. (1990). Broaching and exploring the question of combined group and individual therapy. *International Journal of Group Psychotherapy, 40,* 123–137.

Glatzer, H. (1978). The working alliance in analytic group psychotherapy. *International Journal of Group Psychotherapy, 28,* 147.

Kaplan, H.I., & Sadock, B.J. (Eds.). (1999). *Comprehensive group psychotherapy* (3rd ed.). Baltimore, MD: Williams and Wilkins.

Kauff, P. (1993). The contribution of analytic group therapy to the psycyhoanalytic process. In A. Alonso, & H. Swiller (Eds.), *Group therapy in clinical practice,* pp. 3–28. Washington, DC: American Psychiatric Press.

Kelly, J.A., Murphy, D.A., Bahr, G.R., et al. (1993). Outcome of cognitive-behavioral and support group brief therapies for depressed, HIV-infected persons. *American Journal of Psychiatry, 150,* 1679–1686.

Klein, R.H., Bernard, H.S., & Singer, D.L. (Eds.). (1992). *Handbook of contemporary group psychotherapy.* Madison, CT: International Universities Press.

Leszcz, M. (1992). The interpersonal approach to group psychotherapy. *International Journal of Group Psychotherapy, 42,* 37–62.

MacKenzie, K.R. (Ed.). (1992). *Classics in group psychotherapy.* New York: Guilford Press.

MacKenzie, K.R. (1997). *Time-managed group psychotherapy.* Washington, DC: American Psychiatric Press.

Malan, D.H., Balfour, F.H.G., Hood, V.G., & Shooter, A.M.N. (1976). Group psychotherapy: A long-term follow-up study. *Archives of General Psychiatry, 33,* 1303–1315.

O'Leary, J.V. (2002). The postmodern turn in group therapy. *International Journal of Group Psychotherapy, 51*(4), 473–487.

Pam, A., & Kemper, S. (1993). The captive group: Guidelines for group therapists in the inpatient setting. *International Journal of Group Psychotherapy, 43,* 419–438.

Riess, H. (2002). Integrative time-limited group therapy for bulimia nervosa. *International Journal of Group Psychotherapy,* 1–26.

Riester, A.E., & Kraft, I.A. (Eds.). (1986). *Child group psychotherapy.* Madison, CT: International Universities Press.

Rutan, J.S., & Stone, W.S. (Eds.). (1993). *Psychodynamic group psychotherapy.* New York: Guilford Press.

Scheidlinger, S. (1974). On the concept of "mother-group." *International Journal of Group Psychotherapy, 24,* 417–428.

Spiegel, D., Bloom, J.R., Kraemer, H.C., et al. (1989). Effect of psychosocial treatment on survival of patients with metastatic breast cancer. *Lancet, 2*(8668), 888–891.

Chapter 63

Cognitive-Behavioral Therapy

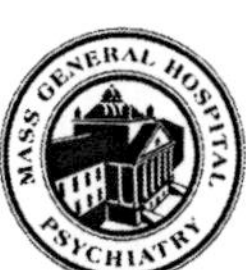

JOHN MATTHEWS, NADINE RECKER RAYBURN, AND MICHAEL W. OTTO

I. Overview and Theoretical Basis

A. **Cognitive-behavioral therapy (CBT) focuses on the interplay of maladaptive behavioral, emotional, and cognitive responses that characterize and perpetuate mental disorders.**

B. **CBT is based on the principles of learning and cognitive theory and uses empirically-based methods to study, develop, and evaluate therapeutic interventions.**

C. **CBT attends to the complex interaction between biology and environment, both in terms of the conceptualization and treatment of psychopathology.** CBT conceptualizations emphasize how certain biological risk factors contribute to disorders. For example, biological processes that influence patients' temperamental predispositions are assumed to be important. In addition, CBT recognizes how changes in emotion, cognition, and behavior have an impact on the central nervous system (CNS). The absence of a clear distinction between somatic and psychological effects of CBT interventions has been shown in research concerning CBT for obsessive-compulsive disorder (OCD). Studies have shown that CBT results in some of the same changes in brain activation that occur when patients respond successfully to pharmacotherapy for OCD.

D. **CBT interventions utilize a variety of techniques.** CBT includes a variety of techniques that modify cognitions, mood, and behavior. A thorough conceptualization of the patients' pathologic patterns, which involve analyzing the interrelated chains of thoughts, feelings, and behaviors, determines the techniques that are used. In addition, when developing a treatment plan, the therapist takes into consideration the individual's clinical state. For example, a severely depressed patient may not be able to employ cognitive techniques; thus, behavioral strategies may be used initially to activate the individual.

E. **CBT has been shown to be highly effective for a variety of disorders.** Over the past two decades, CBT treatment programs have become increasingly specialized. There is currently a wealth of empirical data documenting the efficacy of CBT for many disorders. The efficacy of CBT tends to approximate or surpass that of medication for the treatment of anxiety disorders, eating disorders, and non-psychotic major depression. In particular, there is evidence that treatment gains from CBT are maintained over extended periods.

II. Principles of Cognitive-Behavioral Therapy

A. **CBT conceptualizes a patient's psychopathology in terms of interrelated chains of thoughts, feelings, and behaviors.** This conceptualization is based on a comprehensive assessment conducted during the first few therapy sessions and is modified, as needed, based on new information. The therapist demonstrates to the patient the relationships among distorted thinking, negative emotions, and problem behaviors, and describes how these patterns perpetuate the patient's distress.

B. **CBT uses a collaborative approach.** The therapist and patient work together to determine the goals for therapy, the agenda for each session, the home practice assignments, the frequency of meetings, and how long to continue therapy. The therapist's role is to guide the treatment process based on the patient's needs, priorities, and capabilities. The therapist reinforces responses that represent successive approximations to a patient's goal—an approach called **"shaping."** The evidence suggests that CBT is accessible and acceptable to a wide variety of patients. The use of informational interventions (see below) helps the patient develop independent expertise in understanding the nature of the disorders under treatment and the process of change. In short, the collaborative process of treatment is aimed at **teaching patients to become their own therapists.**

C. **CBT is problem- and goal-oriented.** The therapist assists the patient in identifying the specific problems that brought the patient to therapy, prioritizing which problems are most important and most accessible in a step-wise treatment plan. Identification of goals for treatment and identification of "signposts" for progress are seen as important in helping the patient pursue her or his goals. CBT is also associated with high ratings of **therapy alliance,** perhaps as a consequence of the collaborative therapy environment and the step-wise pursuit of goals. Recent research indicates that patient alliance ratings increase following step-wise goal attainment.

D. **CBT focuses on the modification of thoughts, emotions, and behaviors in the present.** The primary focus of CBT is on the modification of current maladaptive patterns of thoughts, behaviors, and emotions. An examination of the person's learning history may be beneficial in terms of conceptualizing and understanding the relevant patterns underlying symptoms. Historic insight in the psychodynamic sense, however, is not considered to be of central importance in CBT.

E. **CBT is often short-term.** In treating Axis I disorders, CBT is considered to be "brief psychotherapy," which may include 8–20 sessions. For Axis II disorders, the therapy may last 1–2 years. For many disorders, these short-term approaches are associated with long-term maintenance of treatment gains.

F. **CBT also focuses on relapse prevention.** Frequently, the last two or three therapy sessions are devoted to relapse prevention. The therapist encourages the patient to identify potential problem areas that he or she may encounter and to think of possible solutions based on knowledge gained from therapy. The patient is also taught to recognize the early warning signs of relapse and, with some disorders, reminded to schedule booster sessions when needed. A fading schedule of sessions may also help patients enhance therapy skills in the absence of the therapist.

G. **CBT is data-based.** As mentioned earlier, many CBT treatment techniques and packages have been empirically validated, and the body of research on CBT is large and growing. Also, treatment is driven in part by patient self-report data. These data are collected by means of rating scales, diaries, and **home practice assignments.** Cognitive-behavioral therapists view assessment as an ongoing process. Therapist and patient consistently monitor progress and make appropriate adjustments to the treatment if the expected gains are not achieved.

III. Components of Cognitive-Behavioral Therapy (CBT)

A. Goal Setting

The therapist and patient agree on the goals of treatment based on the therapist's conceptualization of the patient's presenting problems. To help the patient achieve his or her goals, the therapist will introduce a range of interventions aimed at facilitating adaptive change.

B. Session Structure

The collaborative and active nature of treatment is underscored in the structure of the session. After opening discussions and review of progress from the last session, patient and therapist frequently choose agenda items for the session. This may involve specific rehearsals, problem-solving reviews, open-ended questions guiding self-discovery around specific topic areas, review of self-monitoring, exposure practice, or other interventions (see below). Near the end of a session, this information may be consolidated into discussions of relevant home practice, rehearsals, or goal pursuit for the interval between sessions. Troubleshooting of anticipated difficulties with regard to the home-practice and/or discussion of the most useful elements of the session help close the meeting.

C. Informational Interventions

Treatment typically begins with informational interventions that are designed to supply the patient with a model of the disorder and the change process. The patient uses this model as a framework for understanding the role of other treatment elements in later sessions and as an impetus to actively engage in a joint treatment effort. The therapist's role in this state of therapy is often characterized as an "expert consultant" or "personal coach." In order to enhance independent learning in CBT, informational interventions may include home reading assignments that further explain the CBT conceptualization and treatment elements.

D. Self-Monitoring

Self-monitoring is a general technique used to help the patient and therapist assess the occurrence or nature of maladaptive behaviors as they occur in the patient's life. Self-monitoring can also be employed in the planning and acquisition of new patterns, with the scheduling and recording of target behaviors or events. In addition, self-monitoring helps patients break experiences into their components, to better understand the role of setting events, thoughts, and emotions in determining behavioral outcomes. Self-monitoring alone is often powerful in helping patients increase desired responses and reduce problem behaviors.

E. Cognitive Interventions

Cognitive techniques are aimed at challenging maladaptive thought patterns, as well as more chronic beliefs (termed, **core beliefs**). They help patients recognize the content of their thoughts, evaluate their accuracy, and guide themselves more effectively. As a central feature of these interventions, patients learn to treat thoughts as hypotheses (or guesses) about the world and to evaluate the validity of these hypotheses.

1. **Introduction to cognitive change.** Approaches to cognitive restructuring differ widely among therapists and theorists, but share in common the goal of helping patients become aware of the nature of their self-talk and the degree to which it influences their affect and behavior.
2. **Self-monitoring of thoughts** in response to situational and emotional cues helps patients identify thoughts as they occur throughout the day. Such monitoring provides a cue for adoption of alternative and more accurate cognitive responses. Patients assess their mood during the process of self-monitoring and

generation of alternative thoughts. This allows them to realize the impact of thinking styles on affect and behavior.

3. **Socratic questioning**—open-ended questions guiding self-discovery—helps patients evaluate the accuracy of their assumptions and perceptions about their self and their experiences.
4. **Negative shifts in mood** provide an excellent opportunity to identify negative thoughts (often termed **automatic thoughts** because of their rapid and habitual nature).
5. **Examination of the evidence** is basic to modifying distorted negative automatic thoughts. The therapist teaches the patient to treat thoughts as hypotheses and to conduct a search for evidence both for and against the hypotheses. The final interpretation is based on the outcome of this "examining-the-evidence" exercise.
6. **Training in the identification of common cognitive errors** enhances a patient's ability to identify faulty thinking processes. Errors in logic present in a variety of forms: dichotomous or all-or-nothing thinking (events are seen in one of two mutually exclusive categories), overgeneralization (a specific event is seen as characteristic of life in general), mind-reading (an individual assumes that others are reacting negatively without obtaining the necessary evidence), catastrophic thinking (negative experiences or events are interpreted as intolerable or in terms of the worst possible outcome), and personalization (an individual automatically assumes responsibility for a negative event without considering other possible contributing factors).
7. **Behavioral experiments** provide patients with a method to examine the evidence for or against thoughts in actual situations. In a behavioral experiment, patients examine their beliefs about and their expectations for events, identify specific predictions, and then examine whether these predictions occur in an actual situation.
8. **Maintaining an accurate perspective on thoughts** may be as important as "restructuring" thoughts. Some treatment approaches focus on increasing attention to life contingencies and values rather than the myriad of self and other expectations that color ongoing experience.

F. Exposure Interventions

Exposures provide patients with real-world experiences by which to become accustomed to avoided (frequently feared) situations. Exposure interventions have served as the mainstay of cognitive-behavioral treatments of anxiety disorders.

1. **Exposure targets maladaptive avoidance.** Exposures help patients alter their emotions, cognitions, and behaviors in response to certain (usually anxiety-provoking or otherwise uncomfortable) stimuli. By breaking maladaptive patterns of avoidance, exposures allow for negative emotional responses to dissipate naturally and to eventually extinguish. In addition, by not prematurely escaping from, or avoiding, uncomfortable situations or stimuli, patients gain the opportunity to adjust inaccurate and unhelpful thoughts and beliefs that perpetuate avoidance behavior.
2. **Exposure is conducted in different modalities.** The nature of the patient's problem and his or her particular patterns of avoidance determine the specific exposure technique and the types of stimuli incorporated. ***In-vivo*** exposures include direct exposure to feared situations, objects, or people. **Imaginal** exposures are a powerful means to confront patients with feared images, memories, or cognitions. **Interoceptive exposure** techniques target patients' fears of their own physiological sensations. With the help of specific procedures, e.g., hyperventilation to induce dizziness, patients systematically confront uncomfortable somatic sensations.
3. **Exposure is usually gradual.** Exposure is typically conducted in a gradual, step-wise fashion. This means that confrontation with the feared object or situation typically proceeds along a hierarchy of personalized, increasingly difficult tasks. However, exposure can also involve the extended confrontation with a strong cue **("flooding").** Most therapists and patients prefer gradual exposure over flooding.
4. **Exposures are frequently implemented in conjunction with cognitive techniques.** In the context of some cognitive-behavioral treatments (e.g., CBT for social anxiety disorder), patients learn to challenge negative thoughts whenever they occur before, during, or after exposure exercises. Hence, exposures provide an excellent opportunity to develop cognitive skills in situations in which these skills are needed most.
5. **Distraction** from fear cues or the use of **"safety behaviors"** (behaviors designed to enhance the feeling of safety during exposure, e.g., carrying water bottles, cell phones, or a pill in the pocket) appear to decrease exposure efficacy. Exposure interventions are enhanced when patients direct their attention to actual outcomes in the feared situation.
6. **Response prevention** helps patients refrain from rituals they use to neutralize fears (e.g., repetitive checking or hand-washing in OCD). Prevention of compulsions allows patients to learn true safety in response to feared events or situations.
7. **Systematic desensitization** is an imaginal exposure procedure where patients are presented with successively more anxiety-provoking stimuli (scenes of feared events). Patients relax after each brief presentation, and move on to more difficult stimuli as they are able to remain relaxed during exposures. Research indicates that relaxation is not necessary for successful exposure therapy.

G. Behavioral Assignments

Behavioral assignments are completed as part of home practice of specific skills.

1. **As noted, behavioral assignments may serve as experiments** to test the validity of negative thoughts and beliefs. The therapist and patient clearly identify the belief to be tested and then collaboratively design an experiment to test the belief. The power of this technique is realized when the patient personally experiences evidence that contradicts the validity of his or her view.
2. **Behavioral assignments may help to reinstate and consolidate normal patterns of behavior.** They ensure that adaptive behaviors get rehearsed independent of the therapist's presence and therefore provide an important tool for ensuring the maintenance of treatment gains.
3. **Behavioral assignments can aid in time-management.** The scheduling of specific activities is useful for dealing with time-management problems and difficulty with prioritizing tasks. The therapist has the patient write down on a grid activities for the week. The therapist may ask the patient to write down for each task ratings for mastery, pleasure, and mood. These ratings provide important data that can be used by the patient and therapist to modify the patient's behavior.
4. **Behavioral assignments can be crucial in helping patients return to valued activities.** In conjunction with self-monitoring, patients may be asked to track pleasurable and productive activities as part of enhancing joy from daily activities.

H. Skill Rehearsal

With the help of in-session rehearsals, therapist and patient ensure that the patient is able to utilize certain skills when they are needed. This may involve modeling of new behaviors by the therapist, role-play, and constructive feedback provided to the patient. In addition, these techniques allow for the activation of specific emotional experiences and may make distressing thoughts and beliefs more accessible. In-session rehearsals are typically followed by behavioral assignments to be completed by the patient in between sessions.

I. Problem-Solving

Active rehearsal of problem-solving helps patients think adaptively about difficult or particularly emotionally-evocative situations. The patient learns to specify a problem, to identify alternative solutions, to examine the pros and cons of each potential solution, to select a solution, to devise a plan for implementation, to implement the plan, and to assess the effectiveness of the results.

J. Contingency Management

Contingency management involves the modification of target behaviors by altering the events following the behaviors. This requires an initial analysis of the target behavior with a close assessment of the events that elicit and follow it. It is important to specify the particular behavior to be changed and the alternative behavior desired. These alternative behaviors should be appropriately rehearsed. Through the application of alternative consequences—e.g., the use of rewards to **reinforce** (increase) a behavior or **punishments** (removing a desired event or adding an aversive event) to decrease a behavior—the desired behavior is strengthened, and the frequency of the undesired behavior decreases.

K. Emotional Acceptance Training

Training in the labeling, acceptance, and tolerance of emotions is increasingly becoming a component of cognitive-behavioral treatment packages. Strategies to enhance emotional acceptance and tolerance vary widely. They range from mindfulness training utilizing meditation, to exposure exercises where patients are asked to note, but otherwise to do nothing to "manage" emotions.

L. Relaxation Training and Diaphragmatic Breathing Training

Training in arousal-reduction procedures was common in many anxiety protocols in the 1970s and 1980s. However, it is increasingly considered to be an unnecessary element for the treatment of many anxiety disorders. Currently, relaxation is used most frequently for generalized anxiety disorder. It also represents a powerful intervention for general stress management, including applications to stress for cardiac risk reduction and other medical conditions. **Progressive muscle relaxation** refers to successive tense-relax procedures to help patients identify tension in specific muscle groups and learn to release that tension on demand. Diaphragmatic breathing training teaches patients to use slow, calming breaths stressing the diaphragm (as opposed to more effortful breaths from lifting the chest upward and outward).

IV. The Application of CBT to Specific Disorders

A. Depression

CBT conceptualizations of depression emphasize self-perpetuating patterns of negative expectations and evaluations, as well as declining contact with pleasurable activities, such as playing a central role in maintaining the disorder. Depressed mood also has an impact on the patient's ability to recall positive experiences and successes and impairs problem-solving abilities.

1. **Treatment**
   a. **Informational interventions.** An important goal of informational interventions in CBT for depression is to help the patient view depression as something external to the self and help her or him prepare for adaptive change. The therapist provides information about the nature of the disorder, common symptoms, and the upcoming treatment interventions. This can also help inhibit the negative self-evaluation in response to symptoms of depression, which is sometimes referred to as "depression about depression."

b. **Activity scheduling.** During the early phase of treatment, a depressed patient may experience significant psychomotor retardation and/or fatigue. Graded activity assignments (focusing on both pleasure and productivity goals) help patients become re-engaged in rewarding activities. These interventions have been found to be efficacious in their own right in treating depression. Treatment packages often combine them with cognitive interventions.

c. **Cognitive restructuring.** Patients learn to use daily thought records in order to systematically challenge their negative views of self, the environment, and the future. Once the negative automatic thoughts are identified, the patient, in collaboration with the therapist, identifies alternative views and searches for the evidence to support them. In addition, it is crucial to identify and correct the dysfunctional core belief system that is responsible for the distorted views of self, environment, and future. The core beliefs are accessed through the discovery of patterns of negative automatic thoughts in given situations. The therapist, along with the patient, identifies the core beliefs by working backward from the cognitive themes observed in the present.

d. **Problem-solving.** Recurrent aversive events or interpersonal interactions may also be targeted with problem-solving training or skills development (e.g., assertiveness training) to enhance a patient's ability to successfully pursue personal goals.

2. **Outcome studies.** In the acute treatment of mild to moderate major depression, the efficacy of CBT is comparable to antidepressants. Evidence is also increasing for the strong efficacy of CBT for severe (but non-psychotic) depression. In preventing relapse, follow-up studies 1–2 years after termination of treatment demonstrate that short-term CBT prevents relapse in the same range as maintenance pharmacotherapy, providing an alternative to long-term pharmacotherapy. In severe cases of depression, combined pharmacotherapy and CBT are a preferred treatment option.

B. Bipolar Disorder

CBT for bipolar disorder is intended to be an adjunct to ongoing pharmacotherapy. It aims to reduce the frequency and severity of both manic and depressive episodes by focusing on medication compliance, elimination of risk factors for future episodes (e.g., biological or psychosocial stressors), and detection of early warning signs for episodes. In addition, CBT for bipolar disorder employs the interventions for major depression described above.

1. **Treatment**

a. **Regularity of the circadian rhythm.** These interventions help bipolar patients monitor and establish regular patterns of sleep, eating, and exercise.

b. **Stress management.** Problem-solving and other stress reduction skills are employed to reduce the risk of future episodes due to interpersonal conflicts and the impact of external stressors.

c. **Early detection.** Patients are instructed to chart their mood on a daily basis in order to become aware of early warning signs of mania and depression.

d. **Compliance.** Educational, motivational, and problem-solving interventions target difficulties patients experience with medication adherence. In addition, cognitive interventions are aimed at identifying and correcting maladaptive beliefs about medication.

2. **Outcome studies.** Empirical evidence from a variety of smaller studies shows that CBT in combination with pharmacotherapy for bipolar disorder is effective in reducing the number and severity of episodes. Future research studies need to confirm these promising results.

C. Panic Disorder

Cognitive-behavioral accounts of panic disorder emphasize the role of catastrophic misinterpretations of anxiety sensations (e.g., "I am having a heart attack," "I am going to lose control") in cueing panic attacks and motivating the avoidance that characterizes the disorder.

1. **Treatment**

a. **Informational interventions.** Patients are provided with a model of the disorder that outlines the "fear-of-fear cycle" characterizing the disorder. Informational interventions commonly include a discussion of the role of thoughts and avoidance patterns in cueing and maintaining panic episodes, as well as a review of the physiological source of panic symptoms.

b. **Cognitive restructuring.** Cognitive interventions aim to correct patients' thoughts and beliefs about the meaning and consequences of the somatic symptoms of panic and anxiety. Common targets include both the tendency to overestimate the probability of negative outcomes, as well as the degree of catastrophe within these outcomes.

c. **Interoceptive exposure.** These exposure exercises target patients' fears of their own physiological anxiety sensations and are commonly implemented in conjunction with cognitive restructuring. With the help of specific procedures, such as running in place, hyperventilating, spinning to re-create feared sensations (e.g., tachycardia, numbness and tingling, dizziness), patients confront feared somatic sensations in a controlled fashion. This provides the opportunity to eliminate fears and anxiogenic responses to these sensations.

d. ***In-vivo* exposure.** Step-wise situational exposures are implemented for patients to gradually overcome their agoraphobic avoidance and re-learn that the once-feared places and circumstances are safe.

e. **Somatic management skills.** These coping skills are helpful in minimizing patients' responses to symptoms and can therefore reduce the likelihood of a panic attack. Skills include diaphragmatic breathing and muscle relaxation training. Recent research suggests that elimination of these strategies in treatment protocols does not reduce overall efficacy, suggesting the importance of exposure and cognitive restructuring interventions as the core efficacy components in treatment.

2. **Outcome studies.** In the past two decades, a great amount of research has emerged in support of the efficacy of CBT for panic disorder. Short-term CBT (often in the range of 12 sessions) is associated with the long-term maintenance of treatment gains, making CBT a particularly cost-effective treatment. It can be applied as an alternative to medication treatment, as a strategy for medication non-responders, or a strategy to replace pharmacotherapy in individuals who wish to eliminate medication use.

D. Social Anxiety Disorder

CBT conceptualizations of social anxiety disorder emphasize self-perpetuating chains of expectations of social failure, negative self-evaluations, increasing anxiety, and avoidance of social situations. Consequently, CBT for social anxiety disorder alters anxiogenic social expectations and exposure to help patients decrease anxiety as part of regular social rehearsal.

1. **Treatment**

   a. **Informational interventions.** These interventions supply the patient with a CBT model of social anxiety. Patients learn about the anxiogenic nature of their thoughts and the role of avoidance in perpetuating their disorder.

   b. **Cognitive restructuring.** Cognitive interventions are aimed at the identification and modification of dysfunctional cognitions that detract from adaptive social performance. Patients learn to identify anxiety-inducing thoughts and learn to "catch" them when they occur in social situations. Monitoring thoughts during spontaneous or planned anxiety experiences (i.e., exposures) facilitates this process. Patients then learn to correct common distortions such as negative expectations of social performance ("My mind will go blank"), distorted evaluations of the self ("I am the only incompetent person around"), distorted expectations and interpretations of the reactions of others ("They will think I am an idiot"). In addition, treatment focuses on adjusting misperceptions about one's ability to cope with a sub-optimal performance and the over-focus on and attentional search for signs of social failure.

   c. **Exposure interventions.** Exposure interventions provide patients with the opportunity to rehearse feared social interactions. They are typically implemented in conjunction with cognitive interventions and are aimed at correcting dysfunctional thoughts, reallocating attention appropriately (i.e., away from signs of social failure), and eliminating overt and subtle avoidance behaviors. Exposures are meant to represent "corrective" experiences that provide the patient with a sense of safety in social situations. Recently developed treatment protocols utilize a group treatment format, which offers the advantage of a ready-made setting (i.e., other group members) for constructing simulated exposure exercises.

   d. **Social skills training.** In social skills training, patients are taught to use adaptive and normative behaviors in a social context. Such training incorporates education about positive social interactions and modeling of target social behaviors by the therapist, followed by role-play rehearsals by the patient. After the role-play, the therapist typically provides corrective feedback. Alternatively, therapist and patient may decide to use videotapes to obtain specific feedback on performance. Research shows that a majority of socially anxious patients possess appropriate social skills but are inhibited to display these skills. Social skills training may therefore be beneficial only for a minority of patients who exhibit actual deficits.

   e. **Interoceptive exposures.** Symptoms of social phobia may resemble those of panic disorder (e.g., increased heart rate, sweating, and dizziness). Consequently, some treatment packages include exposure to the feared bodily sensations, with the goal of reducing performance-related concerns about those sensations.

2. **Outcome studies.** A wide variety of studies provide evidence that short-term CBT results in significant benefits to patients with social anxiety disorder. The effectiveness of CBT approximates that of the most successful pharmacological interventions (e.g., phenelzine and clonazepam). In addition, research suggests that CBT gains tend to be maintained over time and even continue to increase over follow-up intervals.

E. Generalized Anxiety Disorder

CBT conceptualizations of generalized anxiety disorder (GAD) emphasize unrealistic or excessive worry about several life circumstances accompanied by chronic symptoms of anxious arousal. CBT for GAD targets the worry process with the help of cognitive restructuring and symptom management techniques.

1. **Treatment**

   a. **Informational interventions.** Patients learn about the role of maladaptive cognitions in the worry process. Informational interventions also provide patients with a framework for the interventions that will follow.

   b. **Cognitive interventions.** With the help of self-monitoring, patients learn to identify maladaptive cognitions as they occur in the worry process. They evaluate these thoughts logically, examine the evidence and probability for anticipated negative outcomes, and generate alternative explanations of events to challenge catastrophic thoughts. Patients may be assigned specific "worry times" to help them gain control over a constant tendency to worry. Problem-solving training concerning certain recurring worry topics focuses on discriminating between excessive worry and true problem-solving.

   c. **Imaginal exposure.** In some cases imaginal exposure to core worries is implemented in order to decrease patients' anxiety in response to specific concerns.

d. **Somatic management skills.** Relaxation training, diaphragmatic breathing, and biofeedback-assisted procedures are used to decrease physiological arousal that accompanies the worry process. In addition, these skills provide patients with important tools to manage their anxiety in worry-inducing situations.

2. **Outcome studies.** The treatment-outcome literature concerning GAD provides evidence that CBT tends to be as effective as medication (benzodiazepine or antidepressant treatment). However, more research needs to be done to develop effective treatments.

F. Obsessive-Compulsive Disorder

Patients suffering from obsessive-compulsive disorder (OCD) exhibit cycles of intrusive thoughts or concerns followed by ritualistic attempts to reduce the anxiety or discomfort caused by these concerns.

1. **Treatment**

a. **Informational interventions.** Patients are provided with a CBT conceptualization of the disorder that sets the stage for the upcoming treatment components.

b. **Exposure and response prevention.** These interventions are aimed at breaking the chronic cycles of intrusive concerns and anxiety-reducing rituals. Patients are exposed to situations that trigger the intrusive or obsessive thoughts and/or compulsive rituals in a systematic, step-wise manner. Patients are then instructed to resist performing the compulsive ritual in order to break the reinforcing link between the trigger and the compulsive response. Over time, anxiety decreases with repeated exposure to these cues in the absence of compulsive rituals.

c. **Cognitive interventions.** Cognitive interventions may complement exposure and response prevention by enhancing patients' skills for breaking the self-perpetuating cycle of intrusive thoughts and ritualistic responses. These interventions are particularly appropriate for patients who exhibit mental rituals.

2. **Outcome studies.** The treatment outcome literature provides consistent evidence that CBT for OCD is as effective as pharmacotherapy. For patients with severe OCD symptoms, however, a combination treatment of medication and CBT may be the best option.

G. Post-Traumatic Stress Disorder

The CBT conceptualization of post-traumatic stress disorder (PTSD) emphasizes a patient' s disrupted sense of safety in the world as a result of a traumatic event. The perception of chronic danger leads to hypervigilance, arousal, and attempts to avoid situations and cues that are deemed dangerous. CBT interventions are aimed at breaking the connection between trauma-related cues and the severe anxiety and avoidance responses that characterize the disorder.

1. **Treatment**

a. **Informational interventions.** Informational interventions help patients understand the often overwhelming experience of emotional memories linked to exposure to trauma cues. Time is spent helping patients identify cues of the trauma (including a particular emotion, time of the day, or sensory cue). In addition, therapist and patient organize the patient's symptoms within the re-experiencing, avoidance, and arousal domains. This helps patients demystify these experiences and provides an increased sense of control.

b. **Cognitive interventions.** Cognitive interventions target distorted thoughts and beliefs that developed as a consequence of the traumatic event. Treatment for rape, e.g., examines the consequences of rape for beliefs about safety, guilt, esteem, and intimacy. With the help of cognitive interventions, patients correct these assumptions and develop a broader cognitive organization that places the trauma in the proper context of a patient's life and future.

c. **Imaginal exposure.** Exposure interventions are variably described as helping a patient develop a narrative of the trauma, extinguish extreme emotional responses to cues associated with the trauma, and better learn to discriminate between the trauma and current "relatively" safe situations. The procedure involves prolonged "viewing" of the traumatic memory in imagination with thoughts and feelings experienced during the event. With repeated practice, the memory loses its power to provoke extreme distress.

d. ***In-vivo* exposure.** *In-vivo* exposures are implemented in order to help patients eliminate fear and other strong emotions in response to trauma cues. With repeated exposure and appropriate instruction, patients learn to assess the realistic safety of previously emotionally-overwhelming situations.

e. **Emotional regulation skills.** These skills may be applied as a prelude to exposure treatment, to assist patients in the processing of emotions evoked during exposure.

f. **Symptom management skills.** As with the treatment of other anxiety disorders, CBT for PTSD may include breathing and other relaxation techniques in the early stages of treatment.

2. **Outcome studies.** There is evidence that the benefits offered by exposure-based CBT surpass those achieved in medication trials. More research needs to confirm the efficacy of CBT in combination with pharmacotherapy.

H. Specific Phobias

Specific phobias are fear reactions caused by the presence or anticipation of specific events or objects that are not better accounted for by other conditions.

1. **Treatment**

a. **Exposure interventions.** Exposure can be conducted in a variety of formats including *in-vivo* and imaginal exposure, as well as the use of virtual reality technology to enhance the realism of office-based exposure.

b. **Participant modeling.** In participant modeling the therapist exemplifies a behavior (e.g., touching a snake) and encourages the patient to repeat the behavior. Comparable to exposure exercises, participant modeling proceeds along a hierarchy consisting of progressively more anxiety-provoking situations.

2. **Outcome studies.** Exposure-based CBT interventions remain the most efficacious interventions for specific phobias. Recent data on single-session interventions utilizing successive but prolonged exposure (over three hours) have shown long-lasting benefit for specific phobias.

I. Bulimia Nervosa

CBT for bulimia nervosa targets patients' distorted cognitions regarding body image and food, as well as their abnormal eating behaviors.

1. **Treatment**
   a. **Informational interventions.** Psychoeducation emphasizes the medical risks of abnormal eating behaviors and provides information about normal body weight, nutrition, and the effects of dieting on mood.
   b. **Self-monitoring.** Self-monitoring of food intake, binge episodes, and purging facilitates the identification of the triggers and consequences of binge-eating.
   c. **Stimulus-control procedures.** The patient is taught to manipulate certain environmental cues in order to reduce the likelihood of binge episodes. This may involve, e.g., changing one's place of eating. In addition, in order to normalize eating patterns and decrease dietary restraint, balanced meals are scheduled at specific times.
   d. **Cognitive techniques.** Cognitive restructuring addresses beliefs that body shape and appearance determine acceptance. Since eating disorders are often seen as a coping strategy to deal with more fundamental belief systems, therapy may also address the issues of low self-esteem and negative self-image.
   e. **Problem-solving.** This intervention helps patients recognize and implement alternative coping strategies when confronted with the urge to binge.
2. **Outcome studies.** The treatment-outcome literature provides evidence that CBT for bulimia on average eliminates binge-eating and purging in roughly 50% of all patients. The percent reduction in binge-eating and purging is typically 80% or more across patients treated with CBT.

J. Anorexia Nervosa

The main problem areas addressed in CBT for anorexia nervosa include a distorted body image, low weight, and abnormal eating behaviors. The primary goal is to restore weight and normal eating.

1. **Treatment**
   a. **Contingency management.** In the acute phase of treatment, positive and negative reinforcement procedures are frequently implemented to directly manipulate maladaptive eating and weight control patterns.
   b. **Additional interventions,** similar to those for bulimia, also apply.
2. **Outcome studies.** Controlled studies on CBT for anorexia nervosa are rare. However, studies are beginning to emerge that suggest the usefulness of CBT for this disorder.

K. Substance Abuse

A wide variety of approaches have been applied to the CBT of substance abuse.

1. **Treatment elements**
   a. **Motivational interventions.** Motivational interviewing is an empirically supported strategy to enhance engagement in treatment. As compared with efforts to "persuade" patients, motivational interviewing relies on the dispassionate presentation of information and Socratic discussions to help patients clarify and mobilize their own desires for change.
   b. **Functional analysis.** Targets for treatment and enhancement of self-control skills are frequently identified through a functional analysis of patterns leading up to substance use.
   c. **Self-monitoring** procedures may be used to help patients identify cues in the moments leading up to substance use (e.g., self-monitoring cards placed within the cellophane of a cigarette pack).
   d. **Cognitive interventions.** Correction of all-or-none thinking patterns (e.g., "I had one drink, I blew it, so I may as well keep drinking") and other dysfunctional thinking patterns (e.g., " I can't handle stress, I need to use") may be used to help break the chain of use. Alternative cognitive coping strategies and training in emotional tolerance may also be applied to help patients resist both internal cues (negative emotions) and external cues for use (stresses or situations).
   e. **Problem-solving and skills training.** Patients identify alternative ways of dealing with the cues that trigger cravings. In addition, treatment may include the acquisition and training of certain behaviors and skills inconsistent with substance abuse patterns. For example, patients learn to establish contact with people not associated with substance abuse, practice assertiveness skills for refusing drugs or alcohol, and acquire job-hunting and general social skills.
   f. **Contingency management.** To make the consequences of drug use more salient in the moment, treatment contracting of specific consequences (e.g., buying a valued object) for successful abstinence (e.g., as measured by urine drug screens) may be implemented. Couples contracting may engage spouses in the contracting of both negative and positive outcomes relative to use and abstinence, respectively.
2. **Outcome studies.** In general, cognitive-behavioral treatments are among the most effective psychosocial treatments for substance abuse.

L. Psychotic Disorders

CBT for psychotic disorders represents an important adjunct to antipsychotic medication. It addresses several aspects of the psychotic experience, including misunderstandings about impact of the illness on self-esteem, challenging the validity of delusions and hallucinations, assisting in the development of better coping strategies, and identifying triggers and early signs of relapse.

1. **Treatment**
   a. **Informational interventions.** Psychoeducation provides the patient with information about the illness and its treatment and aims to correct misunderstandings about the concurrent pharmacotherapy.
   b. **Cognitive interventions.** These interventions can be aimed at promoting medication adherence by targeting maladaptive thoughts and beliefs that interfere with medication compliance and self-esteem. In addition, cognitive techniques are applied to help patients react adaptively to hallucinations and delusions by testing assumptions about the meaning of voices or the certainty of beliefs.
   c. **Skills training.** Social skills training is designed to promote patients' adaptive social functioning in a wide variety of situations. Skills training can include role-playing, modeling, and contingency management techniques.
   d. **Stress management and problem-solving skills.** These techniques help patients cope with the stressors that frequently precipitate relapse.
2. **Outcome studies.** Early evidence indicates that CBT represents a useful adjunct to medication treatment for psychotic disorders.

M. Personality Disorders

CBT defines personality disorders as pervasive and long-standing maladaptive patterns of behavior which result in distress and impairment of functioning. Consequently, CBT for these conditions tends to be longer-term than those for Axis I disorders.

1. **Treatment**
   a. **Emotional regulation.** Emotional dysregulation represents a common problem of patients with personality disorders. Hence, therapy teaches skills to label, tolerate, and modify emotions.
   b. **Reduction of therapy-interfering behaviors.** CBT for personality disorders places particular emphasis on the therapeutic relationship. Therefore, behaviors that threaten the relationship or the therapeutic process in general (e.g., missing appointments, inability to complete home practices) are addressed immediately and consistently.
   c. **Cognitive interventions.** Patients with personality disorders may view themselves and other people in "black and white" terms. For example, they may describe themselves as "defective" or "totally undesirable," and view others as rejecting and malevolent. Their social interactions consist of extremes, including idealization and rejection. Since personality-disordered patients have a predominance of maladaptive core beliefs, therapy tends focus on belief work.
   d. **Stress management, problem-solving, and skills training.** Many personality-disordered patients exhibit pervasive problem-solving and skills deficits which are addressed with repeated rehearsal of adaptive coping, problem-solving, and interpersonal skills training.
2. **Outcome studies.** There is early evidence supporting the efficacy of CBT for personality disorders.

Suggested Readings

Barlow, D.H. (Ed.). (2001). *Clinical handbook of psychological disorders.* New York: Guilford.

Beck, A.T., Freeman, A., et al. (1990). *Cognitive therapy for personality disorders.* New York: Guilford.

Beck, J.S. (1995). *Cognitive therapy: Basics and beyond,* pp. 1–24. New York: Guilford Press.

Blackburn, I.M. (1989). Severely depressed in-patients. In J. Scott, J.M.G. Williams, & A.T. Beck (Eds.), *Cognitive therapy in clinical practice: An illustrative case book,* pp. 1–24. London: Routledge.

Hawton, K., Salkovskis, P.M., Kirk, L., & Clark, D.M. (1989). *Cognitive behaviour therapy for psychiatric problems: A practical guide.* Oxford: Oxford University Press.

Hofmann, S.G., & Thompson, M. (Eds.). (2002). *Handbook of psychosocial treatments for severe mental disorders.* New York: Guilford.

Kleifield, E.I., Wagner, S., & Halmi, K.A. (1996). Cognitive-behavioral treatment of anorexia nervosa. *Psychiatric Clinics of North America, 19*(4), 715–737.

Mitchell, J.E., & Peterson, C.B. (1998). Cognitive-behavioral treatment of eating disorders. In J.H. Wright, & M.E. Thase (Eds.), *Cognitive therapy,* pp. 107–133. Washington, DC: American Psychiatric Press.

Pollack, M.H., Otto, M.W., & Rosenbaum, J.F. (Eds.). (1996). *Challenges in clinical practice: Pharmacologic and psychosocial strategies.* New York: Guilford.

Chapter 64

Hypnosis

OWEN S. SURMAN, SARA KULLESEID, AND LEE BAER

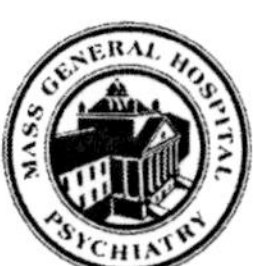

I. Introduction

Hypnosis is a therapeutic modality that has been used, by one name or another, for thousands of years; however, its popularity, as a technique for the treatment of a wide variety of ailments, has fluctuated. Many have attempted to define hypnosis. It is perhaps best understood as **an event or ritual between a hypnotist and hypnotic subject(s) in which both agree to use suggestion to bring about a change in perception or behavior. Hypnosis depends on several things: the dissociative and imaginative abilities (i.e., hypnotic susceptibility) of the subject(s), the motivation of the subject(s), and the relationship between hypnotist and subject(s) (i.e., demand characteristics).** Multiple clinical applications exist for direct suggestions delivered during hypnosis. Hypnosis has also been used as an adjunct to behavior therapy and for memory retrieval.

II. Historical Background

A. The Pre-Mesmer Era

Suggestive therapies have been used since early civilization. Records of their use date back to 2600 B.C.; there are even references to a hypnotic process in the Bible. **Through ritual and ceremony, various healers have used suggestion to ease, if not cure, ailments.** The most important element seems to be the intimate connection made between the subject and the healer.

B. Franz Anton Mesmer (1734–1815) and the Marquis de Puysegur (1751–1825)

1. **Mesmer,** working during the Age of Enlightenment, **is thought to be the originator of what later became known as hypnosis.** In 1766, he **presented his thesis of "universal gravitation"** to the University of Vienna. In it, **he postulated that a fluid contained within all living beings,** as well as in the universe at large, **affected others through gravitational forces.** He called this fluid **"animal magnetism"** and based his model of disease on an imbalance of that fluid in the body. **Mesmer used magnets, literally, to restore equilibrium** to this fluid; later he became convinced that his own animal magnetism could cause fluid movements and therapeutic "crises" in patients. These were distortions in perceptions with a convulsive component, similar to the manifestations of hysteria, that occurred in a hypnotic state. On awakening, many claimed cure. Mesmer saw the importance of the relationship between the magnetizer and the patient, and later called this phenomenon "rapport." In 1784, due to controversy surrounding his work, Mesmer was discredited by an investigative committee of the French Academy of Science which was led by Benjamin Franklin, then a U.S. Ambassador to France. Ultimately, it was decided that the fluid did not exist and that any effects were due to the forces of suggestion.
2. **De Puysegur,** one of Mesmer's disciples, **also practiced magnetism.** His best known patient, instead of exhibiting a convulsive crisis, fell into a type of sleep that he called "artificial somnambulism." In this state, the patient "confessed" worries without apparent subsequent memory of the encounter. This suggested a different state of consciousness with amnestic barriers. **De Puysegur felt that the magnetizer's belief in his/her own ability to heal was what brought about cure.** Others countered this with the belief that this altered state came from the patient—his/her own ability to be suggestible or to internalize the magnetizer's suggestions.

C. James Braid (1795–1860), Jean Martin Charcot (1825–1893), and Hippolyte Bernheim (1840–1919)

1. Through the work of **James Braid,** hypnosis again became integrated into medical practice. **Braid** is said to **have coined the word "hypnosis," from the Greek, *hypnos,* for sleep.** He believed that magnetism resulted in a type of sleep he called "neurypnology." Braid believed that psychological forces within the individual were critical to the process of magnetism.
2. **Charcot** was a noted nineteenth-century French neurologist; he became interested in hypnosis while working with hysterics and epileptics. **He felt hypnosis was a pathologic neurophysiologic state** akin to hysteria. A student of Charcot's, **Pierre Janet,** furthered this theory. Janet thought that the underlying mechanism was a disconnection or "dissociation" from the conscious state, as occurred in hysteria.
3. **Bernheim** challenged these ideas. He felt that hypnosis was not like hysteria. Rather, Bernheim believed that **hypnosis worked through the power of suggestion** and that the effects of hypnosis could be achieved in the waking state. Thus, by the beginning of the twentieth century, two prominent theories of hypnosis co-existed.

D. Sigmund Freud (1856–1939), Milton Erikson (1901–1980), to the Present

1. **Freud** was influenced greatly by his work with Charcot. Freud was an experienced hypnotist; however, he moved to psychoanalysis because of what he considered were the limitations in the technique. **Freud felt**

that hypnosis imposed ideas on a patient which made analysis and critical thinking difficult.

2. **Erikson,** along with his predecessor, **Clark Hull, contradicted Freud, refuting the need to make unconscious processes conscious to achieve change and relief.** They felt that subtle commands or indirect suggestions could make the patient unconsciously change their behavior.
3. The **Hilgards** in the 1950s and 1960s revisited the dissociative theory of Janet with their **"neodissociation" theory; they furthered the concept that the hypnotic process is involuntary,** is not under conscious control, and involves the notion of altered states of awareness. Other theorists took a **"sociocognitive"** stance, in which they discussed environmental cues, social expectations, and motivation as key factors for an individual's undergoing hypnosis. The importance of "role," the focus on performance, and expectations were seen as the powers behind hypnosis. As can be seen by this brief history, the debate has, and continues to center around these two camps.

III. Proposed Mechanisms

There is no consensus on how hypnosis works. The psychological debate continues as outlined above between the dissociation/neodissociation theorists and the sociocognitive theorists. **Whether hypnosis involves an altered state of consciousness or is simply an intense form of role play has been debated.** Hypnosis is viewed by most as idiosyncratic to the individual in a given environmental setting; the ability of subjects to imagine, dissociate, or comply are key to their experience. Indeed, it may be that simpler tasks are due to suggestion and role-play, whereas more complex negative hallucinations, such as ignoring pain, probably involve dissociation or a combination of the two.

As intimated above, it is important to note that **not all subjects are hypnotizable. Levels of hypnotizability tend to fall on a bell-shaped curve.** Several scales have been developed to test hypnotizability (e.g., the **Stanford Hypnotic Susceptibility Scale: Form C** for research use, and the Stanford Hypnotic Clinical Scale for clinical use). A separate measure of subject hypnotic depth is assessed on a numerical scale. Some believe that they can guess a subject's hypnotizability from their capacity for focused attention or creativity. Symptomatic improvement does not require high levels of hypnotizability. The technique should, however, be shaped to the subject's need and cognitive style.

Multiple observations have been made regarding subjects who undergo hypnosis, **including changes in heart rate, respiratory rhythm, muscle tension, blood pressure, and oxygen consumption,** finding them similar to those that occur in other meditative techniques. Changes on the electroencephalogram (EEG) and in the event-related brain potential (ERP) in the cortex have been recorded. In general, it is unclear what can be made of these observations. It is unclear if these are a consequence of the hypnotic state, or are specific to the arousal, or to the cognitive ability, of subjects.

IV. Applications

There is general agreement that hypnosis is an effective intervention in several areas of medicine, including psychiatry. However, the literature is inconsistent in terms of methodology, scope, and focus. Most clinicians ultimately agree that hypnosis should be used as an adjunctive technique in most situations rather than as the sole therapy. **Some of the more widely used and better studied applications of hypnosis are in the areas of pain, asthma, nausea and vomiting, surgical preparation and procedures, eating disorders, phobic disorders, smoking cessation, habit disorders, and wart removal.** This is by no means an exhaustive list. Forensic uses, such as retrieval of memory, have been highly controversial since memory production is notably inaccurate and subject to subtle influences of the hypnotist.

A. Pain

Pain, one of the most common complaints in primary care and general hospital settings, has a strong psychological component. Several studies have indicated that hypnotic suggestions for analgesia can change the relationship between the degree of noxious stimulation received and the pain reported. In addition, for some patients, hypnosis can help control physiological parameters, such as heart rate and blood pressure, associated with pain. When highly hypnotizable patients are tested, they respond best. Neodissociation theorists would argue that the hypnotized subject's brain blocks out information regarding painful stimuli, and makes it unavailable to consciousness; thus it is capable of being ignored.

Children, often the subjects for pain control studies, have been good candidates for hypnosis, likely due to their ability to imagine and to suspend belief. Adult patients under hypnosis have been more tolerant of anxiety and pain in association with cancer, bone marrow transplantation, colonoscopy, angioplasty, wound debridement, arthritis, interventional radiography, dental procedures, and other conditions.

An area of medicine in which hypnosis has been used widely is the treatment of burn patients, especially where pain is associated with the debridement process.

B. Asthma

Anxious asthmatics often overuse their medications and medical services. Since several studies have shown that respiratory symptoms can be produced with non bronchoconstricting agents, and that some patients who are known to be reactive to a bronchoconstricting drug develop bronchospasm, clinical studies employed hypnosis. It was found to be superior to relaxation training alone and to medication control in the reduction of symptoms and medication usage.

C. Nausea and Vomiting

Hypnosis has also been studied in the treatment of nausea and vomiting following surgical procedures, in anticipatory nausea and vomiting associated with cancer medications, and in hyperemesis gravidarum.

D. Surgical Preparation and Procedures

Most patients experience moderate to high anxiety while awaiting surgery. Anxiety can interfere with the success of surgery by impairing post-operative mobilization, nutrition, and adherence. Patients treated with hypnosis prior to surgery had diminished anxiety, and required less anesthesia during the procedure, as shown in several studies. Hypnosis has also been useful for those who cannot have local anesthesia due to an allergic response to the anesthesia itself.

E. Habit Disorders

Hypnosis has often been used in the treatment of habit disorders (e.g., smoking, and compulsive overeating). The results for smoking cessation (20% abstinence rates at 1 year) are no better than are attained with other nonspecific techniques. Weight reduction with hypnosis often fails, or proves transient. It has been said that forcing a reluctant patient to change his or her behavior is no more possible for the hypnotist than it is for the physician, the psychotherapist, or a family member.

F. Other Non-Psychiatric Applications

Hypnosis has been used in gastrointestinal procedures, to allay anxiety, as well as with sufferers of irritable bowel syndrome. Obstetric studies indicate that hypnosis may decrease the time of stage 1 labor. Since there is an obvious similarity between the Lamaze method and hypnosis, this may be a technique employed more often in the future. Research on hypnosis in the field of infection and immunity has led to some interesting findings, such as the effective treatment of warts. Cardiac patients have focused much energy on relaxation techniques and their effectiveness in reducing stress and decreasing cardiac events. However, studies using hypnosis in this population are lacking.

G. Psychiatric Applications

Bulimic patients have been noted to be highly hypnotizable, compared with anorectics. It is unclear whether hypnosis will be useful in this population. Hypnosis has been used in the treatment of phobic disorders as sole therapy, and as an adjunct to cognitive-behavioral therapy. In forensic psychiatry cases, hypnosis has been used in the retrieval of memories; its value is controversial. Most believe that hypnosis is poor at uncovering memories or as an adjunct to psychodynamic work.

H. Research Applications

Hypnosis is also useful as a tool for neuroimaging and research in cognitive neuroscience.

I. Contraindications

The primary contraindication to hypnosis is paranoia; not only are these subjects unwilling to participate, for obvious reasons, but, if a suggestion were made, the patient may forever blame the hypnotist for its presence.

V. Research Findings

Multiple randomized controlled trials have found hypnosis to be a proven, effective treatment for clinical pain (including cancer pain), surgical preparation and recovery, and as an adjunct to cognitive-behavioral treatments (particularly for obesity). In addition, single randomized controlled trials have found evidence for the effectiveness of hypnosis in irritable bowel syndrome and asthma. Higher levels of hypnotic ability (as measured by the Stanford hypnotic scales) are predictive of positive outcome in the hypnotic treatment of asthma, acute and chronic pain, stress-related immunosuppression, and anxiety.

VI. Typical Hypnotic Inductions

It is noteworthy that there is no standard induction of hypnosis: it can be done with an individual or a group; in a hospital setting or on a stage; the amount of time can vary; suggestions can be direct or indirect; inductions can be through verbal or non-verbal (prop, e.g., pendulum) means; and there are many different formulations using imagery, counting, breathing, or combinations of these and others. A typical induction might begin by making sure the subject is comfortable, then having them roll their eyes up and focus on a point above them; asking them to take slow, deep breaths, have them think of their eyelids as getting heavy, then closing, continuing to reinforce relaxation and blowing off tension. At this point, one may ask the subject to imagine a pleasant scene and experience it with as many senses as possible. By raising a hand the subject can indicate they have reached this stage. Using counting (from one to ten, say), the hypnotist can suggest an even deeper state of relaxation, having the subject imagine muscle groups sequentially relaxing. At this point, the hypnotist might indicate that he/she will count to five and the session will end, but that first he/she will give some helpful suggestions. The hypnotist might say that the subject can relax in the future by following this same technique; they will have improved well-being; or other suggestions. The hypnotist may then count of five and have the subject open their eyes, concluding the session.

VII. Conclusions

Hypnosis is a powerful tool, used adjunctively and sometimes solely, for the treatment of a wide variety of medical disorders. It appears that **two types of clinical disorders respond best: those associated with the autonomic nervous system (e.g., anxiety, pain, asthma, possibly irritable bowel), and those related to the principles of classical or operant conditioning (e.g., phobias, nausea, vomiting, and bulimia).** People who are very skilled in hypnosis have found it to be useful in a third class of patients, namely those with dissociative disorders (e.g., multiple personality disorders, and post-traumatic syndromes). Many patients (e.g., those with monosymptomatic phobias) seem to have higher levels of hypnotizability that may contribute to the acquisition and maintenance of their disorder, but conceivably could also be used to cure them.

Physicians have often been wary of using hypnosis in their daily practice. Through exposure and experience to the technique, this could change; if nothing else, it would simply increase physician awareness to the role of suggestion in health care.

Suggested Readings

Benson, H., Frankel, F.H., Apfel, R., et al. (1978). Treatment of anxiety: A comparison of the usefulness of self-hypnosis and a meditational relaxation technique. An overview. *Psychotherapy Psychosomatic, 30*(3–4), 229–242.

Covino, N.A., & Frankel, F.H. (1998). Clinical hypnosis. Personal communication.

Covino, N.A., & Frankel, F.H. (1993). Hypnosis and relaxation in the medically ill. *Psychotherapy Psychosomatic, 60,* 75–90.

Ewer, T.C., & Stewart, D.E. (1986). Improvement in bronchial hyperresponsiveness in patients with moderate asthma after treatment with a hypnotic technique: A randomised controlled trial. *British Medical Journal (Clinical Research Edition), 293*(6555), 1129–1132.

Forbes, A., MacAuley, S., & Chiotakakou-Faliakou, E. (2000). Hypnotherapy and therapeutic audiotape: Effective in previously unsuccessfully treated irritable bowel syndrome? *International Journal of Colorectal Disease, 15*(5–6), 328–334.

Frankel, F.H. (1987). Significant developments in medical hypnosis during the past 25 years. *International Journal of Clinical Experimental Hypnosis, 35,* 231–248.

Fredericks, L.E. (2000). *The use of hypnosis in surgery and anesthesiology: Psychological preparation of the surgical patient.* Springfield, IL: Charles C Thomas, Ltd.

Gruzelier, J.H. (2002). A review of the impact of hypnosis, relaxation, guided imagery and individual differences on aspects of immunity and health. *Stress, 5*(2), 147–163.

Hilgard, E.R., Hilgard, J.R. (1975). *Hypnosis in the relief of pain.* William Kaufmann.

Kirsch, I., Montgomery, G., & Sapirstein, G. (1995). Hypnosis as an adjunct to cognitive-behavioral psychotherapy: A meta-analysis. *Journal of Consulting Clinical Psychologists, 63* (2), 214–220.

Montgomery, G.H., David, D., Winkel, G., et al. (2002). The effectiveness of adjunctive hypnosis with surgical patients: A meta-analysis. *Anesthesia Analgesia, 94*(6), 1639–1645.

Montgomery, G.H., DuHamel, K.N., & Redd, W.H. (2000). A meta-analysis of hypnotically induced analgesia: How effective is hypnosis? *International Journal of Clinical Experimental Hypnosis, 48*(2), 138–153.

Orne, M.T. (1959). The nature of hypnosis: Artifact and essence. *Journal of Abnormal Social Psychology, 58,* 277–299.

Petrovic, P., Kalso, E., Peterson, K.M., & Ingvar, M. (2002). Placebo and opioid analgesia: Imaging a shared neuronal network. *Science, 295,* 1737–1740.

Raz, A., & Shapiro, T. (2002). Hypnosis and neuroscience: A cross talk between clinical and cognitive research. *Archives of General Psychiatry, 59,* 85–92.

Riskin, J.D., Frankel, F.H. (1994). A history of medical hypnosis. *Psychiatric Clinics of North America, 17*(3), 601–609.

Sellick, S.M., & Zaza, C. (1998). Critical review of 5 nonpharmacologic strategies for managing cancer pain. *Cancer Prevention and Control, 2*(1), 7–14.

Spanos, N.P., Radtke-Bodorik, H.L., Ferguson, J.D., & Jones, B. (1979). The effects of hypnotic susceptibility, suggestions for analgesia, and the utilization of cognitive strategies on the reduction of pain. *Journal of Abnormal Psychology, 88*(3), 282–292.

Spanos, N.P., Stenstrom, M.A., & Johnston, J.C. (1988). Hypnosis, placebo, and suggestion in the treatment of warts. *Psychosomatic Medicine, 50,* 245–260.

Surman, O.S. (1979). Postnoxious desensitization: Some clinical notes on the combined use of hypnosis and systematic desensitization. *American Journal of Clinical Hypnosis, 22,* 54–60.

Surman, O.S., Gottlieb, S.K., Hackett, T.P., & Silverberg, E.L. (1973). Hypnosis in the treatment of warts. *Archives of General Psychiatry, 28,* 439–441.

Weitzenhoffer, M., & Hilgard, E.R. (1962). *Stanford Hypnotic Susceptibility Scale: Form C.* Palo Alto, CA: Consulting Psychologist's Press.

Chapter 65

Geriatric Psychiatry

M. CORNELIA CREMENS, LEE E. GOLDSTEIN, AND GARY L. GOTTLIEB

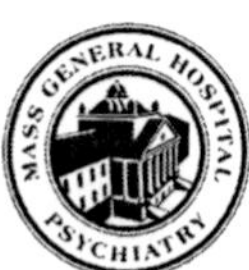

I. Introduction

The elderly population is increasing rapidly; coinciding with this increase is a population that requires greater attention to psychiatric and neuropsychiatric problems.

II. Metabolic Changes Associated with Aging

Determining the appropriate medication in older patients is a complex task.

A. Altered Pharmacokinetics

1. **Hepatic function** in the elderly is **decreased** due to reduced blood flow and cardiac output that results in a lessened first-pass effect. In addition, enzyme activity is reduced; demethylation and hydroxylation are notably effected.
2. **Absorption is decreased** due to reductions in gastric blood flow, acidity, motility, and effective surface area.
3. **Renal excretion is delayed** due to reductions in glomerular filtration rate, tubular excretion, and blood flow.
4. **Protein-binding and albumin levels are diminished.**
5. **The volume of distribution is increased** due to reductions in muscle mass, total body water, and cardiac output. Total body fat increases relative to total body weight; therefore, lipophilic drugs will be diluted due to a greater distribution in peripheral tissues.

B. Central Nervous System (CNS) Changes Associated with Aging

The brain compensates remarkably well for neuronal loss and functional decline. There is **significant age-related loss in neurons, enzymes, neurotransmitters, and receptors, as well as dendritic arborization, and compensatory dendritic proliferation.**

1. **Significant age-related loss of brain-differentiated neurons is permanent;** these cells neither divide nor proliferate; glial cells, however, can divide.
2. Dendritic arborization and compensatory proliferation allow neuronal pathways to maintain contact with other cells despite neuronal loss.
3. **Neurotransmitters and enzymes levels change with age; monoamine oxidase is increased, while acetylcholine and dopamine are decreased.**
4. With advancing age, **receptors decrease in number and increase in their resistance to drug diffusion.**
5. Approximately 10–60% of neuronal cell loss normally occurs in the neocortex, the cerebellum, and the hippocampus; less loss occurs in sub-cortical areas (with the exception of the locus coeruleus). This loss usually does not affect ordinary functions of living or occupational status until after the age of 75 years.

III. Evaluation of the Older Patient

Illnesses often present atypically in older patients; vague complaints, falls, cognitive deficits, functional losses, and behavioral changes are common. Patients often become tolerant of their symptoms and accept discomfort as a function of aging. Physicians contribute to this myth and poorly document atypical findings, thereby missing the diagnosis.

The evaluation begins with observation of the patient as he or she enters the room. The patient's presentation, interaction with the family, and the approach to the physician are critical to the assessment.

A. Conduct a psychiatric assessment that targets affect, behavior, and cognition.

1. **Screening tools can assess cognition.**
   a. The most frequently used screen is the **mini-mental state exam** (MMSE) developed by Folstein and associates (1975).
      i. It is quick and can be easily incorporated into the evaluation process.
      ii. The MMSE is only a screen; it does not fully address the full range of complex neuropsychiatric deficits that can be present.
   b. Other tools currently available may give a more complete picture.
2. **Symptoms of disordered mood and affect** are often subtle in the elderly.
   a. **Sleep** can be increased or decreased.
   b. **Interests** may be decreased.
   c. **Guilt** is often prominent, as are ruminations.
   d. **Energy** may be reduced.
   e. **Concentration** ability may be impaired.
   f. Loss of **appetite** and weight can occur and be harbingers of dementia, depression, or medical illness.
   g. **Psychomotor agitation or retardation** often occurs and can be confused with the manifestations of neurological illnesses, such as Parkinson's disease.
   h. **Suicide** is common in the elderly, with the peak among women between 50 and 65 years old and between 80 and 90 years old in men.
      i. One of every nine suicide attempts in the elderly results in death.
      ii. The risk of suicide in those over the age of 65 years is double that of the U.S. population at large.
      iii. Statistics tend to report suicide following self-inflicted acts and not passive suicides; therefore, suicide in the elderly is probably under-reported.

iv. Predictors of suicide risk include: advanced age; male sex; being separated, isolated, or divorced; having a debilitating illness; and abusing alcohol.

3. **Psychosis (with hallucinations, paranoia, or delusions) is common** in elders with psychiatric disorders.
   a. Hallucinations (visual, auditory, olfactory, gustatory, and tactile) are present in a variety of illnesses, not just psychiatric conditions.
   b. Delirium is highly prevalent in this population.

B. Carry Out a Functional Assessment

1. **Assess activities of daily living** (ADLs) and determine if the patient is capable of transferring independently, dressing him- or herself, bathing and maintaining hygiene, feeding him- or herself, toiletting and using the bathroom, and maintaining bladder and bowel continence.
2. **Assess instrumental activities of daily living** (IADLs), and determine if the patient can live independently, shop for food, cook meals, use the telephone, do light housekeeping, manage medications, handle finances, and arrange transportation.

C. Obtain a complete medical history, and review the medical records. Ask the family to summarize the history of the patient's function over the past several years; if possible have them provide a written summary.

1. Document the history.
2. Perform a mental status examination.
3. Conduct a thorough physical examination, and review the records from the primary care physician (PCP).
4. Conduct a neurological examination.
5. Order an appropriate imaging study (computed tomography [CT] or magnetic resonance imaging [MRI]) if indicated by the history.
6. Obtain an electroencephalogram (EEG) if indicated by the history.
7. Order laboratory tests, after a complete review of records and an evaluation of the patient.

D. Carefully assess the living situation; determine if the:

1. **Patient lives alone,** and is **safe at home.**
2. Patient **lives with the family.**
3. Patient **is dependent on the family.**
4. Patient's **family depends on the elder** for money or other financial benefits.

IV. Depression in the Elderly

A. Diagnosis

The diagnosis of depression in the elderly is **not difficult to make,** but often it is overlooked due to impaired cognition, sadness, and confusion, and to a general decline in function or to a failure to thrive. In addition, medical and neurological complications and side effects of medications can obscure the appropriate diagnosis of any psychiatric illness (see Table 65-1).

B. Impact of Depression

Depression **lowers life-expectancy** in the elderly. **Suicide rates are higher** in the elderly; only 25% of all suicides in the elderly are reported. The suicide rate for white men over the age of 65 is five times greater than that for the general population. Rates increase as isolation increases. Risk factors for suicide are old age; being white male, single, recently widowed, or alcoholic; and having an isolated lifestyle. Late-onset depression is associated with a higher rate of physical illness; **depression also leads to psychiatric hospitalization in half of those who are afflicted.** Approximately 30% of patients with dementia also have major depression; those with a history of stroke, Parkinson's disease, or multiple sclerosis are also vulnerable to depression.

C. Co-Morbidity

1. **Grief and loss** contribute to **depression.**
2. Nearly 60% of depressed patients have **co-morbid anxiety.**
3. Roughly **40% of anxious patients have co-morbid depression related to their medical illness** (e.g., cardiac conditions [such as myocardial infarction—MI], renal failure, cancer, endocrine disturbances, infections) and to neurologic illness (e.g., stroke, Parkinson's disease, cerebral neoplasm, and multiple sclerosis). **It is crucial to realize that undiagnosed medical illness can present as depression.**

D. Epidemiology

Epidemiological studies of the elderly **reveal a 1-month prevalence of all affective disorders of 2.5%.** Depressive

Table 65-1. Common Classes of Drugs Causing Symptoms of Depression

- Analgesics
  - Narcotics
  - NSAIDs
- Antihypertensives
- Antipsychotics
- Anxiolytics
  - Alcohol
  - Benzodiazepines
- Chemotherapeutic agents
  - Antineoplastics
- Sedative-hypnotics
- Steroids
- Diuretics
  - Thiazides
- H_2 blockers

symptomatology is recognized in 10–25% of the elderly, but it is rarely diagnosed. Women have higher rates than men of all types of depression. Major risk factors for depression in the elderly are being female and single (widowed), lacking a social network, and having stressful life events.

1. According to the Epidemiologic Catchment Area (ECA) study, 1–3% of **community elders** are diagnosed with depression.
   a. A 1-month prevalence of those over the age of 65 years revealed:
      i. Major depression is present in 0.7%.
      ii. Dysthymia occurs in 1.8%.
   b. The 6-month prevalence showed:
      i. Men met criteria for depression 0.5–2.2% of the time.
      ii. Women met criteria for depression 3.1–5% of the time.

E. Treatment of Depression in the Elderly (see Table 65-2)

Rapid assessment and treatment of depression helps prevent the onset of "failure to thrive" and progressive deterioration. Factors, such as illness, use of medications, and psychosocial problems, should be addressed, and treatment initiated.

Polypharmacy is a significant problem in the elderly. Therefore, when considering the use of medications it is important to weigh the risks and benefits while monitoring the interactions with other medications prescribed by other doctors. The addition of one new drug can disrupt the tenuous balance of an established drug regimen.

1. **Begin with a complete review of current medications** and include a review of all drugs, including over-the-counter and homeopathic remedies. Ask the patient or family members to bring all the medication bottles and over-the-counter medications.
2. **Propose an initial diagnostic formulation,** and then proceed to a medication trial. Ensure that the **trial is**

Table 65-2. Treatments Recommended for Depression in the Elderly

Drugs	*Dose Range (mg/day)*	*Comments*
Tricyclic antidepressants		
Nortriptyline	10–150	Reliable blood levels, minimal orthostasis, mildly anticholinergic
Desipramine	10–250	
Monoamine oxidase inhibitors		
Tranylcypromine	10–30	Orthostasis (may be delayed), pedal edema, weakly anticholinergic, dietary restrictions needed
Stimulants		
Dextroamphetamine	2.5–40	Agitation, mild tachycardia
Methylphenidate	2.5–60	
Selective serotonin reuptake inhibitors		
Fluoxetine	5.0–60	Akathisia, headache, agitation, gastrointestinal complaints, diarrhea/constipation
Sertraline	25–200	
Paroxetine	5–40	
Fluvoxamine	25–300	
Citalopram	5–40	
Serotonin/norepinephrine reuptake inhibitors		
Venlafaxine	25–300	Increase in systolic BP, confusion, SR formulation is better tolerated
Alpha-2 antagonist/selective serotonin		
Mirtazapine	15–30	Sedation, weight gain
Atypical antidepressants		
Trazodone	25–250	Sedation, orthostasis, incontinence, hallucinations, priapism
Nefazodone	50–600	Pedal edema, rash
Bupropion	75–450	Seizures, less mania/cycling, headache, nausea

time-limited, with clearly identified target symptoms. **Re-evaluate frequently** and give an adequate trial prior to discontinuing a drug. **Avoid drug-drug effects** if possible.

a. **Start with lowest dose possible of a medication and increase it slowly.** In frail, medically ill, or old-old, "start lower, go slower" as age increases.
   i. In the medically ill patient over the age of 80 years, begin with even lower doses and increase them less frequently.
   ii. When side effects appear, discontinue the drug; remember that the elimination half-life is longer and can complicate the effects caused by the addition of a second drug.

b. **Medications for depression**
   i. Evaluate the side-effect profile of a drug and use it advantageously—e.g., induce sedation in a patient with insomnia or weight gain in a patient with significant weight loss.
   ii. Begin one drug at a time, and change one element at a time.
   iii. Treat aggressively when psychosis and suicide are prominent; if depression is life-threatening, consider hospitalization and use of electroconvulsive therapy (ECT).

3. **Re-evaluate** after initiation of a therapeutic trial.
   a. **When symptoms resolve, continue them at the effective dose for at least one year before considering discontinuation of the medication.**
      i. If symptoms have partially resolved, continue the prescription and increase the dose, or add an adjunctive medication to boost the initial response.
      ii. If there is no response, start another medication, possibly even one within the same class.
      iii. Adjunctive medications can be considered if an initial response was noted.
   b. **The question inevitably arises as to when a medication can be discontinued;** remember that the risk of relapse and recurrence is greater in older patients and a trial period off medications may be fraught with complications.
      i. Continue medication for at least 1 year and up to 18 months after a treatment response.
      ii. If there is no contraindication, maintain the medication to prevent recurrence.

F. Psychotherapy is effective, alone or in combination, with medications.

1. Structured individual therapies can be successful alone, but are best when used in combination with medications.
2. Individual therapies include supportive, cognitive, behavioral, interpersonal, and psychodynamic strategies. All modalities have been efficacious among older patients.
3. Group therapy:
   a. Discussion about specific themes can facilitate resolution of issues that may be more difficult to identify (e.g., depression, grief, and anxiety).
   b. Support for patient and/or family may be demonstrated.
   c. Family therapy can:
      i. Deal with conflict resolution.
      ii. Gather information.
      iii. Apply family dynamics.

V. Bipolar Illness

The first onset of mania and hypomania is uncommon in the elderly; most patients with this disorder have had at least one episode earlier in their life. New-onset mania in the elderly should elicit a search for an underlying medical or neurological illness. Complicating the diagnosis of bipolar disorder is a secondary mania due to a medical condition or neurological disorder.

VI. Anxiety

Anxiety is frequently diagnosed in older patients, and symptoms of anxiety are present in 10–20% of older patients. The prevalence is higher in women than in men with a 1-month prevalence of 6.8% in women and 3.6% in men. Anxiety and depression are often associated with physical illness and may present prior to the diagnosis of medical illness. Symptoms of anxiety include worry, fear, apprehension, concern, and foreboding; in addition, there can be somatic complaints of tachycardia, sweating, abdominal distress, and dizziness. **Worries, fears, and concerns tend to center on financial issues, illness, loneliness, dependency, and dementia.** Substances (such as caffeine, ephedrine, and stimulants), can precipitate anxiety in the elderly. Withdrawal from benzodiazepines, alcohol, and barbiturates can resemble anxiety and require aggressive treatment.

Treatment of anxiety in the elderly is similar for younger patients (i.e., with **medications** and/or therapy). **Recently, cognitive-behavioral therapies** have been incorporated more often to avoid the side effects of medications. Benzodiazepines have been used extensively for decades, and judicious use of these medications is effective. However, complications of long-term use of benzodiazepines include daytime somnolence, confusion or cognitive impairment, an unsteady stance or gait, paradoxical effects, memory disturbance, withdrawal, abuse, dependence, and respiratory compromise.

VII. Dementia

Dementia is the most common syndrome of cognitive impairment or decline in the elderly. Dementia involves a chronic and substantial decline in more than two areas of cognitive functioning.

A. Age-associated memory impairment (AAMI) or age-related cognitive decline is common in the elderly.

1. Although patients and family members worry that symptoms of AAMI may be a harbinger of dementia,

these individuals tend not to develop dementia after many years.

a. **Establishing a baseline of cognitive impairments is of benefit** for two reasons.
   i. Future testing will be compared with the original presentation to assess deterioration that has occurred.
   ii. One can strategize and find useful tools to enhance weaker areas and to provide for safety.
b. **Provide for safety when any memory disorder is present.**

B. Dementia tends to present with a chronic persistent decline, albeit subtle, over years. Most dementias have an insidious and progressive course. Of the approximately 4 million patients occupying half the nursing home beds in the United States, approximately 7% carry the diagnosis of Alzheimer's disease (AD).

1. Mild cognitive impairment (MCI) was initially defined as an isolated memory impairment; it was thought to be related to normal aging and not to be progressive. However, recent research reveals that MCI may be a precursor to other dementias. The prevalence of MCI is thought to be double that of Alzheimer's disease as reported in studies of CIND (cognitive impairment, no dementia).
2. **Alzheimer's disease (AD) is a diagnosis that is ultimately made at autopsy.** AD is a clinical syndrome that reflects the rate of amyloid-associated cell death and dysfunction. Abnormal amyloid precursor proteins accumulate and stimulate inflammation; oxidation and tau protein hyperphosphorylation results in cell death. Neurotransmitters abnormalities involved in AD are related to the various nuclei affected by the disease. In the nucleus basalis of Meynert, there is a cholinergic deficit that results in memory loss, poor cognition, apathy, behavioral changes, and hallucinations. In the locus coeruleus, there is a deficit in norepinephrine that leads to disturbed mood. In the raphe nuclei, there is a deficit in serotonin with resultant depression and psychosis.

   The basic criteria for a clinical diagnosis of probable AD are outlined in the NINCDS-ADRDA criteria. **The course is slow; over time there is worsening memory and a decline of other cognitive functions with a clear consciousness.** All other reversible causes are ruled out, and a complete neurological evaluation is essential.

   a. A brief synopsis of the **stages of decline** includes:
      i. No cognitive decline
      ii. Very mild
      iii. Mild, and others now aware of deficits
      iv. Moderate (with clear deficits); the patient may get lost
      v. Moderately severe; requires assistance and reorientation
      vi. Severe; unaware, apathetic, agitated, abulic, violent, with a sketchy memory of the past and marked personality change

Table 65-3. Antipsychotics Commonly Used in the Elderly

Drug/Dose	*Sedation*	*Anticholinergic Potency*	*Extrapyramidal Symptoms (Risk)*	*Equivalency (mg)*
Typical antipsychotics				
Low potency				
Thioridazine (Mellaril) 10–50 mg	High	High	Low	95
Intermediate potency				
Perphenazine (Trilafon) 0.5–5 mg	Medium	Medium	Medium	8
High potency				
Haloperidol (Haldol) 0.25–2 mg	Low	Low	High	2
Thiothixene (Navane) 0.5–4 mg	Low	Low	High	5
Fluphenazine (Prolixin) 0.5–2 mg	Low	Low	High	2
Atypical antipsychotics				
Clozapine (Clozaril) 12.5–300 mg	High	High	Very low	100
Risperidone (Risperdal) 0.5–3 mg	Low	Low	Low-moderate	1–2
Olanzapine (Zyprexa) 2.5–10.0 mg	Moderate	Moderate	Low-moderate	
Quetiapine (Seroquel) 12.5–300 mg	High	Low	Low	
Ziprasidone (Geodon) 20–80 mg	Low	Low	Low	
Aripiprazole (Abilify) 2.0-15.0 mg	Low	Low	Low	

vii. Very severe; unable to communicate, incontinent, with focal neurological signs, needs assistance most of the time

3. **Lewy body disease** (LBD) is often confused with AD; it can complicate the use of medications. **Patients with LBD have more hallucinations and a greater sensitivity to the side effects of neuroleptic medications** than do AD patients (Table 65-3). LBD is characterized by widespread distribution of Lewy bodies in the brainstem, basal forebrain, and cortex.
   a. It is reported to be a fairly common form of degenerative dementia.
   b. it is characterized by fluctuations in cognitive impairment, by transient episodes of marked confusion, by prominent behavioral changes, and by a high incidence of visual/auditory hallucinations and delusions.
   c. Extrapyramidal signs are present as is an exquisite sensitivity to neuroleptic medication.
4. **Frontal lobe dementia** (FLD) manifests prominent symptoms of **disinhibition, self-neglect, and self-destructiveness;** patients are often **unaware or are unconcerned** that any problem or deficit exists. This is often referred to as "Pick's disease."
5. **Vascular dementia usually presents with a stuttering course;** the losses are more focal in the territory of the damage.
6. **Alcoholic dementia** gradually damages the area of the dorsal inferior frontal lobe with symptoms similar to those seen with frontal lobe lesions. When alcohol use is stopped, cognitive losses should stabilize.

C. Medications Used to Slow Cognitive Deterioration (Table 65-4)

Cholinesterase inhibitors are used most frequently to treat the cognitive disturbances in Alzheimer's patients. Recent studies have shown benefit in vascular dementia, as well as other dementias especially with regard to behavioral disturbances. Patients are often less apathetic and are often agitated with reduction of hallucinations.

Table 65-4. Treatments Recommended for Dementia

Drug	*Dose mg/day*	*Dosing*	*Comments*
Aricept	2.5–10	qd	GI complaints, nightmares
Exelon	1.5–12	b.i.d.	Take with meals; nausea, vomiting, and diarrhea
Reminyl	4–24	b.i.d.	Take with meals; nausea, vomiting, and diarrhea

1. Donepezil (Aricept)
2. Rivastigmine (Exelon)
3. Galantamine (Reminyl)

D. Important issues should be **discussed with the family members and caretakers;** education around diagnosis of dementia should include:

1. **Rapid changes in a patient's behavior or cognition**
   a. Consider a medical illness.
   b. Consider the side effects of medication.
2. **Incontinence**
   a. This usually presents late in the progression of the disease.
   b. Evaluate for a medical etiology.
   c. Eventually it may involve both urinary and fecal incontinence.
3. **Driving**
   a. Arrange for alternative transportation.
   b. Hide the car keys or disable the vehicle.
4. **Cooking**
   a. Only cook when supervised.
   b. Remove cabinet knobs.
   c. Turn off the gas and the electricity.
   d. Hide matches.
5. **Smoking**
   a. Smoke only under close supervision.
   b. Remove all smoking paraphernalia (e.g., ashtrays and matches).
   c. Do not smoke in front of the patient.
6. **Firearms**
   a. Remove them from the home.
   b. Keep them locked securely.
7. **Caregiver support**
   a. Day centers
   b. Help, either during the day or overnight
   c. Visiting Nurse Association
   d. Alzheimer's Association (local or national), even if not AD (Alzheimer's Association, 919 N. Michigan Ave, Suite 1000, Chicago, IL 60611; 1-800-272-3900)
   e. Education with pamphlets, books, and videotapes
   f. Support groups
   g. Legal assistance
      i. This is important early in process and prior to a crisis.
      ii. Obtain financial and estate planning.
      iii. Determine future needs and long-term care plans.

VIII. Delirium

Delirium is often under-recognized, under-reported, or inadequately documented by physicians. Signs and symptoms are documented in less than 50% of cases; 10–20% of all hospitalized patients manifest some degree of delirium.

A. Elderly patients are at high risk for delirium.

1. The elderly are at greater risk for delirium due to age-related sensitivity to medications and to co-morbid illnesses.

a. Life-threatening conditions must be treated swiftly and the underlying cause ameliorated. Medical illness is often the culprit, and medications add a second dimension to the problem.
b. Drug-induced delirium can be precipitated by any medication; close scrutiny of all medications is essential.

2. **Presentation of delirium is variable** and therefore it is difficult to diagnose and to determine its etiology accurately.
   a. Clinical features of delirium include a prodrome, a rapidly fluctuating course, a decreased attention span, an altered level of arousal, a psychomotor abnormality, a sleep-wake cycle disturbance, an impaired memory, EEG abnormalities, and affective features of intense anger, fear, sadness, rage, apathy, anxiety, or panic.
   b. **Management of delirium** is complex.
      i. **Accurate diagnosis** is paramount.
      ii. **Treatment of the underlying cause** is required.
      iii. **Elimination of contributing factors** is needed.
      iv. **Supportive care** is helpful, as is maintenance of an adequate fluid balance, nutrition, sedation, rest, comfort, good nursing care, encouragement of a family presence, frequent re-orientation, optimal stimulation, and a well-lit room; appropriate use of eyeglasses and hearing aids are also important.
      v. **Treatment** includes use of high-potency neuroleptics, with attention paid to target symptoms. **Haloperidol** has been the drug of choice, but newer atypical neuroleptics are being used more frequently (see Table 65-3). The starting dose is always the lowest possible dose. **Haloperidol, used intravenously, has the most rapid effect; start with a low dose and titrate upward.** Benzodiazepines may be synergistic with neuroleptics but can disinhibit the patient or cause paradoxical reactions.
      vi. **The course and prognosis** need to be watched carefully, as older patients are at a greater risk for death during the illness and for up to six months after recovery.

IX. Alcoholism

Alcoholism is often overlooked or is minimized in the elderly. The ECA data show that **1% of the elderly have alcoholism.** A life-long pattern of daily use can be a problem and can lead to withdrawal.

A. **Co-morbid illness** (psychiatric, neurologic, and medical) **can obscure an accurate diagnosis.**
   1. A careful history from family, friends, and caretakers is extremely important in this illness characterized by denial.

X. Acute Behavioral Problems

Patients with dementia and delirium can exhibit acute behavioral problems, such as aggression, agitation, rage, wandering, and screaming. These symptoms are difficult to treat; patients are often overmedicated, yet are never successfully relieved of these problems.

XI. Elder Abuse

Elder abuse can present subtly. Family members or caregivers may be overwhelmed. Hotlines are available in every state (in Massachusetts, 1-800-922-2275).

Suggested Readings

Aarsland, D., Larsen, J.P., Lim, N.G., & Tandberg, E. (1999). Olanzapine for psychosis in patients with Parkinson's disease with and without dementia. *Journal of Neuropsychiatry and Clinical Neuroscience, 11,* 392–394.

Alexopoulos, G.S. (1996). Affective disorders. In J. Sadavoy, L.W. Lazarus, L.F. Jarvik, & G.T. Grossberg (Eds.), *Comprehensive review of geriatric psychiatry-II* (2nd ed., pp. 536–592). Washington, DC: APA Press.

Almeida, O.P., Howard, R.J., Levy, R., & David, A.S. (1995). Psychotic states arising in late life. *British Journal of Psychiatry, 166,* 205–214.

Applegate, W.B., Blass, J.P., & Williams, T.F. (1990). Instruments for the functional assessment of older patients. *New England Journal of Medicine, 322,* 1207–1213.

Arnold, S.E. (2001). Contributions of neuropathology to understanding schizophrenia in late life. *Harvard Review of Psychiatry, 9,* 69–76.

Cattell, H., & Jolley, D.J. (1995). One hundred cases of suicide in elderly people. *British Journal of Psychiatry, 166,* 451–457.

Cummings, J.L. (2003). Alzheimer's disease: From molecular biology to neuropsychiatry. *Seminars in Clinical Neuropsychiatry, 8,* 31–36.

Cummings, J.L., Anand, R., Koumaras, B., & Hartman, R. (2000). Rivastigmine provides behavioral benefits to Alzheimer's disease patients residing in a nursing home: Findings from a 26-week trial. *Neurology, 54*(suppl 3), A468.

Davidson, M., Harvey, P., Welsh, K.A., et al. (1996). Cognitive functioning in late-life schizophrenia: A comparison of elderly schizophrenic patients and patients with Alzheimer's disease. *American Journal of Psychiatry, 153,* 1274–1279.

Devanand, D.P., Jacobs, D.M., Tang, M.X., et al. (1997). The course of psychopathologic features in mild to moderate Alzheimer's disease. *Archives of General Psychiatry, 54,* 257–263.

Drevets, W.C. (1994). Geriatric depression: Brain imaging correlates and pharmacologic considerations. *Journal of Clinical Psychiatry, 55*(suppl 9A), 71–81.

Feldman, H., Gauthier, S., Hecker, J., et al. (2001). A 24-week, randomized, double-blind study of donepezil in moderate to severe Alzheimer's disease. *Neurology, 57,* 613–620.

Fernandez, F., Levy, J.K., Lachar, B.L., & Small, G.W. (1995). The management of depression and anxiety in the elderly. *Journal of Clinical Psychiatry, 56*(suppl 2), 20–29.

Jenike, M.A. (1989). *Geriatric psychiatry and psychopharmacology: A clinical approach.* St. Louis, MO: Mosby.

Jenike, M.A., & Cremens, M.C. (1994). Geriatric psychopharmacology. *Psychiatric Clinics of North America, 1,* 125–164.

Jeste, D.V., Eastham, J.H., Larcro, J.P., et al. (1996). Management of late-life psychosis. *Journal of Clinical Psychiatry, 57*(suppl 3), 39–45.

Katz, I.R., Jeste, D.V., Mintzer, J.E., et al. (1999). Comparison of risperidone and placebo for psychosis and behavioral disturbances associated with dementia: A randomized, double-blind trial. Risperidone Study Group. *Journal of Clinical Psychiatry, 60,* 107–115.

Lebert, F., Pasquier, F., & Petit, H. (1994). Behavioral effects of trazodone in Alzheimer's disease. *Journal of Clinical Psychiatry, 55,* 536–538.

Martin, R.L. (Ed.). (1997). Geriatric psychiatry: What's new about the old. *Psychiatric Clinics of North America, 20*(1), 1–268.

McDonald, W.M., & Nemeroff, C.B. (1996). The diagnosis and treatment of mania in the elderly. *Bulletin of the Menniger Clinic, 60,* 174–196.

Mega, M.S., Masterman, D.M., O'Connor, S.M., et al. (1999). The spectrum of behavioral responses to cholinesterase inhibitor therapy in Alzheimer disease. *Archives of Neurology, 56,* 1388–1393.

Newhouse, P.A. (1996). Use of serotonin selective reuptake inhibitors in geriatric depression. *Journal of Clinical Psychiatry, 57*(suppl 5), 12–22.

NIH Consensus Conference. (1992). Diagnosis and treatment of depression in late life. *Journal of the American Medical Association, 268,* 1018–1024.

Oxman, T.E. (1996). Antidepressants and cognitive impairment in the elderly. *Journal of Clinical Psychiatry, 57*(suppl 5), 38–44.

Pande, A., Krugler, T., & Haskett, R. (1988). Predictors of response to electroconvulsive therapy in major depressive disorder. *Biological Psychiatry, 24,* 91–93.

Pollock, B.G., & Mulsant, B.H. (1998). Behavioral disturbances of dementia. *Journal of Geriatric Psychiatry and Neurology, 11,* 206–212.

Rainer, M.K., Masching, A.J., Ertl, M.G., et al. (2001). Effect of risperidone on behavioral and psychological symptoms and cognitive function in dementia. *Journal of Clinical Psychiatry, 62,* 894–900.

Rothchild, A.J. (1996). The diagnosis and treatment of late-life depression. *Journal of Clinical Psychiatry, 57*(suppl 5), 5–11.

Sadavoy, J., Lazarus, L.W., Jarvik, L.F., & Grossberg, G.T. (Eds.). (1996). *Comprehensive review of geriatric psychiatry-II* (2nd ed.). Washington, DC: APA Press.

Sano, M., Ernesto, C., Thomas, R.G., et al. (1997). A controlled trial of selegiline, alpha-tocopherol, or both as treatments for Alzheimer's disease. *New England Journal of Medicine, 336,* 1216–1222.

Shorr, R.I., & Robin, D.W. (1994). Rational use of benzodiazepines in the elderly. *Drugs Aging, 4,* 9–20.

Small, G.W., Rabins, P.V., Barry, P.P., et al. (1997). Diagnosis and treatment of Alzheimer disease and related disorders: Consensus statement of the American Association for Geriatric Psychiatry, the Alzheimer's Association, and the American Geriatrics Society. *Journal of the American Medical Association, 278,* 1363–1371.

Tariot, P.N. (1996). Treatment strategies for agitation and psychosis in dementia. *Journal of Clinical Psychiatry, 57,* 21–29.

Tariot, P.N., Solomon, P.R., Morris, J.C., et al. (2000). A 5-month, randomized, placebo-controlled trial of galantamine in AD. The Galantamine USA-10 Study Group. *Neurology, 54,* 2269–2276.

Weiss, K.J. (1994). Management of anxiety and depression syndromes in the elderly. *Journal of Clinical Psychiatry, 55*(suppl 2), 5–12.

Wilcox, S.M., Himmelstein, D.U., & Woolhandler, S. (1994). Inappropriate drug prescribing for the community-dwelling elderly. *Journal of the American Medical Association, 272,* 292–296.

Work Group on Alzheimer's Disease and Related Dementias. (1997). Practice guideline for the treatment of patients with Alzheimer's disease and other dementias of late life. *American Journal of Psychiatry, 154*(suppl), 1–39.

Young, R.C., & Klerman, G.L. (1992). Mania in late life: Focus on age of onset. *American Journal of Psychiatry, 149,* 867–876.

Zweig, R.A., & Hinrichsen, G.A. (1993). Factors associated with suicide attempts by depressed older adults: A prospective study. *American Journal of Psychiatry, 150,* 1687–1692.

Zyas, E.M., & Grossberg, G.T. (1998). The treatment of psychosis in late life. *Journal of Clinical Psychiatry, 59*(suppl), 5–10.

SECTION V

Special Topics in Psychiatry

Chapter 66

Psychiatric Epidemiology

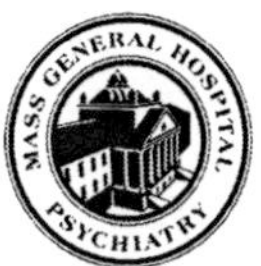

ALBERT YEUNG

I. Introduction

Epidemiology is the study of the distribution and determinants of disease frequency in human populations. It is about observing, counting, and comparing the occurrence of disease between different populations at a given time, between subgroups of a population, or between different periods of a population. Since human disease does not occur at random, systematic investigation of the relationship of disease frequency, and of the characteristics of populations, may shed light on the etiology of the disease. **By providing data on the distribution and frequency of diseases, epidemiological studies help to assess service needs in the community or in special institutions and to describe the natural history of illness.**

To achieve these goals, epidemiological observation studies are conducted with large groups of individuals. The first step is often case recognition. This is especially challenging in psychiatric epidemiology due to the absence of pathognomonic laboratory abnormalities for diagnosing psychiatric disorders.

II. Assessment

A. Case Definition

In 1972, Cooper and colleagues published the U.S./U.K. diagnostic study that demonstrated the variability of diagnosis in psychotic disorders. It highlighted the importance of having explicit operational criteria for case identification. The use of diagnostic criteria as listed in the *Diagnostic and Statistical Manual, Third Edition* (DSM-III) in 1980 represented a great step toward the advancement of the reliability and validity of psychiatric diagnosis.

B. Standardized Instruments for Case Assessment

The clinical interview is generally used to diagnose psychiatric illness. However, differences in personal styles, as well as in theoretical frameworks, may affect the process and the outcome of the psychiatric interview. **To increase inter-rater reliability, a variety of standardized instruments have been used.** The first such instrument was the **Present State Examination (PSE),** which was used in the International Pilot Study of Schizophrenia sponsored by the World Health Organization (WHO). Since the PSE was intended for use by psychiatrists or by experienced clinicians, its use in epidemiologic studies has been limited due to the high volume of subjects involved in such studies. Based on other research instruments, including **the Renald Diagnostic Interview (RDI), the St. Louis criteria, and the Schedule for Affective Disorders and Schizophrenia (SADS),** epidemiologists at the National Institute of Mental Health (NIMH) developed the **Diagnostic Interview Schedule (DIS),** a fully structured interview that could be used by non-clinicians to assess large numbers of subjects according to DSM-III criteria. The DIS has been used extensively in the United States and many other countries for surveys of psychiatric illness. The WHO and the NIMH updated and modified the DIS and developed the **Composite International Diagnostic Interview (CIDI),** which is structurally similar to the DIS and provides both ICD-10 and DSM-IV diagnoses.

C. Reliability

Reliability is the degree to which a measurement produces systematic or reproducible results. Use of explicit diagnostic criteria, a structured assessment instrument, and adequate training of raters, each enhance the reliability of making a psychiatric diagnosis. Reliability is a necessary, but not sufficient, condition for a valid diagnosis. **The kappa statistic (k) is frequently used to measure the reliability between raters** (see Table 66-1). It shows the degree of consistency between raters, with an adjustment of agreement due to chance. An important characteristic of the kappa statistic is that it is influenced by how common the particular condition is in the study sample. When the frequency of the disorder is very low, kappa statistics will be low despite having a high degree of consistency between raters. Therefore, the kappa statistic is not applicable for measuring the reliability for infrequent disorders.

$$\kappa = \frac{P_o - P_c}{1 - P_c}$$

where P_o is the observed agreement, P_c is agreement due to chance, $P_o = (a + d)/n$ and $P_c = [(a + c)(a + b) + (b + d)(c + d)]/n^2$.

D. Validity

An instrument is considered valid if the instrument measures what it is intended to measure. Rater or instrument validity of a psychiatric diagnosis is ideally done by comparison of the tested rater or instrument with a well-known standard of truth. Unfortunately, in psychiatry, there is no absolute measure of a diagnosis. A criterion instrument (rater) is usually chosen as the truth and is used for comparison with the new instrument (rater) (see Table 66-2).

Sensitivity, specificity, positive predictive power, and negative predictive power are frequently used to express the validity of an instrument. Sensitivity is a

Table 66-1. Inter-Rater Reliability

	Rater A		
Rater B	*Disorder Present*	*Disorder Absent*	*Total*
Disorder present	*a*	*b*	*a* + *b*
Disorder absent	*c*	*d*	*c* + *d*
Total	*a* + *c*	*b* + *d*	*n*

measure of the new instrument's ability to detect the true cases of a disorder identified by the criterion instrument. Specificity is a measure of the new instrument's ability to identify the true non-cases identified by the criterion instrument. Higher values of sensitivity and specificity are always desirable. For a given instrument, higher sensitivity is obtained by lowering specificity and vice versa. The only way to improve both sensitivity and specificity without a trade-off is to improve the instrument itself. **Positive predictive power** is the proportion of apparent cases, as detected by the new instrument, that are true cases as determined by the criterion instrument. **Negative predictive power** is the proportion of apparent non-cases, as detected by the new instrument, that are true non-cases as determined by the criterion instrument.

- Sensitivity = $a/(a + c)$
- Specificity = $d/(b + d)$
- Positive predictive rate = $a/(a + b)$
- Negative predictive rate = $d/(c + d)$

III. Measurement of Disease Frequency

A. Prevalence

Prevalence is the proportion of individuals in a population who have a disease at a specific instant; it provides an estimate of the probability that an individual will be ill at any point. Prevalence is determined by the rate at which the disease develops and by the duration of the disease. That is, with the same rate of development, a chronic disease will have a higher prevalence than an acute one. Prevalence rate is more useful for descriptive purposes. It was used to describe the frequency of an illness in a community population. In addition, it reflects service needs:

$$P = \frac{\text{Number of existing cases of disease at a given point in time}}{\text{Total population}}$$

B. Incidence

Incidence quantifies the number of new events or cases of a disease that develop in a population of individuals at risk during a specified time interval. There are two specific types of incidence measures: cumulative incidence and incidence rate. **Cumulative incidence (CI) is the proportion of people who become diseased during a specified period. It is calculated by the equation:**

$$\text{CI} = \frac{\text{Number of new cases of a disease during a given period}}{\text{Total population at risk}}$$

In real life, some people enter a study at different times; others may become lost during the study and no longer available for follow-up. When a person in the study becomes a case, they stop being at risk and no longer contribute to the denominator. **To account for the variable durations for which people are at risk, incidence rate (IR) is used;** this is defined as:

$$\text{IR} = \frac{\text{Number of new cases of a disease in a year}}{\text{Total person} - \text{years of observation}}$$

Table 66-2. Validity of a New Instrument

	Truth (Criterion Instrument Results)		
New Instrument	*Disorder Present*	*Disorder Absent*	*Total*
Disorder present	*a*	*b*	*a* + *b*
Disorder absent	*c*	*d*	*c* + *d*
Total	*a* + *c*	*b* + *d*	*n*

For example, 100 subjects were studied, 2 were lost to follow-up at the end of 6 months, and 8 developed a disease at the end of the sixth month; 90 subjects were disease-free at the end of 1 year. The person-years of observation was (90 × 1 year) + (2 × 0.5 year) + (8 × 0.5 year) = 95 person-years, and IR = (8 persons)/(95 person-years) = 8.42/100 person-years of observation.

Incidence rates are more difficult to calculate than prevalence rates, and require more extensive data collection. Unlike prevalence rates, incidence rates are not affected by the duration of the disease. The incidence rate is more precise when measuring disease rate; it is useful in analytical studies of effects of risk factors.

C. Period Prevalence

The period prevalence rate is used to summarize the number of cases of a disorder that exist at any time during a specified time period. Its numerator includes any existing cases at the start of the period plus any new cases that develop during the time period. For a 1-year period, the annual period prevalence rate is approximately equal to the point prevalence rate [(existing cases)/(population at the start)] plus the annual cumulative incidence rate [(new cases in a year)/(population at risk)].

D. Lifetime Prevalence

The lifetime prevalence rate is a measure of persons considered at a point in time who have ever had the illness under study. It is a useful statistic to describe conditions that remit but often recur, such as major depressive disorder.

IV. Study Designs

A. Descriptive Studies

Descriptive studies describe patterns of disease occurrence in relation to selected variables (e.g., person, place, and time). They utilize census data, vital statistic records, and clinical records from hospitals, or national figures on consumption of goods, oil, or other products. There are **three main types of descriptive studies: correlation studies, case reports or case series, and cross-sectional surveys of individuals.** Data from descriptive studies are useful for public health administrators who plan for health care utilization and resource allocation. They are also valuable for formulation of etiologic hypotheses. However, **descriptive studies in general cannot be used for testing etiologic hypotheses. For hypothesis testing, analytic design strategies (cohort, case-control, or intervention study) are needed.**

B. Cohort Studies

In cohort studies, or follow-up studies, a group of individuals (cohort) is defined on the basis of the presence or absence of exposure to a suspected risk factor for a disease. The rates at which they develop a certain disease or an outcome of interest are measured and compared. By nature of the design, individuals in such a study need to be disease-free at the start of the study. For a prospective cohort study, individuals are followed for a specified period, and their outcome is compared. For a retrospective cohort study, information on risk factors is obtained from records collected in the past at the actual time of the exposure, and the information on disease status is obtained at the time of the study.

Relative risk (RR) is calculated to test for the possible association between exposure and outcome (disease). If the relative risk is greater than 1.0, the exposure is considered to be associated with the disease (see Table 66-3).

$$RR = \frac{a/(a+b)}{c/(c+d)}$$

C. Case-Control Studies

Subjects in case-control studies are selected on the basis of whether they do (cases) or do not (controls) have a particular disease under study. The groups are compared with respect to their proportions of having certain risk factors of interest. A case-control design is usually used for studying rare disorders. **Instead of relative risk, an odds ratio is calculated to detect an association between the risk factor and the disease. If the odds ratio is greater than 1.0, the risk factor is considered to be associated with caseness (see Table 66-3).**

$$\text{Odds ratio} = \frac{ad}{bc}$$

D. Intervention Studies

In an intervention study, the investigator controls the allocation of subjects to different comparison groups and regulates the experimental conditions of each

Table 66-3. Association Between Risk Factors and Disease in Cohort and Case-Control Studies

	New Cases	*Non-Cases*	*Total*
Risk factor present	a	b	$a + b$
Risk factor not present	c	d	$c + d$
Total	$a + c$	$b + d$	$a + b + c + d$

group. Study subjects are randomly assigned to comparison groups and followed over time to observe the outcome (e.g., decreased disease frequency or improved clinical condition, of the intervention). Clinical trials are the most common form of intervention studies. To ensure the comparability between groups and to obtain valid results, intervention studies employ three basic research strategies: randomization, placebo-control, and blinding.

E. The National Co-morbidity Survey (NCS)

1. **Overview. The NCS was the first nationally representative mental health survey in the United States to use a fully structured research diagnostic interview to assess the prevalences and correlates of the DSM-III-R disorders.** It samples widely dispersed subjects that were representative of all people living in households in the continental United States. The survey was done by administering a face-to-face structured diagnostic interview using a modified version of the Composite International Diagnostic Interview (CIDI), a state-of-the art structured diagnostic interview based on the Diagnostic Interview Schedule (DIS) (Robins et al., 1991). Previous validation studies have shown that patients with non-affective psychosis may not be able to report information accurately. In the NCS, respondents with any evidence of schizophrenia or other non-affective psychoses were reinterviewed by experienced clinicians using the Structured Clinical Interview for DSM-III-R, and their diagnoses were based on clinical interviews.

2. **Results. Data from the NCS revealed that the most common disorders are major depression and alcohol dependence.** The next most common disorders are social and simple phobias. As a group, substance use disorders and anxiety disorders are somewhat more prevalent than affective disorders, with approximately one in every four respondents reporting a lifetime substance use disorder and a similar number a lifetime anxiety disorder. Approximately one in every five respondents reported a lifetime affective disorder. The prevalences of other NCS disorders are considerably lower (Table 66-4).

   About one-half of adults in the United States report symptoms that meet criteria for one or more psychiatric disorders during their lifetime. About 30% had at least one disorder in the 12 months prior to the interview. While there is no meaningful gender difference in the overall prevalences of NCS disorders, men were much more likely to have substance use disorders and antisocial personality disorder than women, and women were much more likely to have anxiety disorders and affective disorders than men (with the exception of mania, for which there is no sex difference). The data also show that women in the household population are more likely than men to have non-affective psychosis. One remarkable finding is that most psychiatric disorders have first onsets quite early in life, raising the public health importance of early recognition and treatment of these disorders to prevent protracted courses of the disorders.

Table 66-4. Prevalence Estimates (%) for Specific Disorders

	Lifetime (%)	*12-month (%)*
Major depression	17.1	10.3
Mania	1.6	1.3
Dysthymia	6.4	2.5
Generalized anxiety disorder	5.1	3.1
Panic disorder	3.5	2.3
Social phobia	13.3	7.9
Simple phobia	11.3	8.8
Agoraphobia without panic	5.3	2.8
Alcohol abuse	9.4	2.5
Alcohol dependence	14.1	7.2
Drug abuse	4.4	0.8
Drug dependence	7.5	2.8
Antisocial personality disorder	2.8	—
Non-affective psychosis[a]	0.5	0.3

SOURCE: Adopted from Tsuang, M.T., & Tohen, M. (2002). *Textbook in psychiatric epidemiology* (2nd ed.). New York: Wiley.

[a]Non-affective psychosis = schizophrenia, schizophreniform disorder, schizoaffective disorder, delusional disorder, and atypical psychosis.

V. Epidemiology of Major Psychiatric Disorders

A. Schizophrenia

Prior to the introduction of the DSM-III, the prevalence of schizophrenia was estimated to range from 1–7%. **In a review of recent studies, Jablensky (2000) placed the prevalence rate in the range of 1.4–4.6 per thousand. This downward shift is largely due to the narrowing of the criteria for schizophrenia** in nosological systems published after 1980. Genetic loading is a robust risk factor of schizophrenia (see Table 66-5). **The prevalence of schizophrenia in a monozygotic twin of a schizophrenia patient is 50%; with a dizygotic twin, it is 15%. The prevalence for a child with two schizophrenic parents is 46.3%; for a child with one schizophrenic parent, it is 12.8%.** Other risk factors of schizophrenia include being a member of a lower social class, being unmarried, having birth complications, and being born during the winter months. Studies have also shown that stressful life events, high levels of "expressed emotions" (critical and over-protective behavior and verbalizations toward the family member with schizophrenia), and substance use can precipitate psychotic episodes.

B. Bipolar I Disorder

Bipolar I disorder affects men and women equally. The NCS reported a lifetime prevalence of 1.6% for a manic episode, and a 1-year prevalence for a manic episode was 1.3%. Bipolar I disorder occurs at much higher rates in first-degree biologic relatives of persons with bipolar I disorder than it does in the general population. Family, adoption, and twin studies clearly support the evidence that **bipolar disorder is genetically transmitted.** The lifetime risks of suffering from bipolar disorder in relatives of bipolar probands are 40% to 70% in monozygotic co-twins, 5% to 10% in first-degree relatives, and 0.5% to 1.5% in non-blood-related individuals.

Table 66-5. Prevalence of Schizophrenia in Specific Populations

Population	*Prevalence (%)*
General population	0.3
First-degree relatives of parents of schizophrenic patients	5.6
Children with one schizophrenic parent	12.8
Dizygotic twins of a schizophrenia patient	15.0
Children of two schizophrenic parents	46.3
Monozygotic twins of a schizophrenic patient	50.0

C. Major Depression

Based on the NCS, the 1-year prevalence for major depressive disorder is 10.3%; the lifetime risk for major depressive disorder is 17.1%. Risk factors for major depressive disorder include being female, having a history of depressive illness in first-degree relatives, having prior episodes of major depression or other psychiatric disorders, having a two-week period of two concurrent depressive symptoms, and being divorced.

D. Panic Disorder

The NCS has reported a lifetime prevalence rate of 3.5% and 1-year prevalence rate of 2.3% for panic disorder. Women and persons under the age of 65 are at higher risk of having panic disorder. The differences among Hispanics, non-Hispanic whites, and blacks are small. The only social factor found to be related to panic disorder is a recent history of divorce or separation. Panic disorder most commonly develops in young adulthood; the mean age of presentation is about 25 years, but both panic disorder and agoraphobia can develop at any age.

E. Alcohol Abuse and Dependence

The NCS found that life prevalence rates for alcohol abuse and alcohol dependence were 9.4% and 14.1%, respectively. Yearly prevalence rates for abuse and dependence were 2.5% and 7.2%, respectively. Alcohol dependence is one of the most common psychiatric disorders. Alcoholism was correlated with male gender, younger ages, being separated or divorced, having a low educational level, and low occupational level and income.

Suggested Readings

Agency for Health Care Policy and Research. (1993). *Clinical practice guideline number 5, depression in primary care,* Vol. 1, pp. 1–41. AHCPR Publication No. 93-0551. Rockville, MD: U.S. Department of Health and Human Services.

Cooper, J.E., Kendell, R.E., Gurland, B.J., et al. (1972). *Psychiatric diagnosis in New York and London.* London: Oxford University Press.

Hennekens, C.H., & Buring, J.E. (1987). *Epidemiology in medicine,* pp. 73–100. Boston, MA: Little, Brown.

Jablensky, A. (2000). Epidemiology of schizophrenia: The global burden of disease and disability. *European Archives of Psychiatry of Clinical Neuroscience, 250,* 274–285.

Robins, L.N., Locke, B.Z., & Regier, D.A. (1991). An overview of psychiatric disorders in America. In L.N. Robins, & D.A. Regier (Eds.), *Psychiatric disorders in America,* pp. 285–308. New York: Free Press.

Tsuang, M.T., & Tohen, M. (2002). *Textbook in psychiatric epidemiology* (2nd ed., pp. 343–479). New York: Wiley.

Chapter 67

Statistics in Psychiatric Research

LEE BAER

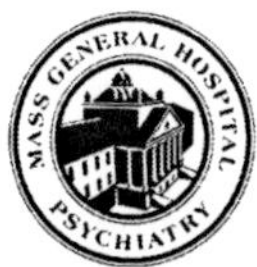

I. Introduction

There are three classes of statistics commonly used in psychiatric research.

A. First, there are statistics used to access how dependable and reproducible an **individual patient's or subject's** score is on a rating scale for a particular characteristic or symptom. These statistics usually refer to the adequacy of a **particular rating scale, diagnostic interview, or laboratory value**. The science of developing and testing the adequacy of these measures is called "psychometrics." Psychometrics of particular rating scales are generally reported in the method section of journal articles.

B. Second, there are statistics used to **describe a group of patients** or subjects on one or more characteristics or symptoms. They are called **descriptive statistics**, since they "describe" the group's distribution statistically. Descriptive statistics like the mean, standard deviation, and frequencies are generally found in the results section of journal articles, and they do not report any p-values.

C. Third, there are statistics used to **draw inferences from one or more groups for the purpose of generalizing to a larger population; they are called inferential statistics.** These commonly compare the means of two or more groups, or examine the relation between two variables within a single group. Inferential statistics are always found in the results section of a journal article and are easy to recognize, because they **always contain at least one p-value** (e.g., $P < .01$) which tells us how likely it is that the findings from our sample will generalize to a larger population.

II. Statistics Relating to an Individual's Score on Some Characteristic ("Psychometrics")

A. Theory

In psychiatry and psychology rarely can we measure directly the characteristics we are really interested in; therefore, we typically rely on a subject's score on either self-report or investigator-administered scales. **Psychometrics is concerned with** how reproducible a subject's score is (i.e., **how reliable is it?**) and how closely it measures the characteristic we are really interested in (i.e., **how valid is it?**).

B. Reliability

1. **Definition. Reliability equals dependability (i.e., the dependability of a score),** the degree to which we can be certain that a measurement can be depended on (i.e., how reproducible is the score?). **For self-rated scales,** such as paper and pencil questionnaires, since there is no rater error to take into account, **the main source of undependability to guard against is differences in the person's self-rating over time.** For example, if a patient completes a depression questionnaire at 3 P.M., how close would his or her score be on the same questionnaire if he/she were to take the same scale at 4 P.M., assuming no change in his/her depression? If the scores were identical, and this were the case for all patients, then the correlation coefficient would be a perfect 1.00 (in this case the correlation coefficient is referred to as the **"reliability coefficient"**).

   For scales or measures administered by a rater, the major question is, "Would this patient get the same score on this depression scale if Doctor A rated him, as if Doctor B rated him?" If agreement was perfect for all patients, then the reliability coefficient would be 1.00. If, on the other hand, there were a random relationship between the scores of the two raters, then the inter-rater reliability would be 0.00.

   Reliability is necessary but not sufficient for a useful scale. Thus, a scale can be perfectly reliable, but have no validity for a particular purpose. For example, every time you ask me my phone number I will give you the same answer (perfect reliability); however, if you attempt to use my phone number to predict my anxiety level, you will find a zero correlation (no validity).
2. **Extremes. If a measure has no reliability (i.e., it is not reproducible), then it has zero reliability. If it has perfect reliability, or repeatability, then it has a reliability of 1.00.**
3. **Rules of thumb. For a continuous measure, this is assessed by the correlation coefficient, and a rule of thumb is generally $r = 0.80$ for adequate reliability. For a binary measure** (e.g., the presence or absence of a disease), **this is often assessed by the kappa coefficient, and a rule of thumb is generally $\kappa = 0.70$.**
4. **Usual notation:** correlation coefficient, r, κ, intraclass correlation coefficient.

C. Validity

1. **Definition. Validity equals usefulness (i.e., the degree of usefulness of a score for a particular pur-**

pose, specifically, the degree to which the test measures what it is supposed to be measuring. The determination of validity usually requires independent, external criteria of whatever the test is designed to measure. For example, if an investigator develops a single question that he/she purports to be a good screening instrument for clinical depression, then patients' responses to this question should relate well to "gold standard" measures of clinical depression, such as structured interviews and well-established rating scales for depression.

2. **Rules of thumb.** There is no real rule of thumb for validity, since there is no one measure. As a bare minimum, however, **the scale should at least be significantly correlated with gold-standard measures for that characteristic.**
3. **Usual notation:** correlation coefficient, ***r*****,** or measures of sensitivity and specificity for a screening instrument.

III. Statistics Used to Describe a Group of Two or More Subjects ("Descriptive Statistics")

A. Theory

Many human characteristics are distributed "normally," that is, if subjects' scores are plotted on a histogram, as the number of subjects gets larger, the distribution will look more and more like a "bell-shaped curve," or "Gaussian distribution." This is convenient, since **any normal distribution can be described very well by two measures: its mean indicates its central point, and its standard deviation indicates its spread. For example, in a normal distribution, about 95% of all scores fall within two standard deviations above or below the mean.**

To make life easier, **researchers usually assume that a characteristic is normally distributed, unless there is strong evidence that this is not true.** For example, gender is a binary (yes/no) variable, so it cannot be normally distributed.

B. Mean (a measure of the CENTER of the distribution)

1. **Definition: the average score of a group of individuals. In a normal distribution, this is the best single estimate of the "true" score of a group of individuals.** The theory is that the mean of a group of individuals represents the "true" score, and the deviation of each individual's score from the mean is caused by random errors.
2. **Usual notation: mean, *X*.**

C. Standard Deviation (a measure of the SPREAD around the mean of the distribution)

1. **Definition: the average spread of each score from the mean of its group. Thus, the smaller the standard deviation, the closer each score is to the mean,** and thus the fewer errors in the scores.
2. **Extremes. If all individuals have the same score, then the standard deviation is zero,** since all scores fall at the mean and there is no error.
3. **Rule of thumb. If the standard deviation is as large or larger than the mean of a group, then there is a large amount of spread in the group, and the mean is probably not an accurate indicator of the group.**
4. **Usual notation: SD, or** (often in tables) **mean ± SD** (e.g., 14.0 ± 7.0 indicates mean = 14, SD = 7.0).

D. Correlation Coefficient (a measure of how two characteristics are related within individuals in the distribution)

1. **Definition: a single number that summarizes the correlation of two measures in a group of individuals. Technically,** the correlation coefficient is **the slope of the line that best fits a scatter plot of two measures** (in standard scores).

   A positive correlation of .33 between rating scales A and B would signify that, if on scale A a subject scores 1 standard deviation above the mean of his group on this scale, then, on average, the same subject's score on rating B will be 1/3 standard deviation (i.e., .33) above the mean for all scores on rating scale B.
2. **Extremes. If two measures are not related** (i.e., knowing one tells you nothing about the value of the other), **then their correlation is zero. If they are perfectly related, then their correlation is 1.00** (if they both change in the same direction), or –1.00 (if they change in opposite directions).
3. **Rules of thumb. The correlation coefficient squared gives the strength of the relation between the two measures.** For example, a correlation between height and nutrition of 0.70 would mean that 49% (i.e., 0.70 × 0.70) of a person's height is determined by his or her nutrition, and thus the other 51% must be determined by other factors.
4. **Usual notation: *r*** (e.g., $r = 0.35$).
5. **Alternatives**
   a. **When very few subjects are available,** or the distributions are markedly different from normality, **the Spearman non-parametric rank correlation test is used to test the association between the ranks of the two groups.**
   b. **When the scores are dichotomous or categorical, the contingency coefficient is used** to test the association between the two groups.
   c. **When we are interested in using one or more measures to *predict* an individual's score on another measure, multiple linear regression is used** (and **upper-case "*R*" is used to represent multiple regression** in place of the lower-case "*r*" used to represent correlation).
   d. When interested in comparing two or more groups on a **set of variables, rather than on a single outcome or de-**

pendent variables, we use either multivariate analysis of variance (MANOVA) or discriminant analysis. (More generally, **univariate tests** assume there is only a single outcome or dependant variable, while **multivariate tests** assume there are two or more outcome or dependent variables to be tested simultaneously.)

e. **When interested in *summarizing* the correlations of many characteristics or rating scales by calculating a few new summary variables (or factors),** principal components analysis or factor analysis is used to summarize a table (or matrix) of correlations.

IV. Drawing Inferences from a Group and Generalizing to a Larger Population ("Inferential Statistics")

A. Theory

An investigator usually assumes that the subjects are drawn randomly from a population in which the characteristic, which is the outcome measure, is normally distributed. Then, **by computing the difference between the means of two samples, or a correlation coefficient, and knowing the sample size these statistics were computed on, their values in the larger population can be estimated (or "inferred") with varying degrees of confidence. The standard degree of confidence in the behavioral sciences is 95%; hence the "95% confidence interval" around a statistic, and the 0.05 *P*-value.**

Note: The statistics described below are those used most commonly when the investigator assumes that the characteristic that is the outcome measure (or "dependent variable," or "end point") is distributed normally (i.e., in a "bell-shaped curve"). If this is not the case, other statistical methods, called "nonparametric" methods, are available (these do not depend on the mean and standard deviation of a sample to draw inferences).

B. Null Hypothesis

1. **Definition. An investigator usually begins with the hypothesis that there is a zero** (or "nil") **difference between two means,** or that there is a correlation coefficient of zero (or "nil") between two measures. **Since statistics cannot prove an hypothesis, we usually phrase the "null hypothesis" and present data showing that it is unlikely to be true; the *P*-value indicates just how "unlikely."**
2. **Usual notation: null hypothesis, H_0.**
3. **Caveat. In *any* very large sample, the null hypothesis is usually rejected.** That is, two groups of individuals rarely have exactly the same mean on any two characteristics; even if they only differ by, say, 0.01 mm, the null hypothesis is not true, and a sample size in the thousands could detect even a tiny difference.

C. *t*-Test

1. **Definition: A test to determine whether the difference between the means of two samples of subjects is likely to be due to chance alone.**
2. **Extremes.** If the difference between two means is zero, the *t*-statistic will also be zero. If all scores in both groups are the same, they both have standard deviations of zero. In this case, the *t*-statistic will be infinitely large.
3. **Usual notation: *t*** [e.g., t(14) = 5.0 indicates that the *t*-statistic with 14 degrees of freedom is 5.0].
4. **Alternatives**
   a. **When very few subjects are available, or the distributions are markedly different from normality, the nonparametric Mann-Whitney *U*-test is used** to test the difference between the mean ranks of the two groups.
   b. **When the outcome measure is survival at various time points, survival analysis is used to determine whether the survival curves of the two groups are significantly different.**

D. Analysis of Variance

1. **Definition: A test to determine whether the difference between the means of *two or more* samples of subjects is likely to be due to chance alone.** The analysis of variance (ANOVA) also tests for interaction effects between factors. For example, if the two factors being tested were drug vs. placebo, and the other factor was young/old, the ANOVA may find that the drug is more effective than the placebo in the young subjects only. **The significance of the analysis of variance is tested by the "*F*-statistic."**
2. **Extremes.** If the difference between two means is zero, the *F*-statistic will also be zero. If all scores in both groups are the same, they both have standard deviations of zero. In this case, the *F*-statistic will be infinitely large (and highly significant).
3. **Usual notation: *F*** [e.g., F(1,20) = 5.0 indicates that the *F*-statistic with 1 and 20 degrees of freedom is 5.0].
4. **Alternatives**
   a. **When only two groups are being compared, and there are no interactions of concern, the *t*-test can be used.**
   b. **When the groups differ on some important variable (e.g., age, education, or baseline illness severity), the analysis of covariance (ANCOVA) is used to statistically adjust for these confounding group differences.**

E. Chi-Square Test

1. **Definition: A test to determine whether the frequencies in each cell of a contingency table are different from the proportions expected by chance. It is most commonly used on a 2 × 2 contingency table, represented as four cells forming a square.**

   A common use is to answer the question: Is there a difference between the occurrence of a given side effect in the drug vs. placebo group? In this case the table is arranged with drug vs. placebo as the

two rows, and side effect vs. no side effect as the two columns. As the difference between the frequency in each cell gets larger, the chi-square statistic also gets larger, and the more significant the result becomes.

2. **Extremes.** If all cells contain exactly the frequencies that would be expected by chance, then the chi-square statistic is zero. If the frequencies differ greatly from chance, the chi-square statistic gets larger and larger. The size of the chi-square statistic is based on the number of cells in the contingency table.
3. **Usual notation:** χ^2 [e.g., $\chi^2(1) = 5.0$ indicates that the chi-square statistic with 1 degree of freedom is 5.0; a 2×2 table has 1 degree of freedom (df)].

F. *P*-Value

1. **Definition: The chance that a positive (i.e., "significant") statistical test represents a false positive finding.** The chance of a false positive finding is called a Type I error, and goes up as the total number of statistical tests increases (it is unrelated to sample size). 1.00 minus a p-value gives the specificity of a statistical test, which is analogous to the specificity of a medical test (i.e., likelihood of not finding a false positive result).
2. **Extremes. If a finding is almost certainly a spurious finding, which would not be reproducible in another sample, the *P*-value will be near 1.00. On the other hand, if the finding almost certainly represents a "true" finding, then the *P*-value will be near zero. A probability can never reach zero, but small *P*-values are represented by several zeros after the decimal point (e.g., $P < 0.00001$).**
3. **Rule of thumb. Most journals require $P < 0.05$ for significance.** If many statistical tests are performed in a study, a more conservative *P*-value should be used.
4. **Notation: either $P <$ (less exact), or $P =$ (exact and preferable).** Also referred to as alpha (α).
5. **Caution: do not be overly impressed by very low *P*-values. Remember that all this tells you is the chance that the difference is probably not zero. Also, remember that, given enough subjects, this is very easy to prove.** Thus, a very low *P*-value does not necessarily indicate a large clinical effect, but instead represents that it is a very reliable effect. Check the effect size (the correlation coefficient squared, or the size of the *t*-statistic) to get an idea of the magnitude of the difference or relation.

G. Statistical Power

1. **Definition:** the likelihood of detecting a true difference or relation between two or more measures. Statistical power is analogous to the sensitivity of a medical test—that is, the higher the sensitivity, the lower the chance of missing a real finding (in statistics, this is referred to as a Type II error, and is most common in studies with small sample sizes).
2. **Extremes.** If a study had no chance of finding a true difference between two drugs (e.g., with only two subjects per group), the power of the study would be nearly zero. If the study had almost no chance of missing a true difference (e.g., comparing the mean height of 10,000 2-year-olds with 10,000 18-year-olds), the power of the study would be nearly 1.00.
3. **Rule of thumb. Power of 0.80 is usually the minimum suggested by statisticians when designing a study.**
4. **Usual notation: power, statistical power, $1 - \beta$ (where β is the likelihood of finding a false negative).**
5. **Caution.** Just as any tiny difference can be found to be significant just by having enough subjects, it is possible to find all but huge differences to be non-significant, simply by having few enough subjects! **Be especially wary of false negatives in studies with few subjects, say less than 25 per group.** Several literature reviews have found that the average behavioral science study has a power of only about 40% to detect a medium-sized effect!

Suggested Readings

Anastasi, A. (1996). *Psychological testing* (7th ed.). New York: Prentice-Hall.

Cohen, J. (1988). *Statistical power analysis for the behavioral sciences* (2nd ed.). Hillsdale, NJ: Lawrence Erlbaum Associates.

Fleiss, J.L. (1986). *The design and analysis of clinical experiments.* New York: John Wiley.

Tabachnick, B.G., & Fidell, L.S. (2001). *Using multivariate statistics* (4th ed.). Neeham, MA: Allyn & Bacon.

Chapter 68

Genetics and Psychiatry

Jordan Smoller and Christine Finn

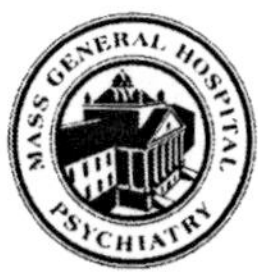

I. Introduction

The impact of genetic research and genetic medicine on psychiatry is growing due to advances in understanding the familial and genetic contributions to common psychiatric disorders and increasing recognition of neuropsychiatric manifestations of genetic and chromosomal disorders.

This chapter reviews both the genetic aspects of psychiatric disorders and psychiatric aspects of genetic disorders.

II. Basic Principles of Genetics and Gene Mapping

A. The Human Genome

The human genome encompasses 23 homologous pairs of chromosomes containing approximately 30,000–40,000,000 genes. The larger portion (> 95%) of chromosomal DNA comprises non-coding DNA sequences. **The chromosomal location of a DNA sequence is referred to as a genetic locus.**

B. Genotypes and Phenotypes

The sequence of nucleotides that make up a gene or an anonymous genetic marker may differ among individuals. **The different forms of a gene or genetic marker are referred to as alleles. Allelic differences are also referred to as polymorphisms and can be used to distinguish the genotypes of different individuals. A genotype refers to the combination of alleles at a given locus. If the two alleles at a locus are the same, an individual is said to be homozygous at the locus; if the alleles differ, the individual is heterozygous. A phenotype is the manifestation (expression) of a set of alleles, or, more generally, the observable expression of a trait.**

C. Genetic Mapping

For the most part, gene mapping studies rely on the phenomena of crossing over and recombination that occur during meiosis. During this process, homologous chromosomes exchange genetic material; thus the gametes formed by meiosis may contain a combination of paternal and maternal chromosomal segments. To the degree that two loci are physically close together on a chromosome, they are unlikely to be separated when recombination occurs (a violation of Mendel's law of independent assortment). Two loci that are not transmitted independently are genetically linked, implying that they reside close together on a chromosome.

D. Genetic Linkage

The degree of genetic linkage reflects the proximity of two loci and depends on the frequency of recombination between them. The distance between two loci can be expressed as a genetic distance (in centimorgans) or a physical distance (in base pairs). Loci that are separated by recombination in 1% of meioses are 1 centimorgan (cM) apart; this corresponds roughly to a physical distance of 1 million base pairs.

E. Psychiatric Phenotypes Are "Complex"

A phenotype may be transmitted in a Mendelian fashion (due to the action of a single major gene) or in a "complex" fashion. Mendelian inheritance patterns include dominant, recessive, and X-linked. **Neuropsychiatric disorders that are due to single major genes include Huntington disease (autosomal dominant), Wilson disease (autosomal recessive), and Fragile X syndrome (X-linked). In the case of Huntington's and Fragile X, the genetic lesion is due to expansion of trinucleotide (triplet) repeat sequences.** Most psychiatric phenotypes, however, are complex traits; they reflect interactions of genetic and environmental factors that may vary among families. This vastly complicates efforts to identify the genetic basis of psychiatric disorders. The genes involved are often referred to as "susceptibility genes" rather than "disease genes" because they increase risk for a disorder without invariably causing it.

III. The Tools of Psychiatric Genetics

Genetic epidemiologists and molecular geneticists rely on a well-defined sequence of study designs to determine whether a disorder has a genetic basis, and then to locate the specific genes that may be involved.

A. Family Studies

Family studies address the first question to be answered: Does the disorder run in families? If relatives of affected probands have a higher risk of the disorder than relatives of unaffected probands, the disorder is familial (proband = the individual through whom a family is ascertained). One index of the strength of familiality is the recurrence risk ratio for first-degree relatives (l_1), defined as the ratio of the risk of the disorder in a first-degree relative of an affected individual to the prevalence in the general population. This ratio can be used to predict the strength of genetic influences on the disorder and the likelihood that gene-mapping studies will have the power to identify the genes involved. Approximate recurrence risk ratios for a variety of psychiatric disorders are presented in Table 68-1. It is important to bear in mind that the size of these risk ratios depends on both

Table 68-1. Genetic Epidemiology of Some Psychiatric Disorders

Disorder	*Lifetime Population Prevalence (approx. %)*	λ_1[a]	*Estimated Concordance Rates*		*Estimated Heritability (Approximate)*	*Selected Linkage and Association Findings*[b]
			MZ	*DZ*		
ADHD	7	2–5	51–58%	31–33%	60–90%	Dopamine transporter; DRD4
Alzheimer's disease (late-onset)	10 (> 65 years)	2	21%	11%	60%	Early-onset: presenilin-1, presenilin-2, amyloid precursor protein Late-onset: ApoE (ε4)
Schizophrenia	1	10	46%	14%	70–89%	Chromosome 6p, 8p, 13q, 22q; dysbindin, COMT, neuregulin 1, G72/G30
Bipolar disorder	1	7–10	62%	8%	60–85%	Chromosome 4p, 18, 21q, 22q; COMT, MAO-A, BDNF, G72/G30
Unipolar depression	5–17	3	23–49%	16–42%	40%	Chromosme 1q, 2q; tyrosine hydroxylase; serotonin transporter
Panic disorder	3	5–7	24%	11%	45%	Chromosome 9q, 13q; COMT, MAO-A
Alcohol dependence	14	3–7	48%	32%	50–60%	Chromosome 1, 4p, 4q, 11p, 16; alcohol dehydrogenase (ADH)

[a]λ_1, recurrence risk ratio for first-degree relatives: the risk of the disorder in a first-degree relative of an affected individual compared to the general population prevalence of the disorder.

[b]With the exception of the findings for Alzheimer's disease, these findings are tentative, and nonreplications of most of these findings have also been reported. This list is illustrative, not exhaustive.

the risk to relatives (numerator) and the base-rate of the disorder (denominator). Even when the relative risk of a disorder is high, the absolute risk to a first-degree relative may be relatively low if the base-rate of the disorder is low. For example, siblings of probands with schizophrenia have a roughly ten-fold increased risk of the disorder compared with an individual randomly drawn from the general population. However, because the population prevalence is approximately 1%, the absolute risk of the disorder for the sibling is only about 10% (with a 90% probability of being unaffected). In contrast, the lifetime prevalence of major depression is approximately 15%, so that even a two-fold increased risk to siblings would be associated with a 30% risk of being affected.

B. Twin and Adoption Studies

It is important to remember that a disorder may run in families for non-genetic reasons. For example, shared environmental experiences may produce the disorder in multiple family members. Twin and adoption studies can be used to separate the contribution of genetic and environmental causes of familial aggregation.

1. **Twin studies compare the concordance rates between monozygotic twins (who are genetically identical) and dizygotic twins (who share on average 50% of their alleles).** A twin pair is concordant if both co-twins have the phenotype. If we can assume that environmental influences on **monozygotic (MZ) twins** are not different from environmental influences on **dizygotic (DZ) twins** (the "equal environments assumption"), then significantly higher concordance rates in MZ twins reflect the action of genes. Nevertheless, an MZ concordance rate that is less than 100% means that environmental factors influence the phenotype. Twin studies can provide an estimate of the **heritability of the disorder, which refers to the proportion of the phenotypic differences among individuals that can be attributed to genetic factors. Heritability refers to the strength of genetic influences in a population, not a particular individual,** and heritability estimates may differ depending on the population studied. Table 68-1 presents heritability estimates for several disorders.
2. **Adoption studies can disentangle genetic and environmental influences on family resemblance by**

comparing rates of a disorder in biological family members with those in adoptive family members. For example, if an adopted child has a genetically influenced disorder, the biological (genetic) parents should have a higher risk of the disorder than the adoptive (environmental) parents. Adoption studies provided the first convincing evidence that genes play an important role in the development of schizophrenia.

C. Modes of Inheritance

Once genes have been implicated in a disorder, segregation analysis is sometimes used to determine the mode of inheritance. This involves fitting various statistical models of inheritance (e.g., dominant, recessive, multi-factorial polygenic) to the observed pattern of disease in pedigrees and determining which modes of inheritance are consistent, or inconsistent, with the observed data. Information derived from a segregation analysis can be used to guide linkage studies (see III.D.3.a) that actually seek to identify the genes involved in the disorder.

D. Molecular Genetics

Molecular genetic methods are used to locate and isolate the specific genes that influence a disorder.

1. The **candidate gene approach examines the inheritance of specific genes that are suspected to be involved in a disorder.** These candidate genes may have been suggested by previous physiologic, pharmacologic, or **gene-mapping studies.** For example, the serotonin transporter gene may be considered a candidate gene for mood disorders because serotonergic function has been implicated in the physiology and treatment of these disorders. Because the pathogenesis of most psychiatric disorders is poorly understood, it may be difficult to identify compelling candidate genes for testing.
2. An alternative approach is to perform a **whole genome scan** in which **linkage is tested for genetic markers spaced at intervals along each chromosome. A marker is a polymorphic DNA sequence whose chromosomal location is known;** it may or may not reside within a gene. The **genome scan approach requires no prior knowledge of the function or location of genes involved in the disorder.**
3. Molecular genetic studies of complex phenotypes, such as psychiatric disorders, are complicated for several reasons. **It may be difficult to accurately classify whether an individual is affected with the disease genotype because there may be phenocopies (individuals who have the disorder for non-genetic reasons), incomplete penetrance (individuals with the disease genotype may not manifest the phenotype), variable expression (the disease genotype may produce a spectrum of phenotypes), and genetic heterogeneity (different genes may independently produce the phenotype). Moreover, the boundaries of psychiatric diagnoses are often uncertain and may not capture the phenotypic features that are under genetic influence. In addition, the phenotype may be the result of many genes rather than of one or a few major genes.** For polygenic disorders, each gene may exert only a weak effect.

   In general, two types of gene-mapping studies may be performed:

   a. **Linkage studies examine whether two or more genetic loci are co-inherited more often than expected by chance.** If individuals who are affected with a disorder within a family tend to inherit the same alleles at a marker locus, this implies that the marker locus is linked to (i.e., is physically close to) a gene that influences the disorder. In classical (parametric) linkage analysis, the **strength of the evidence in favor of linkage is calculated as a LOD (logarithm of the odds) score.** The LOD score compares the likelihood of obtaining the observed genotypes and phenotypes when linkage is present with the likelihood assuming no linkage. Traditionally, **a LOD score of 3 (corresponding to odds of 1000:1 in favor of linkage) has been the threshold for declaring linkage,** but for complex disorders, such as psychiatric illnesses, higher thresholds have been recommended. Traditional LOD score linkage analysis has been most successfully applied when a single major gene is involved and the mode of inheritance (e.g., dominant, recessive) is known. Because these assumptions can rarely be used with psychiatric phenotypes, other (non-parametric) methods, which do not require knowledge of mode of inheritance, are routinely utilized. For example, genome scan linkage analysis may be performed with large numbers of families containing pairs of relatives who are affected. **The affected sibling pair (ASP) method, e.g., examines whether affected siblings share alleles at any marker locus significantly more often than would be expected by chance.** If alleles at a locus tend to be shared by affected sibling pairs, this implies that the locus is linked to a disease gene.

   b. **Association studies examine whether a particular allele of a candidate gene is significantly more common among individuals with a disorder (cases) than among controls without the disorder.** This method led to the finding that the ApoE-ε4 allele is associated with late-onset Alzheimer's disease. Such **case-control association studies can produce false positive results if the ethnic backgrounds of cases and controls differ.** If the case group has a higher proportion of individuals from an ethnic group that happens to have a high frequency of the allele being tested, then that allele will be statistically associated with the disease even though it may play no causal role. **Family-based association studies** avoid this problem by looking at the transmission of alleles within families. However, ascertaining families can be more difficult than ascertaining unrelated cases and controls. With the completion of the Human Genome Project and the identification of all human genes, it may soon be feasible to perform a whole genome scan using alleles of all human genes as "candidates."

c. **Cytogenetic studies.** A third method for identifying the location of a disease gene involves **cytogenetic studies in which psychiatric phenotypes are shown to be associated with chromosomal abnormalities.** For example, a deletion of material from chromosome 22q can result in **velocardiofacial syndrome,** which is associated with a wide range of somatic anomalies, as well as learning disabilities, and behavioral/psychiatric symptoms. An excess prevalence of bipolar spectrum disorders and psychotic disorders among patients with this syndrome has been observed, suggesting that a gene influencing these disorders may lie within this region.

IV. Genetic Aspects of Psychopathology

Evidence for a genetic component of many psychiatric disorders is growing, and gene-mapping studies have begun to identify the location and identity of some of the relevant loci. Unfortunately, many linkage and association findings have been difficult to replicate, emphasizing the **need for caution in interpreting the results of genetic studies.** Some of these findings have undoubtedly been false positives, but non-replication can also be due to inadequate power, differences in diagnosis and phenotype definition, and genetic heterogeneity (different genes acting in different samples). The following summary draws in part on data summarized in the report of the NIMH Genetics Workgroup (1999). **To date, no specific genes have been definitively shown to influence any of the major psychiatric disorders, with the exception of Alzheimer's disease.**

A. Disorders of Childhood and Adolescence

1. **Attention deficit hyperactivity disorder (ADHD)**
   a. **Family studies. ADHD runs in families, and first-degree relatives (parents and siblings) of ADHD probands have a two- to eight-fold higher risk of the disorder than relatives of controls.** Family studies also suggest that ADHD and depression share familial determinants, and that ADHD with conduct or bipolar disorder may be a distinct familial subtype.
   b. **Twin studies and adoption studies. Most heritability estimates for ADHD have ranged from approximately 60% to more than 90%.** Adoption studies have demonstrated that the risk of ADHD is higher among biological relatives than among adoptive relatives of ADHD children.
   c. **Molecular genetic studies.** To date, attention has focused on candidate genes involved in dopaminergic function. Alleles of the dopamine D_2 receptor gene, the dopamine transporter (DAT) gene, and the dopamine D_4 receptor (DRD4) gene have been associated with ADHD. The DAT and DRD4 associations have received support in independent studies.
2. **Autism**
   a. **Family studies. The risk of autism to siblings of affected children is approximately 3–4%, which is more than 75-fold higher than the general population prevalence.**
   b. **Twin studies.** Concordance rates for MZ twins are markedly higher than those for DZ twins, and the **heritability has been estimated to exceed 90%.**
   c. **Molecular genetic studies.** Although it appears to be one of the most heritable psychiatric phenotypes, no genetic loci have yet been convincingly linked to, or associated with, autism. Tentative associations with several genes have been reported, and genome scans have provided suggestive evidence of linkage to loci on chromosome 1p, 2q, 7q, and 16p. Cytogenetic studies have implicated duplications on chromosome 15q in some cases.
   d. A fraction of cases may be due to other genetic disorders, e.g., neurofibromatosis, tuberous sclerosis, and Fragile X.
3. **Tourette syndrome (TS)**
   a. **Family studies. First-degree relatives of TS probands have an 8.7% risk of the disorder, 174-fold greater than the population prevalence.** There is evidence for variable expression of the genetic liability for TS; e.g., relatives of probands with TS have a higher risk of obsessive-compulsive disorder and chronic motor or vocal tics.
   b. **Twin studies.** In one twin study, MZ concordance rates (53%) exceeded DZ concordance rates (8%).
   c. **Molecular genetic studies.** No genetic loci have been convincingly associated with TS. An association with the DRD4 gene has been reported but not established.

B. Dementia: Alzheimer Disease

Of the disorders reviewed here, Alzheimer's disease (AD) is the one in which genetic studies have progressed the furthest, and at least four specific genes have been shown to play a role in the disorder.

1. **Family and twin studies.** The familiality of early-onset (before age 60 years) AD has been well established, and three specific genes influencing early-onset AD have been identified (see below). Late-onset AD is far more common and has a more complex etiology. Having a first-degree relative with AD approximately doubles the risk of AD. A large twin study estimated the heritability of late-onset AD to be approximately 60%.
2. **Molecular genetic studies. Mutations in three genes have been shown to produce *early-onset AD* with an autosomal dominant mode of inheritance.** Together, these genes account for roughly half of early-onset cases of AD:
   a. **Amyloid precursor protein gene on chromosome 21**
   b. **Presenilin 1 gene on chromosome 14**
   c. **Presenilin 2 gene on chromosome 1**

The apolipoprotein E gene (APOE) on chromosome 19 has been associated with *late-onset AD.* There are three common alleles of APOE (ε2, ε3, and ε4) and it is **the ε4 allele that increases risk for late-onset AD.** (APOE-ε2 appears to be associated with a reduced risk of AD.) Unlike the autosomal dominant genes involved in early-onset AD, APOE-ε4 is a susceptibility allele that acts as a risk factor for the disease but is neither a necessary nor sufficient cause. **A primary effect of the ε4 allele is to reduce the age of onset of AD;** individuals with two copies of the allele have the earliest age of onset compared with individuals with other APOE genotypes. Other genes are undoubtedly involved in the etiology of late-onset AD; recent studies indicate that a gene residing on chromosome 12 is linked to AD.

3. **The high risk of AD among individuals with Down syndrome (trisomy 21)** has been attributed largely to triplication of the amyloid precursor protein gene on chromosome 21. Onset of AD in these individuals is typically in the sixth decade of life.

C. Psychotic Disorders: Schizophrenia

1. **Family studies.** Family studies of schizophrenia have repeatedly demonstrated that the **disorder is familial.** Compared with the population lifetime risk of approximately 1%, first-degree relatives have an approximately 10% risk. The risk drops to about 4% for second-degree relatives and 2% for third-degree relatives. This pattern of familial risks is consistent with the hypothesis that between two and five interacting genes may be responsible for most of the genetic liability to schizophrenia. There is evidence for variable expression of the genetic diathesis underlying schizophrenia. For example, Cluster A personality traits are more common in the relatives of schizophrenic probands. **A number of neurobiological phenotypes also appear to be more common among non-schizophrenic relatives of individuals with schizophrenia:**
   a. **Smooth-pursuit eye-tracking dysfunction**
   b. **Neuropsychological deficits (in memory, language, and attention tasks)**
   c. **Abnormal P50 auditory-evoked potentials**
   d. **Structural brain abnormalities**
   e. **Reduced hippocampal *N*-acetyl-D-aspartate (NMDA) levels**

   These phenotypes are sometimes called "intermediate phenotypes" or "endophenotypes" because they may more directly reflect the action of genes than does the clinical phenotype of schizophrenia itself. Incorporating these phenotypes into linkage and association studies may prove critical to unlocking the genetics of schizophrenia.
2. **Twin and adoption studies. The concordance rate for MZ twins (~46%) substantially exceeds that of DZ twins (~14%). The heritability of schizophrenia has been estimated to be 70–89%.** Adoption studies have demonstrated that the prevalence of schizophrenia is significantly higher (approximately four-fold) in biological relatives than in adoptive relatives.
3. **Molecular genetic studies.** Many linkage and association studies of schizophrenia have been reported, and some findings have received support in independent samples. **Some of the strongest evidence to date from genome scan linkage studies has been for regions on chromosomes 5q, 6p, 8p, 10p, 13q, 18p, and 22q.** Cytogenetic studies have also pointed to the region on chromosome 22q implicated in linkage studies. Chromosomal microdeletions in this region have been associated with **velocardiofacial syndrome** (see VI), in which affected individuals appear to have an excess risk of schizophrenia and schizoaffective disorder. Some of these regions contain plausible candidate loci that have been associated with schizophrenia in several studies. These include, e.g., the dysbindin (DTNBP1) gene on 6p, neuregulin 1 (NRG1) on 8p, and catechol-O-methyl transferase (COMT) on 22q. As pointed out earlier, interpreting the results of these studies requires caution; the list of genes with positive associations is expanding, but non-replications are common and none has been firmly established. A promising approach involves the use of intermediate phenotypes directly in linkage and association studies. Among families with schizophrenia, linkage and association have been found between the trait of abnormal P50 auditory-evoked response and a locus on chromosome 15q at the α7-nicotinic receptor gene.

D. Mood Disorders

1. **Bipolar disorder.** As with schizophrenia, studies of bipolar disorder have demonstrated that **genetic factors influence the disorder;** several linkage and association findings have been replicated but not firmly established. It is considered likely that the **inherited susceptibility to bipolar disorder reflects several genes of small effect rather than a single major gene.**
   a. **Family studies. Family studies have consistently demonstrated that there is familial transmission of bipolar disorder. First-degree relatives of individuals with bipolar disorder have an excess risk of both bipolar disorder (seven- to ten-fold) and unipolar depression (two- to five-fold) compared with relatives of unaffected controls; relatives of probands with unipolar depression, however, have an excess risk of unipolar depression but not of bipolar disorder.** Among first-degree relatives of bipolar probands, the range of estimates of the risk for bipolar disorder is approximately 5–10%, whereas the risk for unipolar depression is approximately 10–20%.
   b. **Twin and adoption studies. Concordance rates are substantially higher in MZ twins (39–62%) than in DZ twins (0–9%), and the heritability of bipolar disorder**

has been estimated to be approximately 60–85%. The results of adoption studies have been mixed, although two studies showed higher risk in biological vs. adoptive relatives.

c. **Molecular genetic studies.** Although there have been numerous non-replications of linkage and association findings for bipolar disorder, some linkage results have received support from independent studies, including regions of chromosomes 4p, 13q, 18p, 18q, 21q, and 22q. An early report of linkage to 11p among Old Order Amish families was not supported by subsequent analyses, although the tyrosine hydroxylase gene that maps to this region has been associated with bipolar disorder in some studies. Other candidate genes that have received support in some studies include the genes encoding the serotonin transporter, tryptophan hydroxylase, monoamine oxidase A, COMT, and brain-derived neurotrophic factor (BDNF). Again, however, non-replications have been reported for these and other loci that have been associated with bipolar disorder.

2. **Major depression**

a. **Family studies. Family studies have consistently demonstrated that first-degree relatives of probands with major depression have a higher risk of the disorder (15–22%) than relatives of controls (5–11%).** The recurrence risk ratio (λ_1) for first-degree relatives has ranged from approximately 3. **Certain features of major depression in the proband have been associated with increased familial risk: early-onset, recurrent episodes, long duration of episodes, suicidality, and greater levels of impairment.** Relatives of probands with unipolar depression do not have a substantially increased risk of bipolar disorder.

b. **Twin and adoption studies. Depending on the sample and diagnostic convention used, concordance rates have ranged from 23% to 69% for MZ twins and from 16% to 42% for DZ twins.** The estimated heritability is approximately 40%. The results of four available adoption studies have been mixed, providing modest support for a genetic component.

c. **Molecular genetic studies.** Several linkage studies have been reported, with evidence implicating certain chromosomal regions, including 1q and 2q. Association studies have suggested, but not established, a role for several genes including the serotonin transporter and tyrosine hydroxlase genes.

E. Anxiety Disorders

1. **Panic disorder**

a. **Family studies. The estimated risk of panic disorder to first-degree relatives of affected probands has ranged from about 8% to 31%, significantly higher than the risk to relatives of controls. As with several other psychiatric disorders, early-onset is associated with increased familial risk.** Overall, the recurrence risk ratio for panic disorder is approximately 5.

b. **Twin studies. Concordance rates for panic disorder among MZ twins have ranged from 23% to 73%, compared with 0–17% for DZ twins.** The estimated heritability is approximately 40–45%.

c. **Molecular genetic studies.** Linkage studies have provided preliminary support for findings on chromosomes 1q, 7p, 8q, 9q, 11p, 12q, and 13q, but these await replication. A cytogenetic analysis found strong evidence for an association between a duplication of material on chromosome 15q and phenotypes, including panic/phobic disorders and joint laxity, but this has not been replicated. Unconfirmed associations have been reported for a few candidate genes, including COMT, cholecystokinin (CCK), monoamine oxidase A, and the neurotrophin-3 receptor (NTRK3).

2. **Obsessive-compulsive disorder (OCD)**

a. **Family studies.** Available family studies have yielded mixed results, although **the risk to first-degree relatives of OCD probands has been higher than the population prevalence of the disorder in several studies.** In one case-control family study, the risk was 10.3% for first-degree relatives of OCD probands compared with 1.9% for relatives of control probands. **Early-onset disorder may be more familial.** The risk of tic disorders (Tourette syndrome, and chronic tics) is elevated in a subset of families of OCD probands, suggesting that these disorders can share genetic influences. Conversely, studies have also documented an elevated risk of OCD among relatives of probands with Tourette syndrome.

b. **Twin studies.** Limited available twin data support the hypothesis that obsessional traits and symptoms are influenced by genetic factors, with heritability estimates ranging from 47% to 68%. The heritability of the DSM diagnosis of OCD itself is unclear.

c. **Molecular genetic studies.** An association between OCD and an allele of the COMT gene has been reported in independent samples. Reported associations with the dopamine D_4 receptor, the serotonin transporter, serotonin 1Dbeta receptor, and monoamine oxidase A genes await further replication.

F. Substance Use Disorders

1. **Alcohol dependence**

a. **Family studies.** An overview of family studies indicates that **first-degree relatives of individuals with alcohol dependence have a seven-fold (range 2.5–20-fold) higher risk of the disorder compared with relatives of unaffected individuals.** Susceptibility to alcohol withdrawal symptoms also appears to be familial.

b. **Twin and adoption studies.** Most (but not all) twin and adoption studies of alcoholism have supported the role of genetic influences. Heritability estimates have varied depending on the diagnostic criteria applied, but, among studies demonstrating genetic influence, estimated heritability has ranged from approximately 50% to 60%. Several adoption studies have demonstrated an increased risk of alcoholism among adoptees who have an alcoholic biologic parent.

c. **Molecular genetic studies.** Genome scans have provided evidence of linkage to loci on chromosomes 1, 4p, chromosome 4q (near the alcohol dehydrogenase gene cluster), chromosomes 7 and 11p and 16. As with other psychiatric disorders (see schizophrenia), efforts have been made to identify endophenotypes underlying the disorder. Differences in P3 event-related brain potentials are heritable and have been associated with alcoholism; a recent linkage study found evidence of linkage to loci on chromosomes 2 and 6 using P3 amplitude as the phenotype of interest. Associations between several candidate genes and alcohol dependence have been reported, including an association between genes affecting alcohol metabolism and reduced risk of alcohol dependence. By altering the rate of alcohol metabolism, certain alleles of the alcohol dehydrogenase (ADH) and aldehyde dehydrogenase (ALDH) genes can produce a build-up of acetaldehyde, causing an endogenous disulfiram-like flushing reaction. By discouraging alcohol consumption, these alleles may be protective against the development of alcoholism. A reported association with an allele of the dopamine D_2 receptor (DRD2) gene has been widely studied but remains controversial. More so than with other psychiatric phenotypes, animal models have been used to map genetic loci influencing alcohol consumption, and these should provide crucial clues to the location of homologous human genes.

G. Genetics of Personality and Temperament

An alternative to searching for genes for psychiatric disorders is to identify genes influencing temperament and personality traits. Quantitative variations in these traits reflect individual differences in personality but may also reveal a predisposition to certain Axis I and Axis II disorders. These traits are typically measured with paper-and-pencil tests. Large twin studies have demonstrated that a variety of personality and temperamental constructs are moderately heritable. For example, the heritabilities of neuroticism and introversion-extraversion are approximately 40–50%. An increasing number of gene-mapping studies are reporting evidence of linkage and association between specific loci and personality traits, but, again, none have been confirmed and nonreplications are common. **Widely studied examples include an association of an allele of the DRD4 gene with novelty-seeking, and an association of an allele of the serotonin transporter gene with anxiety-related traits (neuroticism and harm avoidance).**

V. Implications of Psychiatric Genetics

There is reason to be both optimistic and cautious about progress in psychiatric genetic research. **The benefits of identifying and characterizing genes involved in psychiatric phenotypes may include:**

A. An improved understanding of the biological basis of psychiatric disorders.

B. An improved understanding of the role of the environment in psychopathology. Genetic studies are a powerful means for dissecting the role of genes, environment, and gene-environment interactions.

C. An improved basis for defining psychiatric disorders. Genetic studies may validate or challenge diagnostic criteria and diagnostic boundaries among disorders.

D. Improved treatment of psychiatric disorders. The growing field of pharmacogenetics aims to identify genetic factors which predict therapeutic response and liability to drug toxicities. An important goal of this work is to target pharmacologic treatment so as to maximize the likelihood of benefit and minimize the risk of adverse drug effects.

E. The possibility of improved prevention efforts. By identifying the role of environment and gene-environment interactions in psychopathology and by identifying individuals at risk, genetic research may facilitate the development of more targeted and effective prevention measures.

On the other hand, **advances in genetic research may well raise important ethical and social challenges for psychiatrists.** For example, **information about genetic susceptibility could have adverse emotional and financial (e.g., insurability) consequences for some individuals and their families.** Increasingly, psychiatrists will need to have an informed understanding of both the potential benefits and limitations of genetic research.

VI. Psychiatric Manifestations of Genetic Syndromes and Inborn Errors of Metabolism

A variety of genetic syndromes and metabolic illnesses are marked by prominent psychiatric or behavioral symptoms; in some cases these symptoms are the earliest evidence of disease. Psychiatrists must be familiar with physical findings and historical information that may raise suspicions for the presence of genetic illness. Accurate diagnosis may provide opportunities for new treatments or interventions, allow for surveillance of associated medical issues, and help identify other family members at risk. In addition, understanding the causes of psychiatric and behavioral symptoms in disorders where the underlying genetic mechanisms of disease are known may help to shed light on the underlying pathophysiology of psychiatric disorders. **The possibility of a genetic syndrome should be considered in patients with congenital anomalies, comorbid mental retardation or learning disabilities, or a familial pattern of illness that appears Mendelian. Metabolic illness may be associated with a history of food intolerance, decompensation with illness, loss of developmental milestones, seizures or other neurological findings.** Overall, referring a patient for consultation with a geneticist as well as a neurologist can be an important part of the care of psychiatric patients.

A. Disorders Due to Chromosomal Abnormalities

1. Down syndrome (DS)/trisomy 21

a. In the majority of cases, DS is due to **an extra copy of chromosome 21.** It is the **most common *genetic* cause of mental retardation,** occurring on average every 1 in 700 births, with an increased incidence associated with older maternal age (1/385 at age 35, 1/30 at age 45).

b. Common physical features include a **characteristic facial appearance (upslanting), palpebral fissures (eye openings), epicanthal folds, flat nasal bridge, low set ears, protruding tongue), short neck, Brushfield spots on iris, short stature, single palmar crease, congenital heart disease, duodenal atresia, and hypothyroidism.**

c. **Mental retardation is seen in almost all patients, with average IQ in the 25–50 range.** The mental retardation associated with DS is thought to be a static process; **decline in cognition or change in behavior in early or middle adulthood in patients with DS should raise suspicions for possible Alzheimer disease (AD).** AD is thought to be increased in DS patients because the amyloid precursor protein gene (important in the etiology of early-onset AD) is located on chromosome 21. Other psychiatric symptoms include non-specific behavioral issues, depression, and anxiety.

d. Diagnostic testing involves karyotype analysis of chromosomes.

2. Turner syndrome

a. Turner syndrome is due to the **loss of an entire X chromosome and is designated as 45, X.**

b. Patients with this condition are females, and show physical features such as **short stature, excess skin or webbing of the neck, a broad or flat chest, congenital heart defects, hypothyroidism, and gonadal dysgenesis (resulting in infertility and failure to achieve complete secondary sexual characteristics).**

c. Psychiatric symptoms may include delayed social maturation and problems with peer relationships, ADHD, and specific learning disabilities.

d. Diagnostic testing involves karyotype analysis of chromosomes.

3. Klinefelter syndrome

a. Klinefelter syndrome is due to the **addition of an extra X chromosome, and is designated as 47, XXY.**

b. Patients with this condition are males who are, **usually, tall with long legs and a small penis and testes.** Often, these patients first come to medical attention when low testosterone levels interfere with normal pubertal development or cause infertility.

c. Psychiatric symptoms include **average verbal IQ in the 85–90 range, learning disabilities,** ADHD, and possible increased rates of depression.

d. Diagnostic testing involves karyotype analysis of chromosomes.

4. Prader Willi syndrome (PWS)

a. PWS is usually due to the **absence of a critical region on paternally inherited chromosome 15q11-q13,** which may occur by a variety of genetic mechanisms. This area undergoes the process of **imprinting, which is the differential expression of the region based on whether the chromosome is of maternal or paternal origin. (Of note, the deletion of this same region from the maternally derived chromosome results in Angelman syndrome,** which is marked by seizures, severe mental retardation, little to no speech output, abnormal ataxic gait, and characteristic behaviors.)

b. Features of PWS include a characteristic facial appearance (upslanting, almond-shape eyes, thin upper lip, and down-turned mouth), light skin and hair coloring, small hands and feet, small external genitalia, prominent low tone, and failure to thrive in infancy. The **characteristic hyperphagia develops in early childhood,** but may be controlled with use of behavioral techniques started at an early age. These patients are noted to have a high pain threshold, and they rarely, if ever, vomit. The use of growth hormone has been beneficial for the growth and obesity issues seen in these patients, and may also help with behavioral and cognitive aspects.

c. Psychiatric symptoms reported in this condition include obsessive thoughts, compulsions, skin-picking, temper tantrums, depression, anxiety, and psychosis. Patients may show decreased IQ, or specific learning disabilities, accompanied by areas of relative strength (e.g., jigsaw puzzles).

d. Diagnostic testing involves analysis of the critical region for methylation status, or the detection of a microdeletion by fluorescent in-situ hybridization techniques (FISH).

5. Velocardiofacial syndrome/DiGeorge syndrome (VCFS/DGS)

a. VCFS/DGS is due to a microdeletion on one copy of chromosome 22q11, resulting in the loss of up to 60 known and predicted genes. Most cases are sporadic, but it can also be transmitted in a dominant fashion from affected parents.

b. The syndrome occurs in approximately 1 in 4,000 live births.

c. Associated features vary widely, and include a **characteristic facial appearance (broad, squared nasal root, mid-face hypoplasia, short palpebral fissures, small chin), cleft palate, congenital heart defects, thymic aplasia leading to immunological problems, problems with calcium homeostasis due to absent or hypoplastic parathyroid glands, low tone, and scoliosis.** More sublte palatal problems may manifest as velopharygnal insufficiency (nasal speech, speeh difficulties).

d. Psychiatric disorders are common, with 60–75% exhibiting significant symptoms, including psychosis, mood disorders, and anxiety. **Reported rates of schizophrenia and schizoaffective disorder are as high as 25–30%.** In addition, **it is estimated that as many as 2% of schizophrenics may have this condition, undiagnosed, and that rates may be even higher in patients with early-onset schizophrenia.** Learning disabilities, especially non-verbal learning disorder, are common.

e. Diagnostic testing involves detection of the submicroscopic deletion by FISH technique.

B. Autosomal Dominant Conditions

1. **Huntington disease (HD)**
   a. HD is due to an **increased number of "triplet repeats" of the trinucleotide sequence CAG in the *HD* gene on chromosome 4p16.** Repeat length may undergo **expansion from one generation to the next.** The phenomenon of **anticipation is characteristic of triplet repeat disorders, and involves increased severity and earlier onset of illness in subsequent generations.**
   b. Physical findings may include dysarthria and clumsiness early on, followed by a **progressive motor decline of both voluntary and involuntary movements and by the development of chorea. These symptoms are best managed by high-potency neuroleptics, like haloperidol.**
   c. Psychiatric symptoms may be the first presenting features in up to one-third of patients, and may include prominent personality changes early on, with development of **dementia and symptoms of disordered thought and psychosis.** A high suicide rate is reported in these patients.
   d. Diagnostic testing involves **detection of the increased number of CAG triplet repeats in the *HD* gene.**
2. **Tuberous sclerosis**
   a. Tuberous sclerosis is due to a mutation in the *TSC1* gene on chromosome 9q23 or *TSC2* gene on chromosome 16p13.3.
   b. Physical features include a variety of **skin findings (hypopigmented macules, ash leaf spots, shagreen patches, angiofibromas), dental pits, and tumors in different organ systems, including CNS tubers, retinal hamartomas, cardiac rhabdomyomas, and renal angiomyolipomas. Seizures are common.**
   c. Psychiatric findings include PDD and ADHD features.
   d. Diagnosis is usually made on a clinical basis, but diagnostic testing involving mutation analysis of the *TSC1* and *TSC2* genes is available.
3. **Neurofibromatosis type 1 (NF1)/Von Recklinghausen disease**
   a. NF1 is due to a **mutation in the *NF1* gene on chromosome 17q11.2, which is believed to lead to loss of tumor suppressor function.**
   b. Physical findings in NF1 include **abnormalities of skin pigmentation (*café au lait* spots, freckling in axilla or groin), neurofibromas (cutaneous, subcutaneous or plexiform), Lisch nodules on the iris, and bony abnormalities. Acoustic neuromas are found in NF2.** Complications may vary depending on the number, location, and extent of the neurofibromas, and with development of malignant tumors.
   c. Psychiatric symptoms include learning disabilities and ADHD.
   d. Diagnosis is usually made based on clinical features, but confirmatory testing of the *NF1* gene is available and most helpful in families where a mutation has previously been identified.
4. **Williams syndrome (WS)**
   a. WS is due to a microdeletion on one copy of chromosome 7q11, and includes loss of the *elastin (ELN)* gene.
   b. Physical findings include a **characteristic "elfish" facial appearance (broad forehead with narrowing at temples, stellate pattern in iris, short nose with fleshy nasal tip, prominent ear lobes, wide mouth with full lips, and small jaw), short stature, cardiac defects (especially supravalvular aortic stenosis), and connective tissue disease (e.g., joint laxity).**
   c. Psychiatric features included mild-severe mental retardation, ADHD, and anxiety. A friendly personality and good verbal skills are also identifying features of these patients, although their superficial relating abilities may make relationships difficult to sustain.
   d. Diagnostic testing involves detection of the submicroscopic deletion by FISH technique.
5. **Porphyria**
   a. One of the more common types of porphyria is acute intermittent porphyria (AIP) due to mutations in the *hydroxymethylbilane synthase (HMBS)* gene on chromosome 11q23.3, leading to decreased activity of porphobilinogen (PBG) deaminase, part of the heme biosynthetic pathway.
   b. Patients with AIP experience acute **"neurovisceral attacks," marked by abdominal pain and vomiting, generalized weakness, and diffuse body pain. Over time, demyelination may occur. Urine may turn brown or red when left standing from presence of pathway byproducts.**
   c. Psychiatric symptoms are quite variable, and may include a change in mental status or delirium, psychosis, anxiety, and depression. Anecdotally, these patients are often described as having "histrionic" traits, or a distinct personality. **Symptoms are worsened by medications that induce the heme synthetic pathway. Offending medications include those that upregulate the P450 system (e.g., barbiturates, sulfonamides, and alcohol);** the severe reactions that may occur in these patients may cause them to be misdiagnosed as treatment refractory. In addition, hormone changes associated with the menstrual cycle may precipitate attacks.
   d. Diagnostic testing involves the measurement of pathway **by-products in the urine (porphobilinogen, Δ-aminolevulinic acid), or measurement of decreased PBG deaminase in blood.**
   e. Treatment may include medications that suppress heme synthesis, folic acid (a PBG deaminase co-factor), and avoiding offending agents that may precipitate attacks. Supportive care is given during attacks.

C. X-Linked Genetic Syndromes

1. **Fragile X syndrome (FXS)**
   a. FXS is due to an **increased number of triplet CGG repeats in the *FMR1*** gene located on chromosome Xq27.3. It is the **most common *inherited* form of mental retardation.** Although Down syndrome is more prevalent, the great majority of cases of DS are not inherited, as nei-

ther parent carries an extra or abnormal copy of the DS critical region. In contrast, Fragile X is inherited from a mother who passes on the abnormal gene. The syndrome is most often described in males, but findings in carrier females may range from asymptomatic to as severe as affected males.

b. Physical features include a **characteristic facial appearance (large head with long face, prominent jaw and forehead, and large ears), large testes (may not be apparent until puberty), low tone, and connective tissue disease.**

c. Psychiatric symptoms include moderate to severe mental retardation, PDD, ADHD, and mood lability.

d. Diagnostic testing involves **determination of the number of CGG repeats in and methylation status of the *FMR1* gene.**

2. **Rett syndrome (RS)**

a. RS is due to a mutation in the *MECP2* gene on chromosome Xq28.

b. Girls with classic Rett Syndrome appear normal at birth, but experience a **progressive loss of developmental skills associated with acquired microcephaly starting around 18–24 months. These patients are severely mentally retarded. Additional findings include loss of purposeful hand movements (replaced by stereotyped hand movements),** gait abnormalities, seizures, and bruxism. Males with mental retardation and other features have also been found to have *MECP2* mutations, but their characterization requires further study.

c. Psychiatric symptoms include autistic features, anxiety attacks, and screaming fits.

d. Diagnostic testing involves mutation analysis of the *MECP2* gene.

D. Autosomal Recessive Conditions/Inborn Errors of Metabolism

1. **Homocystinuria**

a. Classic homocystinuria is **due to mutations of *cystathionine β synthase (CBS)* gene on chromosome 21q22.3, leading to deficiency of cystathionine β synthase.** Preserved enzymatic activity, and less severe disease, may be seen with the pyridoxine (vitamin B_6)-responsive variant, and other enzyme co-factor deficiencies (folate or B_{12}) may also lead to symptoms. Overall these defects result in problems with conversion of homocysteine to cysteine and remethylation of homocysteine to methionine, resulting in elevated blood homocysteine.

b. **Patients with homocystinuria are normal at birth, with onset of symptoms in childhood.** High levels of homocysteine interfere with collagen cross-linking, resulting in connective tissue disease and disruptions to the vascular endothelium (leading to thrombus formation and potential for vascular events). **Many patients are described as "Marfanoid," with long, thin limbs, high arched palate, scoliosis, arachnodactyly, pectus excavatum, and lens dislocations. In contrast to patients with other connective tissue disease who have hypermobile joints, the joints in these patients may have restricted range of motion.**

c. Psychiatric symptoms include mental retardation, developmental delay, learning disabilities, depression, OCD, and non-specific behavioral problems. Schizophrenia and psychosis may occur at higher rates in these patients.

d. Diagnostic testing involves the use of urine nitroprusside test for disulfides and measurement of **elevated homocysteine and methionine levels in the blood.**

e. **Treatment is centered on providing a diet that is low in methionine** (the precursor to homocysteine) **and supplemented by the vitamin co-factors and cysteine,** which becomes an essential amino acid in these patients.

2. **Wilson disease**

a. Wilson disease is **due to a mutation in the *ATP7B* gene on chromosome 13q14.3-21.1,** leading to decreased levels of copper transporting ATPase 2 and **resultant copper deposition in the CNS and liver.**

b. Physical finding are due to abnormal organ function caused by the copper, and are most prominent in the **liver (jaundice, hepatitis, and cirrhosis) and CNS (movement disorders, dysarthria, and seizures).** Due to copper deposition in the cornea, **many patients may have Kayser-Fleischer rings (brownish-green rings located in the iris),** visible on slit lamp examination.

c. Psychiatric symptoms include **cognitive decline, changes in personality, and mood lability (some with pseudobulbar palsy), and may be the first indication of disease.**

d. Diagnostic testing involves measurement of reduced serum bound copper and ceruloplasmin and elevated urinary copper excretion. Deposition may be visualized by liver biopsy, or neuroimaging. Mutation analysis is available on a limited basis.

e. Treatment consists of **chelation therapy (e.g., penicillamine),** avoidance of copper rich foods (shellfish, liver, chocolate, mushrooms, and nuts), and supplementation with antioxidants. Patients may go on to require liver transplant.

3. **Metachromatic Leukodystrophy**

a. Metachromatic leukodystrophy is **due to deficiency of aryl-sulfatase A,** leading to storage of galactosyl sulfatide (cerebroside sulfate) in the white matter of the central and peripheral nervous systems. There are three forms, presenting in infancy, childhood, and early adulthood.

b. Physical findings include **gait problems and ataxia, difficulty with speech and incontinence and progressive deterioration of the nervous system.**

c. Of note, psychiatric symptoms may be the first presentation of this disorder (especially in the adult variant) and include decline in school performance/cognition, changes in personality and psychosis.

d. Diagnostic testing involves measurement of low aryl sulfatase A levels in blood, elevated urine sulfatides, and characteristic MRI findings that show white matter atrophy.

E. X-linked Recessive Metabolic Conditions

1. **Lesch-Nyhan syndrome**
   a. Lesch-Nyhan syndrome is **due to a deficiency of hypoxanthine-guanine phosphoribosyltransferase (HPRT) with resultant hyperuricemia,** caused by mutations in the *HPRT1* gene located on chromosome Xq26-27.2. Due to its X-linked inheritance, it is described in boys.
   b. Physical findings include **pyramidal and extrapyramidal neurological findings and sequelae of urate crystal deposition in joints, kidney, and bladder.**
   c. **The hallmark of this syndrome is the development of self-injurious and self-mutilatory behaviors (biting lips and fingers, head banging).** Other psychiatric symptoms include developmental delay, aggression, and cognitive impairment.
   d. Diagnostic testing involves the measurement of increased uric acid production and excretion, decreased HPRT enzyme activity, and confirmatory mutation analysis of the *HPRT1* gene.
   e. Treatment is focused on decreasing the amount of uric acid through the use of allopurinol, and behavioral techniques and restraint to manage self-injurious behavior.
2. **X-linked Adrenoleukodystrophy**
   a. X-linked Adrenoleukodystrophy is **due to a deficiency of lignoceroyl-CoA ligase,** caused by mutations of the *ABCD1* gene on chromosome Xq28, **leading to accumulations of very long chain fatty acids (VLCFA) in cerebral white matter and adrenal cortex.** Due to X-linked inheritance, the full syndrome is usually seen in boys, but female carriers may also show symptoms.
   b. Physical findings **include abnormal gait, dysarthria, and dysphagia. Over time, progressive loss of motor skills, vision, and hearing occurs. Sequelae of adrenal dysfunction may occur.**
   c. **The earliest symptoms often result in a diagnosis of ADHD,** but cognitive decline is progressive.
   d. Diagnostic testing involves demonstration of elevated VLCFA in the blood, increased ACTH, and other indications of adrenal dysfunction, as well as characteristic MRI findings. Mutation analysis of the *ABCD*1 gene is available.
   e. **Treatment is focused on correction of adrenal function.** No treatment is available for the neurological sequelae. The use of "Lorenzo's oil" has not proven to be helpful. Bone marrow transplant may be helpful in treating this disease, but high morbidity and mortality associated with this procedure has limited its use.

F. Syndromes Caused by Teratogen Exposure

1. **Fetal alcohol syndrome (FAS)**
   a. FAS involves a spectrum of findings associated with *in-utero* exposure to alcohol; the severity of the syndrome appears to be dose-related, with more severe findings associated with increased alcohol intake and binge drinking. Of note, the possibility of *in-utero* exposure to other drugs must also be considered in patients being evaluated for FAS.
   b. Physical features may include a **characteristic facial appearance (microcephaly, flattened mid-face, epicanthal folds, flat philtrum [the space between nose and upper lip] thin upper lip, and small jaw), pre- and post-natal growth deficiency, and cardiac abnormalities.**
   c. Psychiatric symptoms may include ADHD, prominent oppositional behaviors, depression, and PTSD (due to associated social issues).
   d. Diagnosis is made based on the presence of clinical findings and a known history of alcohol exposure during pregnancy. There is no confirmatory laboratory testing available.

Suggested Readings

Asherson, P.J., & Curran, S. (2001, August). Approaches to gene mapping in complex disorders and their application in child psychiatry and psychology. *British Journal of Psychiatry, 179,* 122–128.

Basset, A.S., Chow, E.W., Waterworth, D.M., & Brzustowicz, L. (2001). Genetic insights into schizophrenia. *Canadian Journal of Psychiatry, 46,* 131–137.

Burmeister, M. (1999). Basic concepts in the study of diseases with complex genetics. *Biological Psychiatry, 45,* 522–532.

Cowan, W.M., Kopnisky, K.L., & Hyman, S.E. (2002). The human genome project and its impact on psychiatry. *Annual Review of Neuroscience, 25,* 1–50.

Estrov, Y., Scaglia, F., & Bodamer, O.A. (2000). Psychiatric symptoms of inherited metabolic disease. *Journal of Inherited Metabolic Disorders, 23,* 2–6.

Faraone, S., Tsuang, M., & Tsuang, D. (1999). *Genetics of mental disorders: A guide for students, clinicians, and researchers.* New York: Guilford Press.

Folstein, S.E., & Rosen-Sheidley, B. (2001). Genetics of autism: Complex aetiology for a heterogeneous disorder. *Nature Reviews Genetics, 2,* 943–955.

Gene Clinics. Available *www.geneclinics.org.*

Hattori, E., Liu, C., Badner, J.A., et al. (2003). Polymorphisms at the g72/g30 gene locus, on 13q33, are asssociated with bipolar disorder in two independent pedigree series. *American Journal of Human Genetics, 72*(5), 1131–1140.

Hettema, J.M., Neale, M.C., & Kendler, K.S. (2001). A review and meta-analysis of the genetic epidemiology of anxiety disorders. *American Journal of Psychiatry, 158,* 1568–1578.

Kendler, K. (1993). Twin studies of psychiatric illness. *Archives of General Psychiatry, 50,* 905–915.

McGuffin, P., Tandon, K., & Corsico, A. (2003). Linkage and association studies of schizophrenia. *Current Psychiatry Report, 5*(2), 121–127.

Moldavsky, M., Lev, D., & Lerman-Sagie, T. (2001). Behavioral phenotypes of genetic syndromes: A reference guide for psychiatrists. *Journal of the American Academy of Child and Adolescent Psychiatry, 40,* 749–761.

Online Mendelian Inheritance in Man (OMIM). Available *www.ncbi.nlm.nih.gov/omim.*

Plomin, R., DeFries, J., McClearn, G., & Rutter, M. (1997). *Behavioral genetics* (3rd ed.). New York: W.H. Freeman.

Report of the NIMH Genetics Workgroup. (1999). Genetics and mental disorders. *Biological Psychiatry, 45,* 559–602.

Rutter, M., & Plomin, R. (1997). Opportunities for psychiatry from genetic findings. *British Journal of Psychiatry, 171,* 209–219.

Selkoe, D.J., & Podlisny, M.B. (2002). Deciphering the genetic basis of Alzheimer's disease. *Annual Review of Genomics and Human Genetics, 3,* 67–99.

Sklar, P., Gabriel, S.B., McInnis, M.G., et al. (2002). Family-based association study of 76 candidate genes in bipolar disorder: BDNF is a potential risk locus. Brain-derived neutrophic factor. *Molecular Psychiatry, 7*(6), 579–593.

Sullivan, P.F., Neale, M.C., & Kendler, K.S. (2000). Genetic epidemiology of major depression: Review and meta-analysis. *American Journal of Psychiatry, 157,* 1552–1562.

Chapter 69

Psychiatry and the Law III: Malpractice and Boundary Violations

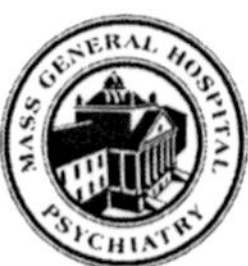

RONALD SCHOUTEN

I. Overview

The law related to malpractice litigation has had a significant effect on the practice of modern psychiatry. This chapter reviews the legal basics of malpractice litigation, some major topics in malpractice, and the important area of boundary violations.

II. Malpractice Law

A. Malpractice cases are part of the general field of personal injury or tort law. There are two types of torts:

1. **Intentional torts** (e.g., sexual contact with a patient, physical assault on a patient, fraud, or misrepresentation). Malpractice insurance covers intentional torts (e.g., sexual misconduct) only when the intentional act is part of standard practice (e.g., restraint of a patient).
2. **Unintentional torts or negligence.** This is the basis for most malpractice claims.

B. In order to prove a malpractice claim, a plaintiff (the party who claims to have been injured and who is seeking damages) must establish the four elements of a malpractice claim—the 4 Ds:

1. **The defendant was derelict in his responsibilities.** This can be established either by showing that the treating clinician departed from, or ignored, the standard of care, or by establishing that the treating clinician was negligent in the manner in which he or she followed the standard of care.
2. **The defendant had a specific obligation or duty to the patient.**
   a. **The general duty of physicians is to possess and employ such reasonable skill and care as are commonly had and are exercised by respectable, average physicians in the same or similar community.**
   b. **Specialists are held to a higher standard of performance because they hold themselves out to the community as having special expertise.** A physician who holds him- or herself out as an expert in a specific area will be judged according to this higher standard, regardless of the actual credentials.
   c. **The "school rule." Practice in accordance with the standards of a recognized school of thought or training will be judged according to the standards of that school to which the defendant physician is a member.** For example, cognitive-behavioral therapists should be judged according to the standard of care for that school of treatment, not according to a psychoanalytic standard of care. However, all clinicians that hold themselves out to the public as being qualified to diagnose and treat illnesses are held to the same basic standard of care with regard to safety, assessment, and conduct. For example, a psychiatrist cannot excuse himself from failing to diagnose his patient's myocardial infarction on the basis that he does not prescribe medication and only does psychotherapy.
   d. **Duty to consult. Physicians have a duty to get consultation when the limits of the physician's knowledge and experience have been exceeded.**
3. **The dereliction of duty is the direct cause of an injury.** Direct causation has two separate components:
   a. A mechanical notion assessed by the **"but for" rule, i.e., "but for" the negligent behavior, the injury would not have occurred.**
   b. **Proximate or legal cause: the harm that occurred was a "reasonably foreseeable" consequence of the negligent action.** In proving causation, a plaintiff may invoke the evidentiary concept of *res ipsa loquitur* (the thing speaks for itself) when the cause of injury to the plaintiff was under the sole control of the defendant and the defendant alone has knowledge of the injurious event. In such cases, the presumption is that the defendant was responsible for the injury and the defendant must rebut that presumption.
4. **Damages must be proven.** Unless harm is shown to have occurred, the malpractice suit will not succeed, even if there was negligent performance of a duty. **Damages can be of three types:**
   a. **Economic damages** (e.g., lost earnings, cost of medical treatment for the injury)
   b. **Physical damages** (e.g., loss of a bodily function)
   c. **Emotional pain and suffering**

III. Selected Malpractice Issues

A. Abandonment: the unilateral termination of the doctor-patient relationship, by the doctor, without consent or justification, where the termination results in harm to the patient.

1. **Justification can arise in a variety of circumstances;** e.g.,
   a. No-show patients
   b. Assaultive or abusive patients
   c. Non-compliant patients
2. **When it is necessary to terminate the relationship, claims of abandonment can be avoided by providing**

a referral to another clinician or agency, access to emergency coverage, and medications between the time of termination and the time of the appointment with the new treater.

3. **Abandonment allegations can arise when the physician is absent for vacation or conferences and fails to provide coverage or provides substandard coverage.** These allegations can be avoided by providing adequate coverage during absences. **The physician is responsible for ensuring that the coverage is competent and available.** For example, a physician may be held liable if harm occurs to a patient during his or her absence and he/she knows or should have known that the covering physician was incompetent.

B. Vicarious liability is the imposition of liability on one party for the negligent acts of another.

1. **Under the doctrine of *respondeat superior* (let the master answer), the "master" (employer) may be held liable for the negligent acts of a second person, the "servant" (employee), committed within the scope of the employment.**
   a. **A master,** for these purposes, **is one who has direct authority over the servant,** as evidenced by the power to hire or fire and veto power over the servant's decisions.
   b. **A consultant is distinguished from a master or employer by being outside the direct line of responsibility for the acts of the second person,** having no direct authority over the second person, and offering advice and direction on a "take it or leave it" basis.
2. This concept applies to the supervision of residents as well as to the supervision of non-physicians.
3. **The physician who signs prescriptions or disability forms as the attending physician for patients he or she did not evaluate may be held to the same level of responsibility as if he or she had personally evaluated the patient.**

C. Confidentiality

1. **Confidentiality is the physician's duty to hold matters revealed by the patient in the course of treatment in confidence from unauthorized third parties.**
2. There are a number of **exceptions to this general duty,** including:
   a. **Emergency.** This is defined as **a situation when failure to breach confidentiality would result in a serious (e.g., life-threatening) deterioration in the patient's condition.**
   b. **Waiver of the duty by the patient or other appropriate decision-maker.**
   c. **When the patient is temporarily or permanently incompetent,** information may be released about the patient in order to provide care to the patient. However, when a substitute decision-maker is identified, permission should be obtained from the decision-maker before information is to be released about the patient.
   d. Various state and federal laws provide exceptions to confidentiality, such as permitting **release of information during civil commitment proceedings, malpractice cases related to the treatment, bill collections, and litigation in which the patient puts his or her mental status at issue.**
   e. **Breaches of confidentiality may be required by statute or case law,** such as obligations to report child abuse or neglect or the duty to take steps to protect third parties from harm threatened by a patient (see below).
3. **In the normal course of treatment, information about a patient may be shared with a limited group of individuals without getting the express permission of the patient. These are generally held to include the patient, co-treaters, consultants, supervisors, and facilities to which the patient is being admitted or transferred. Before information is released to family members, referring clinicians, lawyers, or law enforcement, the patient's express permission should be obtained.**
4. **In all cases where confidentiality is to be breached, it should be breached to the least extent possible and with the patient being aware.**
5. **The Health Insurance Portability and Accountability Act (HIPAA) is a federal statute that imposes a number of requirements on the disclosure of information and the protection of patient privacy in clinical care and research.** The details of these requirements, which first became effective in April 2003 and apply to "covered entities," are beyond the scope of this chapter. The reader should be aware of the basic confidentiality/privacy requirements, regardless of whether he or she is a covered entity, as these are likely to become standard requirements. These basic requirements include notifying the patient of privacy rights and policies, obtaining from the patient written acknowledgment of having received those rights, keeping track of releases of patient information, and providing reasonable safeguards to protect the privacy of patient records, e.g., locked cabinets. Detailed information about the privacy provisions of HIPAA can be found at http://www.hhs.gov/ocr/hipaa/privrulepd.pdf.

D. The Duty to Protect Third Parties: The *Tarasoff* Legacy

1. **Breach of confidentiality is ethically permissible when there is a need to protect the patient or third parties:** "Psychiatrists at times may find it necessary, in order to protect the patient or the community from imminent danger, to reveal confidential information disclosed by the patient" (Principles of Medical Ethics with Annotations Especially Applicable to Psychiatry, Section 4, Annotation 8).
2. The general concept is that there is a basic duty to protect a potential victim if a therapist knows or should

know of a patient's potential for substantial harm to an identified or a readily identifiable individual.

3. The key case in this area is *Tarasoff* v. *Regents of the University of California,* 551 P. 2d 334 (1976).
   a. Holding: "When a therapist determines, or pursuant to the standards of his profession should determine, that his patient presents a serious danger of violence to another, he incurs a serious obligation to use reasonable care to protect the intended victim from such danger."
   b. **Implications of the *Tarasoff* decision**
      i. Psychotherapists and patients have a special relationship that makes the therapist uniquely liable for some actions of the patient.
      ii. It is not necessarily a duty to warn the intended victim or law enforcement, which would require a breach of confidentiality, but it is a duty to protect that can be fulfilled through a variety of other actions on the part of the treater.
      iii. **The duty that was established by *Tarasoff* was to an identified victim, although subsequent cases expanded the duty to broader classes of individuals and in some cases to individuals who might be in a "zone of danger" around an intended victim.**
   c. Although the duty to protect third parties has been rejected by courts and legislatures in several states, the duty saw a rapid expansion in many jurisdictions. As a result, a number of states passed statutes that placed some limitations on the duty. **The American Psychiatric Association (APA) developed a model statute that provides for liability to third parties for the acts of a patient when:**
      i. The patient communicates an explicit threat to identified victim(s) with apparent intent and ability to carry out the threat, and reasonable steps are not taken.
      ii. The patient has a known history of physical violence, the therapist has a "reasonable basis to believe that there is a clear and present danger that the patient will attempt to kill or inflict serious bodily injury against a reasonably identified victim or victims," and reasonable steps are not taken.
      iii. Reasonable steps are defined as one or more of the following:

         - Warn the potential victim or victims.
         - Notify law enforcement in the area.
         - Arrange for voluntary hospitalization.
         - Take appropriate steps to commit.

E. The National Practitioner Bank

1. Authorized by **the Health Care Quality Improvement Act of 1986 (HCQIA),** the database applies to physicians, dentists, and other health care practitioners.
2. **It requires mandatory reporting of:**
   a. **Payments made to satisfy malpractice claims** (including settlements)
   b. **Adverse privilege actions taken by health care entities**
   c. **Actions taken on licensure**
3. The practitioner who is reported must be notified and given an opportunity to respond.
4. Hospitals are required to query the databank for information on each physician, dentist, or other health care practitioner appointed to staff or granted clinical privileges.
   a. Other health care facilities may query.
   b. Malpractice insurers may not directly query.

IV. Boundary Violations

A. An Introduction to Professional Boundaries

1. **Boundaries** between doctors and patients **provide a set of rules and expectations that allow the patient to develop trust in the physician and know what to expect from the relationship.**
   a. **Boundary crossings** involve minor, but potentially important, blurring of the boundaries.
   b. **Boundary violations** involve more clear-cut transgressions of the accepted boundaries between doctor and patient.
2. **What constitutes a boundary crossing or violation is determined both by the nature of the action and by the setting in which it occurs.** For example, in a rural area it might be appropriate for the family doctor to spend time with patients at a social gathering, while the same socializing for a doctor in an urban practice might be considered a boundary crossing.
3. The maintenance of professional boundaries has been the subject of both ethical and legal proscriptions. **The basic principle of these limitations on physician behavior is that physicians have a fiduciary duty to their patients. This duty is to put the best interests of the patient ahead of the physician's interest.**
   a. The Hippocratic Oath includes admonitions about maintaining appropriate boundaries, including maintaining confidences and avoiding sexual relations. **In 1989, the American Medical Association Council on Ethical and Judicial Affairs passed an ethical rule that prohibits physician-patient sexual contact, regardless of specialty.**
   b. **Physician-patient sexual contact and other forms of physician exploitation of patients are the basis for discipline by physician registration authorities in all states.**
   c. **The APA** has adopted an ethical guideline that **declares it is unethical for a psychiatrist to have a sexual relationship with a former or current patient.**
   d. **A number of states have enacted laws that make it a *criminal offense* for a physician to have a sexual relationship with a patient.**
      i. Statutes vary as to whether they classify doctor-patient sexual contact as a misdemeanor or a felony. Some statutes distinguish between first and repeated offenses.

ii. While many of the statutes criminalize psychotherapist-patient sexual contact, the term psychotherapy is broadly defined in some statutes as "the professional treatment, assessment, or counseling of a mental or emotional illness, symptom, or condition." Thus, many of these statutes would apply to primary care physicians who treat psychiatric illness.

iii. Statutes also differ with regard to how they define "patient," and whether and when the prohibition applies.

B. Selected Boundary Issues

1. **Business dealings between doctor and patient**
   a. **The physician-patient relationship is fundamentally a business relationship.** The terms of the contract are that the physician receives a fee in return for helping the patient with medical problems. The arm's-length nature of the relationship allows the physician to be objective in his or her dealings with the patient.
   b. **Involvement in other business dealings can detract from the distance, objectivity, and empathy necessary for the physician-patient relationship to succeed and is discouraged except under special circumstances;** e.g., the psychiatrist lives in a small community where the patient operates the only hardware store. Even in this limited situation, the psychiatrist would be well advised to find another store in a neighboring town.
2. **Social (non-sexual) relationships with patients**
   a. In certain settings (e.g., small towns), social contact between physician and patient is unavoidable. Confidentiality and cordiality without undue familiarity can allow these treatment relationships to succeed.
   b. **Close friendships between physician and patient can compromise the physician's objectivity and lead to errors in judgment because of the physician's emotional involvement.** The same principles apply here as apply in the context of physicians treating family members.
3. **Sex in the treatment relationship**
   a. As indicated earlier, sexual relations with patients has been the subject of great attention in legal and ethical circles. The reasons why physicians get involved in these relationships vary. They include predatory sexual behavior by physicians seeking to take advantage of the patient, as well as infatuation on the part of physicians who are vulnerable because of their own life circumstances. Some patients may be seductive, or at least engage in behavior that may be interpreted by the physician as seductive. Nevertheless, **it is always the physician's responsibility to maintain appropriate boundaries. Failure to do so is *always* the fault of the physician.**
   b. Sex with patients in the guise of treatment constitutes fraud and misrepresentation, and may provide the basis for criminal prosecution in some states and civil litigation in all states.
   c. Sexual relationships with patients in many cases result from the disparity in power and authority between doctor and patient. Such relationships are inherently coercive and without consent.
   d. Patients who have had sexual relationships with their physicians often suffer significant harm as a result. Such injury becomes a justifiable basis for a lawsuit against the physician. **While involvement in a sexual relationship with a patient constitutes an intentional tort that would ordinarily not be covered by malpractice insurance, courts have held that it represents a mishandling of the transference and countertransference in the treatment relationship, thus putting it within the realm of malpractice.**

Suggested Readings

Bisbing, S.B., Jorgenson, L.M., & Sutherland, P.K. (1996). *Sexual abuse by professionals: A legal guide.* Charlottesville, VA: Michie Company.

Gabbard, G.O. (1994). *Sexual misconduct. Psychiatric update, Vol. 18.* Washington, DC: American Psychiatric Press.

Gabbard, G., & Nadelson, C. (1996). Professional boundaries in the physician-patient relationship. *Forum, 17*(2), 7–8.

Gutheil, T.G., & Appelbaum, P.A. (2002). *Clinical handbook of psychiatry and the law* (3rd ed.). Baltimore, MD: Lippincott, Williams & Wilkins.

Prosser and Keeton on Torts (5th ed.). (1984). St. Paul, MN: West Publishing.

Chapter 70

Psychiatric Consultation to Medical and Surgical Patients

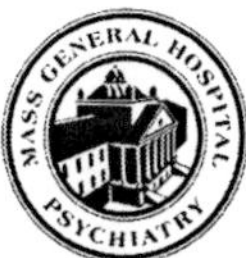

JOHN QUERQUES, THEODORE A. STERN, AND NED H. CASSEM

I. Overview

A. Functions of Consultation-Liaison (C-L) Psychiatry

C-L psychiatry is a branch of psychiatry that entails:

1. **Consultation to medically and surgically ill hospitalized patients**
2. **Enhancement of non-psychiatric clinicians' awareness of affective, behavioral, and cognitive disorders**
3. **Education of students and clinicians of all disciplines about the psychosocial and psychiatric aspects of medical care**
4. **Research at the interface of medicine, surgery, neurology, and psychiatry**

B. History of C-L Psychiatry

1. Rooted in psychosomatic medicine and psychobiology, C-L psychiatry has gradually widened its arena from the medical wards of large general hospitals in the 1930s, to critical-care units, to specialized centers that provide care for patients with cancer, human immunodeficiency virus (HIV) infection, and transplanted organs.
2. The mid-1970s marked a growth phase for the field, fueled by the return of the medical model and the provision of grant money by Dr. James Eaton, then the director of the Psychiatric Education Branch of the National Institute of Mental Health, for the establishment of new C-L services and research activities.
3. Whereas in the early 1970s only three-quarters of all psychiatry residency programs even offered an experience in C-L psychiatry, today such rotations are required.
4. Recently, the American Psychiatric Association and the American Board of Psychiatry and Neurology have recognized C-L psychiatry as a subspecialty and will be awarding certificates for Added Qualifications in Psychosomatic Medicine.

II. Epidemiology

A. Prevalence of Psychopathology among the Medically Ill

1. **The frequency of psychopathology in the general-hospital population ranges from 10% to 50%,** depending in large part on the type and severity of underlying medical or surgical illness.
2. Since **psychiatric co-morbidity prolongs length of stay, increases costs, and worsens the course of medical illness,** prompt recognition and treatment are essential.

B. Rates of Psychiatric Consultation

1. Despite the high frequency of psychiatric disturbance in general hospitals, in general, **the rate of referral for psychiatric consultation is estimated to be only 3–5%.**
2. Rates of psychiatric consultation vary across institutions based on differences in patient population, length of stay, nature and severity of illness, and personal style of referring physicians and consulting psychiatrists.
3. At the Massachusetts General Hospital (MGH), approximately 6% of all hospital admissions are seen by a psychiatrist.

C. Reasons for Psychiatric Consultation

1. Reasons for which consultation is requested typically **involve affective, behavioral, and cognitive derangements.**
2. Common requests include:
   a. Evaluation of depression and suicidal ideation
   b. Management of patients who have interpersonal difficulties with care providers or who fail to cooperate with the medical-surgical team
   c. Evaluation of decision-making capacity
   d. Evaluation of delirium and dementia

III. Diagnostic Features and Differential Diagnosis

A. Categorization of Psychiatric Problems

Diagnoses assigned by psychiatric consultants fall into one or more of the following categories:

1. **Psychiatric presentations of organic disease** (e.g., hypothyroidism with depressive features)
2. **Psychiatric complications of organic disease or its treatment** (e.g., steroid-induced psychosis)
3. **Psychiatric reactions to organic disease or its treatment** (e.g., adjustment disorder after a diagnosis of cancer)
4. **Organic presentations of psychiatric disease** (e.g., depression with multiple somatic complaints)
5. **Co-morbid independent psychiatric and medical illness** (e.g., schizophrenia and coronary artery disease [CAD])

B. At the MGH, the most common diagnoses given by psychiatric consultants are depression, delirium, anxiety, substance abuse, personality disorder, various pain syndromes, and dementia.

IV. Principles of Psychiatric Evaluation of Medical-Surgical Patients

A request for consultation may belie a problem within the patient, among the medical-surgical staff as individuals, and, as a whole, between patient and staff. An effective consultant recognizes the importance of each of these forces and considers each in an accurate formulation of the problem.

A. Speak directly with the consultee to define the reason for the consultation and to establish its urgency.

1. While the "real" reason for the consultation may not be obvious from the stated request, it may be discerned from a conversation with the consultee.
2. The consultant is most helpful when he or she understands the consultee's question or concern and then specifically addresses that issue throughout the consultative process.

B. Review the current and pertinent portions of the old record.

C. Review the patient's medications, including those taken at home and those ordered in the hospital. Be vigilant for recently added and discontinued agents that may bear on the current mental status.

D. Gather collateral information from family, friends, and staff without becoming an advocate of these sources' points of view or opinions. Maintain an open mind and avoid premature closure.

E. Interview the patient and perform a mental status examination (MSE).

1. Anticipate:
   a. An atmosphere less formal and rigid than in the outpatient setting
   b. The sights, smells, and sounds of a medical or surgical ward
   c. Frequent interruptions by nurses, other staff, and family
   d. The presence of roommates
   e. The requirement for flexibility in timing and format
   f. The goal to be not only diagnostic but therapeutic
   g. A review of the patient's medical issues early in the interview
   h. An appropriate use of humor
   i. Defense mechanisms activated against fear, anxiety, and mistrust

F. Do the appropriate physical and neurologic examinations.

G. Write a brief, jargon-free note that emphasizes impressions and recommendations and plans for treatment. Because these sections are the most important to the consultee, it is especially critical to be clear and specific in these sections.

1. In the medical record, avoid "note wars," criticism of the consultee, and accusations of shoddy work. If the consultee chooses a therapeutic course equally appropriate to the consultant's preferred choice, an indication of agreement in the chart may be more prudent than rigid insistence on the consultant's preference.
2. The consultation note includes all of the elements of a standard psychiatric note plus:
   a. **A two-sentence summary of the patient's medical and psychiatric history, the reason for admission, and the reason for consultation.** For example, a 75-year-old man with a history of CAD, hypertension, and depression was admitted to the medical service for evaluation of substernal chest pain thought to be secondary to myocardial infarction. Psychiatric consultation is requested to assess the safety of continuing tricyclic antidepressant therapy.
   b. **A brief summary of the present medical illness, test results, and hospital course** that demonstrates a basic appreciation for the medical issues material to the consultation rather than rehashes data already present in earlier notes.
   c. **A brief description of the patient's typical patterns of response to stress and illness.**
   d. **Relevant physical and neurologic examinations.**
   e. **Relevant current and past laboratory results.**
   f. **Differential diagnoses** listed in order of decreasing likelihood. An indication that the patient's symptoms are not attributable to a certain psychiatric disorder may be very helpful.
   g. **Recommendations or plans** listed in order of decreasing importance:
      i. **Diagnostics** (laboratory tests, neuroimaging, projective testing, neuropsychological testing)
      ii. **Therapeutics** (biological, psychological, social, and behavioral)
         - For medications, include dose, route of administration, and frequency. The consultee should be able to transcribe recommendations for medications directly onto the order sheet.
         - Anticipate and address problems that may appear later. For example, for a delirious patient who is currently calm, the consultant may recommend that a neuroleptic agent be given should the patient become agitated in the future.
   h. **An indication that the consultant will provide follow-up.**
   i. **The consultant's printed name and phone or beeper number.**

H. Speak with the consultee, nurses, and other relevant staff about your findings, opinion, and treatment proposal, highlighting the rationale and anticipated outcome of your recommendations. This step is especially important when diagnoses or recommendations are crucial or controversial (e.g., when a pre-operative patient is found to have the capacity to refuse surgery).

V. Treatment

A. Treatment should proceed along multiple lines: biological, psychological, social, and behavioral.

1. **Biological.** When prescribing psychotropic agents for patients who are taking other medications for medical illnesses, the consultant must be vigilant for:
   a. **Drug-drug interactions.** Numerous medicines, including many psychopharmaceuticals, are metabolized in the liver by the cytochrome P450 enzyme system. Many psychiatric medications inhibit this enzymatic pathway and thus raise serum levels of concomitantly administered drugs. (See chapter 51 for a detailed discussion of these interactions.)
   b. **Protein binding.** Some psychopharmacologic agents are highly protein-bound. These drugs may displace other protein-bound medicines and thus raise their serum concentrations, potentially to dangerous levels. (See chapter 51 for a detailed discussion of these interactions.)
   c. **Side effects.** Certain adverse effects that medically healthy patients tolerate may be troublesome or dangerous for patients undergoing treatment for active medical illness. These side effects may worsen the medical problem or the side effects of other treatments. For example, the gut-slowing effect of tricyclic antidepressants may worsen post-operative ileus.
2. **Psychological. Psychotherapy with hospitalized, medically ill patients is brief, focused on the here-and-now and the practical.** The consultant's goal is to identify and bolster patients' innate defenses to help them better cope with illness and hospitalization and to explain these coping strategies to the medical-surgical team. To be an effective therapist, the consultant must appreciate the variable stresses that different diseases engender, as well as the universality of the experience of **uncertainty** (in diagnosis, treatment outcome, and prognosis), and **grief** (over disfigurement, disability, or imminent death). Consultants may instruct patients in the use of **relaxation techniques, guided imagery,** and **hypnosis** to quell anxiety and reduce stress.
3. **Social.** Consultants help the medical-surgical team and patient make decisions about:
   a. End-of-life care (e.g., do-not-resuscitate [DNR] and do-not-intubate [DNI] decisions)
   b. Disposition to an appropriate living situation (e.g., home with visiting nurses, skilled nursing facility, or nursing home)
   c. Short-term disability after a protracted illness or hospitalization
4. **Behavioral. Explanation for the medical-surgical staff of patients' natural coping styles helps the treatment team better understand and care for patients.** For example, an electrical engineer with obsessive-compulsive traits feels out of control when he is admitted to the coronary care unit (CCU) with chest pain. He questions the team frequently because information helps him to feel more in control, even though the team considers his questions bothersome and they begin to avoid him. If the CCU team understands this patient's defensive structure, they will be less hostile toward him, answer his questions appropriately, and provide him with information before he asks for it. The consultant may suggest that the patient decide the times of medication administration or physical therapy (e.g., within an hour or so of the usual time) to help the patient feel more in control. For patients who are agitated or likely to hurt themselves or others, the consultant may recommend physical restraints and/or constant observation.

B. **A key element of effective therapeutics is the provision of periodic (usually daily) follow-up visits** until the patient is psychiatrically stable, is discharged, or dies. This allows the consultant to:
   1. Gather further history from patient, family, friends, previous treaters, and other collateral sources.
   2. Supplement findings of the initial MSE, which provides only a cross-sectional snapshot of a patient's mental functioning at a given time, with longitudinal data.
   3. Refine diagnoses.
   4. Monitor treatment and recommend appropriate changes.
   5. Engage in ongoing dialogue with the consultee and other staff.

C. **"Signing off" of stable cases is acceptable, but the consultant should be prepared to resume follow-up should matters destabilize,** as many neuropsychiatric disturbances wax and wane.

D. **Consultants should be prepared to transfer patients who are psychiatrically unstable to an inpatient psychiatric unit once their medical and surgical issues are resolved.** Patients who require psychiatric follow-up but can safely go home should be referred for outpatient care.

E. Consultants may be called upon to complete medical certificates for patients incapable of making medical decisions for themselves and who require guardianship.

VI. Conclusions

A. **The C-L psychiatrist is an expert in the affective, behavioral, and cognitive disturbances of hospitalized medically or surgically ill patients, with skill in rapid assessment and in biological, psychological, social, and behavioral treatments.**

B. **First and foremost a competent and thorough physician, the C-L psychiatrist takes a panoramic view of the patient, the disease, and the interrelationships between the two.**

C. **The effective C-L psychiatrist addresses the needs of both the patient and the medical-surgical team.**

D. Accessibility, excellent communication skills, and tolerance for unpredictability are essential attributes.

Suggested Readings

Bronheim, H.E., Fulop, G., Kunkel, E.J., et al. (1998). The Academy of Psychosomatic Medicine practice guidelines for psychiatric consultation in the general medical setting. *Psychosomatics, 39*, S8–S30.

Ford, C.V. (1996). Introduction. In J.R. Rundell, & M.G. Wise (Eds.). (1996). *The American Psychiatric Press textbook of consultation-liaison psychiatry*, pp. xix–xxi. Washington, DC: American Psychiatric Press.

Garrick, T.R., & Stotland, N.L. (1982). How to write a psychiatric consultation. *American Journal of Psychiatry, 139*, 849–855.

Goldman, L., Lee, T., & Rudd, P. (1983). Ten commandments for effective consultations. *Archives of Internal Medicine, 143*, 1753–1755.

Hackett, T.P., Cassem, N.H., Stern, T.A., & Murray, G.B. (1997). Beginnings: Consultation psychiatry in a general hospital. In N.H. Cassem, T.A. Stern, J.F. Rosenbaum, & M.S. Jellinek (Eds.), *Massachusetts General Hospital handbook of general hospital psychiatry* (4th ed., pp. 1–9). St. Louis, MO: Mosby.

Kontos, N., Freudenreich, O., Querques, J., & Norris, E. (2003). Consultation psychiatrist as effective physician. *General Hospital Psychiatry, 25*(1), 20–23.

Kornfeld, D.S. (2002). Consultation-liason psychiatry: Contributors to medical practice. *American Journal of Psychiatry, 159*, 1964–1972.

Kunkel, E.J.S., & Thompson, T.L. (1996). The process of consultation and organization of a consultation-liaison psychiatry service. In J.R. Rundell, & M.G. Wise (Eds.), *The American Psychiatric Press textbook of consultation-liaison psychiatry*, pp. 13–23. Washington, DC: American Psychiatric Press.

Lipowski, Z.J. (1983). Current trends in consultation-liaison psychiatry. *Canadian Journal of Psychiatry, 28*, 329–338.

Lipowski, Z.J. (1996). History of consultation-liaison psychiatry. In J.R. Rundell, & M.G. Wise (Eds.), *The American Psychiatric Press textbook of consultation-liaison psychiatry*, pp. 3–11. Washington, DC: American Psychiatric Press.

McIntyre, J.S. (2002). A new subspecialty. *American Journal of Psychiatry, 159*, 1961–1963.

Pasnau, R.O, Fawzy, F.I., Skotzko, C.E., et al. (1996). Surgery and surgical subspecialties. In J.R. Rundell, & M.G. Wise (Eds.), *The American Psychiatric Press textbook of consultation-liaison psychiatry*. Washington, DC: American Psychiatric Press.

Popkin, M.K. (1995). Consultation-liaison psychiatry. In H.I. Kaplan, & B.J. Sadock (Eds.), *Comprehensive textbook of psychiatry* (6th ed., pp. 1592–1605). Baltimore, MD: Williams and Wilkins.

Chapter 71

Coping with Medical Illness

HELEN G. KIM AND DONNA B. GREENBERG

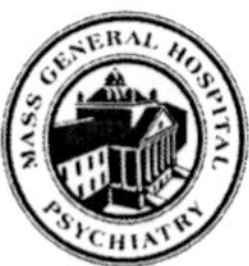

I. Introduction

How does one patient with hemophilia become a daredevil sportsman while another fearfully obsesses over the possibility of a fatal bleed? Why does one patient respond to the same disease differently than another? **Psychiatrists are frequently asked to see patients facing medical illness. Whether initiated by overwhelmed staff or by distraught patients, these consultations require careful psychiatric assessment, thoughtful ego lending, timely dynamic interpretations, and support of needed defenses.** Faced with physical illness, patients may feel damned by fate or divine intervention. Psychiatrists can help patients bear these threats to their bodies, mobilize personal and social resources, and overcome maladaptive defenses.

II. Aspects of Coping

A. Psychological Factors

Similar to the elegant feedback loops that maintain physiological homeostasis, patients have mechanisms to maintain psychological balance. When confronted by physical illness most patients revert to well-worn patterns of stress response. Medical illness can overwhelm these customary coping strategies, resulting in emotional imbalance manifested by anxiety, fear, guilt, despair, or anger. Ultimately patients achieve a new psychological homeostasis. For some, this represents an adaptive progression toward acceptance and mobilization of resources. For others, these crises evolve into maladaptive responses, such as embittered defeat, unyielding denial, or treatment non-compliance.

1. **Coping skills may be adaptive in one situation but self-sabotaging in another.** By classifying these coping mechanisms as "skills," Moos and Tsu (1977) and others have emphasized that **coping can be taught and used flexibly** and **psychological defenses are not innately pathologic.**
   a. **Denying or minimizing the seriousness of one's condition.** An obese woman may welcome unexplained weight loss and delay medical evaluation rather than interpret it as a possible harbinger of an underlying malignancy. After a teenager is told by her neurosurgeon that her cervical injury has left her paraplegic, she may lament missing her senior prom rather than grieve the loss of ever walking. Denial protects both patients from intolerable emotions. However, in the first case, denial delays crucial treatment, while in the second, it merely allows her time to assimilate her physical losses.
   b. **Isolation of affect** can be highly adaptive in helping a patient overcome immediate challenges posed by physical illness (e.g., a patient may keep appointments or follow-through with medical tests in a matter-of-fact unemotional way).
   c. **Intellectualization.** A patient may seek information to offset the helplessness engendered by disease. The physics professor with prostate cancer may focus on the results of scientific studies as the only means of restoring control. As with other coping skills, intellectualization can be highly adaptive if an obsessive search for information does not compromise sensible care.
   d. **Requesting reassurance and support** from family, friends, and health care providers can help counter feelings of isolation and helplessness.
   e. **Learning illness-related procedures,** such as how to administer insulin or how to develop the right strengthening exercises, may help to restore a sense of control and effectiveness.
   f. **Setting concrete limited goals,** such as a time to reveal the diagnosis of human immunodeficiency virus (HIV) infection to specific individuals, a special event, or certain physical tasks (e.g. running a race), can help a patient to identify manageable goals amidst seemingly overwhelming obstacles.
   g. **Rehearsing alternative outcomes.** The process of anticipating difficulties and creating alternative strategies can make it easier to conquer demoralizing tasks. For instance, a hard-driving business executive might recognize that resuming her hectic work schedule after a myocardial infarction would undermine recovery. Rather than wait for a resurgence of angina, she could proactively resume a reduced work schedule.
   h. **Finding meaning.** For one person, a hip fracture following a car accident may seem like punishment from an unjust god. Someone else might re-frame the trauma as an opportunity to reassess priorities and to re-define life goals.
2. **Character traits** shape the significance of disease for individual patients. These factors include age, intelligence, cognitive and emotional development, ego strength, object relatedness, and defensive style. For instance, an individual with a poor sense of self might adamantly deny his symptoms and depend excessively on health professionals. A more integrated, mature patient might rely more on gathering information to quell fear and anxiety and be able to rely on physicians with more flexibility.

Table 71-1. Biopsychosocial Components of Illness Dynamics

Psychological components
Personality traits
Ego mechanisms
Object relatedness
Stage of life during illness
Medical history
Past psychiatric history
Physician-patient relationship
Biological components
Nature and severity of disease process
Physical integrity of the patient
Genetic endowment
Response to pharmacotherapy
Medical history
Social components
Family relationships
Personal history
Family medical history
Cultural factors

SOURCE: Green, S.A. (1985). *Mind and body: The psychology of physical illness.* Washington, DC: American Psychiatric Press.

3. **The developmental moment** plays an important part in a patient's ability to cope with disease. A back injury in an adolescent male may undermine his developmentally appropriate urge to assert independence. His adolescent coping resources may be more limited than the resources of a 70-year-old with the same injury. On the other hand, injury at a later age brings its own challenges, including greater physical frailty and reminders of one's mortality.
4. **Catastrophic fears** evoked by physical illness can become manifest as anxiety, depression, fear, or treatment non-compliance. Direct questions about a patient's greatest fears can identify specific areas of vulnerability. For instance, loss of life may not necessarily be a foremost concern for a patient with terminal illness. Rather, an individual may fear loss of certain faculties, such as sexual function, sight, speech, or continence. The scope of catastrophic fears often includes the following:
   a. Loss of bodily integrity (e.g., colostomy, amputation, hysterectomy)
   b. Loss of power and dignity (e.g., weakness, incontinence)
   c. Abandonment or loss of intimacy (e.g., cognitive or emotional unavailability to loved ones)
   d. Loss of control (e.g., dependency on medications for health and survival)
   e. Loss of mental alacrity or memory (e.g., after stroke, dementia)
5. **Grieving**
   a. Coping with physical illness involves a grieving process. While the specific meaning of illness is peculiar to each patient, one should at least expect the patient to mourn his previous state of health. Psychiatrists can hear out and acknowledge denial, anger, bargaining, depression, and acceptance as stages of grief described by Kubler-Ross (1969). Patients may experience these stages at one time or another, and in no particular order as they work through their loss.
   b. **Unresolved grief** refers to feelings of loss that prevent the patient from accepting the illness. A person may be stuck in depression, hopelessness, anger, and helplessness, and may withdraw socially and curtail outside activities. These self-imposed limitations can extend far beyond the necessary restrictions of physical illness. If anger is unresolved, a patient may blindly seek retribution from physicians or family members for impositions caused by their physical illness. For instance, rather than grieve and accept the loss brought on by his illness, an individual may devote himself to baseless malpractice lawsuits (as if money could restore some sense of wholeness in the wake of physical illness).

      Unresolved grief can also lead to non-compliance with medical treatment. For example, a woman with complete remission of breast cancer after mastectomy and radiation may convince herself that she has conquered her illness and no longer needs her physicians. Such unyielding denial may lead to a Pyrrhic victory over cancer as she misses signs of recurrence that insidiously progress to metastatic disease. Here, denial may be her downfall.
   c. Green (1985) characterized the most abnormal psychological responses as denial, anxiety, anger, depression, and dependency. While each of these reflects a normal emotional response to grief, rigid denial, overwhelming anxiety, severe depression, or excessive dependency may be associated with regression or psychological stagnation rather than adaptation to the new reality.

B. Biological and Illness-Related Factors

1. **Symptom meaning.** Hand tremors can be a minor nuisance for a truck driver, but a devastating threat to self-identity for a concert violinist. **To determine the significance of a particular symptom, the psychiatrist must appreciate an individual's developmental stage, personal history, and defensive style.** Different symptoms often have a psychological meaning disproportionate to their actual prognostic importance. For instance, a disfiguring facial burn may have more psychological impact than a chronically progressive disease, such as diabetes. **Different diseases often have different impacts, depending on whether they**

are painful, disfiguring, disabling, or in a body region with special significance (e.g., face, prostate, breast).

2. **Nature and severity of disease.** HIV infection will convey a different meaning to a 22-year-old college senior than a 65-year-old retiree, even if both have the same viral load and require the same medications. Each has certain strengths and psychological vulnerabilities that will affect his experience of illness.
3. **Recovery from illness** may impose stress on a patient. Transfer from the intensive care unit to a general medicine floor may evoke relief in some who interpret it as a sign of recovery or outrage in others who rail against their physicians' perceived disregard.
4. **Disease complications** may undermine habitual coping mechanisms. For instance, dementia may hinder a surgeon's defenses of intellectualization and sublimation as he comes to terms with his failing memory and worsening tremor. Physiological problems (e.g., electrolyte imbalance, anemia, or hypoxia) may also impair cognition and coping.
5. **Psychiatric complications and co-morbidity** may accompany physical illness and interfere with recovery and treatment compliance. Despair and anxiety may naturally accompany the emotional response to physical illness. However, major depression, generalized anxiety disorder, or any Axis I condition should never be dismissed as "appropriate" responses and, therefore, unnecessary to treat.
6. **Treatment-related factors**
   a. **Patients must cope not only with disease but also with medical treatment.** A diabetic patient's response to needing insulin may range from intransigent denial to consuming obsessiveness. Behind such disparate defenses may lie similar fears of disability; however, one patient's denial may lead to premature blindness and lower extremity amputation, whereas another's fastidiousness may effect a better long-term course consistent with tightly controlled diabetes.
   b. Special treatment environments (e.g., the dialysis unit, intensive care unit, or even the doctor's waiting room) may present unique challenges to particular patients. Unfamiliar routines and separation from loved ones may evoke intolerable feelings of inadequacy, doubt, and failure.
   c. **The response of health professionals can influence a patient's ability to cope with illness.** A patient may feel intimidated by the perceived power of his physicians. In addition, patients may be stressed by the involvement of multiple physicians with no one asserting primary responsibility in what the Balints called a "collusion of anonymity." Whether a patient asks for a second opinion, pain medication, or a bill, he may shy away from confronting his physician directly for fear he will withdraw care or provide suboptimal treatment.

C. **Social factors** involved in illness dynamics include relationships with family, friends, health care providers, and the wider community. Physical illness can further tax chronically unstable interpersonal relationships, as well as strain empathic, constant ones. Studies have shown that the **quality of social supports can affect a patient's experience of illness as well as his long-term course.**

III. Psychiatric Assessment

A. Establish the Patient's Concerns

Psychiatrists must consider what has precipitated a patient's interest in seeking psychiatric consultation. Patients may have a range of worries, including pain, weakness, separation from family, confinement in a hospital, certain medical tests or procedures, and financial strain. **Common immediate concerns** of patients with physical illness include:

1. **Dealing with physical symptoms and incapacitation.**
2. **Dealing with the hospital environment and special treatment procedures.**
3. **Negotiating confusing health care systems and consulting with multiple health care providers.**
4. **Preserving a reasonable emotional balance.** Physical illness evokes a myriad of distressing feelings, such as self-blame, anxiety about an uncertain prognosis, alienation from loved ones, and resentment at health care providers for not "saving" them. Psychiatrists can help patients contain these feelings and experience them in non-destructive, tolerable aliquots.
5. **Preserving a satisfactory self-image.** Self-identity may evolve as a by-product of coping with medical illness. Patients must incorporate changes in physical functioning and appearance into their self-identity. The corporate lawyer awaiting a heart transplant must contend with the narcissistic injury of illness and dependency. Part of this evolving self-identity includes establishing goals and expectations. For this lawyer, coping with illness may involve allowing others to assist him and re-defining work and family roles.
6. **Coping with uncertainty** may be the biggest challenge for many patients.
7. **Preserving relationships with family and friends.** Psychiatric assessment should include an inventory of relationships that may facilitate or hinder coping. Family and friends may respond to a patient's illness in a way that leaves the patient feeling supported or completely alienated. In addition to re-defining one's own self-image, patients must often adapt to changing roles within a family system.
8. **Managing financial problems if one is unable to work and is forced to pay medical expenses.**

B. Personality Types in Medical Management

Understanding different personality traits can help psychiatrists anticipate a patient's strengths and vulnerabilities when coping with medical illness. Kahana and Bibring (1964) described the following personality types to characterize the basic needs, fears, defenses, and adaptive behaviors that influence a patients' experience of illness. These simplistic paradigms are presented in modified and extreme form to help psychiatrists detect subtler versions in their patients.

1. **The dependent, demanding personality.** This patient may unconsciously cling to physical illness as the only concrete evidence that he deserves love and attention. While the patient may demand multiple consultations and tests, the diagnosis and extensive medical attention is a bittersweet victory. It is based on the fundamental premise that he is in fact defective. The illness resonates painfully with the patient's unconscious belief that he is irrevocably damaged and unworthy. His dependency on others for protection is reminiscent of the helpless infant, wholly dependent on the mother. Health care providers inevitably disappoint the patient with less than perfect maternal love. The patient is left with feelings of anger, depression, helplessness, and hopelessness. Disappointment and rejection are an inevitable part of this patient's experience of illness as he alienates health care providers with his cloying requests for advice and reassurance.
   a. **The illness experience.** The anxiety accompanying illness may reflect this patient's unconscious wish for abundant care, as well as his fear of abandonment and starvation. Illness may provide the regressive pull toward an earlier, secure state of infantile helplessness. The patient's solution to these intense wishes and fears may be to become overly dependent on his physician and unquestioning of any medical recommendations. On the other hand, the patient may resist these unconscious feelings and become overly independent, help-rejecting, or embittered.
   b. **Treatment implications.** Health care providers should communicate their readiness to care for the patient with respect and compassion. For the acutely ill patient, tending to the patient's basic physical comfort becomes extremely meaningful in the context of his heightened dependency. The patient's consuming presence and insatiable demands may evoke countertransference feelings of frustration and fury. When the patient's demands become excessive, health care providers should gently set clear limits to mitigate the patient's experience of limits as punitive and rejecting.
2. **The orderly, controlled personality.** The orderliness and predictability that organize a patient's world can make him seem admirably disciplined and conscientious, and, at other times, annoyingly rigid and obstinate. This heightened insistence on rules and compliance may have its roots in parental intolerance of the child's lack of control over behavior, feelings, or bodily function. An emphasis on thoughts over feelings leads to the repression of undesirable impulses and the development of inflexible attitudes. Under stress, this patient may impress others with his reliance on rational, linear thought, and thorough accumulation of information. However, these attempts at cognitively organizing stressful situations belie this patient's core feelings of ineffectuality and chaos.
   a. **The illness experience.** Physical illness threatens the control and self-discipline that define a patient's existence. He may respond with redoubled efforts to suppress intolerable emotions. His health care providers may experience him as opinionated and unyielding in his attitude. The patient's persistence in fact-gathering and educating himself about his illness may come at the expense of dealing with the illness on a more intimate level. Flashes of rage, fear, and despair may break through this patient's rigid defenses only to be readily sequestered by his reflexive and protective self-restraint.
   b. **Treatment implications.** Giving this patient information about his illness will help bind his anxiety. The goal is to help sustain his cognitive armor with information to prevent the terrifying loss of control that he experiences with illness. This patient would likely welcome active participation in his treatment (e.g., logging his caloric intake or changing his own dressings). Acknowledgment of his conscientiousness and discerning mind may support his sense of control and bolster his belief that he is doing all he can to contain the threat of illness.
3. **The dramatizing, emotionally involved, captivating personality.** This patient may strike the physician as charming, fascinating, imaginative, dramatic, flirtatious, or enticing. Such a patient's intense and engaging interpersonal style stems from his yearning for singular devotion from his health care providers. Often this patient will reject same-sex physicians, who may seem like uncaring, threatening rivals. With opposite-sex physicians, however, this patient can become a caricature of certain gender stereotypes (e.g., the fearless, brute male or the helpless damsel in distress).
   a. **The illness experience.** To this patient, physical illness may feel like a public advertisement that he is in fact defective, weak, and unattractive. The narcissistic injury of physical illness may tap into a patient's fear of losing power, bodily integrity, or his unique physical appeal. In striving to quell his anxiety, this patient embarks on dramatic demands for admiration and attention, or at times assumes a nonchalant disregard for the serious implications of his disease. When overt attempts at securing attention and reassurance fail, this patient may also paradoxically become overly glib and concede too readily to procedures or recommendations.
   b. **Treatment implications.** Health care providers could offer directed questions about the specific fears driving his anxiety and the persistent requests for attention. To help this patient cope with illness, clinicians could offer consistent encouragement, along with explicitly stated interpersonal boundaries.

4. **The long-suffering, self-sacrificing patient.** This patient's personal narrative is filled with stories of disappointment, failure, and tragedy. This patient may outwardly lament his misfortune yet precipitate his own misfortune by unconsciously placing himself in harm's way. He may arouse in others uneasy sympathy rather than praise as he flaunts his self-sacrifice and suffering in an exhibitionistic and immodest way. This patient may have experienced a repressed childhood marred by parental intolerance of anger in the child along with corporal punishment, which he may have experienced with both pleasure and pain. As a child he may have found that physical illness prevented his parents from casting aspersions and may have even garnered him more love and attention.
   a. **The illness experience.** This patient unconsciously assumes that self-sacrifice and suffering must be the cost for all the love and acceptance he yearned for as a child and now as an adult. The physician may resent this patient's use of his physical illness as unconditionally entitling him to limitless love. The physician may also find the patient intolerable in his disregard of any encouragement or sign of improvement.
   b. **Treatment implications.** Self-pitying statements are this patient's invitation to others to acknowledge his pain and sacrifices. Countering the patient's defeatism with encouragement may seem dismissive and unempathic. The physician may have to present medical treatment as yet another burden the patient must bear for others rather than as a means to alleviating pain and achieving health.
5. **The guarded, querulous patient.** The world is a lonely place for this patient. He may see himself as the victim of other's thoughtless disregard or vengeful cruelty. He may feel that tragedy, insult, and injury shadow only him. In his world, disappointment, oppression, and exploitation at the hands of others are inevitable. Self-loathing, which fuels his sense of victimization and helplessness, gets reassigned to others.
   a. **The illness experience.** Periods of sickness may push him toward the well-oiled pit of paranoia that colors his perceptions and leaves him alone in the world. He may become even more guarded, quarrelsome, and suspicious as he blames others for his medical illness.
   b. **Treatment implications.** Clear descriptions of the short- and long-term view of his diagnostic work-up and treatment may mitigate his perception of health care providers as manipulative and reckless. The physician should strive to be courteous without getting either overly involved or distant. Confronting his paranoid and baseless suspicions will further alienate him and drive him from treatment. Health care providers could try to empathize with his aloneness in the world and ally with his heightened sense of helplessness and victimization in the setting of physical illness. Rather than reinforcing his suspicions or refuting them outright, one could acknowledge that, for the patient himself, the feelings are very real.
6. **The patient with the feeling of superiority.** Arrogance and condescension shield this patient from his own shame and insecurity. Although this patient may come across as confident and smug, his grandiosity may be his only defense.
   a. **The illness experience.** For the narcissistic patient, physical illness may affront his sense of perfection and invulnerability. He may insist on seeing only the most eminent physician, for who else could be worthy of understanding so complex and interesting a person. No matter how real or inflated his perception of his physician, however, over time he may need to outdo him, dwell on his faults, and belittle his interventions.
   b. **Treatment implications.** Challenging his narcissism and entitlement may further alienate this patient. In the service of providing good medical care, one should support his needed defenses by understanding his need to believe in the unique competence of his primary physician.
7. **The patient who seems uninvolved and aloof.** Within his solitary world, this patient may actually use aloofness to defend against his perceived frailty and inner emptiness. He may have an early life marred by repeated disappointments that taught him to avoid investing emotions in any relationships.
   a. **The illness experience.** This patient may experience physical illness as an intrusion on his static and solitary world. Illness may also force him to interact with others (e.g. health care providers) in a way that feels oppressively intimate and leaves him feeling exposed. He may deal with anxieties evoked by illness with renewed denial and familiar defenses of social isolation and emotional distance.
   b. **Treatment implications.** This patient's aloofness and eccentricities can be understood as his solution to intolerable fear, anxiety, and vulnerability, rather than as intentional sleights. Health care providers can limit demands on him for social involvement but insist that he not withdraw completely. It is also important to offer reassurance and support without expecting the gratifying warmth and indebtedness of other patients.

C. Coping Capacity

Directed and timely questions can rapidly determine a patient's style of coping, vulnerabilities, adaptive traits, and cognitive flexibility. Weisman (1978) described a screening tool to assess a person's coping strengths (Table 71-2). He described good copers as flexible, resourceful, optimistic, practical, and good at identifying pressure points and at finding solutions. Bad copers include those that deny the reality of their problems or paradoxically overwhelm their physicians with descriptions of their embittered defeat and suffering. Other screening questions include:

1. What has bothered you most about this illness?
2. How has it been a problem for you?
3. What have you done or what are you doing about the problem?

Table 71-2. Assessment of Coping Capacity

The problem: What has been the most important problem you've had to face since your illness began? How has your illness affected people closest to you?

The strategy: What did you do about it?

- Seek more information (rationalization/intellectualization)
- Talk with others to relieve distress (shared concern)
- Laugh it off; make light of the situation (reversal of affect)
- Try to forget or put it out of your mind (suppression)
- Do other things to distract yourself (displacement)
- Take firm action based on present understanding (confrontation)
- Accept, but find something favorable to deal with (redefinition)
- Submit, accept the inevitable (fatalism)
- Do something, anything, however reckless or impractical (acting out)
- Negotiate feasible alternatives (if X, then Y)
- Reduce tension by drinking, eating, or taking drugs
- Withdraw into isolation
- Blame someone or something (externalize)
- Seek direction from an authority and go along (compliance)
- Blame yourself, sacrifice, or atone (self-pity/surrender)

The resolution: How did it work for you (or is it working)?

- No resolution or relief
- Uncertain, indefinite, doubtful
- Qualified, limited resolution
- Specific, definite resolution; good relief

SOURCE: Adapted from Weisman, A.D. (1978). Coping with illness. In T.P. Hackett, & N.H. Cassem (Eds.), *Massachusetts General Hospital handbook of general hospital psychiatry*, pp. 264–275. St. Louis, MO: Mosby.

4. What has been the most difficult thing you've had to face until now?
5. What did you do then?
6. Whom have you relied on most in the past?
7. Who do you expect will be most helpful to you now?
8. In general, how do things usually turn out for you?
9. What do you dread the most about this illness?

IV. Other Interventions

A. **Psychotherapy (e.g., supportive, psychoeducational, interpersonal, cognitive, or dynamic therapy) can be life- and spirit-saving in the face of medical illness.** Patients can clearly benefit from therapy that addresses **practical issues related to their physical illness.**

B. **Medically ill patients may also benefit from relaxation techniques, hypnosis, family therapy, self-help groups, and spiritual supports.**

V. Conclusions

Physical illness can undermine one's identity or effect permanent changes in appearance and bodily function. The personal significance of disease depends on highly subjective factors, such as developmental stage and character traits. Psychiatrists are uniquely qualified to appreciate the medical aspects of disease while facilitating a patient's adaptation to the challenges and uncertainty of illness.

Suggested Readings

deRidder, D., & Schreurs, K. (2001). Developing interventions for chronically ill patients: Is coping a helpful concept? *Clinical Psychology Review, 21*(2), 205–240.

Green, S.A. (1985). *Mind and body: The psychology of physical illness.* Washington, DC: American Psychiatric Press.

Hamburg, P. (1989). Bulimia: The construction of a symptom. *Journal of the American Academy of Psychoanalysis, 17,* 131–140.

Heijmans, M.J. (1998). Coping and adaptive outcome in chronic fatigue syndrome: Importance of illness cognitions. *Journal of Psychosomatic Research, 45*(1), 39–51.

Kahana, R.J., & Bibring, G.L. (1964). Personality types in medical management. In N.E. Zinberg (Ed.), *Psychiatry and medical practice in a general hospital.* New York: International Universities Press.

Kubler-Ross, E. (1969). *On death and dying.* New York: Macmillan.

Lazarus, R.S., Averill, J.R., & Opton, E.M. (1974). The psychology of coping: Issues of research and assessment. In G. Coelho, D.A. Hamburg, & J.E. Adams (Eds.), *Coping and adaptation.* New York: Basic Books.

Moos, R.H., & Tsu, V.D. (1977). The crisis of physical illness. In R.H. Moos (Ed.), *Coping with physical illness.* New York: Plenum.

Stuber, M.L. (1996). Psychiatric sequelae in seriously ill children and their families. *Psychiatric Clinics of North America 19*(3), 481–493.

Weisman, A.D. (1978). Coping with illness. In T.P. Hackett, & N.H. Cassem (Eds.), *Massachusetts General Hospital handbook of general hospital psychiatry,* pp. 264–275. St Louis, MO: Mosby.

Chapter 72

Treatment Decisions at the End of Life

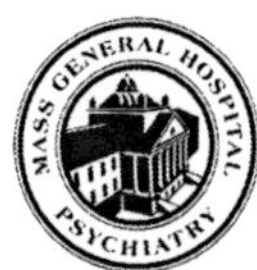

BRAD REDDICK, REBECCA W. BRENDEL, AND NED H. CASSEM

I. Introduction

Through the advancement of medical technology and practice, the human lifespan has grown. This has created fertile ground for opportunities and for conflicts. For centuries, medicine as a discipline has followed two age-old credos: **"first do no harm"** (*primum non nocere*) and **"above all relieve suffering."** It is within the final chapter of a person's life that **medicine stands at the crossroads between these two statements** (Cassem, 1999).

At no other point in the care of the patient are the unique skills, knowledge, and nurturance of the physician more important than in the process of a patient's dying. **The physician who has long-term knowledge of the patient and the patient's family can play an important role in increasing the quality of life for the dying patient. The psychiatrist's primary goals are to ensure optimization of palliative care and to assist the patient and the family in the dying process.** This process is one that requires a multi-dimensional or multi-axial understanding of the patient and his environment and the sometimes complex ethical issues that can arise.

II. The Psychophysiological Process of Dying

As disease pre-empting, death is often that which consumes or destroys the body; **dying patients may interpret even the slightest bodily changes as heralding demise.** Frequently, patients will experience fear with these bodily changes, but more often fear occurs long before these changes take place.

A. Psychiatric Consultation

Requests for **psychiatric consultation at the end of life,** by patients and their caregivers, **occur most commonly for major depression, substance abuse, delirium, organic brain syndromes, personality disorders, pain syndromes refractory to treatment, and difficulties with grieving.**

Other common causes for consultation with a psychiatrist include an inability to accept the diagnosis, and/or manifestations of pathological denial.

In treating the dying patient, **the role of the psychiatrist** is no different than it is with other patients; the aim is to diagnose and to treat. Often the psychiatrist can facilitate treatment, as well as communication between the patient, the family, and caregivers, by modeling qualities most helpful for the patient and sought in caregivers.

B. Qualities Sought in Caregivers

These qualities include being competent, concerned, comforting, cheerful, and consistent. In addition, one should be able to communicate, to have children present, and to facilitate cohesion of the family.

III. Goals for Treatment at the End of Life

The aim is to keep patients feeling like themselves for as long as possible (Saunders, 1978). This goal allows for reconciliation and resolution of conflicts with loved ones and pursuit of remaining hopes (Kubler-Ross, 1969). Kubler-Ross described stages of dying that consisted of denial and isolation, anger, bargaining, and acceptance, which may occur in any order. **Goals for an "appropriate death"** (Hackett and Weisman, 1962) are as follows:

1. **To be pain free.**
2. **To operate on as effective a level as possible within the constraints of disability.**
3. **To satisfy remaining wishes consistent with ego ideals.**
4. **To recognize and resolve residual conflicts.**
5. **To yield control to persons who are trusted.**

IV. Hospice Care of the Terminally Ill

Hospice care seeks to allow the dying patient to live to the limit of his or her physical strength, social relationships, and mental and emotional capacity. The average patient is enrolled in hospice care about 1 month before death, with provisions for home nursing, family support, spiritual guidance, pain treatment, and medication, as well as medical care.

The World Health Organization (WHO) defines hospice or palliative care as "total care of patients whose disease is not responsive to curative treatments," seeking to aggressively minimize the patient's burdens while maximizing quality of life.

V. Psychiatric Co-morbidity and Terminal Illness

A. Major Depression

The more progressively ill a person becomes, the more likely he or she is to develop major depression. Many have shown the heightened suffering such depression generates when it occurs in the terminally ill. As is true for depression in other stages of life, careful detection and aggressive treatment are essential. When depressed, patients make more restricted advance directives and change them after achieving remission (Ganzini et al., 1994). The wish to end one's life prematurely frequently accompanies depression. Breitbart and co-workers (1996), in a study comparing terminally ill patients with suicidal thoughts with those without suicidal thoughts, found the primary difference to be the presence of depression in those with suicidal thoughts. A similar study by Chochinov and colleagues (1995) discovered that, of those enrolled in a Winnipeg palliative care unit who wished to hasten death, 62% met diagnostic criteria for major depression. **In the dying patient, suicidal ideation should never be accepted as "understandable." Rather, it demands the same thoughtful examination as when it occurs in any other circumstance.**

A substantial contribution to depression in the terminally ill is made by the physical loss that occurs with declining health, body disfigurement, and loss of social roles. Frequent visits and discussions are essential to facilitate the patient's working through the grieving process.

B. Anxiety

Anxiety frequently arises or worsens at the end of life. This anxiety is not limited to the patient, but can occur within the families, friends, and caretakers of those facing death.

The most common fears associated with death are:

1. Death will resemble the dying of a friend or relative with the same disease.
2. Death will result in a loss of control and helplessness.
3. Death will cause physical pain, injury, or suffocation.
4. Feelings of guilt (being bad) will arise.
5. Death will lead to abandonment.

The anxious patient frequently is unaware of what it is about death that is so frightening, although memories of personal loss and associations to illness may provide clues. Most often anxiety relates to a patient's developmental history; anxiety surfaces as fear of loss of control or helplessness (e.g., unresolved dependency conflicts) or fear of abandonment (e.g., maternal bonding difficulties) arises. It is crucial that the physician explore with the patient fears of isolation, abandonment, anticipated suffering, and separation from loved ones.

C. Delirium and Dementia

As terminal illness progresses, cognitive difficulties are common and interfere with the quality of time spent with family, friends, and caretakers. Diagnosis and treatment of these difficulties are outlined in chapters 6, 7, 9, and 36.

D. Personality Style and Developmental Concerns

As interpersonal relationships are the most important supporting force for patients at the end of life, **maladaptive personality features and defense mechanisms** associated with personality disorders and mental retardation **can interfere with the patient's ability to attain comfort from these relationships.** Dependency on others, can be especially difficult for the patient at the end of life. Re-framing dependency on others, as an opportunity for loved ones to give something back to the patient instead of being a burden, is often helpful. Patients with terminal illness and co-morbid narcissistic or borderline character pathology are at great risk for treatment confounds, such as poor communication with caretakers, inadequate pain management, and failure to resolve interpersonal or familial conflicts. This is in part due to the negative feelings aroused in the caretakers of borderline and narcissistic patients, as well as the borderline and narcissistic patients' propensity to feel victimized and to distrust those involved in their care. When negative emotions arise in the clinician and/or when the treatment team is divided, a personality disorder should be suspected.

Psychodynamic understanding of the patient's style of coping and personality structure can guide the psychiatrist to convert caretakers' negative countertransference towards the patient into useful data that informs the team as to how they can best help the patient through the process of dying. Close work with family and the many members of the patient's treatment team is essential when working with character-disordered patients.

VI. Psychosocial Considerations

The end of life does not occur in a vacuum; rather, **multiple life and environmental stresses and supports interplay in a way that can both facilitate and complicate treatment at the end of life.**

A. Family

The importance of the presence of family in helping patients resolve long-standing conflicts, and providing a context for remembering (and grieving) life and an opportunity to give to younger generations, cannot be emphasized enough. **Psychiatrists can aid both the patient and the family by encouraging reconciliation, by sharing of emotions and memories, and by creation of specific plans of the family** (e.g., wills, funeral or memorial services, or trips), and construction of memorabilia (e.g., photo albums).

B. Work Relationships

Similar to family relationships, **relationships at work can help create the sense of a life lived meaningfully.** Mobilization of colleagues and friends can do much toward this aim. Involving those whose relationships centered around recreational activities and participation in self-help groups can be another source for support and personal understanding. The patient's faith and relationship with their religious figure(s) are also essential.

C. Religion and Faith

Koenig and colleagues (1995) demonstrated the benefits of reliance on religious faith for coping as a means of reducing cognitive symptoms of depression associated with the end of life. Conversations about death provide the opportunity to explore the patient's beliefs and thoughts about an afterlife. Careful exploration of the patient's attitudes, thoughts, beliefs, and hopes regarding God and religious faith is crucial. Terminally ill patients can benefit from psycho-educational groups; they can improve mood, reduce anxiety, and allow for the use of adaptive coping skills. Significant prolongation of life has been demonstrated in patients with breast cancer and melanoma involved in psycho-educational groups (Spiegel et al., 1989; Fawzy et al., 1993).

VII. Ethical Decisions at the End of Life

As advances in medicine proliferate, so do our abilities to sustain life and to prolong the dying process. Although the potential for increased suffering exists, it is not necessary. **Careful consideration should be given to preserve patient autonomy and to optimize palliative care;** when exercised, suffering can be reduced and the dying process can be facilitated without prematurely ending it. With these advances, **issues pertaining to euthanasia, substituted judgment, and treatment futility remain tender.** In considering management of a patient at the end of life, ethical decisions regarding treatment remain both important and challenging.

A. Legal Issues

Several court rulings have provided guidelines for considering ethical issues at the end of life. The Supreme Court's ruling in the case of Nancy Cruzan established several basic tenets, which help to resolve decisions about incurable illness.

1. Competent patients have the right to refuse treatment.
2. Nutrition and hydration are included among medical treatments, such as artificial ventilation and pressor agents, that a competent patient can refuse.

In addition to rulings outlined in the Cruzan case, several principles serve as guidelines when considering ethical decision-making at the end of life.

B. First, Do No Harm

What is in the patient's best interest is the primary aim, and includes limiting treatments that may prolong or intensify suffering in the setting of terminal illness.

C. The will of the patient, rather than the health of the patient, is supreme. Preserving patient autonomy at the bedside is important for any caretaker. It involves providing ample information and detail regarding diagnoses, treatments, and the potential outcomes of these treatments. An autonomous choice is made when a competent informed patient expresses the preferences. Such decision-making is a process, and is made through thoughtful dialogue with the patient, the family, and the primary caretakers. **In communicating facts, physicians should be mindful of how their own feelings about death and dying may influence their interpretation of the medical situation to the patient or family.** The SUPPORT study in 1995 found that less than half of terminally ill patients have had discussions with their physicians about cardiopulmonary resuscitation (CPR). **Physicians are poor at predicting their patient's preferences and underestimate their patient's perceptions of quality of life.** There are many potential confounding factors which may allow for any stated preference to change. **The following is a list of important questions that are raised when assessing a patient's stated preference:**

1. **Are psychiatric issues, such as depression and personality styles, being addressed which may interfere or color a patient's stated preference?**
2. **How is the patient perceiving his or her social supports?**
3. **What is the patient's world view?**
4. **Have the patient's stated reasons for wanting to die been explored?**
5. **Have the dynamics of the patient-doctor relationship been explored?**
6. **Are all symptoms being treated aggressively?**

The 1995 SUPPORT study found that half of the terminally ill patients who died in the hospital were in severe pain. Concomitant substance abuse is a risk factor for the undertreatment of pain.

D. All decisions involving medical ethics begin with the best facts available. Important facts include the diagnosis, prognosis, treatment options, reversibility of the illness, and the potential benefit or harm associated with each treatment. Talking with the patient and family regarding their questions and exploring their concerns is the natural result of sharing these essential facts. **The process of exploration is best accomplished in a quiet room, at a time set aside for this purpose, while sitting down.** Care should be taken not to confront initially when denial is utilized in response to factual information. **When denial is utilized as a defense initially, waiting for the patient's defenses to adapt in the context of repeated interviews is preferred before confronting the patient.** When discussing life-sustaining measures, it is helpful for the family and patient to know that treatments (e.g., mechanical ventilation) may help clarify potential for recovery, and may be tried until it is clear that health can no longer be restored.

E. When the patient is not competent, treatment decisions rely on either advance directives or an appointed power of attorney. Competence is a legal concept that is presumed in a patient's exercising choice. Conditions which may affect competence include medical illnesses producing delirium, mood disorders (e.g., depression), and dysfunction of thought, as occurs in psychotic disorders. **An advance directive is designed to**

extend a patient's autonomy; it contains the patient's expressed wishes for what should be done when the patient becomes incompetent or appoints a surrogate (health care proxy) who will express the wishes of the patient as if he or she were competent. The advance directive is composed when the patient possesses competence. Hospitals are now required by law to inform and ask patients about advance directives. Should the patient be alert but incompetent, substituted judgment rather than prior stated wishes should be the guide. In the absence of an advance directive, both the physician and the patient's close relatives must together provide substituted judgment with the patient's best interest. Should the patient be incompetent but alert (e.g., psychotic depression), guardianship should be considered.

F. **When is treatment limited? The physician should question any treatments that possess risks that outweigh potential benefits.** Patients who suffer from an irreversible and progressive illness (e.g., cancer) are particularly at risk for receiving needless burdensome treatments. Competent patients with both irreversible and reversible illness have the right to refuse any treatment, including life-sustaining treatments (e.g., hydration and nutrition). In the setting of irreversible coma, the standard medical recommendation to family would be to stop life-sustaining treatment. In the event that there is no family available, standard medical practice would be to allow the patient to die, understanding the inevitability of death and the futility of further treatment. When a patient has a functioning brainstem with a loss of cortical function (i.e., is in a permanent vegetative state), the American Academy of Neurology recommends that all life-sustaining treatment be withdrawn due to lack of medical benefit to the patient.

G. **Futile Treatment**

A particular problem arises when, **in the setting of irreversible illness, coma, or a persistent vegetative state, the family wishes that "everything be done,"** but **potential harm of continued life-sustaining measures exists.** Although **a physician is under no obligation to provide futile or harmful treatment,** the definition of ***futility* is under debate and is an area of focus for medical ethics.** The approach to such a problem begins with determination of futility. Various ways of examining and enhancing the quality of the communication with the family may lead to at least a partial agreement between the treating physician and the family. To fully appreciate the quality of communication with the family, an honest assessment of the working alliance with the patient and family is important. It is most helpful to review clinical information with the patient and the family in a manner that is free of jargon, is clear, and is open to follow-up questions. **A thoughtful assessment of family dynamics may uncover potential conflicts and issues among family members which confound clear communication** (as is true when faced with any ongoing ethical dilemma). A consultation with an ethics committee or legal counsel can provide further assistance and a fresh perspective.

VIII. Physician-Assisted Suicide and Euthanasia

For many, the topic of physician-assisted suicide is both actively debated and controversial. In struggling with this question it is helpful to review existing policies, standards of practice, and study observations.

The majority of states explicitly outlaw assisted suicide, although there have been two court rulings in the United States striking down such laws. **Most professional organizations,** such as the American Medical Association and the American Geriatric Association, **have issued statements against physician-assisted suicide. Beyond the policy, psychiatrists who are asked to hasten death for the dying patient must seek to understand what underlies the patient's wish to die.** Often careful, gentle questions can illuminate this understanding, and highlight ways in which the physician can improve in caring for the dying patient. Further questioning will uncover co-existing depression and disabling anxiety for which active treatment is both available and mandatory. Far too often ongoing despair is related to undertreatment of pain. **Those with concomitant substance abuse and personality disorders are especially at risk for sub-optimal pain management.** Aggressive and comprehensive palliative care should make requests for euthanasia rare. Unwillingness on the part of the physician to comply with requests from a patient for euthanasia should not result in the physician's abandoning the patient in treatment. **Ample use of narcotics to treat pain and to promote comfort is not euthanasia; knowing that a patient desires death should never result in withholding pain medication for fear of suicide.**

Suggested Readings

Appelbaum, P.S., & Grisso, T. (1988). Assessing patient's capacities to consent to treatment. *New England Journal of Medicine, 319*, 1635–1638.

Block, S.D. (2000). Assessing and managing depression in the terminally ill patient. *Annals of Internal Medicine, 132*(3), 209–218.

Breitbart, W., Rosenfeld, B.D., & Passik, S.D. (1996). Interest in physician assisted suicide among ambulatory HIV-infected patients. *American Journal of Psychiatry, 153*, 238–242.

Cassem, N.H. (1990). Depression and anxiety secondary to medical illness. *Psychiatric Clinics of North America, 13*(4), 597–612.

Cassem, N.H. (1999). The person confronting death. In A. Nicoli (Ed.), *The Harvard guide to psychiatry* (3rd ed., pp. 699–734). Cambridge, MA: Harvard University Press.

Chochinov, H.M. (2000). Psychiatry and terminal illness. *Canadian Journal of Psychiatry, 45*(2), 143–150.

Chochinov, H.M., Wilson, K.G., Enns, M.E., et al. (1995). Desire for death in the terminally ill. *American Journal of Psychiatry, 152,* 1185–1191.

Council on Scientific Affairs, American Medical Association. (1996). Good care of the dying patient. *Journal of the American Medical Association, 275,* 474–478.

Fawzy, F.I., Fawzy, N.W., Hun, C.S., et al. (1993). Malignant melanoma. Effects of an early structured psychiatric intervention, coping, and affective state on recurrence and survival 6 years later. *Archives of General Psychiatry, 50,* 681–689.

Ganzini, L., Lee, M.A., Heintz, R.T., et al. (1994). The effect of depression treatment on elderly patients' preferences for life sustaining medical therapy. *American Journal of Psychiatry, 151,* 1631–1636.

Hackett, T.P., & Weisman, A.D. (1962). The treatment of the dying. *Current Psychiatric Therapy, 2,* 121–126.

Kim, S., & Flather-Morgan, A. (1998). Treatment decisions at the end of life. In T.A. Stern, J.B. Herman, & P.L. Slavin (Eds.), *The MGH guide to psychiatry in primary care.* New York: McGraw-Hill.

Koenig, H.G., Cohen, H.J., Blazer, D.G., et al. (1995). Religious coping and cognitive symptoms of depression in elderly medical patients. *Psychosomatics, 36,* 369–375.

Kübler-Ross, E. (1969). *On death and dying.* New York: Macmillan.

Leeman, C.P., Blum, J., & Lederberg, M.S. (2001). A combined ethics and psychiatric consultation. *General Hospital Psychiatry, 23*(2), 73–76.

Report of the Quality Standards Subcommittee of the American Academy of Neurology. (1995). Practice parameters: Assessment and management of patients in the persistent vegetative state. *Neurology, 45,* 1015–1018.

Saunders, C. (Ed.). (1978). *The management of terminal illness.* Chicago, IL: Year Book Medical Publishers.

Spiegel, D., Bloom, J.R., Kraemer, H.C., et al. (1989). Effect of psychosocial treatment on survival of patients with metastatic breast cancer. *Lancet, ii,* 888–891.

Sullivan, M.D. (1998). Treatment of depression at the end of life: Clinical and ethical issues. *Semin Clinical Neuropsychiatry, 3*(2), 151–156.

SUPPORT Principal Investigators. (1995). A controlled trial to improve care for seriously ill hospitalized patients: The study to understand prognoses and preferences for outcomes and risks for treatments (SUPPORT). *Journal of the American Medical Association, 274,* 1591–1598.

World Health Organization. (1990). *Cancer pain relief and palliative care: Report of a WHO expert committee.* Geneva: WHO.

Chapter 73

Organ Transplantation

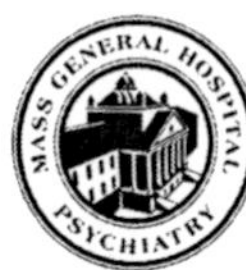

LAURA M. PRAGER, JOHN K. FINDLEY, AND OWEN S. SURMAN

I. Introduction

Organ transplantation has become a reasonable and often successful intervention for patients with end-organ failure. Organs currently transplanted include the heart, lungs, liver, kidney, pancreas, and small intestine. With advances in immunosuppressive therapy and in techniques for organ procurement, transplant recipients are living longer and more productive lives. Psychiatrists or other mental health professionals are involved in many stages of the transplantation process ranging from selection of candidates and their pre-operative evaluation to short- and long-term post-operative management of both recipients and their families.

II. Overview of Transplantation

A. Limitations on Transplantation

All efforts at transplantation are limited by the potential for allograft rejection, by the side effects of immunosuppressive medicines used to manage that rejection, and by the risks of infection inherent in any immunocompromised host.

B. Availability of Transplantation

Availability is limited by:

1. An insufficient supply of transplantable organs.
2. The financial cost of surgery and medications

C. Source of Transplanted Organs

The principle source of transplant organs in the United States is cadaveric, usually brain dead, donors. Brain death is determined by hospital-specific criteria, usually requiring examination by a neurologist, intensivist, or surgeon. Diagnostic tests used to support a diagnosis of brain death may include an apnea test, an electroencephalogram (EEG), a transcranial doppler, a cerebral blood flow scan, or an arteriogram. Clinical criteria for brain death include:

1. Fixed and dilated pupils
2. Absent reflexes
3. Unresponsiveness to external stimuli
4. Apnea

D. Living Donors

Scarcity of cadaveric organs has prompted consideration of related or "Good Samaritan" (unrelated) living organ donors.

1. These options are currently available for kidney, liver, and lung transplantation at some centers in the United States.
2. Living donor transplantation is more common in other countries, such as Japan, where religious or cultural ideology prohibits the use of cadaveric organs.
3. Potential donors undergo a comprehensive psychological evaluation, as well as a medical work-up in order to determine motivation and to ensure autonomy, informed consent, and absence of coercion.
4. Living donor lobar liver transplantation carries the potential for high risk to the donor. The National Institutes of Health (NIH) and the American College of Transplant Surgeons are currently studying this procedure and creating a registry that would allow for centralization of morbidity and mortality data.

E. United Network for Organ Sharing

In the United States, The United Network for Organ Sharing (UNOS) is the non-profit corporation, endowed by Congress and reporting to the Department of Health and Human Services, that regulates the allocation of organs.

1. UNOS has the power to enforce its policies as federal regulations
2. UNOS is divided into two branches:
   a. Organ Procurement and Transplant Network (OPTN)
   b. Scientific Registry
3. The OPTN divides the country into eleven distinct geographic regions and allocation of organs is done by local priority.
4. The radius of distribution for each organ is dependent on the vulnerability of that organ to ischemic injury and the time required for air transport of the available organ.
   a. Donor hearts are limited to a 500-mile radius as they require transplantation within 4 hours of procurement.
   b. Lungs can live outside of the body for only 6 hours.
   c. Kidneys can tolerate 48 hours of hypothermic perfusion and may be transported across the continent.
5. The length of the waiting list for each organ differs among geographic regions.
   a. Time spent waiting is the primary determining factor for kidney transplantation candidates and the only determining factor for a lung transplantation candidate.
   b. Acuity of illness confers priority for heart and liver candidates.
   c. Pediatric candidates for kidneys and livers take precedence over adult candidates.
   d. Full HLA compatibility confers priority for kidney transplantation.
   e. Ventilatory support is a contraindication to transplantation for potential lung candidates but confers priority status to heart and liver candidates.
   f. Sepsis is a contraindication to transplantation for all solid organ candidates.

III. Recipient Selection

A. Ethical/Medico-Legal Considerations

The process by which patients are selected to receive an organ for transplantation has been the topic of continuous debate since the first successful kidney transplant between monozygotic twins was done by Murray in 1954. Three precepts serve as a template:

1. Rights-based approach that includes all candidates who wish to be included
2. Utilitarian-based approach in which worth to society is a criterion for candidacy
3. Medically-based approach that offers candidacy to those who can physically benefit from transplantation

B. Selection Process

Once a candidate has been chosen, several criteria must be met:

1. Tissue matching—all candidates must have appropriate ABO blood group compatibility
2. Negative urinary drug screening for ethanol, recreational drugs, and cotinine
3. Negative human immunodeficiency virus (HIV) and hepatitis B (HBV) tests
4. Psychological evaluation to determine presence of disabling psychiatric symptoms, such as acute psychosis, suicidal or homicidal ideation, active substance abuse, dementia, and history of multiple suicide attempts
5. History of compliance with medical regimens

IV. Psychiatric Screening

Psychiatric assessment and management of candidates for organ transplantation requires a thorough understanding of the unique problems faced by this patient population. Not all transplant teams have psychiatric consultants. Psychologists and/or social workers may do psychosocial assessments at some centers. These evaluations should include a social service review and incorporate additional consultative expertise, e.g., substance abuse, if indicated.

A. Pre-Transplant Psychiatric Evaluation: Pre-transplant evaluation of candidates requires recognition of common psychological symptom clusters and syndromes. Informed consent, teaching, and pre-operative management help ensure compliance with the requirements of transplant teams and thus more favorable post-operative outcomes. Unfortunately, there are no uniformly accepted psychiatric guidelines for acceptance or rejection of transplant candidates. Sometimes evaluation of candidates may differ among transplant centers based on what degree of risk the transplant team is willing to assume. Factors that complicate pre-transplant evaluation include a lack of reliable and predictive data re: "suitability for transplant." The objectives of the psychiatric evaluation include:

1. Screening potential recipients for the presence of significant Axis I diagnoses (e.g., mood, anxiety, and psychotic disorders, as well as substance abuse) and Axis II diagnoses (e.g., involving personality disorders), and cognitive impairment that might complicate management or interfere with one's ability to comply with treatment recommendations.
2. Determining whether a given candidate will be able to collaborate with the transplant team in a joint effort to optimize medical care both pre- and post-transplant. This includes assessment of motivation, compliance with previous recommendations by other caregivers, availability of social supports, and history of perseverance in the face of adversity.
3. Educating about the risks and benefits of transplant.

B. Pre-Existing Psychiatric Syndromes

Many psychiatric disorders are common in the transplant candidate population. Some are pre-existing conditions, some arise due to the stress inherent in the patient's lengthy period of waiting for transplantation, and others are more characteristic of patients with a particular type of end-organ failure. Common syndromes include:

1. Encephalopathy
   a. Hepatic encephalopathy results from the liver's inability to clear toxins from the gastrointestinal tract and the bloodstream.
   b. Uremic encephalopathy may result in significant neuroendocrine effects and seizures. It can be secondary to renal failure and/or to the so-called "dialysis disequilibrium."
   c. Cardiac failure may induce encephalopathy if it results in changes in the cerebral circulation. Risk for delirium is increased in patients who require left ventricular assist devices or intra-aortic balloon pumps.
   d. Pulmonary disease often causes delirium due to hypoxia or hypercapnia.
2. Adjustment disorders are common to all forms of end-organ failure.
3. Depression is associated with an increased risk of pre-operative morbidity.
4. Anxiety is exceedingly common in patients with cardiac or pulmonary failure. It may be generalized, or phobic, or be characterized by panic attacks.

V. Treatment Strategies

As in other areas of psychiatry, treatment plans are multifaceted and usually consist of a combination of psychopharmacologic interventions and psychotherapeutic techniques. With encephalopathic patients, medical management is essential.

A. Psychopharmacology

Psychopharmacologic agents can and should be used when indicated. Choosing a medication regimen for a potential transplant recipient with end-organ failure can be challenging. Many medicines, depending on their route of metabolism, will require dose adjustments based on the presence of renal or hepatic failure. A good rule of thumb is to "start low and go slow."

1. Antidepressants
   a. Selective serotonin uptake inhibitors (SSRIs), e.g., fluoxetine, sertraline, paroxetine, citalopram, are the first choice because of their benign side-effect profile and anxiolytic effects. Rarely, they may cause hyponatremia and the syndrome of inappropriate antidiuretic hormone secretion (SIADH).
   b. Bupropion is more stimulating than other antidepressants but also appears to have a benign side-effect profile. It can also be helpful to patients who are struggling to remain abstinent from tobacco products.
   c. Tricyclics are no longer a first-line choice because of their potential for cardiac (quinidine-like) effects. However, they can be helpful in low doses for neuropathic pain.
2. **Anxiolytics**
   a. Benzodiazepenes can be invaluable in the management of anxiety although some transplant teams are unwilling to use them because of their addictive potential. Shorter-acting agents, e.g., lorazepam and oxazepam, are preferable. Alprazolam can be problematic because of its potential for rebound symptoms that are often indistinguishable from the symptoms of anxiety themselves. Many long-acting agents, e.g., diazepam, have active metabolites that can accumulate, particularly in patients with hepatic dysfunction.
3. **Neuropletics.** Patients with chronic psychotic disorders can and should be maintained on their existing antipsychotics. Low-dose neuroleptics can be helpful in ameliorating anxiety, particularly in patients who cannot take benzodiazepines because of the risk of abuse.
4. **Mood Stabilizers**
   a. Patients who require mood stabilizers, such as lithium, valproic acid (Depakote), or carbamazepine (Tegretol) can be maintained on them prior to transplant. Lithium levels will need to be adjusted for the patient with renal failure as valproic acid and carbamazepine will be for patients with hepatic failure.
   b. Gabapentin (Neurontin) can be particularly helpful in the management of steroid-induced mood lability.
   c. Valproic acid stimulates the cytochrome P450 enzymes and has the potential to effect immunosuppressive medications.
5. **Stimulants.** These agents can be used as adjuncts for the treatment of depression.

B. Psychotherapy

Psychotherapeutic interventions are often extremely important as candidates for transplant have a wide variation in their coping styles and the strength of their support networks. Patients usually do best with supportive, cognitive, or behavioral approaches. Even the one-time psychiatric pre-transplant evaluation can serve as a good opportunity for listening and for validation of a patient's hopes and concerns. Common issues raised include:

1. Loss of occupational status with secondary financial pressures
2. Guilt over lack of ability to perform at pre-morbid level of functioning
3. Change of role within the family system
4. Cognitive blunting or impairment
5. Inability to perform sexually
6. Denial of the progressive nature of disease

C. Substance Abuse Counseling

This is essential for those who are struggling to remain abstinent. It is inappropriate for the transplant team to monitor the patient (with urine toxicological screens) although many lung transplant programs do check cotinine levels. Such patients are better served by a referral to a substance abuse treatment program.

VI. Care of the Post-transplant Patient

A. Short-Term Care

Post-operatively, some patients recover rapidly and are able to leave the hospital within a 1–2 weeks. Others are less fortunate and can spend many weeks in an intensive care unit (ICU) before being transferred to the floor or to a rehabilitation facility. Patients can manifest the following:

1. Organic brain syndromes
   a. Etiologies of delirium include medication effects or medication withdrawal, metabolic changes, and infection. In the post-transplant patient, they are most commonly caused by immunosuppressive medication.
   b. Cyclosporine, FK-506 (Tacrolimus), and prednisone toxicity can produce a wide variety of neuropsychiatric symptoms that include seizures, sensorimotor changes, psychosis, delirium, and central pontine myelinosis.
   c. Heart transplant patients are at risk for intra-operative cerebral ischemia that can cause psychosis in the early post-operative period.
   d. Management requires an accurate assessment of the patient's mental status, a hunt for the etiology, and treatment of the underlying disorder if possible. Judicious use of neuroleptics can ameliorate the symptoms.
2. Depression can result from:
   a. Medications, such as beta-blockers, or benzodiazepines
   b. Infection, particularly from cytomegalovirus (CMV)
   c. Rejection
   d. Recurrence of pre-morbid symptoms
   e. Chronic pain
3. Anxiety can follow:
   a. Direct medication effects, particularly from high-dose steroids, cyclosporine, and FK 506 (Tacrilomus)
   b. Withdrawal from sedative-hypnotics
   c. Weaning from the ventilator
   d. Pain or anticipation of pain

e. Anticipatory anxiety surrounding potential for rejection of the allograft
f. Medical dependence, with symptoms occurring in the setting of leaving the hospital and losing medical supports

B. Long-Term Follow-up

Transplant patients exchange one set of problems, those of end-organ failure, for another set of problems, those that attend the side effects of immunosuppressive medications, rejection of the allograft, and progression of systemic disease. Pre-morbid vulnerabilities can easily resurface in the setting of unmet expectations.

1. Depression may be related to:
   a. Medication effects
   b. Frequent medical setbacks
   c. Bodily changes (such as weight gain, acne, hirsutism), which are caused by steroids
   d. Persistent weakness
   e. Reaction from family members who may either demand too much too soon or be unable to see the patient as less dependent and/or more capable
2. Anxiety can re-emerge in response to:
   a. Side effects of medication
   b. Anticipation and worry about allograft rejection
   c. Concern regarding inability to live up to the expectations of self or others
   d. Separation from caregivers (particularly members of the transplant team) and loss of other, tangible supports such as dialysis or oxygen tanks
3. Substance abuse can also re-emerge even after the patient has had years of sobriety.
4. Non-compliance with medication regimens deserves an assessment for depression and suicidality, as well as an exploration of possible causes of anger at, and disappointment with, the treatment team.

VII. Treatment Strategies

Long-term care of the transplant patient can be guided by the same principles used pre-operatively. A combination of psychopharmacologic and psychotherapeutic intervention usually works best.

A. Psychopharmacologic Treatment

Psychopharmacologic treatment is complicated by the neuropsychiatric side effects of the immunosuppressive medications and by the risk for multiple drug interactions.

1. **Cyclosporine (CYA)** is a widely used immunosuppressive. Adverse effects include nephrotoxicity, hypertension, neurotoxicity, hypomagnesemia, hyperkalemia, hyperlipidemia, osteoporosis, and gastroparesis. It can increase lithium absorption and lead to higher lithium levels. It is metabolized in the liver by the cytochrome P450 enzyme system. Carbamazepine, valproate, and phenobarbital may decrease its levels through hepatic induction. SSRIs could increase its levels through inhibition of cytochrome P450 enzyme system, but that has not been demonstrated. Nefazodone, however, is a source of significant competitive inhibition.
2. **FK506 (Tacrolimus)** is also a frequently used immunosuppressive, often used as a "salvage" therapy for patients who fail CYA. It can also cause neuropsychiatric symptoms, such as headache, insomnia, tremor, and visual hallucinations. It, too, is metabolized through the cytochrome P450 isoenzyme system, and its blood levels will likely be affected by the SSRIs. Again, while this has not been demonstrated, caution is advised when adding antidepressants to regimens that include Tacrolimus. Blood levels may be effected by concominant treatment with nefazodone.
3. **OKT3** is a monoclonal antibody that is used to treat rejection. It has neuropsychiatric side effects that include delirium, tremors, seizures, and, sometimes, aseptic meningitis.
4. **Corticosteroids** continue to be a mainstay of immunosuppressive regimens, and most transplant patients remain on them (at lower and lower doses) for the rest of their lives. They have numerous side effects (including weight gain with fat distribution, easy bruising, osteoporosis, and hirsutism), as well as a tendency to cause emotional lability, hypomania, mania, irritability, and depression. Patients often manifest rapid-cycling and can become psychotic. Benzodiazepines, such as clonazepam, or mood stabilizers, such as gabapentin, can be extremely helpful in ameliorating these uncomfortable symptoms. Antipsychotics may also be of benefit. Weight gain should be a concern when atypical antipsychotics are used.

B. Psychotherapeutic Interventions

1. The transplant patient can also benefit from **supportive therapy.** Pre-morbid issues, such as anxiety or depression, often thought to be a product of the end-organ failure, may not go away but may recur in a slightly different form. Other issues that may emerge include:
   a. **Discussion about one's curiosity** about the donor and a wish to meet and thank the family.
   b. **Fantasies about the donor organ** that can cause personality changes within the recipient.
   c. **Sadness over loss of the native organ** and concerns about what might have happened to the missing body part.
   d. **Worry** that one is not taking full advantage of the "second chance" offered by transplantation.
   e. **Rebirth phenomena** that can be conceptualized as a celebration of a chance for a new life.
   f. **Body image change** associated with immunosuppressive medication; patients often complain about side effects of prednisone, such as weight gain, hirsutism, acne, and tremor.

VIII. Conclusion

The patient with end-stage organ failure who is approaching transplant has few alternatives. These patients are disabled and often desperate. Prompt recognition and treatment of psychiatric illness can significantly impact the quality of life for these patients. Post-transplant patients face different but equally daunting challenges. Early recognition and treatment of psychiatric symptoms can often bolster compliance with medical regimens, prevent complications, and improve the likelihood of a favorable outcome.

Suggested Readings

Burdick, J.F., DeMeester, J., & Koyama, I. (1999). Understanding organ procurement and the transplant bureaucracy. In L.C. Ginns, A.B. Cosimi, & P.T. Morris (Eds.), *Transplantation,* pp. 875–896. Medford, MA: Blackwell Science.

Colon, E.A., Popkin, M.K., Matas, A., et al. (1991). Overview of noncompliance in renal transplantation. *Transplant Review, 5,* 175–180.

Dew, M.A., Roth, L.R., Schulberg, H.C., et al. (1996). Prevalence and predictors of depression and anxiety-related disorders during the year after heart transplantation. *General Hospital Psychiatry, 18* (suppl), 48–61.

Levinson, J.L., & Olbrisch, M.E. (2000). Psychosocial screening and selection of candidates for organ transplant. In P.T. Trzepacz, & A.F. DiMartini (Eds.), *The transplant patient,* pp. 21–41. Cambridge: Cambridge University Press.

Surman, O. (1999). Psychiatric considerations of organ transplantation. In L.C. Ginns, A.B. Cosimi, & P.T. Morris (Eds.), *Transplantation,* pp. 709–724. Medford, MA: Blackwell Science.

Surman, O. (2002). The ethics of right lobe liver transplantation. *New England Journal of Medicine, 344*(14), 1038.

Trzepacz, P.T., Gupta, B., & Di Martini, A.F. (2000). Pharmacologic issues in organ transplantation: Psychopharmacology and neuropsychiatric medication side-effects. In P.T. Trzepacz & A.F. DiMartini (Eds.), *The transplant patient,* pp. 187–213. Cambridge: Cambridge University Press.

Chapter 74

Chronic Mental Illness

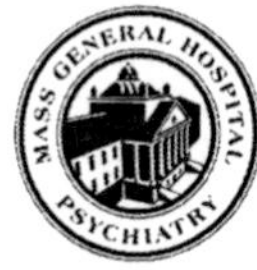

ALICIA POWELL AND DONALD C. GOFF

I. Introduction

A. Definition

Chronic, severe mental illness is characterized by persistent disabling psychiatric symptoms or by severely impaired function. Frequently, this population is labeled as the severely and persistently mentally ill.

B. Scope of the Problem

1. Several events **in the 1950s, including the development of antipsychotic medications and new commitment laws, led to dramatic changes (i.e., deinstitutionalization) in the treatment of the severely and persistently mentally ill. The 1960s brought the Community Mental Health Center Program as an alternative to state hospitalization, as well as new federal programs (Supplementary Security Income [SSI], Social Security Disability Insurance [SSDI], Medicaid, and Medicare health benefits).** Thousands of formerly hospitalized mentally ill persons were discharged to live in the community. Unfortunately, most communities lacked sufficient resources to provide adequate care for these patients.
2. **The prevalence of mental illness is higher in cities and in lower-class neighborhoods.** This is largely due to the drift of chronically ill patients toward urban environments, where aftercare for formerly institutionalized patients has typically been concentrated. Many chronic psychiatric patients experience homelessness at some time during the course of illness.
3. **Direct and indirect costs associated with schizophrenia in the United States were estimated at $33 billion in 1990; treatment of schizophrenia accounted for almost 3% of all health care expenditures.**

C. Demographics

1. **Between 1955 and 1985, the state hospital resident population decreased by 80%, from 559,000 to 110,000.**
2. **The lifetime prevalence of schizophrenia is 0.85%; the incidence of schizophrenia is about 0.4 per 1,000 population per year.**
3. **Roughly one-third to one-half of homeless persons in the United States suffer from schizophrenia, although such estimates remain controversial.**

II. Assessment of the Chronically Mentally Ill

A. Features of the Interview

1. **Be aware of interpersonal space.** Individuals with chronic mental illness, especially when paranoia is present, may require a larger space to feel safe. Be sure to ask the patient whether he or she is comfortable. Do not hesitate to rearrange the seating if you believe it will help put the patient at ease.
2. **Emphasize and clarify issues of confidentiality.** This reassures most patients, especially paranoid or homeless persons who feel disempowered.
3. **Minimize interruptions,** in treatment situations, if possible. The chronically mentally ill patient appreciates promptness and your undivided attention as much as any higher-functioning patient.

B. Special Considerations in History-Taking

1. The chronically mentally ill patient may have difficulty recalling the experience of symptoms, making it necessary to **obtain history from additional sources.** Ask the patient questions such as, "Who else would remember what you were going through before that hospitalization?" or "Who has seen you at your most depressed?" to elicit the best outside sources.
2. **Don't neglect the medical history.** Place special emphasis on a history of head injury and seizures. The severely and persistently mentally ill often neglect their medical problems. Therefore, it is important to ask about the patient's last physical examination, and, if necessary, to obtain a review of systems.
3. **Ask about sexual activity,** especially when interviewing a woman of childbearing age. This is important because many psychotropics are teratogenic. Many of these patients underestimate the risks of sexually transmitted disease.
4. **Substance abuse or dependence frequently co-exists with severe mental illness.** It is wise to begin your inquiry with questions about more socially accepted addictive substances (e.g., nicotine and caffeine), and then work your way up to other drugs (e.g., alcohol, marijuana, cocaine, opiates, psychostimulants, hallucinogens, barbiturates, benzodiazepines, and inhalants).
5. **The social history of these patients should include information regarding where the patient sleeps at night, who else resides with the patient, what the educational level of the patient is,** whether he or she has served in the armed forces, and what is the major source of the patient's income. **Asking about their history of violence, both as perpetrator and as a victim, is important** for diagnostic, as well as for safety, reasons.

C. The Mental Status Examination

1. During the interview, **make mental notes about the patient's hygiene, attire, speech, attitude, and eye**

contact, as well as any abnormalities of movement, such as tremor, bradykinesia, or odd mannerisms. At times you can obtain valuable information by asking the patient questions about the patient's attire, e.g., "How did you choose to wear this unusual piece of clothing today?" Be sure to include any noteworthy features in your presentation of the patient.

2. **Use a gradual, gentle approach when asking about psychotic symptoms.** Some patients are relieved to learn that their symptoms can be understood as a result of an extreme form of normal brain activity. For instance, when asking about visual hallucinations, the interviewer might compare them to the experience of "dreaming while you're awake."
3. Since a key concern of board examiners is to determine the candidate's ability to assess a patient's safety, **one should remember to ask the patient about current thoughts of suicide or homicide, or about command hallucinations, thought control by outside forces, a history of violence, and possession of weapons.** Recent evidence suggests that psychiatric patients are more likely to commit violent acts than are those in the general population, and that the prevalence of schizophrenia in samples of murderers is consistently 5 to 20 times higher than it is in the general population.

III. Diagnostic Issues

A. Socioeconomic Factors

Socioeconomic factors often complicate diagnosis. What may be seen as hypervigilance in some is just plain "street smart" for a homeless patient. Paranoia can be complicated by social isolation, or by a lack of a private space due to homelessness.

B. Negative Symptoms

Negative symptoms of schizophrenia include apathy, social isolation, poverty of thought or speech, flattening of affect, and neglect of hygiene. Negative symptoms profoundly impair an individual's ability to function and to engage in treatment; these symptoms can also alienate family members and caregivers. The diagnosis of co-morbid depression and/or the presence of medication side effects can also be complicated by negative symptoms.

C. Co-morbid Medical Illness

Since psychotic symptoms can occur in many medical and psychiatric illnesses, **one should inquire about the onset of symptoms in relation to the use of new medications or substances, physical illness, depression, mania, or flashbacks of traumatic experiences.** Be particularly careful to rule out a medical etiology with any new, sudden onset of psychotic symptoms, or when psychotic symptoms begin after the age of 50 years.

IV. Treatment Strategies

A. Pharmacologic

1. General considerations to maximize compliance
   a. When choosing medications for this population, remember that **once-a-day dosing is most convenient for the patient** and is the schedule usually used by these patients.
   b. **Cost of medication is an important consideration.** Although most patients have medication insurance coverage that requires only a small co-payment for each prescription, even this amount may be a burden for a patient, especially when multiple medications are prescribed and the patient is on a fixed income.
   c. Bear in mind that **certain medication side effects (e.g., diarrhea and frequent urination) are problematic in the patient who has limited access to rest rooms and laundry facilities;** sedation can compromise a patient's need for self-protective vigilance, is very difficult for homeless persons to tolerate, and can lead to discontinuation of treatment.
   d. **If the resources are available, monitored dosing (supervised dosing at the patient's group residence or daily dosing at the community mental health clinic) can facilitate compliance.**
   e. In patients taking antipsychotics, **consider using a depot preparation of haloperidol or fluphenazine** if the patient has no contraindications to using these medications. Depot neuroleptics can also be used to "back up" a daily antipsychotic pill regimen.
2. **The atypical antipsychotic clozapine (Clozaril) has been shown effective in the treatment of the disabling negative symptoms of schizophrenia;** effective treatment often enables patients to reach a higher level of functioning.

B. Non-Pharmacologic

1. **The severely and persistently mentally ill person may be best cared for by an assertive community treatment team,** also known as a Program for Assertive Community Treatment (PACT), or by a Community/Continuous Treatment Team (CTT). These programs are based upon a model which provides intensive support for a patient by a community-based team available 24 hours a day, 7 days a week. Program staff work long-term with patients, families, and agencies in the community to support patients and to help avert hospitalization. Each patient has an identified staff member who coordinates services. When a patient is hospitalized, the team remains directly involved in treatment planning and in discharge preparations. Randomized clinical trials of such programs demonstrated benefits in clinical status, social functioning, medication compliance, employment, and in quality of life, as well as in reduced rates of hospitalizations when compared with conventional outpatient treatment.

2. **The severely and persistently mentally ill patient being treated in the community is often involved with multiple providers,** including case managers, outreach workers, residential staff, social workers, and primary care physicians. Frequent contact between providers may seem time-consuming, but diligent communication enhances treatment and helps to avoid costly and time-consuming hospital stays or other emergency treatment.
3. **Some communities offer respite or short-term crisis management units** that help divert a patient from a prolonged hospitalization when only a brief crisis intervention is necessary. When possible, one should avoid a prolonged, debilitating, and isolating hospitalization to maintain function and connections in the community.
4. **Day treatment also plays an important role in the treatment of the severely and persistently mentally ill;** they provide structure in a safe setting, opportunities to socialize with others, psychoeducational groups, and at times can coordinate vocational training.
5. **Although supportive psychotherapy alone is inadequate treatment for schizophrenia, it can be helpful when combined with medications.** Emphasis should be placed on establishing and maintaining an alliance, fostering compliance with medication and other treatment, helping the patient cope with stressors, and assisting with reality testing.
6. Cognitive-behavioral treatments are under-studied in the severely and persistently mentally ill, but **recent work with cognitive approaches demonstrates efficacy in teaching social skills and reality testing.**
7. **Education and support for a patient's family has been shown to significantly improve the course of the illness.**

V. Conclusion

Care of the severely and persistently mentally ill is one of the most difficult and costly of all health-related problems in this country. During the second half of the twentieth century, the approach of long-term custodial care in state psychiatric hospitals gave way to community mental health models which improved the quality of life for many patients. The future of care for the chronically mentally ill will increasingly incorporate less costly care delivered by a variety of providers. Recent developments of atypical antipsychotics, with fewer debilitating side effects should help this population attain a higher level of function.

Suggested Reading

Goff, D.C., & Gudeman, J.E. (1999). The person with chronic mental illness. In A.M. Nicholi, Jr. (Ed.), *The Harvard guide to psychiatry,* pp. 684–698. Cambridge, MA: Belknap Press of Harvard University Press.

Chapter 75

Domestic Violence

B. J. Beck

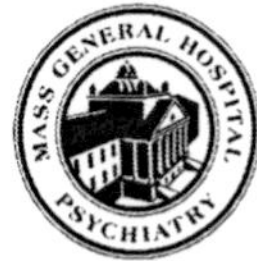

I. Introduction

A. Definition

Domestic violence, as used in this chapter, is synonymous with partner violence, spouse abuse, wife-beating, battering, and violence in intimate relationships. Domestic violence is the **intentionally violent or controlling behavior of a currently, or previously, intimate partner of the victim.** The goal of the violence is to **coerce, assert power, and maintain control** over the victim. Examples of coercive or violent behaviors include, but are not limited to, any combination of the following:

1. **Actual or threatened physical injury**
2. **Sexual assault**
3. **Psychological or emotional torment**
4. **Economic control**
5. **Social isolation**

B. Overview

Hardly a new problem, **evidence of domestic violence spans the millennia and is seen in all cultures and segments of society.** The public health implications of this endemic problem include injury, physical and mental disability, death, increased health care costs, and lost wages and productivity, and the long-term effects on children who witness violence. Victims' and health care providers' attitudes toward violence are among the barriers to disclosure and detection—the necessary first steps for intervention. **Victims who leave their batterers are at a 75% greater risk (than those who stay) of being murdered by their batterer;** this fact underscores the victim's vulnerability and the complex nature of successful interventions.

II. Epidemiology

A. Prevalence

In the United States, 3–4 million women each year are abused by a partner or by a former partner. Domestic violence is repetitive, and escalates over time.

1. **Women are 6 times more likely than men to be victims of partner violence.**
2. 90% of abusive relationships involve men who abuse their female partners. Some women are violent towards their male partners, frequently in self-defense.
3. 30–50% of all married couples experience some episode of physical violence.
4. **Almost 10% of homicides involve a spouse killing a spouse.**
5. Women are more often assaulted, raped, or murdered by current or former partners than by strangers.
6. Although less well studied, **same-sex couples appear to experience domestic violence as often as heterosexual couples.**
7. **In the medical setting, abused women account for:**
   a. **22–35% of women who present to an emergency room (ER) for any reason**
   b. Up to 40% of women in the ER for non-motor-vehicle trauma
   c. 14–28% of women attending general medical clinics
   d. 16–23% of women seen for routine prenatal care
   e. Over 50% of the mothers of abused children
8. **In the psychiatric setting, abused women account for:**
   a. **25% of women who present for emergency psychiatric services**
   b. **33% of women who attempt suicide**
   c. 50% of women in psychiatric outpatient services
   d. 64% of women on psychiatric inpatient units

B. Risk Factors for Victims

Although no socioeconomic, educational, professional, ethnic, racial, or religious affiliation bestows immunity to domestic violence, certain women are at greater risk, including those who:

1. Are single, separated, or divorced
2. Have recently applied for a restraining order
3. Are between the ages of 17 and 28 years
4. Are poor
5. Abuse alcohol or drugs
6. Have partners who abuse alcohol or drugs
7. Are pregnant and have been abused before
8. Have excessively jealous or possessive partners

C. Risk Factors for Perpetrators

Despite the heterogeneity of abusers, certain men have an increased risk of violence, including those with:

1. Antisocial personality disorder
2. Depression
3. Youth
4. Low income
5. Low educational level

III. Clinical Presentation

A. Victims of domestic violence represent a broad spectrum of the population. There is no predisposing, or diagnostic, pre-violence personality structure. **The one thing victims have in common is a violent partner.**

1. **Over time, chronic physical and emotional abuse leads to a sense of worthlessness, shame, and incompetence.**

2. **Victims who present to the health care (or legal) setting may appear passive, dependent, unstable, and "somatic."**
   a. **Social isolation, economic control, and threats** (toward the victim, her children, family, or pets) may **render the victim totally dependent** on her abuser. **This is a consequence of the abuse,** not the cause of it.
   b. Victims of domestic violence **may not look abused,** i.e., they may not initially present with injuries or have physical evidence of abuse. They often **present with behavioral or somatic complaints.**
   c. **Addiction, depression, anxiety, post-traumatic stress, and eating disorders are associated with abuse.**
   d. Domestic violence has also been **associated with intractable abdominal pain, chronic headaches, pelvic pain, and musculoskeletal problems.**

B. **Perpetrators of domestic violence** also come from all walks of life. However, perpetrators may **have certain pre-battering cultural or developmental experiences and personality traits in common.** Once the violence has begun, perpetrators often share similar behavioral patterns.
1. Perpetrators have often **witnessed or experienced violence in their families of origin.**
2. Violent men have often been **violent in previous relationships.**
3. They are often **immature, needy, dependent, nonassertive men with fragile self-esteem and intense feelings of inadequacy.**
4. **"Insanely jealous" and untrusting,** they cannot tolerate even the least hint of autonomy, **and must dominate or control their partners.**
5. Many perpetrators **abuse alcohol, or alcohol and drugs.** Although they may attribute their violence to the influence of these substances, victims indicate that **violence is not dependent on the perpetrator's recent substance use or intoxication.**
6. **Abusers often minimize or deny the violence; they may blame the victim for provoking the violence.**
7. **Excessively concerned with outward appearances,** perpetrators are **often socially congenial and able to successfully conceal their violence** from friends and professional contacts.
8. Abusive men often appear **more credible and intact than their victims, whom they portray as prone to exaggeration and emotional instability.**

IV. The Nature of Violent Relationships

A. **The violence does not start at the beginning of the relationship.**
1. **A non-assaultive prodrome** may include gradual control over the partner's activities, finances, or family, social, or professional contacts.
2. **Initial overtures may seem caring and exceptionally considerate** (e.g., dropping the partner off at work and picking her up afterward; multiple phone calls during the day; offering to support the partner or giving her spending money; accompanying her to health care appointments).
3. A **pattern of control and dependence** gradually develops.
4. Often a **major event in the couple's life** (e.g., marriage, pregnancy, or the birth of a child) **precipitates actual violence.**
5. The couple's **response to the initial episode** of violence may be shock and abhorrence, rationalization, and a firm **belief that it is an isolated incident** never to be repeated.

B. **The cycle of violence is repetitive and often predictable.**
1. **Violence may involve weapons** (guns, knives, clubs), **shoving, punching, kicking, burning, forced sex, or the forced use of drugs or alcohol.**
2. **Violence escalates over time,** with increased frequency and severity. It may be **life-threatening. Presence of a firearm greatly increases the risk.**
3. Because **the motivation is to exert control over the victim, physical abuse is often accompanied by emotional abuse, humiliation, intimidation, threats, or coercion.**
   a. **Emotional abuse** includes putting the victim down (especially in front of others), calling her names, playing mind games or making her think she's crazy, making her feel guilty or bad about herself.
   b. **Humiliation** may involve treating her like a servant, making her beg, forcing her to perform degrading or illegal acts.
   c. **Intimidation** may involve using certain looks or gestures to incite fear, destroying the victim's property, brandishing weapons, driving recklessly, or abusing/torturing pets.
   d. **Threats** of violence, murder, suicide, abandonment, loss of children, or harm to a family member may be terrifying.
   e. **Coercion** is used to keep the woman in the relationship, to conceal the abuse, or to drop charges. Perpetrators may threaten the victim with psychiatric commitment, deportation, Welfare or legal actions.
4. **Children may witness parental violence,** or be coopted by the abuser to relay messages. Victims may be made to feel guilty about their children or to fear losing them. Visitation may be used to further torment the victim.
5. **Violence is often followed by a period of extreme contrition and reconciliation.** The remorseful batterer may bestow gifts and affection on the victim, while vowing never to strike her again. In turn, the victim may feel sorry for her assailant and guilty for having provoked him. **They may both feel hopeful that "this is the last time."**

6. **Remorse is followed by a tension-building phase that inevitably culminates in another outburst of violence.** The anticipation during the tension-building phase may be so stressful that some women seek to induce the violence to get it over with.

C. **Deterrents to leaving a violent relationship** include the consequences of repeated battering, the dynamics of violent relationships, and the reality of inadequate support systems.

1. **Shame, humiliation, and feelings of worthlessness** keep women in abusive relationships. They are repeatedly told, and may begin to believe, that they get what they deserve, and that they cannot expect anything better.
2. **Fear of real and perceived danger** to herself, her children, family, or friends restricts the victim's ability to leave. Batterers may coerce their partners into staying with just such threats. Fear of being homeless, indigent, and unable to care for their children also keeps women from leaving.
3. **Financial dependence** is calculated to keep women in the control of the abuser. She may have no knowledge of, nor access to, family assets. She may have been prevented from working outside the home. The abuser may even have taken control over any money the victim did have.
4. **Isolation** from family, friends, community supports, health care and legal professionals, and educational opportunities make the abuser the victim's single contact with the outside world. She may feel hopeless to find assistance, or even be believed if she tries to escape.
5. **Intermittent reinforcement of apologies, gifts, and affection** give the victim recurrent hope that things will change. Many **victims do not want to end the relationship; they want to end the abuse.**
6. **Unsuccessful prior attempts** are potent deterrents to future attempts. When women have been blamed, not believed, or not supported by family, police, physicians, or social agencies, they have little incentive to risk the real danger of another attempt to leave.

V. Evaluation

A. **Screening for violence should be a routine part of every psychiatric evaluation and every general medical assessment.** Many patients will not volunteer information, but will respond to empathic, nonjudgmental questioning.

1. Male and female patients should be asked about *their own* violence, as well as whether anyone else is (or has been) hurting them. **A simple question (Have you been hit, kicked, punched, or otherwise hurt by someone within the past year? If so, by whom?) will identify over 70% of women in violent relationships, as detected by lengthier screening tools** (Feldhaus et al., 1997). Patients should also be asked about violence in previous relationships, and sexual assault. **Partner rape is often part of domestic violence.**
   a. Patients must be asked these questions alone, in private (confidential) settings. **Partners, family members, or friends should never be used as interpreters.**
   b. Asking about abuse in the presence of a violent partner not only inhibits the patient from responding truthfully, but puts her at increased risk.
2. There are **multiple barriers to screening and detecting domestic violence.**
   a. **Provider factors** include **time constraints, lack of training, inadequate supports** (e.g., security, social services, interpreters), **and lack of suspicion or awareness.** Especially when patients are known socially, are highly educated, professional, or of high socioeconomic status, physicians may be **embarrassed, or feel it insulting, to ask about abuse.** They may feel **helpless to "fix" the situation, or frustrated** by a past experience in which the victim would not leave her batterer. They may simply be uncomfortable thinking or talking about violence.
   b. **Patient factors** include the effects of chronic abuse: **shame, fear, worthlessness, hopelessness, depression, anxiety, dissociation, or numbness.** Women may **feel they won't be believed or that they will be blamed.** They may **fear not only increased violence, but destitution** if the batterer leaves them, or is jailed.
   c. **Certain groups (e.g., illegal aliens, those addicted to illegal drugs) are particularly disenfranchised and may fear legal retaliation.** Victims from **certain cultural or ethnic groups** may feel they will shame not only themselves, but their entire extended families. The **chronically mentally ill or cognitively limited** victim may not know how to talk about battering. **Abused men may be especially ashamed** to admit they are victims; they may also **fear counter-allegations** from their partners. **Gay and lesbian victims may not feel safe to divulge their sexual orientation,** let alone their abuse, to the health care system.

B. **The medical history** may hold clues to previously unsuspected abuse.

1. **Multiple unscheduled, or ER, visits, multiple traumas, "accidents," or unusual injuries** with unlikely explanations are cause for suspicion of abuse. **Multiple, unexplained, somatic complaints** (headaches, abdominal, pelvic, musculoskeletal pains) should also trigger more careful, confidential questioning. **Alcohol and drug addictions** are common sequelae of abuse.
2. **Patients who disclose current or past abuse** should be asked about the **first episode, the worst episode, and the last episode.** If there are children in the family, the **victim should be asked whether the children have witnessed or experienced violence.** Most states have mandatory reporting requirements for physicians who suspect child abuse or neglect, and patients should be advised of this.

C. A thorough physical examination should be performed, and carefully documented, by a knowledgeable and empathic general physician. The medical record may become important legal evidence.

1. Care should be taken to **document any injuries, including signs of sexual trauma,** using diagrams, sketches, or photographs. **A screening neurologic examination** should note any focal findings or suggestions of acute or repeated head trauma.
2. The **mental status exam** should be equally thorough. **Thoughts of suicide, or homicide,** should be asked directly. Signs and symptoms of **anxiety, hypervigilance, autonomic arousal, flashbacks, depression, apathy, dissociation, numbness, and psychosis** should be explored and carefully documented.

D. The psychiatric differential diagnosis of victims of domestic violence includes **adjustment disorders** (early on), **depression** (with or without psychotic symptoms), **anxiety disorders** (generalized anxiety, panic, post-traumatic stress), **dissociative disorders** (especially in victims with histories of childhood physical or sexual abuse), **eating disorders, substance-related disorders, and mental disorders due to acute or repeated head trauma.**

1. **Repeatedly traumatized patients may *appear* personality-disordered** (e.g., paranoid, borderline, avoidant, dependent), but **Axis II diagnoses are not appropriate,** unless the clinician has pre-battering knowledge of the victim's personality structure.
2. **Pre-existing or persistent psychiatric disorders** (e.g., bipolar disorder, schizophrenia) **are predictably exacerbated** in chaotic, violent living situations. If the abuse is not detected, these patients may be assumed to be non-adherent to their medication or treatment programs. Their medications may be inappropriately adjusted.

VI. Treatment Considerations

A. The detection of violence is the beginning of treatment.

1. **Physicians should not gauge their success by when or whether the victim leaves the batterer.** Leaving is a very high-risk proposition and needs to be carefully planned out. The patient needs to know the physician's care is not dependent on her leaving. The victim is the best judge of when she is prepared and when it is safe for her to leave.
2. **It is not the physician's sole responsibility** to intervene, or "fix," the abusive relationship. They should, however, **know appropriate resources** in their area (e.g., hotlines, shelters, advocacy groups, and emergency numbers) and be able to refer the patient as necessary.
3. **It is the physician's responsibility to take the patient seriously, to document carefully, and to assert that:**
   a. **Violence is unacceptable and criminal.**
   b. **The victim does not deserve to be hurt in any way.**
   c. **The victim did not bring this on herself.**
   d. **It is not the victim's fault; the perpetrator is unequivocally responsible for his actions.**

B. Risk assessment must rely heavily on the victim's own appraisal of the immediate situation (e.g., how afraid she is right now, what she believes to be the immediate danger). However, **patients may minimize their concerns** to their doctor, or may not think clearly in this stressful situation. They should be asked about the **presence of guns, escalating frequency or severity of threats or violence, or new violence outside the relationship.**

C. Developing a safety plan includes an assessment of the patient's social and financial supports, coping strategies in the past, the outcome of any previous attempts to leave or disrupt the violent pattern, the patient's current level of function at home or work, and the status of children in the home. Details of the plan include mobility, phone and car access, safe destination, and timing. Other safety concerns exist for women who are sexually assaulted in their relationships, including prevention, detection, and/or treatment of sexually transmitted diseases or pregnancy.

D. Treatment of primary psychiatric disorders should avoid the use of benzodiazepines or sedating medications, if at all possible. Victims should not be further dulled, or impaired, in their ability to anticipate, flee, or protect themselves (or their children). Iatrogenic addiction is a real though lesser, concern.

E. Mandated reporting of suspected abuse of children, elders (60 years or older), or the disabled should be carefully considered, and carried out in a manner that does not put the victim at greater risk.

VII. Conclusion

A. Domestic violence is common, under-reported and life-threatening. It escalates over time, and is motivated by the need to exert control over the victim. Although the victims are predominantly women, domestic violence is a public health problem that cuts across all segments of society. **Screening for violence should be part of every general medical or psychiatric evaluation.** Victims may not voluntarily disclose their abuse, but will often open up to empathic questioning. The physician who detects abuse need not "solve" the problem but should re-frame the violence as unacceptable document clearly, and make appropriate referrals. There are many deterrents to the victim leaving her batterer, including increased risk of murder. Victims of domestic violence need to know their physician